*Multiphasic Health
Testing Services*

BIOMEDICAL ENGINEERING AND HEALTH SYSTEMS

Advisory Editor:
JOHN H. MILSUM, University of British Columbia

L. A. Geddes and L. E. Baker
Principles of Applied Biomedical Instrumentation

George H. Myers and Victor Parsonnet
Engineering in the Heart and Blood Vessels

Robert Rosen
Dynamical System Theory in Biology

Stanley Middleman
Transport Phenomena in the Cardiovascular System

Samuel A. Talbot and Urs Gessner
Systems Physiology

Morris F. Collen
Hospital Computer Systems

Israel Mirksy, Dhanjoo N. Ghista, and Harold Sandler
Cardiac Mechanics: Physiological, Clinical and Mathematical Considerations

Richard S. C. Cobbold
Transducers for Biomedical Measurements:
Principles and Applications

Marshall M. Lih
Transport Phenomena in Medicine and Biology

Morris F. Collen
Multiphasic Health Testing Services

Multiphasic Health Testing Services

Edited by

Morris F. Collen, B.E.E., M.D.
Director, Medical Methods Research
The Permanente Medical Group
Oakland, California

Foreword by
Lester Breslow, M.D., M.P.H.

A Wiley Medical Publication
John Wiley & Sons
New York ● London ● Sydney ● Toronto

Library of Congress Cataloging in Publication Data:

Main entry under title:

Multiphasic health testing services.

(Biomedical engineering and health systems)
(A Wiley medical publication)
    Includes bibliographical references and index.
    1. Multiphasic health screening. I. Collen, Morris
Frank, 1913–   [DNLM: 1. Multiphasic screening.
QY40 M959]
RA427.6.M84   614.4′4   77-22969

ISBN 0-471-16509-3

Printed in the United States of America

10 9 8 7 6 5 4 3 2 1

*For better health through personal
preventive medical services by MHTS.*

*Dedicated to Bobbie Collen, Sidney Garfield and Cecil Cutting
without whose support MHTS would not have happened.*

Multiphasic Health Testing Services

The ideal protocol for health,
For wellness is one's greatest wealth,
Is paying good attention to
Health habits sound, performed life through;
And periodically seek
A health appraisal which can speak
To status of each person who
Can then well learn what he should do.

For this a service systemized
To test well-being, programized
With multiphasic tests all geared
To find for each who has appeared
The status of his health profile
And what to do for best life style;
Has automated history
And tests of physiology.

Computer data then collate,
Provide report by scheduled date
For doctor's thorough physical
From head to toe, naught mystical,
But carefully determine state
And patient's health evaluate.

The systemized MHTS
Is answer to, and can say yes
If one needs any special care
Of which we all require a share
To give each one protection good
From birth to aging years that should
Be well enjoyed as man's birthright;
Such checkups can most illness fight.

F. Bobbie Collen

1977

Contributors

Constance M. Allen, M.D., Department of Pediatrics, Kaiser-Permanente San Francisco Medical Center, 2200 O'Farrell Street, San Francisco, California 94115

F. Bobbie Collen, R.N., M.Ed., Formerly, Education Director, Health Center, Kaiser-Permanente Oakland Medical Center, 280 West MacArthur Boulevard, Oakland, California 94611

Morris F. Collen, B.E.E., M.D., Director, Department of Medical Methods Research, The Permanente Medical Group and the Kaiser Foundation Research Institute, 280 West MacArthur Boulevard, Oakland, California 94611

Lou S. Davis, M.A., Formerly, Manager, Computer Center, Department of Medical Methods Research, The Permanente Medical Group and the Kaiser Foundation Research Institute, 280 West MacArthur Boulevard, Oakland, California 94611

James H. Duncan, B.S.I.E., Senior Systems Analyst and Evaluator, Department of Medical Methods Research, The Permanente Medical Group and the Kaiser Foundation Research Institute, 280 West MacArthur Boulevard, Oakland, California 94611

Gary D. Friedman, M.D., M.S., Assistant Director, Epidemiology and Biostatistics, Department of Medical Methods Research, The Permanente Medical Group and the Kaiser Foundation Research Institute, 280 West MacArthur Boulevard, Oakland, California 94611

Michael D. Gahar, Formerly, Systems and Procedures Supervisor, MHTS, Department of Medical Methods Research, The Permanente Medical Group and the Kaiser Foundation Research Institute, 280 West MacArthur Boulevard, Oakland, California 94611

Sidney R. Garfield, M.D., Founder, Kaiser-Permanente Medical Care Program, Consultant, Department of Medical Methods Research, The Permanente Medical Group and the Kaiser Foundation Research Institute, 280 West MacArthur Boulevard, Oakland, California 94611

Robert L. Harrington, M.D., Formerly, Chief, Department of Psychiatry, Kaiser-Permanente Santa Clara Medical Center, Currently, Physician-in-Charge, Kaiser-Permanente San Jose Medical Offices, 5755 Cottle Road, San Jose, California 95123

Dankward Kodlin, M.D., M.P.H., Formerly, Senior Biometrician, Department of Medical Methods Research, The Permanente Medical Group and the Kaiser Foundation Research Institute, 280 West MacArthur Boulevard, Oakland, California 94611

Henry R. Shinefield, M.D., Chief, Department of Pediatrics, Kaiser-Permanente San Francisco Medical Center, 2200 O'Farrell Street, San Francisco, California 94115

Abraham B. Siegelaub, M.S., Biostatistician, Department of Medical Methods Research, The Permanente Medical Group and the Kaiser Foundation Research Institute, 280 West MacArthur Boulevard, Oakland, California 94611

Krikor Soghikian, M.D., M.P.H., Assistant Director, Health Services Research, Department of Medical Methods Research, The Permanente Medical Group and the Kaiser Foundation Research Institute, Chief, Division of Preventive Medicine and Health Center,

Kaiser-Permanente Oakland Medical Center, 280 West MacArthur Boulevard, Oakland, California 94611

Vicki Surdez, R.N., Formerly, Information Systems Analyst, Department of Medical Methods Research, The Permanente Medical Group and the Kaiser Foundation Research Institute, 280 West MacArthur Boulevard, Oakland, California 94611

Stephen L. Taller, M.D., Physician Supervisor, Nurse Practitioner, Health Evaluation Section, Kaiser-Permanente Oakland Medical Center, 280 West MacArthur Boulevard, Oakland, California 94611

Joseph F. Terdiman, M.D., Ph.D., Senior Biomedical Information Scientist, Department of Medical Methods Research, The Permanente Medical Group and the Kaiser Foundation Research Institute, 280 West MacArthur Boulevard, Oakland, California 94611

Edmund E. Van Brunt, M.D., Assistant Director, Medical Data Systems, Department of Medical Methods Research, The Permanente Medical Group and the Kaiser Foundation Research Institute, 280 West MacArthur Boulevard, Oakland, California 94611

Foreword

In *Multiphasic Health Testing Services*, Collen and his associates have written the most definitive work on the subject to date, summarizing their 25-year experience with the technology at the Kaiser-Permanente Medical Center in Oakland, California. For some years now the group's development and studies of multiphasic health testing have inspired its application throughout the world. Dozens of visitors to the Oakland center have, upon return to their own countries, initiated similar enterprises. This book will serve as a guide to the further evolution of the technology.

Multiphasic health testing arose from the confluence of several streams of development in American medicine, midway in the twentieth century. Prominent among these was the recognition that chronic disease had become a major health problem, and that one approach to its control was to find the conditions that lead to chronic illness early in their development so that treatment could be more effective. This approach was termed "secondary prevention" in order to emphasize that even though the disease process had started, it would often be possible to prevent the progress of disease to disability and death; and to differentiate this approach from "primary prevention," namely, averting the conditions entirely.

A second element in the origin of multiphasic health testing was the rapid growth of medical technology following World War II and its application to determining abnormalities in the biologic structure and functioning of individuals. Advances in blood chemistry, cytology, diagnostic radiology, serology and other techniques were coupled with electronic and other engineering developments to make multiphasic health testing feasible.

Third was the drive toward efficiency. Always a feature of American industry, a high degree of efficiency was going to be necessary to bring whatever benefits health testing could offer to the mass of people. The nation obviously could not afford "secondary prevention" on a mass scale with blood chemistry being performed as it was prior to 1950 and cytology performed only by pathologists, or with searches for early signs of chronic diseases carried out one by one. It was necessary to develop automation, utilize personnel so as to achieve maximum productivity at the highest level of competence, and organize screening for several conditions simultaneously.

Kaiser-Permanente in Oakland was only one of the several places where multiphasic health testing was tried about 1950. Why did it take root there? Probably one little-appreciated reason was that Morris Collen was both a physician and a graduate engineer; an internist and head of the medical service at the institution, and interested and capable in instrumentology as well. This favored his immediate and comprehensive grasp of the potential of the technology. It also enhanced his ability to form and lead the interdisciplinary team that was necessary for its development. Even more important, perhaps, was the nature of the Kaiser Health

Plan—a large, prepaid medical service based on group practice. In that milieu, which is oriented to health care for large groups of subscribers, the idea of disease prevention in medicine could really flourish and the resources for multiphasic health testing could be assembled. Two essentials were thus present: an institutional framework that was both impelled toward and supportive of its development; and an individual, a highly competent leader.

It may be of interest to note that the dynamic interrelationship between multiphasic health testing and the group practice of medicine with disease prevention–health maintenance as a prepaid service is continuing. For example, a construction trades union in Hawaii negotiated in 1974 a new feature for its health plan: a periodic health maintenance examination. Then the group arranged with its health service organization (Blue Shield) to provide the examinations through physician group practices which would have the capability to organize efficient, high-quality services.

The implications of the latter for the future of medical care to the group may be readily appreciated, especially if one accepts the viewpoint of Sidney Garfield. He sees multiphasic health testing as the entry point and organizing focus for medical care. It is the element for initial contact of the patient, for determining the patient's immediate needs, and for periodic guidance to the patient services that are provided.

If one accepts that function for multiphasic health testing in medical care at present, one may consider its role in the future. During the past quarter-century, a new approach to preventive medicine and, in fact, a new focus for health care as a whole has been emerging, deriving largely from experience with screening for early disease. This new focus is on the physiologic, anatomic, chemical, immunologic, bacterial and behavioral *condition* rather than on clinically defined disease as the basis for therapeutic action. It is increasingly possible to maintain periodic surveillance of the important biologic parameters in human function—growth and decline—and to correct those abnormalities likely to lead to disability and premature death. Thus, for example, periodically we now: measure blood pressure and treat persons with slight elevations, rather than allowing hypertensive heart disease to develop; examine the cervical epithelium for dysplasia or carcinoma-in-situ and manage the patient accordingly, rather than allowing invasive disease to develop; consider the immunologic status of persons under care, and take steps to bring it to the optimum for health; measure blood cholesterol, and seek to bring that blood constituent to a healthful level; test for and treat venereal infections if found; ascertain the cigarette-smoking and alcohol consumption patterns of people, and persuade them to adopt habits that are conducive to good health. These are, of course, merely illustrative of an important trend in medicine. Many more examples could be given.

This emphasis on surveillance of and treating conditions related to health, rather than awaiting the patient's appearance with symptoms that may lead to diagnosis and treatment, offers a basis for *the preventive medicine of the future*. In the future the epidemiologist may link up with the basic medical scientist as much as or more than with the clinician to formulate what will be done in the coming period of preventive medicine.

In that endeavor multiphasic health testing will have a prominent part.

LESTER BRESLOW, M.D.

Los Angeles, California

Series Preface

"To love
is not to gaze steadfast
at one another:
it is to look together
in the same direction"

St. Exupery, *Terre des Hommes*

The provision of good universal health care has only just become a social imperative. Like such other interlocking systems as transportation, water resources, and metropolises, the recognition of the need to adopt a systems approach has been forced upon us by the evident peril of mutual ruin resulting if we do not. The required systems approach is necessarily interdisciplinary rather than merely multidisciplinary, but this always makes evident the very real gulf between disciplines. Indeed, bridging the gulf requires much more time and patience than necessary just to learn the other discipline's "language." These different languages simultaneously represent and hide the whole gestalt associated with any discipline or profession. Nevertheless sufficient bridging must be achieved so that interdisciplinary teams can tackle our complex systems problems, for such teams constitute the only form of "intelligence amplification" that we can presently conceive.

Fortunately the existence of urgent problems always seems to provide the necessary impetus to work together in the same direction, using St. Exupery's thought, and, indeed, as a result of this to understand and value each other more deeply.

This series started with its emphasis on biomedical engineering. It illustrates the application of engineering in the service of medicine and biology. Books are required both to educate persons from one discipline in what they need to know of others, and to catalyze a synthesis in the core subject generally known as biomedical engineering. Thus one set of titles will aim at introducing the biologist and medical scientist to the quantitatively based analytical theories and techniques of the engineer and physical scientist. This set covers instrumentation, mathematical modelling, signal and system analysis, communication and control theory, and computer simulation techniques. A second set for engineers and physical scientists will cover basic material on biological and medical systems with as quantitative and compact a presentation as is possible. The omissions and simplifications necessitated by this approach should be justified by the increased ease of transferring the information, and more subtly by the increased pressure this can bring to bear upon the search for unifying quantitative principles.

A second emphasis has become appropriate as society increasingly demands universal health care, because the emphasis of medicine is now rapidly shifting from individual practice to health care systems. The huge financial burden of our health care systems (currently some 8% of GNP and increasing at about 12% per year) alone will ensure that engineers will be called upon, for the technological content is already large and still increasing. Engineers will need to apply their full spectrum of methodologies and techniques, and, moreover, to work in close collaboration with management professionals, as well as with many different health professionals. This series, then, will develop a group of books for mutually educating these various professionals so that they may better achieve their common task.

Multiphasic Health Testing Services focuses on an increasingly important area of our health care system, as this system faces the responsibility of providing universal, accessible, equitable and portable care at an acceptable cost. On one level, MHTS involves a major interfacing between technology and medicine in deciding what to measure routinely and then implementing these decisions with efficient, automated machines. On a second level, MHTS must achieve personal acceptance in interfacing its automated processes with the largely ambulatory and usually non-ill clientele for this service. On a third level, MHTS must work satisfactorily with the various payors for its services, mostly third parties. It is on this level that the ultimately crucial questions about the cost-effectiveness of MHTS in terms of a nation's health care must be answered. The answers must include in their scope the developing trends towards much greater emphasis on the prevention of illness and promotion of health relative to the care of the acutely ill.

This book has developed from the many years of research, development and practice devoted to MHTS by Morris Collen in particular, and by his colleagues, especially within the Kaiser-Permanente Health Plan. It therefore is able to combine theory and practice in a very important way.

JOHN M. MILSUM

Vancouver, British Columbia

Preface

Man is very fortunate to have inherited a body in which the various physiological systems (nervous, cardiorespiratory, gastrointestinal, locomotor, endocrine-metabolic, etc.) have remarkable homeostatic capabilities for early detection and self-correction of undesirable variations from the normal state. Eventually the aging process, harmful environmental agents, and the vicissitudes of life produce excess strain on these natural self-correcting mechanisms so that everyone at one time or another develops an abnormality and becomes sick. Thus, chronic disease and disability are especially common in the middle-aged and the elderly. It appears rational that the earlier one can identify in any physiological system a significant trend away from its normal state which might result in an abnormality sufficient to produce symptomatic disease and associated disability, the easier it should be to reverse this trend for correctable conditions and normalize the abnormality, thus hopefully preventing or at least postponing the disease and the disability. In essence, this is the premise on which the practice of preventive medicine for personal health care is based.

Given that personal preventive health care is a desirable objective, it then becomes important to consider methods for improving both the efficiency of the process of providing preventive health care, and the effectiveness of such care in preventing disease and disability. In this book, multiphasic health testing services (MHTS) is presented and described as one systemized approach for providing personal preventive health care, and its effectiveness and efficiency is considered. MHTS primarily systemizes the general clinical examination which always has been the traditional approach to the health evaluation of a patient. MHTS can serve as the keystone to personal preventive health maintenance through efficiently furnishing high quality health examinations, which can be repeated through life in accordance with each individual's risks. In this book, health checkups are recommended every year or two for those over age 40 and less frequently for younger adults.

Multiphasic health testing is diverse and flexible in its applications, can be cost-effective in achieving specified objectives, and is responsive to systems planning and to monitoring of quality and efficiency. Industry marketing analysts have projected multiphasic health testing to have a great market potential. It can be anticipated that in the future every community of 100,000 or more will have at least one multiphasic health testing center.

The history of the introduction of technological innovations in medicine has shown that in health care it often takes five to 25 years for a newly developed technique to be widely applied. We believe that with the emerging concept of "health care as a right" and with government support of Health Maintenance Organizations (HMOs), the time for MHTS has arrived.

Preventive medicine is the key to the future health of mankind. MHTS is an efficient method to achieve better health through personal preventive medicine. It can serve to provide periodic health examinations to help guide each person along a personal pathway to improved health status.

Although there are now several hundred operational MHTS programs in the world, the most extensive experience and research in this field for the past 25 years has been in the Kaiser-Permanente Medical Center in Oakland, California. Accordingly, this book is based primarily on the 25 years of the personal experience of a large team that has engaged in continuing research, development and operation of MHTS. Its current state of development could not have been achieved but by the cooperative efforts of many devoted people.

MORRIS F. COLLEN

Oakland, California

Acknowledgments

During these past 25 years, Sidney Garfield was the first to integrate multiphasic services into a prepaid health care program and later was the first to advocate its use as the primary entry mode to a health care delivery system. Cecil Cutting was the first medical director to actively foster and support MHTS. Edmund Van Brunt was the first "physician supervisor" of an automated multiphasic health testing service. Krikor Soghikian was the first to add to a multiphasic testing program the adjunctive preventive health maintenance services, and Bobbie Collen was the first to add organized health education services. Henry Shinefield and Constance Allen were the first to add pediatric MHTS, in the San Francisco Kaiser-Permanente Medical Center. Nicholas Cummings was the first to develop an automated psychological test for MHTS; and Robert Harrington was the first to develop a comprehensive mental MHTS in the Santa Clara Kaiser-Permanente Medical Center. Stephen Taller was the first to integrate online nurse practitioner physical examinations into a MHTS. Lou Davis was the first to computerize a MHTS and the first to develop software for a comprehensive lifetime MHTS data base. Leonard Rubin was the first chief of data processing for a MHTS and Joseph Terdiman was the first MHTS data base manager. Michael Gahar was the first to completely flowchart and document the standard operating procedures for a MHTS. Robert Richart and James Duncan were the first to evaluate the impact of MHTS on a total health care delivery system. Robert Feldman was the first to use a MHTS for clinical-epidemiological research in diabetes and Bernard Resnick the first to use it for renal research. John Cutler was the first epidemiologist to evaluate patient outcomes from MHTS and Gary Friedman was the first to use a MHTS data base for extensive epidemiological research. Savitri Ramcharan was the first to guide thousands of visitors from all over the world on tours through a MHTS. A. B. Siegelaub was the first biostatistician to develop age-sex specific normal values for a population from its own MHTS data base. Dankward Kodlin was the first to use a MHTS data base for extensive computer-aided diagnosis studies.

The success of the Oakland and San Francisco Kaiser-Permanente MHTS programs is due to the combined efforts of all the above and, in addition, to its Oakland and San Francisco medical department physicians without whose continuing support and cooperation these multiphasic programs could not function. Through the years, the major responsibilities for the day-to-day operations of the MHTS were carried out by physician supervisors Edmund Van Brunt, Harold Stocker, Krikor Soghikian, Robert Feldman and Derek Crawford; and by nurse supervisors Muriel Thompson and Anna Menke. The administrative support of Joseph Sender, Robert Cella, and Lester Hollander in the Kaiser-Permanente Oakland Medical Center and of John Smillie, Bruce Sams, Harry Caulfield, Lee Harris, and Matthew Janin in the Kaiser-Permanente San Francisco Medical Center is gratefully acknowledged.

The research and developmental activities of the Oakland MHTS program have, since 1960, been supported in part by the Kaiser Foundation Research Institute and by several grants from HEW (CH 05-8, CD 00142, HSM 110-70-407, HS 00288). Robert Thorner, Archer Copley, Raymond Hofstra, Eleanor Smith, and Paul Sanazaro were each of inestimable value in their visionary outlook for the potentialities of MHTS and in their help and guidance as project officers for the various HEW grant projects. Lester Breslow was always helpful in providing encouragement and inspiration.

The editor acknowledges the innumerable important contributions to MHTS from the many workers in the field and from other multiphasic screening and testing programs. We have all learned from each other that there are many ways to operate a successful MHTS and there are still so many improvements which are needed. The continuing criticisms of MHTS by physicians, medical administrators, public health executives, and epidemiologists have been humbling and challenging, yet problems should be looked upon as opportunities.

The editor wishes to express his deepest personal gratitude to the Kaiser-Permanente Medical Care Program as a whole in providing the remarkably ideal and unique environment for the birth and growth of MHTS—perhaps nowhere else in the world could this have been possible.

The editor is indebted to Bobbie Collen for her encouragement and material assistance in editing and proofreading; to Irene Mahoney, Beryl Cummings and Jean Shrewsbury for their indefatigable typing and retyping; and to John Wiley's personnel with whom it is always a pleasure to work.

MORRIS F. COLLEN

Contents

History of MHTS

Morris F. Collen

A. INTRODUCTION

Over the past 45 years multiphasic health testing services (MHTS) has evolved as a systemized approach that attempts to provide health examinations efficiently. The concept of health checkups is not new, as for decades the practice of periodic health examinations has been recommended generally. In order to decrease the costs of providing such examinations, some of the principles and methods of systems engineering have been applied in multiphasic health testing. A gradual evolution through the various historical steps of screening, mass screening, multiphasic screening, automated multiphasic screening, and multiphasic testing has arrived finally at automated multiphasic health testing services.

B. PREVENTIVE MEDICINE AND HEALTH EXAMINATIONS

More than 100 years ago Horace Dobell, M.D., was apparently the first to introduce the concept of periodic health examinations. He published, in London, *Lectures on . . . the Prevention of the Invasion and Fatality of Disease by Periodical Examinations,*[1] from which the following is an extract:

> I am perfectly convinced, from my own observation and experience in practice, that patients never think of consulting their doctors till these conditions of impaired general health have advanced far enough to have been developed into some form of disease; that thousands and thousands of people, believing themselves to be in health, are nevertheless undergoing these early, occult, and evasive states of defect in the physiological state; and that such persons may be considered to be in health, not only by themselves, but by any one accustomed to associate with them, even though it be a physician, and that even if they submit to a medical examination, as ordinarily conducted, they may be declared to be in health.
>
> I wish, then, to propose as the only means by which to reach the evil and to obtain the good, *that there should be instituted, as a custom, a system of periodical examination, to which all persons should submit their children.*
>
> Such an examination must include an inquiry into the family history, to learn the hereditary constitution; into the personal history, to learn all the previous diseases that have been passed through, and the habits and vicissitudes of life; into all the conditions of life surrounding the individual; into the condition of the organs and functions of the body; into the state of the secretions and fluids of the body by analysis and microscopical examinations, and so forth.
>
> The examination should be reported in writing; and, after due consideration, such advice must be given as a careful judgment may dictate, for the future conduct, pursuits, and habits of the patient, with a view to correcting any defects or tendency to defects in the organism. Advice must also be given as to the means of removing any vestiges of disease that have been detected, or if they are not removable, advice as to the best way of overcoming their influence or of averting their increase. To this must be added precautions to be adopted in certain contingencies which, according to the judgment of the case, appear probable.
>
> If such a plan as I have here proposed were to be faithfully and conscientiously carried out by the present and rising generation of well-educated studious medical men, I think no one can doubt, after a careful consideration of the subject, that immense benefit would be conferred upon the public.

President Theodore Roosevelt ordered routine physical testing for army officers in 1908. In 1922 the House of Delegates of the American Medical Association[2] encouraged county medical societies to declare to the public that their members were prepared to conduct periodic health examinations, and in 1925 the Association published a manual of suggestions for the conduct of such examinations.[3] However, for the next twenty years periodic health examinations did not become popular, probably because of their cost and because physicians were not oriented to the concept of personal preventive health maintenance.

In 1921 the Metropolitan Life Insurance Company published in its Statistical Bulletin the following report[4] on the value of periodic health examinations: "For more than seven years the Metropolitan Life Insurance Company has made it possible for policy-holders in its Ordinary Department to obtain, without cost, a physical examination and the other health services offered by the Life Extension Institute. Between February 1914 and July 31, 1921, this Company has authorized nearly 95,000 physical examinations through this agency. . . . The outstanding feature of the experiment is that there has been a saving of life corresponding to 28 percent of the expected mortality in the short five-year period. It was to demonstrate the life-saving possibilities of such health work that this activity was begun. It has been established to the satisfaction of this Company that periodic medical examination is justified by the benefit in added life expectancy to the policy-holders examined. It is hoped that other agencies will see the value that follows from annual physical examinations and all that goes with that type of life conservation." (This study will be referred to again in Chapter Eighteen, D.)

Roemer[5] in 1945 advocated that the "concept of preventive services to the individual is to consider as preventive a health service rendered to the presumably normal person. Once a specific disorder has been detected, its correction, while preventive of future difficulties, would arbitrarily not fall under this concept. Because the most basic preventive approach, taking its origin in environmental sanitation and control of acute communicable disease, required organized community action, the province of prevention has been left largely to government agencies of public health. In contrast to this attack on 'disease in the mass,' the approach to the individual has been almost entirely within therapeutic confines and in the hands of the private medical practitioner." Roemer took inventory 30 years ago of known preventive measures and estimated their cost as a part of an organized group medical service. He suggested that the most economical program would be a "health center" form of operation with salaried physicians providing periodic examinations directed toward the early detection of the commonest diseases in the age and sex group of the particular individual; thus, the actual unit cost of each of several tests provided at the same time would be less than if each were carried out as an independent operation at a separate time. Roemer stated that the keystone of the entire preventive program would be the periodic examinations of the presumably normal individual. He suggested that from the public health point of view the periodic examinations could be systemized according to the age, sex, occupational status, income level, race, geographical location of the persons involved and that a physician medical examination should be integrated with the several special diagnostic tests provided in a periodic health examination so that significant disorders could be sought for clinically (i.e., by the physician) that could not be detectable by the laboratory tests.

C. THE INTRODUCTION OF SCREENING TESTS

Screening as a public health measure in the United States is an old established procedure. It began before 1900 with the screening of immigrants by the Marine Hospital Service in order to identify those with significant disease who might become a burden to the country. This process was extended to screen communities for communicable diseases. As communicable diseases gradually diminished in importance, the Public Health Service expanded its attention to screening for chronic noncommunicable diseases.

In order to decrease the costs of examinations to large numbers of people, screening techniques were developed consisting of simple, quick, and often only approximate tests that could, with reasonable accuracy, sort out persons likely to have the disease targeted for detection.

Beginning in 1930, mass screening techniques were applied by the U.S. Public Health Service for the case detection of syphilis and tuberculosis.[6] The miniature x-ray photofluorographic technique for mass radiography for pulmonary tuberculosis and mass serology for detecting latent syphilis permitted health agencies to economically screen large populations for these diseases. In fact, routine premarital serology testing is still procedural in the United States.

Petrie and his associates[7] exploited the full capabilities of mass screening techniques in Atlanta, where between 1945 and 1950 more than one million residents voluntarily took multiple health screening tests. From 7 to 14 testing stations, mostly in mobile units, often moved daily to locations convenient for examining large numbers of people (80 to 100 persons per hour), testing for heart disease and tuberculosis (photofluorographic chest x-rays), syphilis (venereal disease research laboratories "VDRL" test), hemoglobin (Phillips-Van Slyke copper sulphate specific gravity test), blood sugar (Anthrone method), height and weight, and oral and dental conditions. In 1952 Petrie applied the term "multiphasic screening" to his program.

In Oxford, Mass. in 1947 Wilkerson and Krall[8] carried out a diabetes detection program based upon screening tests for elevated blood sugar and glycosuria, referring suspicious cases to the community physicians for diagnostic evaluation.

Breslow[9] in 1949 reported a heart disease screening program carried out in Los Angeles, where miniature chest x-ray films were interpreted specifically for the presence of cardiac abnormality and approximately one percent of adults were found to have heart disease previously unknown to themselves that required the care of a physician.

D. THE INTRODUCTION OF MULTIPHASIC SCREENING

In 1948 Breslow[6] first introduced the term "multiphasic screening" (semantically derived from the Minnesota Multiphasic Personality Inventory) and applied it in San Jose, Calif.,[9] as an extension of the mass screening technique. Since tuberculosis, syphilis, diabetes, and heart disease had been proven to be detectable in the general population on a mass scale, and since it was not uncommon for a group of people to be surveyed for tuberculosis and then surveyed again a few months later for syphilis or diabetes, the multiphasic survey was conceived to combine several of these tests in one package. Breslow proposed that such a combination would be more economical and efficient for each person screened, yielding him and the physician to whom he was referred much more useful information concerning his health status than would be obtained from any single test, while costing little more in time lost from occupation. Breslow felt that the sponsoring agencies would save time and money by administering a single health education campaign, record system, and followup service for a screening program embracing several diseases rather than approaching each one separately.

With these considerations in mind, the Santa Clara County Medical Society, the San Jose City Health Department, and the California Department of Public Health undertook a multiphasic survey among the industrial employees of four San Jose establishments. Their conclusions were that the results in case finding were considerably greater than those of the customary screening for a single disease.

It was immediately recognized by some in the medical profession that multiphasic screening had a potential application for periodic health examinations. As early as 1948 an editorial in the *Journal of the American Medical Association* suggested that "in contrast to periodic health examinations, these screening procedures are capable of a very wide application; they are relatively inexpensive per person tested, and they require relatively little time on the part of physicians."[10]

Chapman[11] in 1949, as Chief of the Division of Chronic Diseases in the Bureau of State Services of the U.S. Public Health Service, actively supported the concept of multiphasic screening. Mass testing of the population already included chest x-rays for tuberculosis, the serological test for syphilis, blood and urine sugar tests for diabetes, and hemoglobin testing for anemia. Vision and hearing were already routinely tested in school, and the taking of blood pressure was routine in physicians' offices. Chapman suggested that it was logical now for public health administrators to ask: "Why not combine as many of these tests as practical into a battery of tests, reduce the overall cost of administering them, and thereby encourage universal usage?" Chapman advocated multiphasic screening because he saw that it made "an undeniable appeal to the individual who may be ill, to the physician, to the public health worker, and to the taxpayer." For the individual patient with chronic disease he thought it could lead to early control; for the physician he felt it would bring patients who ordinarily might not come until definite signs and symptoms had developed. To the public health officer he believed it would provide an opportunity to increase the quantity of tangible services at a lower cost of personnel and dollars. To the taxpayer he thought it should reduce the number of days of hospitalization and the costs of care for persons with chronic diseases.

In 1950 Ryder and Getting[12] reported the historic action of the Council of the Massachusetts Medical Society, which in May 1949 voted to establish five pilot multiphasic clinics (called Health Protection Clinics) to offer health examinations under the auspices of the district medical societies in cooperation with the community hospitals and other interested groups. It was recommended that the findings of these examinations be reported to the family physicians. In December 1959 the New England Center Hospital became the first operational multiphasic clinic in Boston with a self-screener history and a broad battery of screening tests for a variety of disease categories, including heart disease, hypertension, diabetes, tuberculosis, cancer, syphilis, nephritis, vision and hearing defects, and nutritional status. A ten-minute physical examination by clinic physicians was also included, since it was the intent of the Medical Society to evaluate screening and to determine whether or not the physical examination revealed disease that was missed by the history of clinical tests. Pelvic examinations and Papanicolaou smears for cervical cancer were provided to all women over age 35. They subsequently reported[13] that for 1,252 persons screened, approximately two-thirds of the detected conditions could be found without the assistance of a physician. They concluded: "Because of our experience we are convinced that multiple screening will prove to be a valuable program for both the patient and the physician to whom he is referred."

In 1950 Bugbee,[14] the executive director of the American Hospital Association, suggested that hospitals should include multiphasic screening clinics as part of their services. Chapman[15] reported the same year that multiphasic screening programs had been initiated in Indianapolis and in Richmond.[16] On the basis of these early experiences he suggested some principles for multiphasic screening:

> (1) Multiple screening tests should be specific, they should be relatively inexpensive, and none should take more than three minutes to perform.
>
> (2) Multiple screening tests are not designed to diagnose disease. They are designed to screen out of the apparently well population those in whom the index of suspicion is high.
>
> (3) These screening procedures are meant to channel people with early, undiagnosed chronic disease or disability to their physicians early enough to stabilize, if not actually to correct, the disease. Many of the late complications usually can be prevented if diagnoses are made early.
>
> (4) Multiple screening programs are designed to utilize to the maximum extent nonmedical personnel. Physicians in the screening line increase the risk of confusing screening with diagnosis, and they increase the overall cost of this relatively inexpensive type of operation.

Mountin[17] in 1950, as Assistant Surgeon General and Associate Chief of the Bureau of State Services of the U. S. Public Health Service, expressed alarm that the demand for multiphasic screening programs was growing faster than could be met by the resources of public health organizations. "Its seeming simplicity and economics," he observed, "have captured the imagination of public health administrators and the general public alike," especially for detection of chronic diseases. He cautioned that multiphasic screening might be adopted as a routine public health practice before some basic questions were answered and before adequate safeguards were employed. Multiphasic screening was "just one rung of a ladder" and must be followed up by diagnosis and treatment. Mountin felt that followup measures for the chronically ill would be inadequate for large numbers of patients and that new relationships would need to be developed with physicians, hospitals, and community resources for followup care. He saw a need for better criteria for selecting the specific tests for screening and the appropriate screening levels to be used. He warned that since the specificity and sensitivity of many of the screening tests had yet to be fully established, "too many persons are referred for definitive diagnosis when, in fact, they did not have the disease in question— the so-called false positives—and many persons who should be referred for further services are passed over—the so-called false negatives." He warned that unconfirmed and borderline referrals might irritate members of the medical profession as well as the patient. Smillie[18] similarly attacked multiphasic screening on the basis of poor quality testing.

Mountin's and Smillie's warnings were well founded as to the need for adequate followup and for accurate screening tests with good sensitivity and specificity.

Samis[19] in 1951 reported on multiple screening programs being planned for Mount Sinai Hospital in New York City and Gallinger Municipal Hospital in Washington, D.C. He went so far as to suggest that multiphasic screening might be the "keystone of preventive medicine." He considered it to be the logical extension of the mass screening technique for a single disease, "based on the fundamental concept in preventive medicine that early detection, early diagnosis and adequate treatment can accomplish substantial reduction in disability and deaths from significant diseases."

Some industrially oriented multiphasic screening programs were developed in the late 1940s for the Tennessee Valley Authority and the Phillips Petroleum Company, and in the early 1950s one was offered for lease to any industry by Robertson of Asheville, N.C.[20]

In 1951 the first multiphasic screening project within a comprehensive prepaid health plan was initiated in the Kaiser-Permanente Medical Care Program. Based upon the favorable experience of Breslow with multiphasic screening surveys in California, the International Longshoremen's and Warehousemen's Union joined with Kaiser-Permanente Health Plan to set up temporary screening facilities in the union hiring hall on the San Francisco waterfront, and 3,994 men were tested between June 18 and November 30, 1951.[21]

Encouraged by the success of this experience, the Executive Committee of The Permanente Medical Group approved on November 20, 1951, the establishment of a permanent multiphasic screening program in Kaiser-Permanente's Oakland Medical Center and on January 15, 1952, in the San Francisco Medical Center.[22] These were supervised and conducted by the same physicians who furnished the physical examinations, treatment, and followup care, as an integral part of the group practice, prepaid, comprehensive medical care plan. Both of these MHTS programs have continued to operate to this day. In each program, from 1951 to 1964, patients received the following multiphasic screening procedures during a 60-minute appointment period: completion of a health questionnaire form; measurement of height, weight, and blood pressure; screening tests for urine albumin and blood hemoglobin; blood or urine sugar as collected one hour after ingestion of 100 gm of glucose; a serologic test for syphilis; chest x-ray; and a lead one electrocardiogram.

Women over 35 years of age were referred to the gynecology department for examination of the breasts and pelvic organs and a cytologic examination of a smear of the cervix. Men and women over 40 years of age were referred for sigmoidoscopy examination.[23]

Patients were then requested to return a few weeks later for an appointment with an internist in the Kaiser-Permanente medical department who reviewed the health questionnaire, obtained any pertinent additional history, performed a physical examination, appraised the laboratory screening tests, and then reviewed with the patient his health status. Any necessary followup visits or additional consultations were then arranged by the physician.

This program operated from 5:30 to 8:30, Monday through Friday evenings after regular office hours, using the physicians' vacant outpatient offices and the regular clinic x-ray and laboratory services. From 50 to 70 patients were processed each evening in each facility and they were directed from station to station by a series of directional signs. Women were examined Monday, Wednesday, and Friday evenings and men on Tuesday and Thursday evenings. In the first full year of operation in 1952 a total of 9,403 patients were examined in the two MHTS programs.

In 1951 a President's Commission on the Health Needs of the Nation[24] recommended periodic health examinations as a means of chronic disease control and suggested that multiphasic screening be used to detect disease early.

In 1956 a Commission on Chronic Illness[25] again reviewed chronic disease screening and listed conditions for which it considered screening tests were then applicable; these included (1) pulmonary tuberculosis, (2) visual defects including glaucoma, (3) hearing defects, (4) syphilis, (5) diabetes mellitus, (6) cancer of the skin, mouth, rectum, breast, and cervix, (7) hypertensive disease, and (8) ischemic heart disease. The commission recommended periodic multiphasic screening for these conditions.

In the late 1950s and early 1960s considerable criticism of multiphasic screening developed, primarily because of (1) the poor quality of screening tests (that is, they were qualitative sorting tests rather than quantitative measuring tests) and (2) the lack of effective medical followup of positive screenees. Most physicians who were engaged in fee-for-service practice viewed multiphasic screening as an intrusion in the traditional physician-patient relationship. In 1955 the American Medical Association reported[26] that only in 15 of 33 surveys reviewed were such followup data available. These problems emphasized the need for improved quantitative tests and the affiliation of multiphasic programs with physician groups. Nevertheless, in 1955 the American Medical Association initiated the offering of health examinations to its physicians at its annual meetings; and in 1961, through its Section on Pathology and Physiology, continued to offer typical multiphasic health testing examinations at its annual meetings.

Although physicians traditionally advocated periodic health examinations, most continued to be opposed to the introduction of multiphasic techniques. However, some clinicians aggressively supported health examinations using multiphasic screening. White[27] as early as 1952 had pointed out that in the traditional role of the physician as healer and therapist the search for disease in its earliest presymptomatic stages represented a new form of medical activity. He advocated that the medical profession view each patient as an individual with a chief complaint or medical problem and as a person to be screened for unsuspected chronic disease. This additional task of screening, White concluded, could be provided most economically by packaged laboratory facilities such as multiphasic screening programs.

It was primarily through the support of physicians in group practice, both prepaid medical and industrial, that multiphasic screening was to mature into a useful health care delivery technology in the United States. In 1959 Roberts[28] comprehensively reviewed the literature, which revealed that periodic health examinations were beginning to be increasingly advocated and provided in industrial medicine. He summarized the practice that was often being adopted: to examine persons under age 30 every third year, those between 30 and 40 every second year, and those over 40 every year. (See Chapter Sixteen.)

In the early 1960s multiphasic screening was first exploited on a large scale when Jungner, in Sweden, carried out on 100,000 people in Varmland county a multiphasic screening program, characterized primarily by an extensive battery of biochemical tests.[29,30,44] At the same time Paul Hall first used multiphasic screening for the routine admission of patients to the Serafimer Hospital in Stockholm.

In 1960 the American Public Health Association strongly endorsed multiphasic screening, and in 1961 the U. S. Public Health Service established the Chronic Diseases Division, which began to provide grants to establish and evaluate multiphasic screening programs.

E. THE INTRODUCTION OF MULTIPHASIC HEALTH TESTING SERVICES

The advent of electronics and automation into medicine provided the opportunity to improve and augment screening techniques so that not only more tests but more accurate and quantitative measurements could be used. The terms "automated multiphasic screening" and "automated multiphasic health testing" were introduced in 1964 by the Oakland Kaiser-Permanente medical group[32] as an expanded concept of utilizing automated and semiautomated electronic and mechanical equipment to determine automatically whether there was sufficient likelihood of disease present to warrant further specific diagnostic testing. In this context the term "automated" applied to the computer processing (by statistical methods, algorithms or decision rules) of the patient test data so as to automatically sort out the positives from the negatives. The mere employment of automated equipment or a computer is not considered sufficient to satisfy the concept of automated multiphasic screening.

In 1963–64, with the partial support of a grant from the U.S. Public Health Service, the multiphasic screening programs operational in the Kaiser-Permanente Oakland and San Francisco medical centers since 1951 were replaced by the first automated multiphasic screening programs dedicated to better health through preventive medicine (Figure 1-1). In the first year over 35,000 patients[33,34] were processed (Table 1-1). The two programs have operated continuously since that date and in ten years have provided a total of 500,000 examinations.

Table 1-1. Total Numbers of Multiphasic Checkups Given, Kaiser-Permanente Oakland and San Francisco, 1964–1973

	Oakland		San Francisco		Totals	
Period	Exami-nations	Cumu-lative	Exami-nations	Cumu-lative	Exami-nations	Cumu-lative
7/64–6/65	18,438	18,438	17,281	17,281	35,719	35,719
7/65–6/66	21,538	39,976	21,805	39,086	43,343	79,062
7/66–6/67	22,515	62,491	21,108	60,194	43,623	122,685
7/67–6/68	23,879	86,370	22,158	82,352	46,037	168,722
7/68–6/69	23,260	109,630	20,868	103,220	44,128	212,850
7/69–6/70	22,974	132,604	20,348	123,568	43,322	256,172
7/70–6/71	26,703	159,307	24,022	147,590	50,725	306,897
7/71–6/72	28,886	188,193	23,944	171,534	52,830	359,727
7/72–6/73	30,640	218,833	24,414	195,948	55,054	414,781

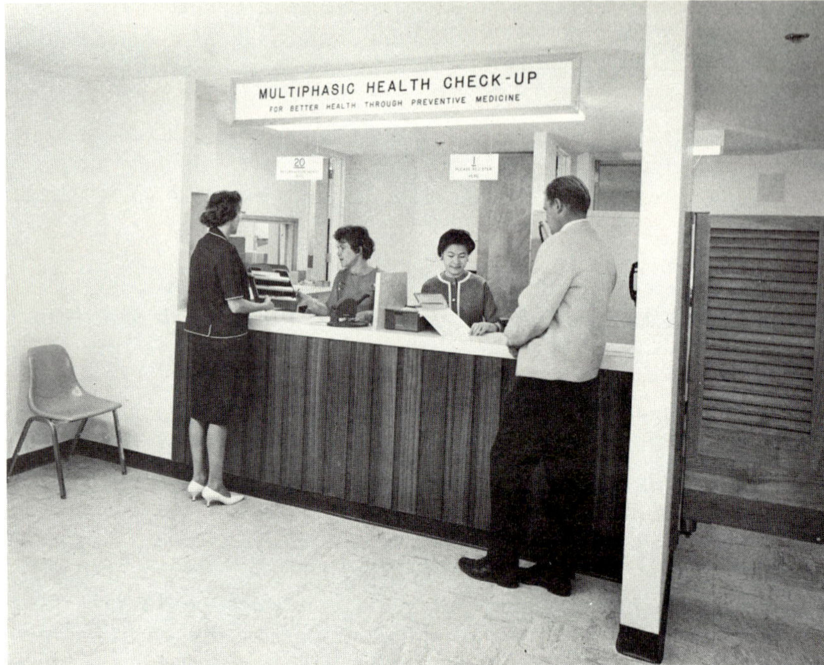

Figure 1-1.   First registration station for Oakland MHTS.

(These services will be considered in detail in later chapters; a contemporary description is given in Chapter One, F, and selected data analyses from this MHTS data base are presented in Chapter Nineteen.)

As all qualitative screening tests were replaced by quantitative standard clinical laboratory methods, and as patients began to be referred periodically by their physicians for evaluation of changes in their health status or for monitoring of the status of chronic diseases, the term "automated multiphasic health testing" (AMHT) replaced "automated multiphasic screening." This introduction of more accurate quantitative testing was a primary objective, meeting one of the important criticisms from physicians about earlier screening programs. The introduction of automatic computer sorting of those needing followup tests was also of benefit.

In 1964 the multiphasic health checkup consisted of three parts:[35]

(1) the automated multiphasic health testing (AMHT) program (a battery of tests and procedures),

(2) a physical examination by an internist, and

(3) a group of specialty physician examinations, including a gynecological examination (with cervical smear for cancer detection) and a sigmoidoscopy.

In this form it took two to three hours and included the following:

(1) Electrocardiogram (six leads) and phonocardiogram (at apex and base), simultaneously graphed on paper by a direct-recording, multiple-channel Sanborn optical oscillograph (Figure 1-2).

(2) Table-tilt cardiovascular test (80° tilt in 35 seconds; pulse and blood pressure recorded supine and one minute after tilt) (Figure 1-3).

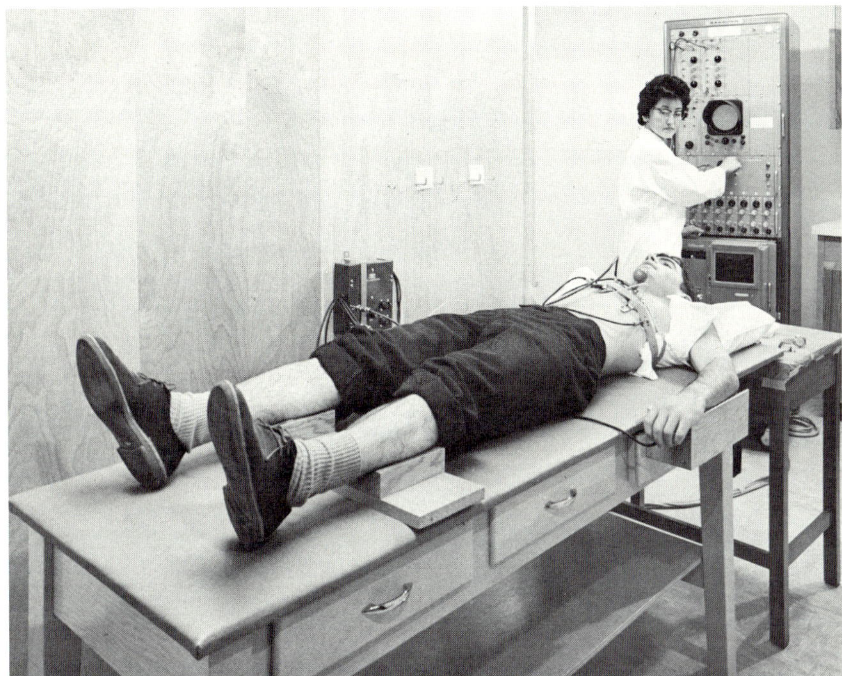

Figure 1-2. First multichannel Sanborn ECG machine and specially constructed table with built-in electrodes for extremities.

(3) Height, weight, and other body measurements, recorded by an automated anthropometer with direct punched-card output (Figure 1-4).

(4) Chest x-ray (70 mm minifilm) (Figure 1-22).

(5) Breast x-ray (cephalocaudal and lateral views in women) (Figures 1-5 and 1-6).

(6) Visual acuity (modified Sloan chart) and pupillary escape test (an unsustained pupillary light reflex occurring in retinal or optic nerve disease).[60]

(7) Ocular tension (measured by Schiotz tonometer) (Figure 1-7).

(8) Retinal photograph (of left eye) (Figure 1-8).

(9) Timed vital capacity (one second and total) by the Gaensler-Collins spirometer (Figure 1-9).

(10) Pain reaction test (a modified Libman test, measured as pain tolerance to increasing pressure on Achilles tendon) (Figure 1-10).

(11) Hearing test (for six frequencies by a Rudmose-Bekesy automated audiometer) (Figure 1-25).

(12) Self-administered health questionnaire form (present and past history). In addition, a set of 207 medical questions on prepunched cards were sorted by the patient so that the "yes" responses could be automatically produced for computer processing (Figure 1-26).

(13) Personality appraisal questionnaire (a modified MMPI type of test with 155 psychological questions sorted by the patient as in item (12) above.

(14) At this station patients could receive tetanus toxoid immunization (Figure 1-11).

(15) Eight blood chemistries performed within 12 minutes by a multichannel

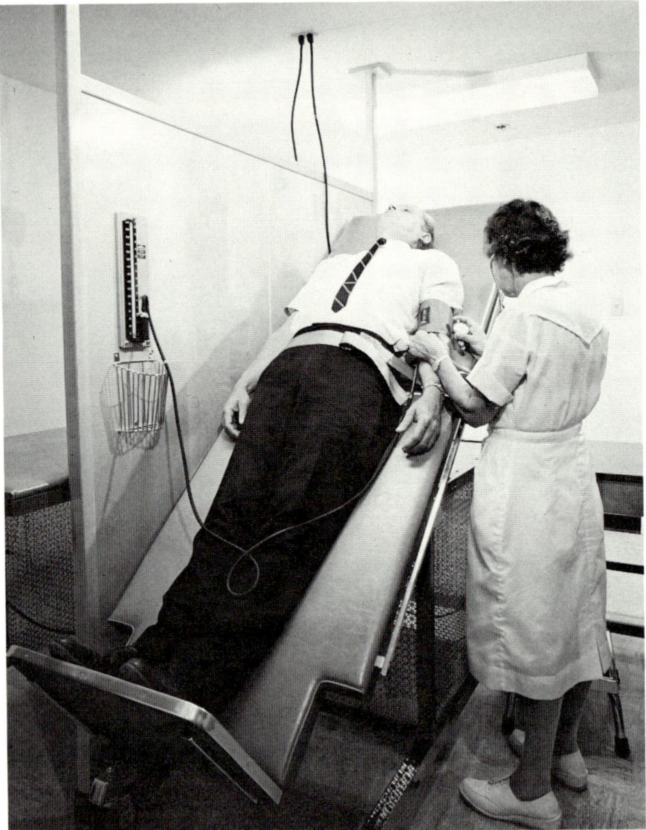

Figure 1-3. Tilt table research test station.

Technicon AutoAnalyzer with direct punched-card output (Figure 1-12), including: (a) serum glucose (one hour after 100 gm glucose), (b) serum creatinine, (c) serum albumin, (d) serum total protein, (e) serum cholesterol, (f) serum uric acid, (g) serum calcium, (h) serum transaminase (SGOT).

(16) Blood hemoglobin and white cell count automatically measured.

(17) Blood group (ABO).

(18) Serological (VDRL) test for syphilis.

(19) Blood rheumatoid factor (latex test).

(20) Urinalysis for: (a) urine pH, glucose, protein, and blood by enzyme paper strip tests (Figure 1-17); and (b) urine bacteria by a four-hour triphenyltetrazolium chloride culture of midstream specimen).

(21) In accordance with programmed online "advice" rules, additional tests and followup appointments with physicians were arranged by means of an IBM 1440 computer (Figure 1-13) before the patient left. All test results were stored for summary report printout.

The planners of this first automated multiphasic health testing program realized that a large number of accurately performed chemical tests might now be included at a low cost, since single-channel automated chemical analyzers invented by Skeggs were now available from Technicon Corporation. In 1964 a proposal was

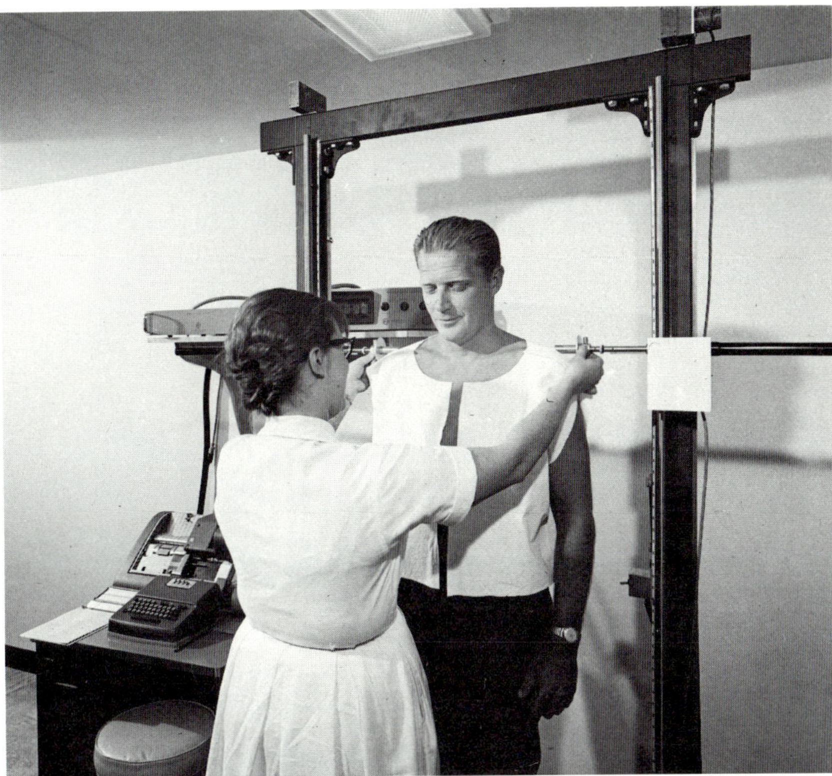

Figure 1-4. Automated anthropometer for somatotyping.

made to Whitehead, the President of Technicon, that he fabricate a multichannel automated chemical analyzer. Mr. Whitehead asked how much money was available for project development and was told there was $25,000 for the chemistry tests. He said he guessed that would have to be all right, and so the first prototype multichannel AutoAnalyzer was built, installed, and tested in the Oakland MHTS. After a few months an improved model was installed in San Francisco, and later a similar machine replaced the prototype in Oakland. These two first-generation multichannel AutoAnalyzers then operated as production machines for five years (Figure 1-12). The advent of the AutoAnalyzer provided a great impetus to panel chemistry tests for biomedical profiling and multiphasic health testing.

A difficult decision was whether to include mammography as a routine multiphasic procedure, until a woman in San Francisco was found to have a clearly positive mammogram for which none of the surgeons could palpate any lesion in the breast. Finally one of them biopsied the area that looked suspicious on the x-ray, and the biopsy was found to be positive for carcinoma (Figure 1–6). Henceforth, there was no question in the minds of the San Francisco physicians that screening mammography had its place in the multiphasic package of tests, and the subsequent experience was reported by Griesbach and Eads.[36]

Another problem was the vomiting and near-shock produced in an occasional patient drinking hypertonic glucose, when 75 to 100 gm of that solution was introduced as the challenge dose for the glucose tolerance test in screening for diabetes mellitus. This problem was resolved through serendipity. Someone acci-

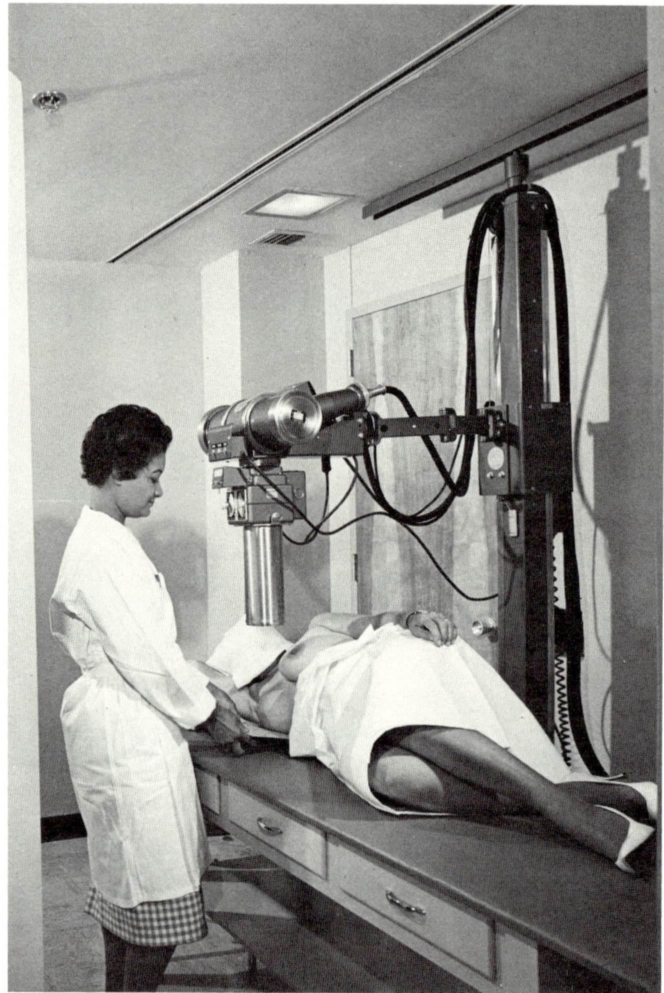

Figure 1-5. First mammography (Continental x-ray) test station in Oakland MHTS. Breast cancer detection by x-ray mammography.

dentally tasted a bottle of 7 UP that had been standing opened for several hours and discovered that warm, flat 7 Up was very similar to the glucose challenge dose. When a soft drink dispensing machine (Figure 1-14) was modified to chill and carbonate the glucose solution, the cases of nausea and vomiting disappeared.

Because of low frequency of parathyroid tumors, it was often asked why serum calcium should be tested for in the multiphasic laboratory. One day a patient came into the emergency room of the San Francisco hospital in a coma and died a few days later. An astute pathologist did a postmortem blood calcium, found it elevated, and then dissected out a parathyroid tumor. At the subsequent clinical-pathological conference he dramatically announced that if this patient had had a multiphasic examination in the previous year, he would still be alive. After that no one in the San Francisco medical center questioned doing multiphasic blood calciums.

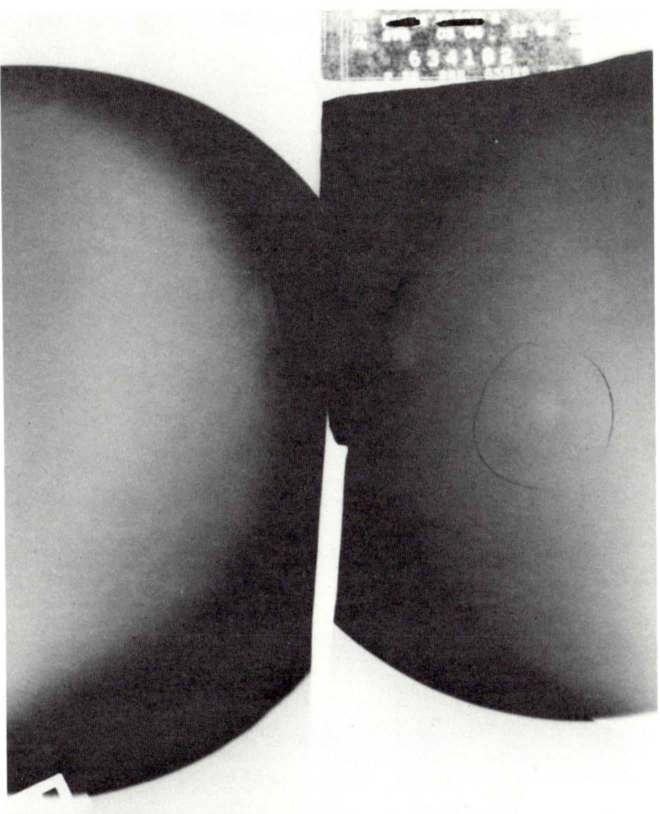

Figure 1-6. First breast cancer, not clinically palpable, detected in San Francisco MHTS.

An extraordinary event that occurred on a West Coast visit by Congressman Fogarty, who was then very influential in supporting medical research, gave MHTS some favorable publicity in Washington, D.C. After touring the Oakland multiphasic program, Fogarty stood in the computer center (Figure 1-13) watching the computer print out online advice rules, when one of the patient's reports showed a very high white cell count; the patient apparently had leukemia, previously unknown. The Congressman was greatly impressed; two days later he phoned from Washington to confirm whether the patient did have leukemia. This rare event could not have happened at a better time.

The importance of patient privacy was demonstrated early in the MHTS program when a prominent journalist, in his zeal to comprehend the full scope of the new concept, requested a multiphasic checkup for himself. He widely proclaimed his planned visit. Naturally, the multiphasic personnel attempted to treat him in a routine manner, like the other patients, yet they all knew this ''very important person'' was being examined. To everyone's everlasting embarrassment the computer reported out for this person a positive VDRL serological test for syphilis. It turned out to be a biologically false positive, but the lesson had been painfully learned. Henceforth it was established—and this rule has never been broken—

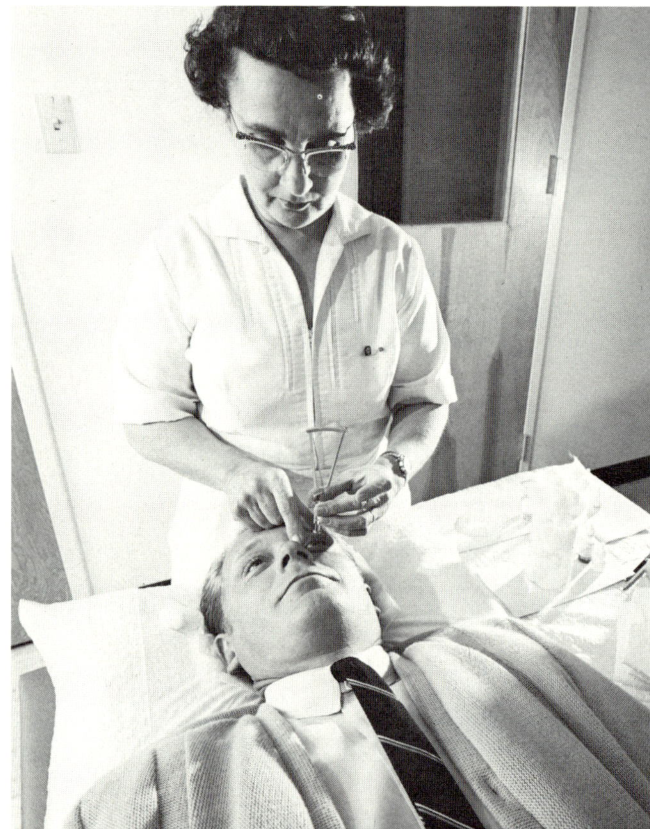

Figure 1-7.   First ocular tension measurements by Schiotz tonometer.

that anyone wishing to have a multiphasic checkup must arrange directly with the appointment clerks for his examination and that such booking information must be treated as confidentially as other patient data.

In the first Kaiser-Permanente multiphasic screening program in Oakland in 1951 a physician was at the last station reviewing all the online test results so that he could immediately arrange secondary and followup tests when indicated. The monotony of this task was so great that after a month or two no staff physician would accept it. Accordingly, medical resident physicians and the hospital internes were hired, but the responsibility not to overlook abnormalities while checking so many routine repetitive monotonous test results eventually overwhelmed them. This task was then discontinued for 12 years until automated computer-assisted MHTS permitted automatic review of test results by programmed decision rules. This is an excellent example of how the computer can and should replace a human for certain routine, repetitive, exacting, high-volume tasks. In the Kaiser-Permanente Oakland and San Francisco MHTS programs the computer, in the ten years between 1965–1975, provided this online review of multiphasic tests for about one-half million patients.

Overcoming the traditional opposition from physicians to multiphasic testing was something of a problem even within the Kaiser-Permanente program. Internists trained in traditional medicine felt that only the physician can determine

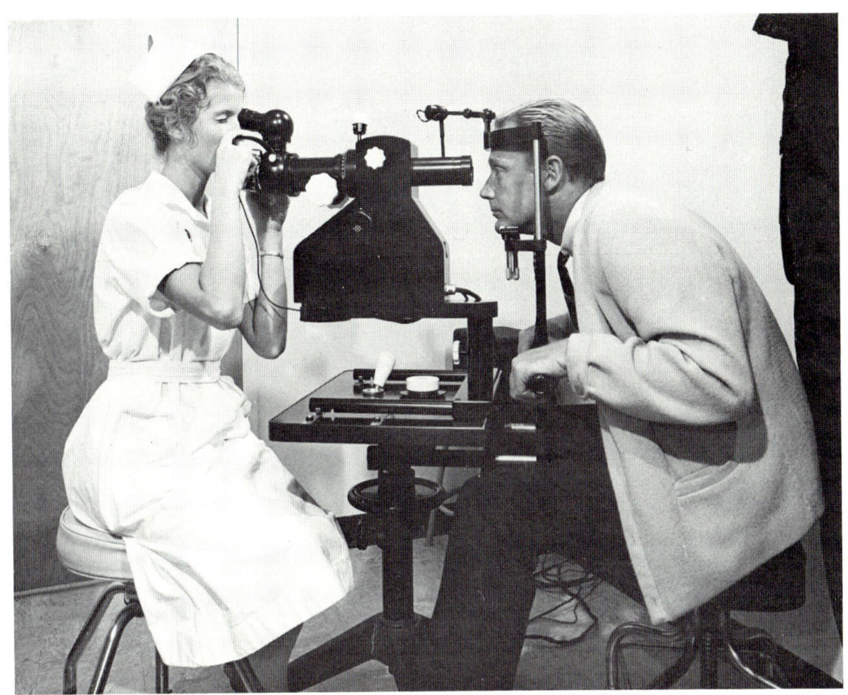

Figure 1-8. Retinal photography included as a research station to evaluate its clinical utility.

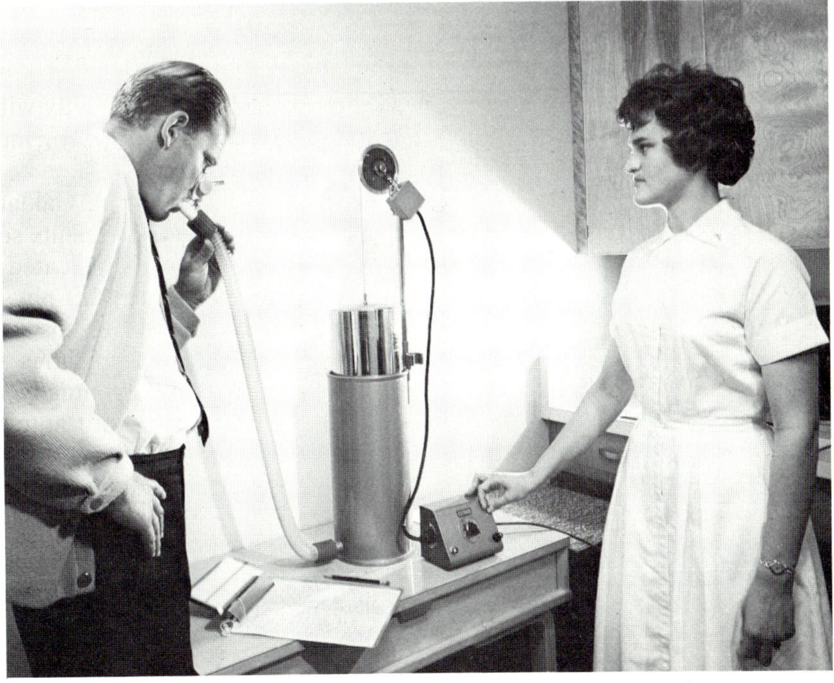

Figure 1-9. First timed vital capacity test with the Gaensler-Collins spirometer.

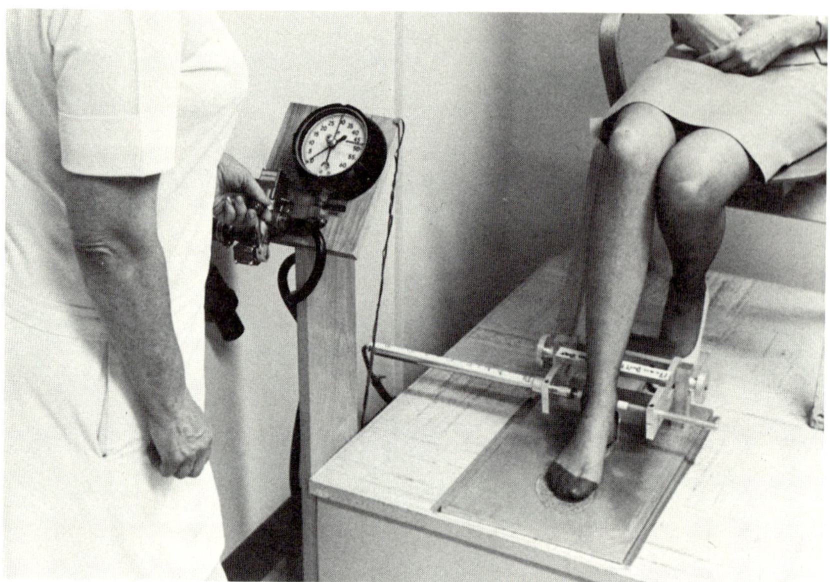

Figure 1-10. Pressure tolerance test for research studies on pain threshold.

what tests should be done for each patient. When, however, after a year's experience with the program, physicians in the Oakland medical department, who controlled the professional aspects of the multiphasic program, were given the option to terminate the program by secret ballot, they voted to continue it. Many Oakland and San Francisco Permanente physicians felt that multiphasic testing might increase the expense of medical care by generating secondary followup testing for (1) false positives, (2) borderline abnormal test results that they were not sure how to manage, and (3) early asymptomatic disease for which they had no effective treatment. On the other hand, a cost analysis presented at a formal meeting of the medical partnership in the late 1960s demonstrated that if the Oakland and San Francisco multiphasic programs were discontinued, the expenses of the medical group would increase by about $500,000 a year. Opposition reached a crisis on one occasion when the Oakland clinic medical director announced his decision to close down the multiphasic health checkup program. Fortunately for the program this decision was vetoed by Kaiser-Permanente's executive director. The continued support of forward-looking Kaiser-Permanente executives and of Kaiser Foundation Health Plan representatives, who found the membership and the public to be enthusiastic about the multiphasic checkups, carried the program through this difficult period.

In 1962 a Multiphasic Evaluation Study was initiated by the Kaiser-Permanente Medical Care Program in Oakland and San Francisco, sponsored in part by the U.S. Public Health Service and the Kaiser Foundation Research Institute. This project has continued to evaluate the effectiveness of periodic health examinations utilizing the MHTS approach. (See Chapters Seventeen and Eighteen.) During 1962–64 the study design for this project was formulated by an Advisory Committee composed of L. Breslow, J. Clausen, G. Dantzig, H. Jones, B. Milmore, L. Moses, J. Neyman, E. Scott, R. Stallones, A. Weissman, and J. Yerushalmy.

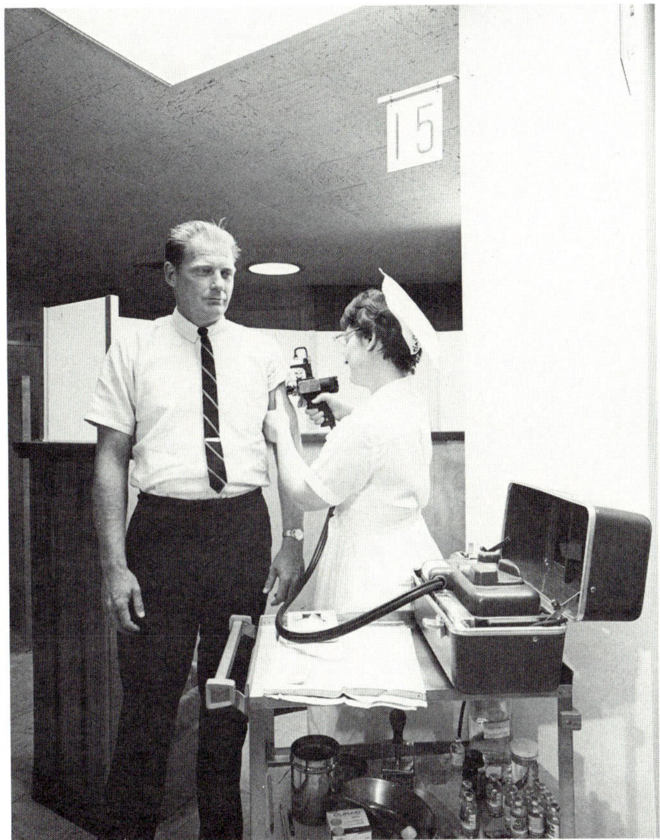

Figure 1-11. Tetanus toxoid immunization with the Hypospray gun.

After publication of the early results of the Multiphasic Evaluation Study, showing that automated multiphasic health testing was economical and efficient and that it did yield some patient outcome benefits (see Chapters Seventeen and Eighteen), opposition within the Kaiser-Permanente programs ceased, and multiphasic programs were begun in other of its centers including those in the Los Angeles, Hawaii, and Cleveland areas.

In industry, the gradual emergence of interest in automated multiphasic testing was manifested by a series of ten annual meetings arranged by the U.S. Public Health Service from 1958 to 1969. This Periodic Health Examination Group represented medical directors of several major American industries, U.S. Public Health Service officers, large medical group practices, and providers of health examinations. Information was exchanged on both the process and results of periodic health examinations. (See also Chapter Sixteen.) A Periodic Health Examination Cooperative Research Project continued some of these evaluations.[37]

In 1963 two comprehensive bibliographies were published—the first by Siegel[38] with 152 abstracts on periodic health examinations and the second by Mandel and Lillick[39] listing 250 references from 1960–1964 on health maintenance, periodic health examinations, and multiphasic screening.

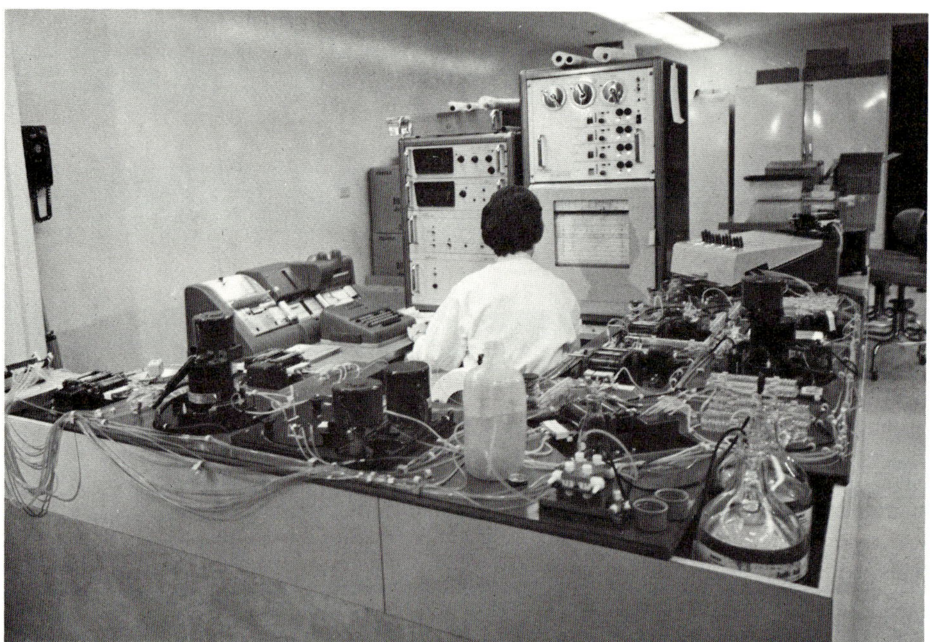

Figure 1-12. First automated eight-channel multichannel chemical analyzer (Technicon) interfaced with automated IBM card punch in the Oakland MHTS.

In 1966 a special committee of the U.S. Senate held extensive hearings on multiphasic screening.[40] These resulted in publication of abstracts[41] but no Senate legislative action.

The first books on multiphasic screening were published in 1968. Wilson and Jungner[42] published an excellent review of the subject for the World Health Organization, and Sharp and Keen[43] edited a series of papers reviewing the contemporary experience with the use of multiphasic screening for early diagnosis.

Automated multiphasic health testing received considerable impetus from a series of joint meetings of physicians and engineers arranged by Devey of the Engineering Foundation[44] in the late 1960s. In addition to the Engineering Foundation Research Conferences,[45] several symposia on MHTS were sponsored in the late 1960s and early 1970s by the Society for Advanced Medical Systems (SAMS)[46] and by the International Health Evaluation Association (IHEA).[47] The annual Technicon Symposia, initiated in 1965, also stimulated biomedical chemical profiling and chemistry panel testing for multiphasic programs.[48]

By 1968 organized medicine recognized the increasing importance of multiphasic testing by establishing the Intersociety Committee on Multiphasic Health Screening, which included ten major national medical groups as well as the American Medical Association.

In 1970 Sanazaro, then the Director of the HEW's National Center for Health Services Research and Development, sponsored a series of workshops that resulted in the publication of *Provisional Guidelines for AMHTS*,[49] a major milestone in providing definitions, guidelines for operation and test selection, and suggestions of further areas for research. Watts, the general chairman of this

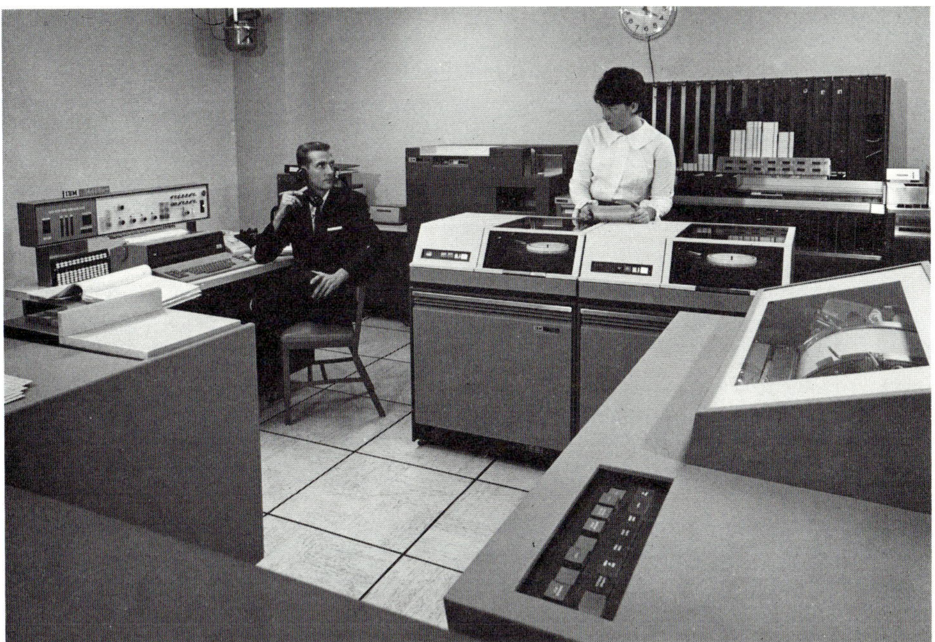

Figure 1-13. First IBM 1440 computer to provide data processing to both Oakland and San Francisco MHTS.

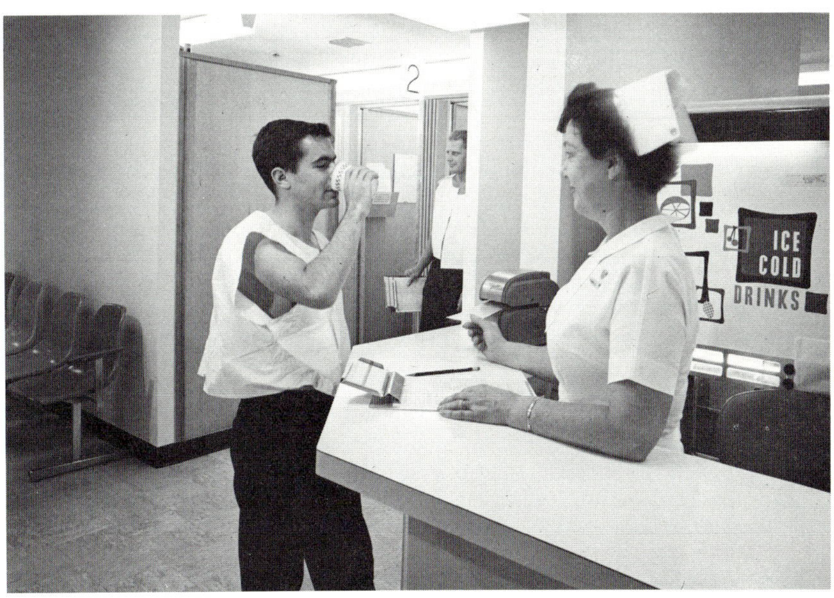

Figure 1-14. First automated glucose solution dispenser.

governmental advisory committee, expanded the concepts of automated multiphasic health testing to include adjunctive services. He recommended the term "automated multiphasic health testing and services" (AMHTS), since he felt the automated multiphasic principle clearly could be extended beyond testing to include programs for instruction and management of patients, under the direction of the patient's physician.

Watts felt that AMHTS had "promise of substantially increasing the capacity and reach of the pluralistic health care delivery system as it exists in the United States. When wisely and economically used, AMHTS should not only increase the quantity but also improve the quality and efficiency of medical and other health care services rendered to the citizens of this Nation. It is inevitable and also desirable in these times, when the expectations and demands for health care services have so far outstripped the capabilities of relatively scarce resources to deliver them, that the many potential uses of AMHTS will be explored, tested, and more widely applied."

Watts suggested:

> If one can view AMHTS as a planned course or series of events or procedures, programmed in advance and utilizing allied health personnel and automated instrumentation, through which various categories of persons who may or may not be patients under medical care are processed, in order to accomplish some medical or health-related purpose, then it becomes possible to appreciate how important an adjunct to medical and health care this can become. Briefly, AMHTS has the potential to do for the pluralistic health care delivery system of this Nation what programmed services and automation have done for much of its business and industry when these were faced with similar rising expectations and had inadequate resources with which to meet the new demands.
>
> While AMHTS can and will still be used to screen hitherto unreached segments of the population with a view to bringing additional individuals who need health care into the delivery system, this is clearly not enough. A parallel and perhaps even greater need to use AMHTS to augment available resources for delivery of patient care services to whatever extent may be feasible deserves to receive equal or even greater attention. And it should be added that there can be other highly desirable by-products to the uses of AMHTS. For example, its proper use can establish an accurate health data base for a given population. Also, there is reason to hope that by using AMHTS to detect disease early not only will patients benefit but the cost of remedy may be less.

He concluded:

> This then is what AMHTS is. It can and should be used to augment the capabilities of both public health and patient care services in order to enable the health care delivery system to "handle the increased traffic." Care must always be exercised to be certain that AMHTS be used only to improve the quantity, quality, and efficiency of needed services and that they do not simply add to the complexity and cost of health care without adding benefits which are in fact worth the additional cost.

The U.S.P.H.S., meanwhile, had awarded four contracts to initiate a formal study of the automated multiphasic health testing concept under the direction of Eleanor Smith.[50] As a result four Adult Health Protection Centers were established under (1) Constantine in Rhode Island Hospital with the State Health Department, Providence, (2) Krumbiegel in the City Health Department, Milwaukee, (3) Barbaccia at Tulane University, School of Medicine, New Orleans, and (4) Gitman in Brookdale Hospital Center, Brooklyn.

Although it was not unusual for some MHTS programs to incorporate physical examinations performed by physicians on site, in 1969 in the Kaiser-Permanente Oakland medical center a team of four specially trained nurse practitioners (under physician supervision) began to provide complete physical examinations online— that is, to patients immediately after their completion of the battery of multiphasic tests. (See Chapter Ten.)

In 1970 Garfield advocated a new concept of a medical care delivery system that used MHTS and physical examinations provided by nurse practitioners to triage patients into health care, preventive care, or sick care. (See Chapter Fifteen.)

In December 1971, after twenty years of experience, the Kaiser-Permanente program officially formulated and published the following advice to its health plan members:[52]

> For repeat periodic health checkups, after an initial such examination, healthy robust young adults in their twenties can wait an interval of three years or more. On these examinations, your doctor may have available or he may request certain laboratory or x-ray examinations, in addition to the physical examination. These findings are recorded in your medical record and serve as a basis for comparison at the time of later examination. If everything is within normal limits, your doctor may assure you that you can wait three years or more for your next checkup. If he finds something that requires more frequent attention, even though it is not a serious threat to your health, you will be advised to return as frequently as needed.
>
> Of course, if you do not feel entirely well or if you have any symptoms or other changes which disturb you, you should see a doctor. In this case, you should ask for an examination for medical diagnosis and care, rather than asking for a periodic ''checkup.''
>
> For healthy young adults in their thirties, periodic checkups at about two or three year intervals are recommended, after the initial checkup. If you are in your forties, an examination about every eighteen months or two years is recommended. If you are in your fifties, sixties, or older, your Permanente doctor can tell you how often to return. If everything was normal the last time and you feel healthy and full of zest, an annual checkup is recommended.
>
> Again, any deviation from an active enjoyable state of health should be an indication for diagnostic evaluation, rather than waiting a specified time for the next periodic health checkup.
>
> An exception to the above advice is for women in the childbearing age or older. Sexually active women should have an initial series of pelvic examinations and necessary tests about annually until the doctor recommends longer intervals between examinations. Although it is desirable to have this limited special examination, a complete overall medical checkup at the same time is unnecessary. You can also learn from your doctor (or from the exhibits at the Health Center in Oakland) about self-examination of your breasts for lumps.
>
> In summary, your doctors feel that it is in the best interest of your continued good health that you should have an initial complete examination on joining the Health Plan. As long as you enjoy robust positive health it is not necessary to have an *''annual''* checkup. Of course, if you wish, you are entitled to request such periodic checkups. However, many healthy young persons don't wish to take time out to see the doctor when they are full of vim and vigor. The other

side of the coin is that you should seek care when you notice any changes in your well-being; specifically, you should not wait until the next time your physical checkup is due.

Schoen[53] provided an *AMHT Program Directory, International 1972–73,* which detailed some specifications of about 200 operational MHTS programs. In 1971 Gelman[54] published an extensive study of the relevant literature on MHTS including its practice and evaluation.

In 1972 the American Medical Association published a comprehensive *Statement on Multiphasic Health Testing*[56] in which it reviewed the status of MHTS programs and advocated that multiphasic testing "should be integrated into the health care system in a manner that will assist the physician in the management of his patients." It prescribed ethical principles and provided guidelines for establishing and operating MHTS.

In 1973 Wynder[55] sponsored a "forum" on multiphasic health testing in the *Journal of Preventive Medicine. The Lancet* published a series of articles on multiphasic screening in Volume ii from October 5 to December 21, 1974.

In 1973 the Health Maintenance Organization (HMO) Act was passed in the United States to encourage organized systems of health care linked to prepayment, with a positive emphasis on preventive medicine. This was expected to encourage MHTS programs within HMOs, but the recession of 1974–75 inhibited the development of HMOs, though they began to emerge in 1976.

In 1975 HEW's Fogarty International Center sponsored a National Conference on Preventive Medicine, and Task Force III, chaired by Breslow, compiled detailed recommendations for periodic health evaluations for both children and adults.[58] (See Chapter Two.)

The provision of regular health examinations for children was accepted more readily than for adults. In 1900 compulsory school examinations were first established in Pennsylvania and Massachusetts. In 1967 the first automated multiphasic screening program specifically for children, designed by Shinefield and his associates,[57] was initiated in the Kaiser-Permanente San Francisco medical center. (See Chapter Fourteen.) However, it was not until 1972 that the Department of Health, Education, and Welfare in Washington established the program called Early and Periodic Screening Diagnoses and Treatment (EPSDT) to screen millions of school children throughout the United States. In 1975 a preventive health program, Child Health and Disability Prevention, was legislated in California, requiring that youngsters beginning school receive a prior multiphasic health testing examination. The law specified that each child was to receive a health history, physical and dental examination, hearing and vision assessment of growth and development, a check for tuberculosis, diabetes, anemia, and sickle cell trait when indicated, and immunization against measles and rubella, diphtheria, whooping cough, and tetanus.

F. THE CURRENT STATUS OF THE KAISER-PERMANENTE MHTS

The Kaiser-Permanente automated multiphasic health testing services program, operational in the Oakland medical center since 1964, served as a model for many of the MHTS programs that followed. It also served as the research and developmental center for trying out and evaluating many test phases for MHTS. Over a ten-year period the following tests were evaluated and discontinued for the reasons given:

(1) Phonocardiography. Insufficient sensitivity.[59]

(2) Tilt-table cardiovascular test to measure pulse and blood pressure before and after upright tilt to 70° (Figure 1-3). Not clinically useful.

(3) Pulse-wave velocity test to correlate velocity of propagation of the arterial pulse wave with the condition of the vessel wall. Not clinically useful.

(4) Somatotyping by multiple body measurements (Figure 1-4). Not clinically useful.

(5) Skinfold measurements. Of value in nutritional research but not clinically useful.

(6) X-ray of abdomen and back. Useful for detection of many asymptomatic clinically important abnormalities, but expensive to the point that it was not cost-effective.

(7) Pupillary escape test (''swinging flashlight test''). Detected some retinal or optic nerve disease,[60] but too infrequently to be cost-effective.

(8) Skull echograms. Demonstrated feasible as a screening test for deflections of the falx cerebri, but the condition was found to be too rare.

(9) Supraorbital thermography for cerebrovascular disease. Insufficiently sensitive and not cost-effective.

(10) Retinal photography (Figure 1-8). Excellent for recording retinal abnormalities but relatively insensitive for detection and too costly; also, it was too difficult to standardize diagnostic interpretations.

(11) Thermography for breast cancer detection. Less sensitive than mammography.

(12) Achilles reflex relaxation time to screen for thyroid disorders. Insufficient sensitivity and specificity.

(13) Pressure tolerance test to detect patients with high pain thresholds (Figure 1-10). Not successful.[61]

(14) Neuro-mental questionnaire—a modified MMPI type of psychological test. Useful for classification of research patients but not acceptable for clinical application.

(15) Immunization procedures for tetanus, smallpox, etc. Very cost-effective, but were transferred to the preventive health clinics as being more suitably located there (Figure 1-11).

(16) Medical history questionnaires in a variety of methods, including check lists, sort cards, portable punch cards, and interactive terminals (Searle Medi-Data). With all its limitations, the sort card method is still the most cost-effective in our program (Figure 1-26).

(17) Urine cultures on women. Discontinued after 10 years, since the treatment of asymptomatic bacteriuria was not demonstrated to be clinically effective.[62]

(18) Blood tests. Many were evaluated and discontinued as not being sufficiently sensitive or clinically useful, including vitamin C, trace metals (lead, cadmium, zinc, copper, arsenic, nickel, chromium, lithium, manganese, cobalt, and mercury), ABO blood grouping, latex agglutination (rheumatoid factor) test, serum albumin and total protein, serum iron and total iron binding capacity, SGPT, total lipids and β-lipoproteins.

The following brief description of the Oakland MHTS in 1976 represents the contemporary battery of tests considered most useful from a clinical viewpoint. (Subsequent chapters give more details.)

When a person makes an appointment for a multiphasic health checkup, he is sent printed instructions on how to prepare for it. He begins his multiphasic examination, which will take two to three hours, by presenting himself at the reception desk for registration. (A patient registers approximately every two minutes. Up to 220 patients are scheduled each day, of whom about 90 percent keep their appointments. Appointments for women are alternated according to age under and over 47 to accommodate the mammography schedule. Prior to each appointment the patient is mailed a reminder, together with an information sheet briefly describing each examination phase and giving directions for a standard meal to be eaten at home two hours in advance. A medical history questionnaire also has been included for the first examination.)

When the patient arrives, the receptionist identifies him, selects his deck of prepunched cards, and verifies the data on the identification card (Figure 1-15). She puts the deck of prepunched cards into a card holder attached to a clipboard, in which she also places an interval history form, which she instructs the patient to fill out whenever he has a few minutes to spare between tests.

The length of time since the patient has eaten a recommended standard test meal is noted, and the patient is sent to the clinical laboratory where samples are collected for blood and urine analysis. Twelve blood chemistry determinations are simultaneously performed by an automated chemical analyzer (Technicon), and the values for alkaline phosphatase, total bilirubin, calcium, cholesterol, creatinine, glucose, lactic dehydrogenase, potassium, sodium, transaminase (SGOT), urea nitrogen, and uric acid are punched directly into cards (Figure 1-16). Blood hemoglobin, red and white cell counts, and red cell indices are automatically measured (Coulter counter) and also punched into cards. A serological (VDRL) test for syphilis is performed. A freshly voided urine specimen, collected midstream, is analyzed for pH, glucose, protein, and blood by paper-strip enzyme tests, and these results are marksensed onto a card (Figure 1-17).

The patient is then directed into a dressing cubicle, where he undresses to the waist and puts on a disposable paper gown (Figure 1-18). When the patient, wearing a paper gown, arrives at the electrocardiography station, he is directed to lie on a table, electrodes are applied, and the electrocardiogram is recorded using a multichannel polygraph (Figure 1-19).

Since a computer program that accurately compares an ECG to a prior ECG is not yet available, the polygraph paper tracing is sent, with the electrocardiogram report marksense card, to the cardiologist, who records the appropriate interpretation by marking it with a special high-carbon marksense pencil. The next day the cards are returned to the computer center, where the marks on them are sensed by a reproducing machine that punches a hole corresponding to each mark, thus converting the marked cards into machine-readable cards.

Blood pressure is measured with automated equipment that produces direct punched-card output. A cuff is wrapped around the patient's upper arm and automatically inflated to a high pressure; then it is allowed to deflate at a standard rate, while the systolic and diastolic pressure are recorded (Figure 1-20).

The patient's weight and height are then determined, the readings being recorded by manual keypunching into the anthropometry test card.

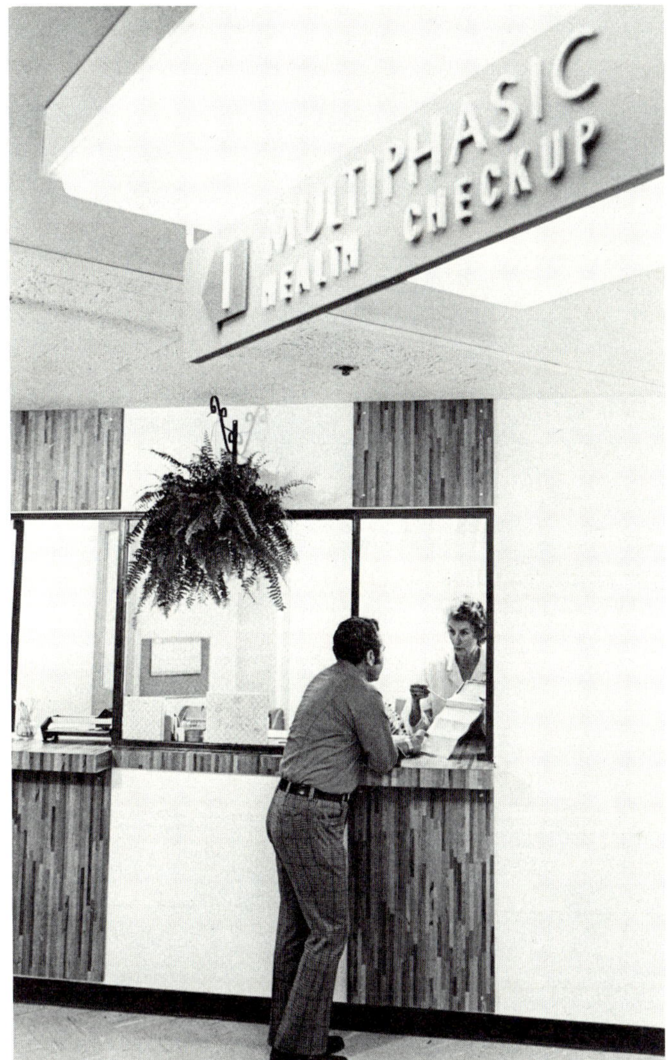

Figure 1-15.   Present registration area in Oakland MHTS.

Next the patient's ventilatory function is measured with a flow meter (Figure 1-21) which records the one- and two-second forced expiratory vital capacities, total vital capacity, and the peak flow measurements directly into the punched card. The test is repeated three times, and the computer program selects the best of the three tests.

At the following station the patient receives a 70 mm posterior-anterior chest x-ray (Figure 1-22), which is subsequently read by the radiologist who records his interpretation on a marksense card. The cards are returned to the computer room for data processing.

All women over age 47 receive an x-ray examination of the breast for detection of possible cancer (Figure 1-23). Cephalocaudad and lateral-tangential views of

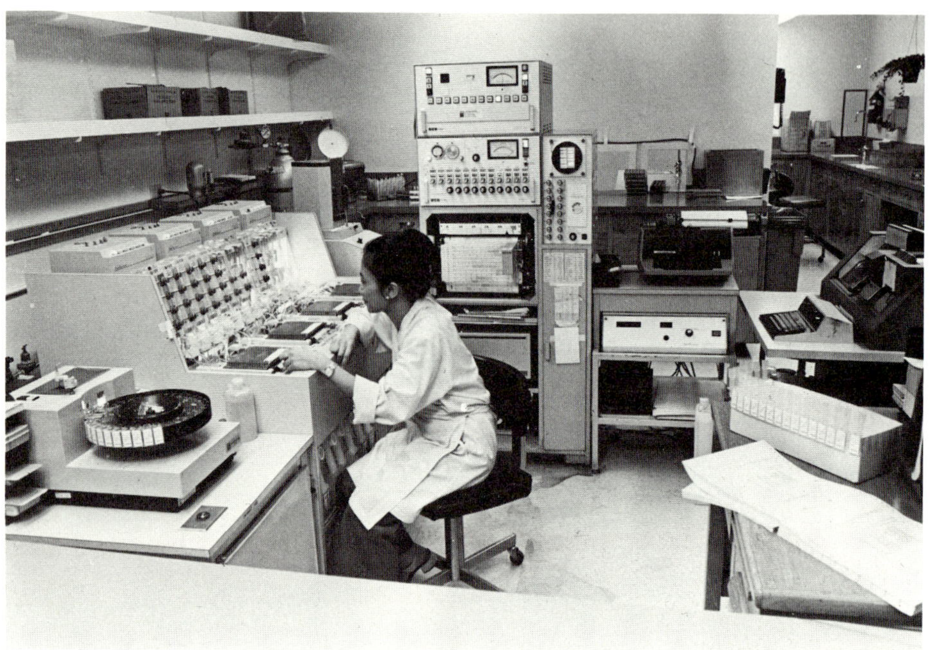

Figure 1-16. Present 12-channel automated chemical analyzer (Technicon) in Oakland MHTS, interfaced with original card punch shown in Figure 1-12.

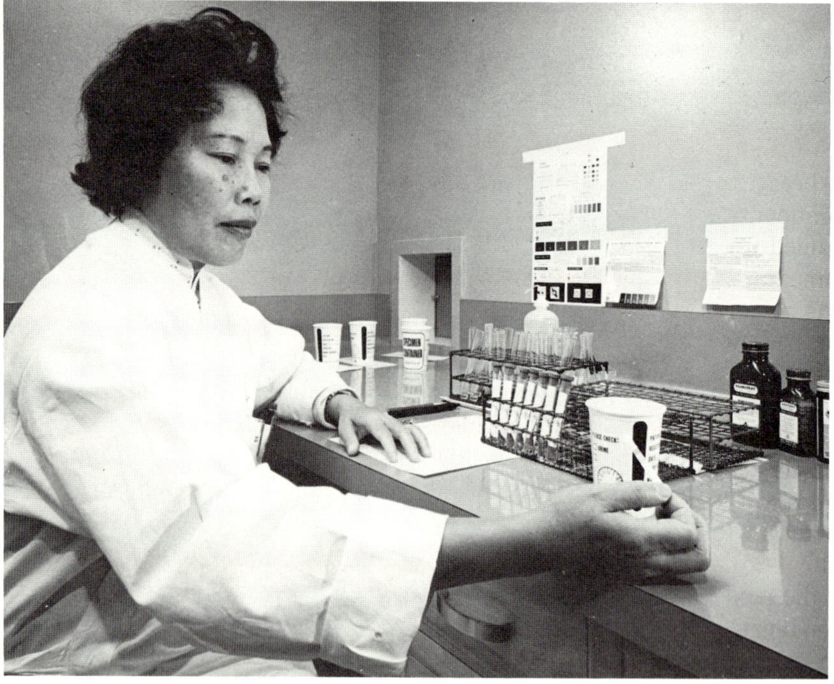

Figure 1-17. Urinalysis performed by paper-strip enzyme tests (Ames) and results marksensed on patients' cards.

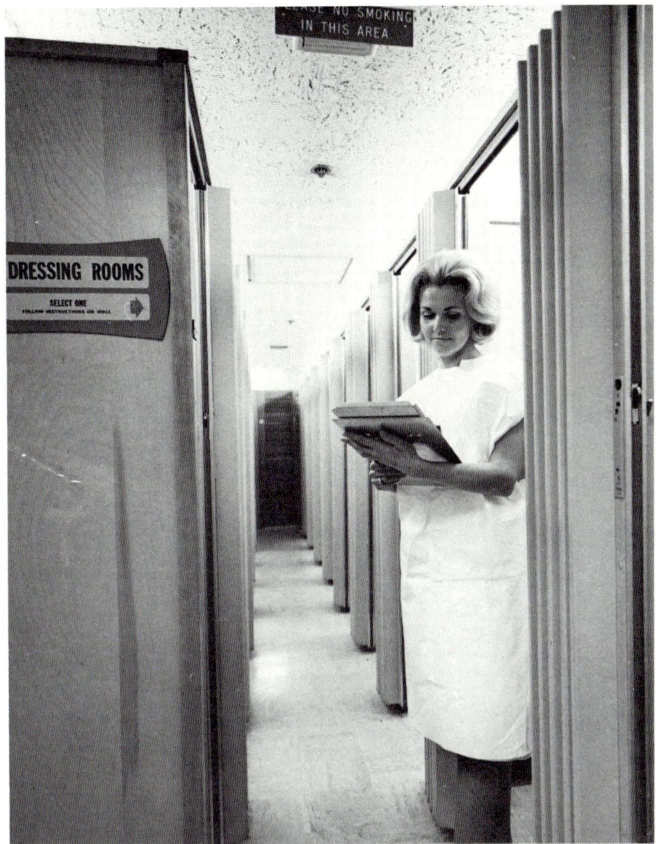

Figure 1-18.   Patient with disposable paper gown emerging from dressing booth carrying cardholder-clipboard.

each breast are taken. Since mammography requires about 10 to 12 minutes, appointments are alternated according to age, so that only every other woman is scheduled for this procedure; or else two mammography stations can be used. Mammograms are subsequently read by the radiologist, who records his interpretations on marksense cards.

The patient then returns to the dressing booth and dresses.

Next the visual acuity is tested by chart reading, and ocular tension is automatically determined by an instrument that measures the deflection of the cornea by a puff of air (Figure 1-24).

Hearing acuity is tested with an automated audiometer, and the graphed readings are transferred by the technician to a marksense card. A group of six patients are tested simultaneously, each seated in an acoustically tiled cubicle (Figure 1-25).

At the next station the medical questionnaire form that the patient received at station one to complete during waiting periods is audited by a nurse. The patient is given another inventory-by-systems medical questionnaire, which he answers by sorting as "yes" or "no" a set of cards prepunched for computer input (Figure 1-26) or by indicating multiple-choice responses on portable punch cards (Figure 1-27). (See also Chapter Sixteen, B.1, and Figure 16-1.)

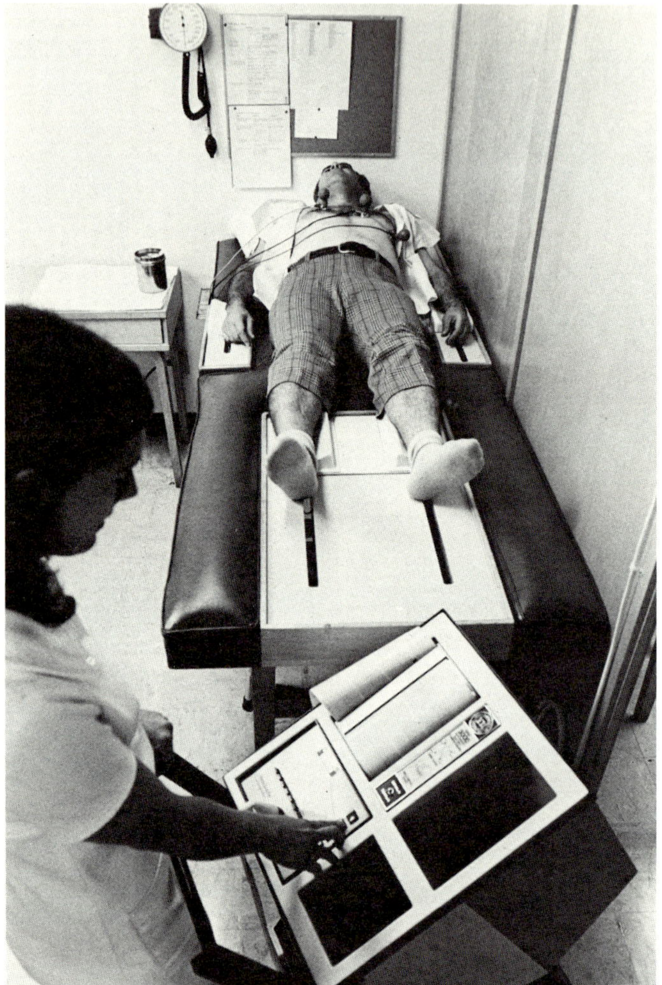

Figure 1-19.   Current multichannel electrocardiograph cart (Marquette).

At the last MHTS station the patient returns the medical questionnaires and the packet of cards on which, whenever possible, his test results were directly recorded by punching or marksensing, so as to permit their immediate introduction into the data processing system (Figure 1-28). While he waits, the online punched cards are read into the computer by a remote, job entry, card reader terminal. The computer processes all online test data before the patient leaves the MHTS laboratory and provides "advice rules" as to any indicated repeat tests or urgent followup appointments.

The majority of the patients now receive a complete physical examination (including pelvic examination and cervical smear for females) by a certified nurse practitioner under supervision of a physician (Figure 1-29). (See Chapter Ten.) The remainder receive a followup appointment with their physician for the physical examination.

Within 20 days the computer processes all offline test results and provides a final printout MHTS report for the physician (or nurse practitioner). Figure 1-30

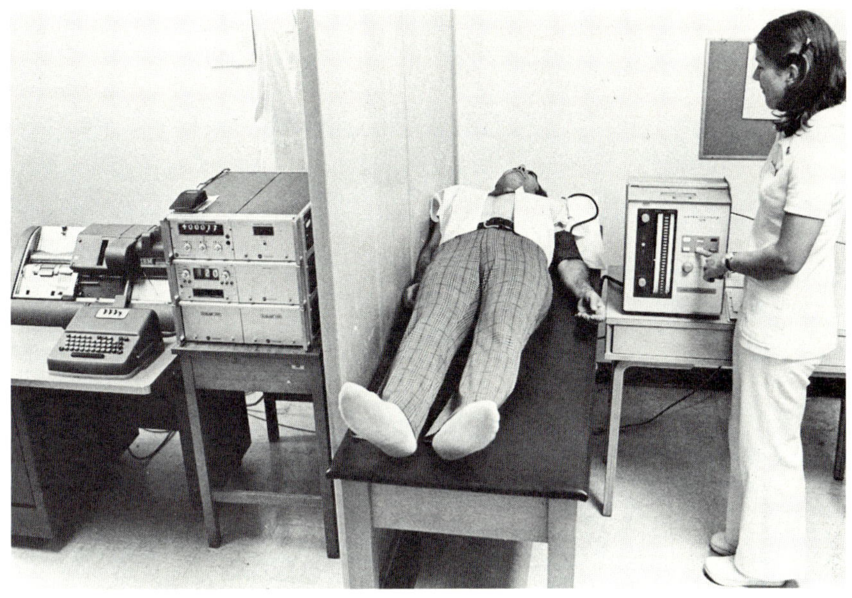

Figure 1-20. Current automated blood pressure instrument (Arteriosonde) interfaced to card punch.

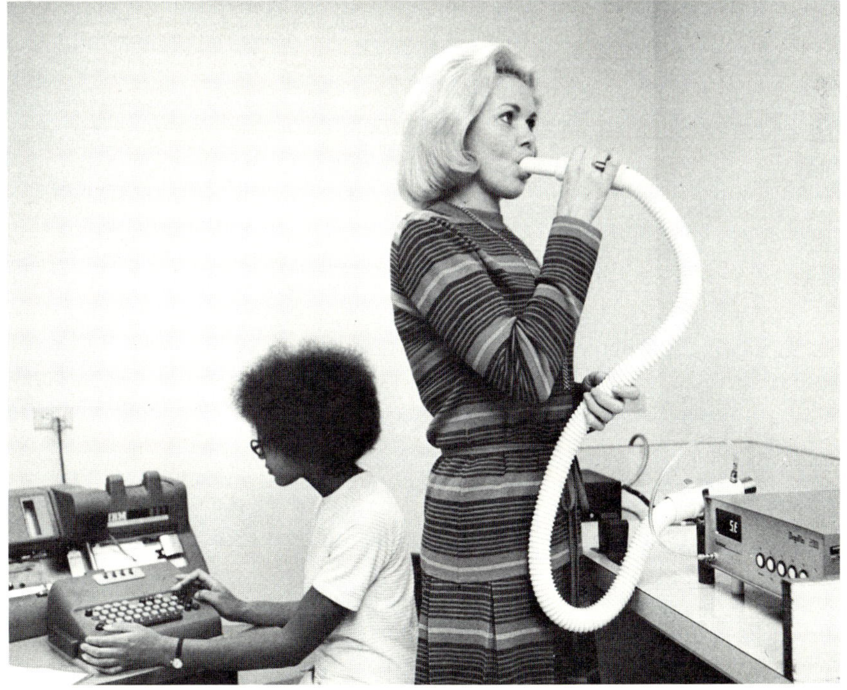

Figure 1-21. Flow meter spirometer (Digiflo) interfaced to card punch.

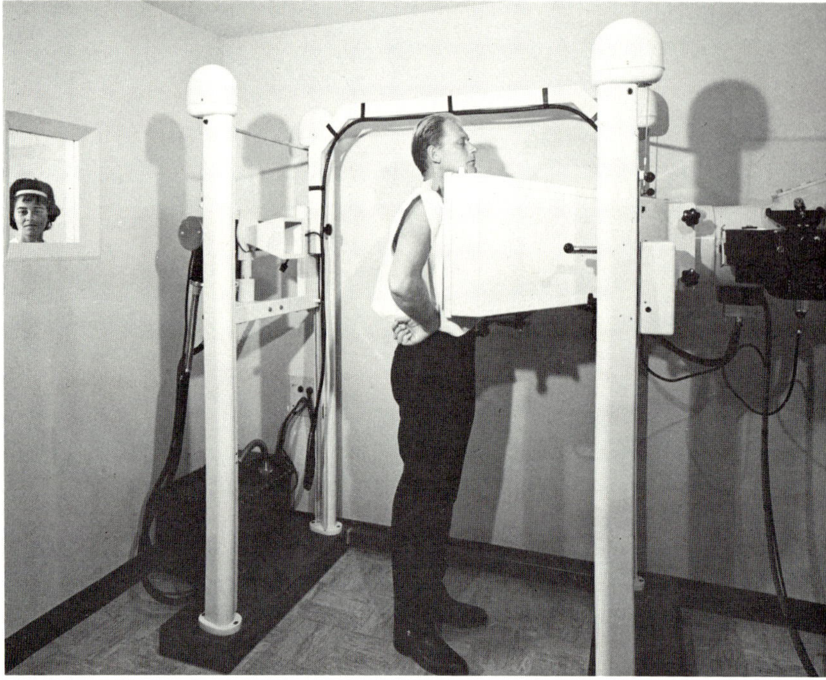

Figure 1-22.   Chest x-ray (Odelca) providing 70 mm roentgenograms.

shows an example of one of several evolutions of a final MHTS report. Referrals for necessary followup care are then arranged by the physician or nurse.

G.   THE CURRENT WORLDWIDE STATUS OF MHTS

Although it still contains some controversial aspects, the MHTS concept is now widely accepted for a great variety of preventive medical care applications in many countries. Many governments and their health departments are now officially advocating health centers which, if systematized for large population groups, will eventually tend to accept some modification of the multiphasic health testing services approach. In the United States, many of these are sponsored by the community, by prepaid or fee-for-service physician groups, or by industrial medical programs. Some are operated by union or welfare agencies or by armed services. They are mostly organized for adults but some are for children; they are generally located in urban areas but may be contained in mobile units for rural areas. They are essentially preventive medicine programs for disease detection, disease monitoring, health surveillance, and health appraisal, but they are also used for determination of the individual's and community's health status, for physical capacities analysis by industry or the armed services, for entry to medical care, for establishing an individual's health profile or a population data base for health services research and development, and for the teaching of community and preventive medicine. Some MHTS programs are small and very selective for specified high-risk groups; some are large and provide a uniform comprehensive battery of tests to all. Most provide periodic examinations at intervals according

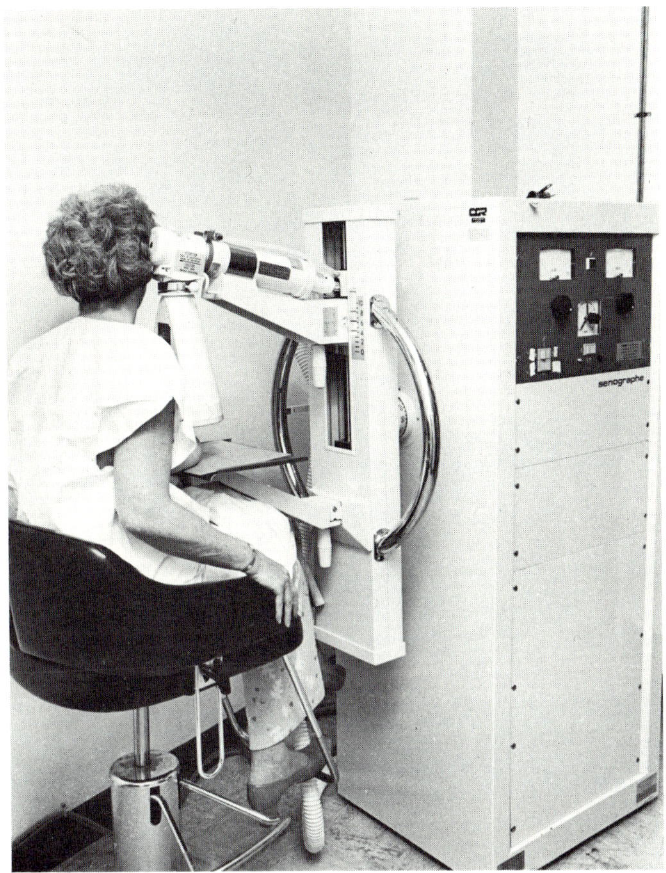

Figure 1-23. Current mammography (Senograph) machines for breast cancer detection.

to age, health-hazard risk factors, or the individual physician's recommendation rather than annually. Most that have survived have been an integral part of some health care system.

Computer-supported MHTS programs are now widespread throughout the developed countries of the world. As of 1975 there were about 325 in the United States, about 40 in Japan, about 30 in Europe, and a few in Australia, Asia, Canada, and Latin America. Many of the comments made below on specific programs are based upon personal visits to these countries.

A registry of automated multiphasic health testing programs published in 1973[53] listed 26 in California, 21 in New York, 13 in Illinois, and 11 in Michigan. Other states had less than 10 each.

Japan has placed a high priority on MHTS for industry health examinations. During the late 1960s hundreds of Japanese physicians visited the Oakland Kaiser-Permanente MHTS program. By 1975 there were 10 programs in Tokyo, five in Osaka, and one or two in additional cities for a total of more than 40. Some of these centers have the most advanced computer technology in the world, using time-sharing, data base management systems to compare current patient data to those from prior examinations. The programs of Japan's well-designed mobile MHTS units include routine gastrointestinal x-ray examinations.

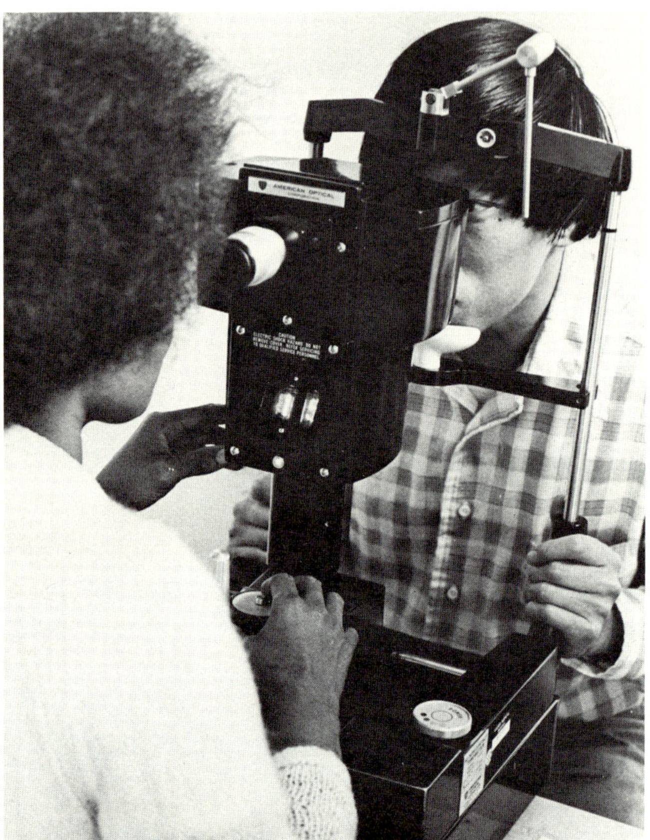

Figure 1-24.   Current instrument (American Optical) for measuring ocular tension.

France has a number of evolving MHTS programs. Although a Social Security law passed in 1947 which permits every person one health checkup every five years, the first and the largest MHTS was started in 1971 in Nancy modeled after the Oakland Kaiser-Permanente multiphasic center. This program, supported entirely by Social Security, provided free checkups to the immediate community of 200,000 people around Nancy at the rate of 1,250 examinations per month. The French Social Security System is planning additional MHTS programs in Paris, Marseilles, Rennes, Tours, Bordeaux, Toulouse, and other major French cities.

Sweden was one of the pioneers in multiphasic health testing. Hall at the Serafimer Hospital in Stockholm was the first to use multiphasic testing for hospital admissions, and Jungner did the first large regional multiphasic screening program in the Varmland project. Sweden's Surgeon General Linroth was the first to use an MHTS for military screening, examining 60,000 Swedish Armed Forces conscripts yearly. (See Chapter Sixteen.)

MHTS programs have begun in Germany, and one is in operation in Vienna.

A National Health Act came into force in Finland in 1972, establishing Health Centers with the primary responsibility of providing health checkups, health maintenance, and health education. The MHTS concept is being considered.

The Swiss government's health insurance was revised in 1974 to allow adults

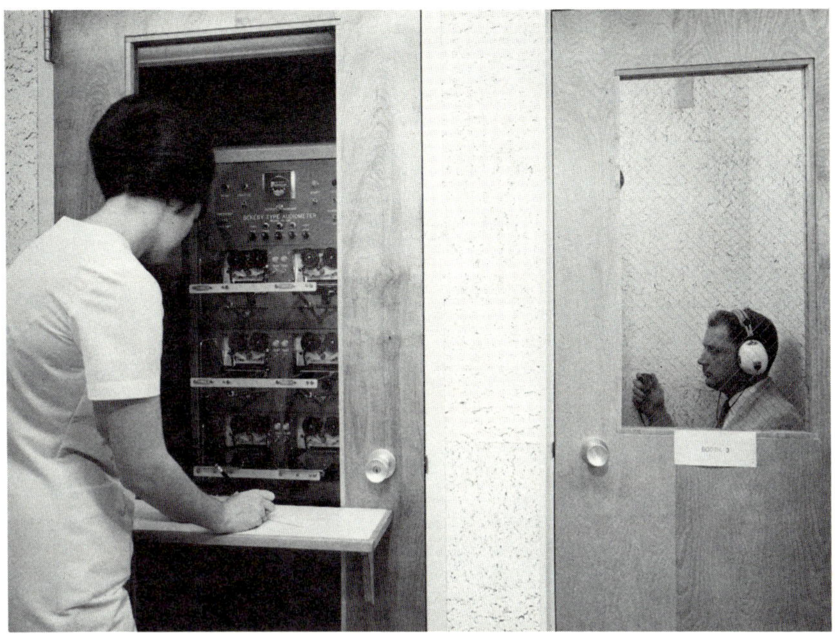

Figure 1-25. Automated audiometer (Rudmose-Bekesy) for simultaneous testing of hearing acuity of six patients.

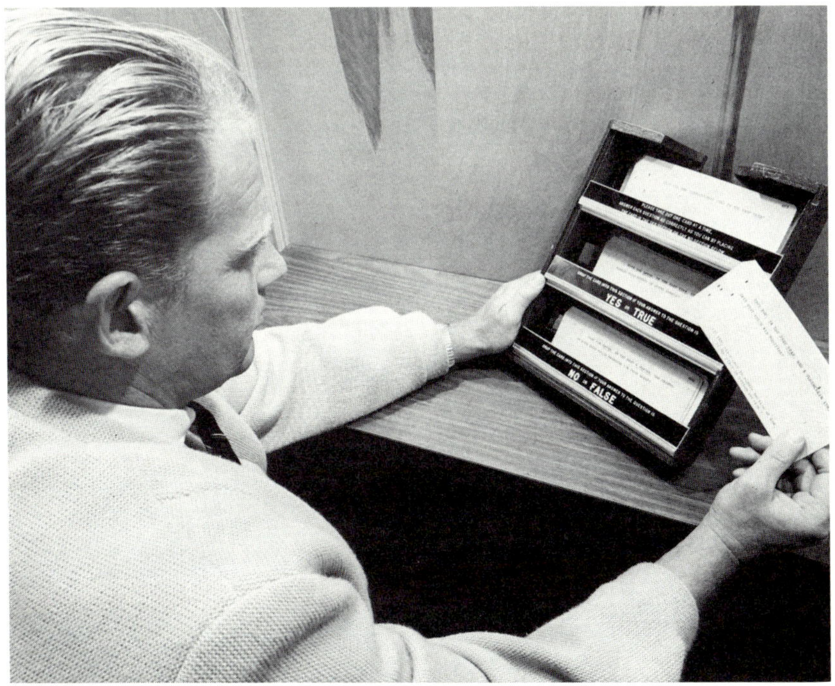

Figure 1-26. Obtaining a self-administered medical history by sorting prepunched questionnaire cards. (See also Figure 20-38.)

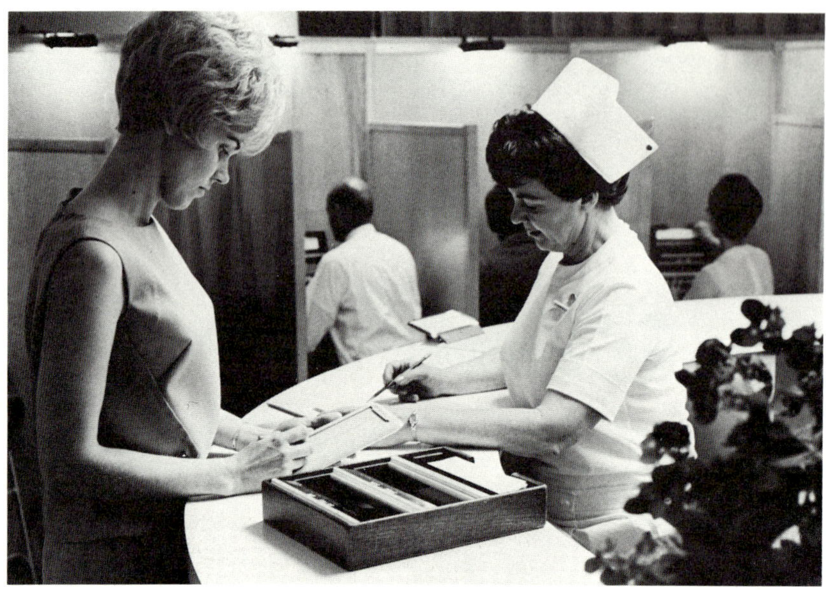

Figure 1-27. Nurse reviewing medical history checklist and patient using portable punch cards. (See also Figure 16-1.)

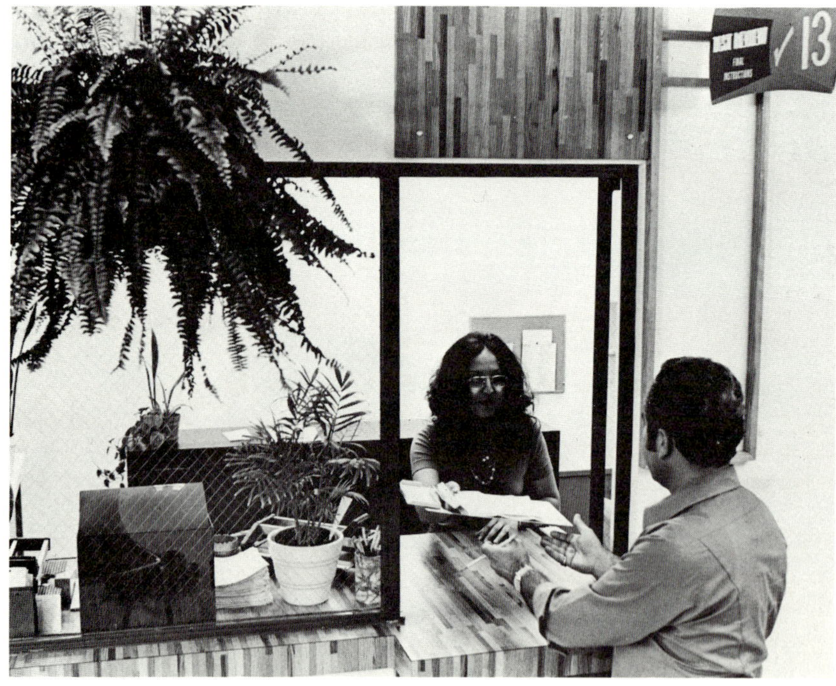

Figure 1-28. Final test review and referral for followup station.

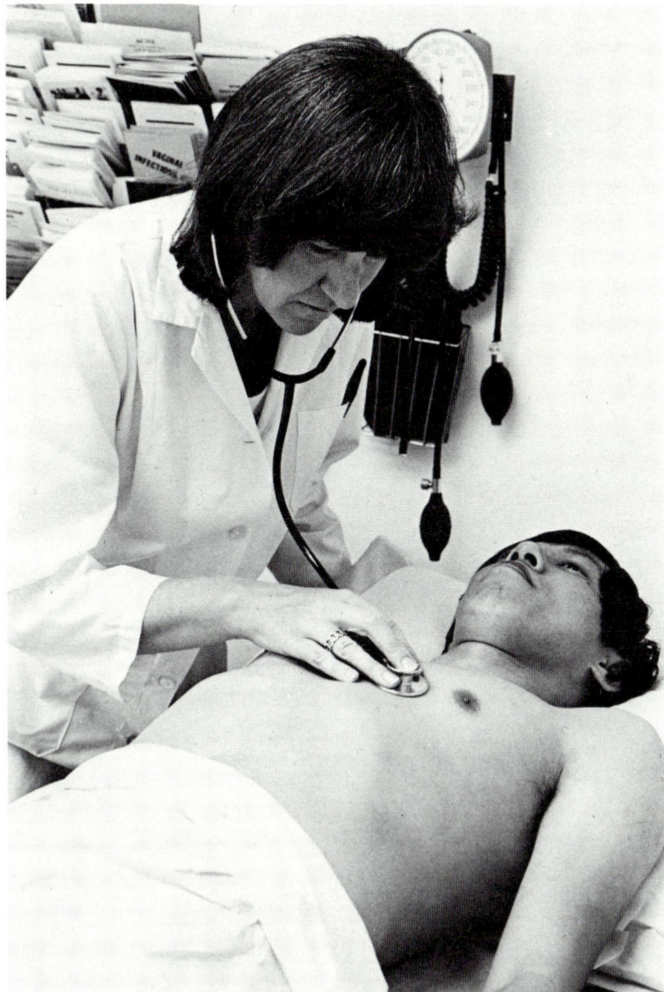

Figure 1-29. Nurse practitioner giving physical examination.

to obtain periodic health examinations, but systemized MHTS were not yet planned.

In Italy four MHTS programs are operational, two in Milan, one in Montecatini, and one in Rome; and Mase, Scientific Head of their National Institute for Health Insurance (INAM) is planning a large health evaluation center in Rome.

In Titograd, Yugoslavia, a pilot MHTS for evaluative purposes was initiated in collaboration with U.S.P.H.S. support in 1969. In the Soviet Union, although several official visits to the Kaiser-Permanente MHTS have occurred for the purpose of initiating more preventive health care in the U.S.S.R., no MHTS programs have yet been instituted.

In England the National Health Service does not support a single health evaluation program, because the official policy is to wait until there is agreement among physicians on the value of multiphasic health testing. British epidemiologists

```
                    PERMANENTE MEDICAL GROUP - OAKLAND
           DUPLICATE REPORT - MULTIPHASIC HEALTH CHECKUP (MHC)  -   5/20/69

TEST,PATIENT                    RETIRED                  S.F. DR. SMITH
MR: 2258590 J1      AGE 50      FEMALE      WIDOWED          LAST MHC  6/16/68


                            SUMMARY OF REPORT
           ************************************************

          (TEST)                   (NORMAL)    (THIS EXAM)
          CIRCULATORY:
  **      B.P.SUPINE(GODART): 90-159/ 50- 89     164/100      1
          HEMATOLOGY:
  **      HEMOGLOBIN GM.:         12.0- 16.0        9.2
  **      MHC MCMCG:              26.0- 34.0        20.6
  **      MCHC %:                 32.0- 38.0        25.6
  ¬       BLOOD CHEMISTRY:
  **      GLUCOSE 1 HR MG%:     UNDER-   263        332
  **      GLUCOSE 2 HR MG%:     UNDER-   150        164
  **      VDRL:                      NEG           POS
  **      QUANTITATIVE VDRL:                       RRWWWN
          URINE:
  **      GLUCOSE:                   NEG           MED
  **      CLINITEST:                 NEG           3+
  **      ACETONE:                   NEG           POS

  ** BREAST X-RAY:  FIBROCYSTIC DIFFUSE CHANGES
  ** HEARING:       CLINICALLY IMPAIRED HEARING LEFT

     PATIENT RECEIVED FOLLOWING (ADVICE RULE) DIRECTIONS:
        700-REQUEST PT.RET. AMS LAB FOR 2-HR SERUM SUGAR
        801-NOTICE SENT TO PHYSICIAN: CONSIDER EARLY APPTMT.

  *     IN PAST YEAR SPELLS OF WEAKNESS OR PARALYSIS OF ARMS OR LEGS
  *     IN PAST YEAR BLURRING OF EYESIGHT LASTING OVER A FEW MINUTES
  *     IN PAST YEAR ANY LOSS OF HEARING WHICH IS STILL PRESENT
  *     IN PAST 6 MONTHS OFTEN HAD PAIN IN THE EAR
  *     IN PAST 6 MONTHS 2 OR MORE NOSE BLEEDS NOT FROM INJURY OR A COLD
  *     IN PAST YEAR COUGHED UP ANY BLOOD




TND = TEST NOT DONE   PRT = PAT. REFUSED TEST   TNI = TEST NOT INDICATED
BND = BLOOD NOT DRAWN  UNSAT = TEST UNSATISFACTORY   - = DATA NOT AVAILABLE
NSA = NO SIGNIFICANT ABNORMALITY
 * = PATIENT ANSWERED YES ON THIS MHC AND NO ON LAST MHC
** = CONSIDER POSSIBLE ABNORMAL           ¬ = NOTE        242-11:47:03
```

Figure 1-30a. Multiphasic health checkup final report computer printout.

generally oppose MHTS on the basis that for some conditions (especially chronic diseases) it is difficult to evaluate to what extent early detection alters the natural history of the disease. (See Chapter Eighteen.) Despite this, private groups have set up multiphasic health testing programs in London and Lancashire.

England's negative view has had an effect on Canada, which has MHTS centers in Montreal and Toronto; and on Australia, which has centers in Sydney and in Melbourne.

In Latin America, health evaluation programs are operational in Mexico City and are being established in Buenos Aires, Sao Paulo, and Rio de Janiero.

```
              PERMANENTE MEDICAL GROUP - OAKLAND
       DUPLICATE REPORT - MULTIPHASIC HEALTH CHECKUP (MHC)  -  5/20/69

TEST,PATIENT                    RETIRED                  S.F. DR. SMITH
MR: 2258590 J1      AGE 50      FEMALE      WIDOWED          LAST MHC  6/16/68


       (TEST)                 (NORMAL)    (THIS EXAM)  (LAST MHC)   (RANGE  2 MHCS)
                                                        (1968)      (1967-1966)
       HEIGHT  IN.:                         63.8        64.0        63.5 - 63.9
       WEIGHT  LB.:                        133.5       132.0       131.5 -133.5
       TRICEPS SKINFOLD MM.:  UNDER- 43.0   23.0        18.0        19.0 - 20.0
       CIRCULATORY:
  **    B.P.SUPINE(GODART): 90-159/ 50- 89 164/100     154/104  135-144/ 86- 98
       RAD. PULSE SUPINE:       60-    95    68          76          66 -    74
       RESPIROMETRY:
       FEV 1 SEC   L.:        OVER-  1.2     2.1         2.0         1.9 -  2.3
       FEV 2 SEC   L.:                       2.4         2.5         2.2 -  2.6
       TOTAL FEV   L.:        OVER-  2.1     2.8         2.7         2.5 -  2.9
       PEAK FLOW   L.:                       4.1         4.0         3.9 -  4.4
       ACHILLES REFLEX MS.:   250-   400     290         270         280 -  310
       HEMATOLOGY:
       WBC /CU MM.:           3500-12000    7700        6600        5500 - 7700
       RBC MILLIONS/CU MM.:    4.0-   5.5    4.5         TND         TND -    TND
  **    HEMOGLOBIN GM.:       12.0-  16.0    9.2        11.2        13.1 - 13.9
       HEMATOCRIT:            35.0-  49.0   36.0         TND         TND -   TND
       MCV CU MICRONS:          80-   100    80          TND         TND -   TND
  **    MHC MCMCG:            26.0-  34.0   20.6         TND         TND -   TND
  **    MCHC %:               32.0-  38.0   25.6         TND         TND -   TND
  ¬    BLOOD CHEMISTRY:
       POTASSIUM MEQ/L:        3.0-   5.0    3.7         TND         TND -   TND
       CALCIUM MG%:            8.0-  10.5    9.9         9.5         9.0 - 10.8
  **    GLUCOSE 1 HR MG%:     UNDER-  263    332         234         212 -  247
  **    GLUCOSE 2 HR MG%:     UNDER-  150    164          -          -  -   -
       BUN  MG.:              UNDER- 22.0  15.2(C)       TND         TND -   TND
       CREATININE MG%: .      UNDER-  1.4    .9(C)        .9          .8 -  1.2
       URIC ACID MG%:          2.0-   7.3   3.5(C)       TND         2.2 -  5.4
       BILIRUBIN TOT MG%:     UNDER-  1.5    .9          TND         TND -   TND
       ALK PTASE KA UNITS:    UNDER- 15.0    6.0         TND         TND -   TND
       SGOT RF UNITS:         UNDER-   40   36(C)        25          23 -   38
       SGPT RF UNITS:         UNDER-   50   25(C)        TND         TND -   TND
       CHOLESTEROL MG%:         90-   330  275(C)        200         195 -  220
  **    VDRL:                   NEG          POS        NEG         NEG -   NEG
  **    QUANTITATIVE VDRL:                  RRWWWN
       BLOOD GROUP:                           O


¬ ONE-HOUR SERUM CHYLOUS:     (C) INDICATES TEST MAY BE AFFECTED
¬ ONE HR BLOOD DRAWN 20 MINUTES LATE    TWO HR BLOOD DRAWN 22 MINUTES LATE






** = CONSIDER POSSIBLE ABNORMAL          ¬ = NOTE
SEE LAST PAGE FOR DESCRIPTION OF ADDITIONAL FOOTNOTES         CONTINUE
```

Figure 1-30b.

In the Middle East, an MHTS was being installed in 1975–76 in Saudi Arabia and in Tel Aviv.

In the underdeveloped countries of the world numerous factors, including lack of trained medical and technical personnel, inhibit successful delivery of health services, and MHTS is applicable to such areas only with extensive modifications, including low-cost intermediate technology to meet the specific needs of such populations. In these areas, where data for health planning is often inadequate, MHTS could obviously provide a valuable data base for such planning.

In general, the international picture for MHTS is optimistic. Considering the common economic problems of the world in 1974–77 and the time required for

```
TEST,PATIENT              MR 2258590    ACE 50    FEMALE    MHC    5/20/69  PAGE 2

        (TEST)                 (NORMAL)   (THIS EXAM)  (LAST MHC)  (RANGE  2 MHCS)
                                                        (1968)      (1967-1966)


     URINE:
       PH:                                    6            7          7 -     7
**     GLUCOSE:               NEG            MED          NEG        NEG -   NEG
**     CLINITEST:             NEG            3+            -          - -  -
**     ACETONE:               NEG            POS           -          - -  -
       PROTEIN:               NEG            NEG          NEG        NEG -   NEG
       BLOOD:                 NEG            NEG          NEG        NEG -   NEG
       URINE BACILLI:         NEG            NEG          NEG        NEG -   NEG


     CHEST X-RAY:    NO SIGNIFICANT CHANGE FROM PRIOR X-RAY
            1968:    NO SIGNIFICANT CHANGE FROM PRIOR X-RAY
**   BREAST X-RAY:   FIBROCYSTIC DIFFUSE CHANGES
            1968:    NO SIGNIFICANT CHANGE FROM PRIOR X-RAY
     ECG:            NO SIGNIFICANT CHANGE FROM PRIOR ELECTROCARDIOGRAM
            1968:    NO SIGNIFICANT CHANGE FROM PRIOR ELECTROCARDIOGRAM
**   HEARING:        CLINICALLY IMPAIRED HEARING LEFT
            1968:    CLINICALLY IMPAIRED HEARING LEFT
     VISUAL ACUITY:  L.E. 20/40 OR BETTER, R.E. 20/40 OR BETTER
            1968:    L.E. 20/40 OR BETTER, R.E. 20/40 OR BETTER
     OCULAR TENSION:LEFT EYE NORMAL, RIGHT EYE NORMAL
            1968:    LEFT EYE NORMAL, RIGHT EYE NORMAL


     PATIENT RECEIVED FOLLOWING (ADVICE RULE) DIRECTIONS:
        700-REQUEST PT.RET. AMS LAB FOR 2-HR SERUM SUGAR
        801-NOTICE SENT TO PHYSICIAN: CONSIDER EARLY APPTMT.


        PATIENT ANSWERED YES TO THESE QUESTIONS ON THE MHC 1969 FORM:
        HAD BAD REACTION OR SENSITIVITY TO SULFA DRUGS
        IN PAST 6 MONTHS BAD HEADACHES NOT HELPED BY ASPIRIN, EMPIRIN, ETC
*       IN PAST YEAR SPELLS OF WEAKNESS OR PARALYSIS OF ARMS OR LEGS
*       IN PAST YEAR BLURRING OF EYESIGHT LASTING OVER A FEW MINUTES
        IN PAST YEAR ANY TIMES WHEN YOU WERE CROSS-EYED OR WALL-EYED
*       IN PAST YEAR ANY LOSS OF HEARING WHICH IS STILL PRESENT
*       IN PAST 6 MONTHS OFTEN HAD PAIN IN THE EAR
*       IN PAST 6 MONTHS 2 OR MORE NOSE BLEEDS NOT FROM INJURY OR A COLD
*       IN PAST YEAR COUGHED UP ANY BLOOD
        IN PAST YEAR HAD ANY ASTHMA




     TND = TEST NOT DONE    PRT = PAT. REFUSED TEST    TNI = TEST NOT INDICATED
     BND = BLOOD NOT DRAWN    UNSAT = TEST UNSATISFACTORY   - = DATA NOT AVAILABLE
     NSA = NO SIGNIFICANT ABNORMALITY
     * = PATIENT ANSWERED YES ON THIS MHC AND NO ON LAST MHC
     ** = CONSIDER POSSIBLE ABNORMAL          ¬ = NOTE
```

Figure 1-30c.

diffusion of innovations in technology, the general acceptance of MHTS in the developed countries of the world can be considered good.

H. THE FUTURE OF MHTS

Although the only predictable certainty for the future is that there will be unpredicted changes, futuristic thinking and long-range planning can help us avoid unnecessary surprises. In the early 1970s some business advisers had predicted a great surge of demand and sales for MHTS vendors. By 1976 a more realistic reappraisal envisioned a gradual increase in the numbers of MHTS programs as health professionals and the public accept and apply the full capabilities of this systematic mode of health evaluation. The public want such periodic health examinations because (1) they wish to follow the model set by their leaders (presidents, generals, industrial executives, etc.) who all have checkups at least annually; (2) the higher socioeconomic classes are more health conscious and can afford periodic health checkups; and (3) many primary care physicians recommend periodic health examinations to their patients.

Some of the automated multiphasic programs implemented in the early 1970s were owned and operated by individual entrepreneurs, often pathologists, not associated with a group of referring physicians. Most of these failed within a year or two, demonstrating the need for an MHTS to be integrated with primary medical care services. MHTS functions best within an organized system of medical care. With the implementation of the Health Maintenance Organization (HMO) Act of 1974, it can be predicted that most HMOs will use some modification of the MHTS approach to provide health evaluations to their defined populations. Accordingly, most MHTS programs in the future will probably be associated with HMOs, medical groups, medical foundations, or other organized systems of health care delivery.

Some of the slowness of MHTS growth during 1973–76 was due to the generally poor economic situation throughout the United States and Europe and to questioning by antitechnology forces. Although the past few generations have believed in the increasingly beneficial effects of technological progress, a few years ago some observers began asking whether in its side effects upon the environment and upon people technology might be doing more harm than good. Florman[63] critically reviewed the recent antitechnology movement and concluded that technologists, like all other experts, do make mistakes and should try to learn from them to plan more effectively; that there are no simple solutions to most of man's problems; and that technology should not become a convenient scapegoat. As Meadows and associates pointed out in *The Limits to Growth*,[64] many of man's problems are not caused by technology and may not be helped by technology; in fact, their model suggested "the basic behavior mode of the world system is exponential growth of population and capital, followed by collapse" and that "when we introduce technological developments that successfully lift some restraint to growth or avoid some collapse, the system simply grows to another limit, temporarily surpasses it and falls back"; and they conclude that continuing technological developments are absolutely vital to the future of human society. Even Toffler[65] in his projections of "future shock," which technology could help induce, pointed out the essential part being played by technology in the emerging increased individualism. He projected that a "super-industrial" society will permit evolution of diverse technological bases, more varied occupational specialties, and different life styles within the same society. He emphasized that technology has provided low-cost, mass-produced individualized clothing and even customized automobiles.

Similarly, MHTS technology has evolved so as to provide low-cost health examinations for all, so that every individual may now obtain a high-quality comprehensive medical checkup at a cost he can afford. Based upon the experi-

ence of the Kaiser-Permanente program, it is predictable that as health maintenance organizations (HMOs) increase throughout the United States, about one-
fourth of adults served by those HMOs will have a health checkup each year by a
systemized multiphasic approach.

Huntley[66] predicts that the application of MHTS "will occur in primary care
generally; in the prehospitalization evaluation of elective admissions of all sorts,
especially surgical admissions; and in the periodic medical reassessment of the
chronically ill and aged who are receiving either institutional or home care."

Garfield (see Chapter Fifteen) envisions the future health care delivery system
beginning each patient's entry workup with a comprehensive multiphasic health
evaluation to determine his health and sick care needs and employing periodic
repeat multiphasic examinations to monitor his health status and update his
medical data base in the MHTS computer, so as to keep him on his own personalized pathway for optimal health throughout life.

Increasing public expectations and demands will aggravate the physician shortage and increase the numbers of allied health professionals using MHTS technology in trying to meet these demands. As primary (first-contact) care, health
maintenance, and personal preventive medicine become more important in
medicine of the future, MHTS will become more central in health service systems.
Periodic redesign and continual functional improvement will be needed in all
phases of MHTS to achieve improved instrumentation for physiological and
biochemical measurements and more effective data acquisition from patients (for
history) and from personnel (for examination findings). MHTS will need to continually add new tests and procedures, including stress tests to detect earlier any
failing bodily response systems. It will need to accomodate new generations of
automated chemical analyzers using micro methods and providing more tests for
each patient with better quality control. In addition, the increasing use of online
computing will permit more protocolized triage by nurses and more complex
advice rules to provide secondary testing for borderline and false positives.
Microprocessors will probably handle acquisition and conversion of data at each
phase and then transmit them to a minicomputer that contains the patient's
current data file. MHTS will require access to a large computer that contains a
continuing-through-time medical data base for each patient, permitting trend
analyses and earlier detection of significant variations from prior values and
individually established normal values. Telecommunication will be needed from a
large central MHTS in a medical center to smaller MHTS in the satellite health
centers. The central computer will be able to advise programmed selective screening for each patient in accordance with prior test results and known health hazards
and risk factors, suggest likely diagnoses and protocolized management, and
thereby improve the cost effectiveness of health testing. Increasing automation
and computerization have introduced a new era to personal preventive medicine
and health care delivery. It is difficult to foresee the limits to further applications
of MHTS.

We are developing from an industrial society to a technological society. Prior
generations, involved in an industrial revolution, devoted their new machines and
factories to exploiting natural resources and to improving productivity and output.
This generation is entering a technological revolution in which prime efforts will
be devoted to exploiting scientific knowledge to improve the quality of life through
better health, better communication, and better control of environment. A

technological society emphasizes problem solving by systems analysis and systems engineering. MHTS fits very well into this trend.

REFERENCES

1. Dobell, H. *Lectures on the Germs and Vestiges of Disease and the Prevention of the Invasion and Fatality of Disease by Periodical Examinations.* London: J. & A. Churchill, 1861.

2. Dodson, J. M. "The American Medical Association and Periodic Health Examinations." *Am. J. Pub. Health* 15(1925):599–601.

3. *A Manual of Suggestions for the Conduct of Periodic Examinations of Apparently Healthy Persons.* Chicago: American Medical Association, 1925.

4. "The Value of Periodic Medical Examinations." *Statistical Bulletin, Metropolitan Life Ins. Co.,* 2(1921):1.

5. Roemer, M. I. "A Program of Preventive Medicine for the Individual." *Milbank Memorial Fund Quarterly* 23(1945):209.

6. Breslow, L. "Historical Review of Multiphasic Screening." *Prev. Med.* 2(1973):177–196. "Multiphasic Screening Examinations—An Extension of the Mass Screening Technique." *Am. J. Pub. Health* 40(1950):274–278.

7. Petrie, L. M., Bowdoin, C. D., and McLoughlin, C. J. "Voluntary Multiple Health Tests." *J.A.M.A.* 148(1952):1022–1024.

8. Wilkerson, H. L., and Krall, L. P. "Diabetes in a New England Town." *J.A.M.A.* 135(1947):209 and 169(1959):910–914.

9. Canelo, C. K., Bissel, D. M., Abrams, H., and Breslow, L. "A Multiphasic Screening Survey in San Jose." *Calif. Med.* 71(1949):409.

10. Editorial: "Streamlining Health Examinations." *J.A.M.A.* 137(1948):244.

11. Chapman, A. L. "The Concept of Multiphasic Screening." *Pub. Health Reports* 64(1949):1311.

12. Ryder, C. F., and Getting, V. A. "Preliminary Report on the Health Protection Clinic, Massachusetts Department of Public Health." *N. Eng. J. Med.* 243(1950):277–280.

13. Getting, V. A., and Lombard, H. L. "The Cost and Evaluation of Multiple Screening Procedures." *N.Y. State J.M.* (1952):2605.

14. Bugbee, G. "Can Hospitals Adopt It?" *Hospitals, J.A.H.A.* 24(May 1950):28.

15. Chapman, A. L. "Multiple Screening for a Variety of Diseases." *Hospitals, J.A.H.A.* 24(1950):37.

16. Holms, E. M., Bowden, P. W., and Stone, J. H. "Mass Multiple Test Screening." *New Jersey Pub. Health News* 31(1950):315–319; and *J. Venereal Dis. Inform.* 31(1950):151–155.

17. Mountin, J. W. "Multiple Screening and Specialized Programs." *Public Health Reports* 65(1950):1359–1368.

18. Smillie, W. G. "Multiple Screening." *J.A.M.A.* 145(1951):1254–1256; and *Am. J. Pub. Health* 42(1952):255–258.

19. Samis, S. M. "Multiphasic Screening May Be the Keystone of Preventive Medicine." *The Modern Hospital* 77(1951):92.

20. Collings, G. H., et al. "Multiphasic Health Screening in Industry." *J. Occup. Med.* 14(1972):437–496.

21. Weinerman, E. R., Breslow, L., Belloc, N. B., Waybor, A., and Milmore, B. "Multiphasic Screening of Longshoremen with Organized Medical Followup." *Am. J. Pub. Health* 41(1952):1552–1567.

22. Collen, M. F., and Linden, C. "Screening in a Group Practice Prepaid Medical Care Plan." *J. Chronic Dis.* 2(1955):400–408.

23. Molofsky, L. C., and Hayashi, S. J. "Proctosigmoidoscopy as a Routine Part of a Multiphasic Program." *Am. J. Med. Sc.* 235(1958):628–661.

24. *Building America's Health.* A Report to the President by the President's Commission on the Health Needs of the Nation. Vol. 1. Washington, D.C.: U.S. Govt. Print. Off., 1951.

25. *Chronic Illness in the United States*. Vol. 1. *Prevention of Chronic Illness*. Commission on Chronic Illness. Cambridge, Mass.: Harvard Univ. Press, 1957.

26. American Medical Association. *A Study of Multiple Screening*. Chicago: A.M.A. Council on Medical Services, 1955.

27. White, B. V. "Practical Diagnosis in Preventive Geriatrics." *Geriatrics* 7(1952):87.

28. Roberts, N. J. "The Values and Limitations of Periodic Health Examinations." *J. Chron. Dis.* 9(1959):95–116.

29. Jungner, G., and Jungner, I. "A Pilot Study on Mass Screening with Application of a Chemical Test Battery." Regional Com. for Europe of WHO, 14th Session, Prague, Sept. 1964.

30. *The Värmland Survey*. Translation by Sargent, G. Socialstyrelsen Redovisar 23. Stockholm, 1971.

31. *Chronic Disease and Rehabilitation: A Program Guide for State and Local Health Authorities*. New York: Am Public Health Assoc., 1960.

32. Collen, M. F., Rubin, L., Neyman, J., Dantzig, G. B., Baer, R. M., and Siegelaub, A. B. "Automated Multiphasic Screening and Diagnosis." *Am. J. Pub. Health* 54(1964):741–750.

33. Collen, M. F. "Periodic Health Examinations Using an Automated Multitest Laboratory." *J.A.M.A.* 195(1966):830–833.

34. Collen, M. F. "The Multitest Laboratory in Health Care of the Future." *Hospitals, J.A.H.A.* 41 (1967):119–125.

35. Collen, M. F. "Multiphasic Screening as a Diagnostic Method in Preventive Medicine." *Method. Inform. Med.* 4(1965):71–74.

36. Griesbach, W., and Eads, W. "Experience with Screening for Breast Carcinoma." *Cancer* 19(1966):1548–1550.

37. Roberts, N. J., et al. "Mortality Among Males in Periodic Health Examination Programs." *N. Eng. J. Med.* 281(1969):20–24.

38. Siegel, G. S. *Periodic Health Examinations*. Abstracts from the Literature. U.S.P.H.S. Publication 1010. Washington, D.C.: U.S. Govt. Print. Off., 1963.

39. Mandel, W., and Lillick, L. *Bibliography on Diseae Detection*. Berkeley: Calif. State Dept. of Health, 1963.

40. *Detection and Prevention of Chronic Disease Utilizing Multiphasic Health Screening Techniques*. Hearings before the Subcommittee on Health of the Elderly by the Special Committee on Aging. U.S. Senate. Washington, D.C.: U.S. Govt. Print. Off., 1966.

41. Chadwick, D. R. *Multiphasic Screening for the Chronic Diseases*. Pub. Health Serv. Publ. No. 1779. Washington, D.C.: U.S. Govt. Print. Off., 1968.

42. Wilson, J. M. G., and Jungner, G. *Principles and Practice of Screening for Disease*. WHO Public Health Paper No. 34. Geneva, 1968.

43. Sharp, C. L., and Keen, H. *Presymptomatic Detection and Early Diagnosis*. London: Pitman Med. Pub. Co., 1968.

44. Berkley, C., Devey, G. B., et al. *Automated Multiphasic Health Testing*. Proceedings of Engineering Foundation Research Conferences. New York: Engineering Foundation, 1970.

45. *Automated Multiphasic Health Testing*. Proceedings of Engineering Foundation Research Conferences. New York: Engineering Foundation, 1971.

46. Davies, D. F. ed. *Health Evaluation, An Entry to the Health Care System*. New York: Intercontinental Medical Book Co., 1973.

47. *Proceedings of the Symposia of the International Health Evaluation Association, 1971–1972; 1973–1974*. IHEA.

48. *Automation in Analytic Chemistry*. Technicon Symposia, Mediad, Inc., White Plains, N.Y., 1968.

49. *Provisional Guidelines for Automated Multiphasic Health Testing and Services*, Vol. 1, N.T.I.S. PB 195 654; Vol. 2, N.T.I.S. PB 196 000, 1970.

50. Smith, E. F. "The Utilization of Multiphasic Screening in Public Health Centers." *J. Occup. Med.* 11(1969):364–368.

51. Garfield, S. R. "The Delivery of Medical Care." *Scientific American* 222(1970):15–23.

52. Smillie, J. "Planning for Health." *Kaiser Foundation Hospitals* 4(Dec. 1971):2.

53. Schoen, A. V. *AMHT Program Directory, International 1972–73.* 3 ed. Burbank, Calif.: Bioscience Pub., 1973.

54. Gelman, A. C. *Multiphasic Health Testing Systems: Reviews and Annotations.* H.E.W. Health Services and Mental Health Adm. HSRD 71-1, 1971.

55. Wynder, E. L., Collen, M. F., et al. "Multiphasic Health Testing Forum." *Prev. Med.* 2(1973):175–301.

56. *Statement on Multiphasic Health Testing.* Chicago: A.M.A. Department of Community Health, 1972.

57. Allen, C., Metz, J., and Shinefield, H. "Test Development in the Pediatric Multiphasic Program." *Pediat. Clin. N. Amer.* 18(1971):169–178.

58. Breslow, L., et al. "Theory, Practice and Application of Prevention in Personal Health Services." Pages 257–359, in *Preventive Medicine USA.* New York: PRODIST, 1976.

59. Klatsky, A., Bolomy, A., and Siegelaub, A. "Auscultation of the Adult Heart by Machine." *New Eng. J. Med.* 279(1968):230–234.

60. Levatin, P., Prasloski, P. F., and Collen, M. F. "The Swinging Flashlight Test in Multiphasic Screening for Eye Disease." *Canad. J. Ophthal.* 8(1973):356–360.

61. Woodrow, K., Friedman, G., Siegelaub, A., and Collen, M. F. "Pain Tolerance: Differences According to Age, Sex and Race." *Psychosom. Med.* 34(1972):548–556.

62. Resnick, B., Cella, R., Soghikian, K., Lieberman, A., and Weil, E. "Mass Detection of Significant Bacteriuria." *Arch. Int. Med.* 24(1969):165–169.

63. Florman, S. C. "In Praise of Technology." *Harper's Magazine,* Nov. 1975, 53–72.

64. Meadows, D. H., Meadows, D. L., Randers, J., and Behrens, W. W. "Technology and the Limits to Growth." Chapter IV in *The Limits to Growth.* New York: Universe Books, 1972.

65. Toffler, A. *Future Shock.* New York: Random House, 1970.

66. Huntley, R. R. "Role of Automated Multiphasic Screening in Future Patterns of Health Care." *Bull. N.Y. Acad. Med.* 45(1969):1383–1387.

CHAPTER TWO

Concepts and Objectives

Morris F. Collen

A. CONCEPTS

In this chapter the word "concept" is used to represent the general ideas or notions surrounding multiphasic health testing services (MHTS); "principles" applies to basic guiding rules for MHTS; and "objectives" means specific aims.

The basic concept of MHTS is to provide a systems engineering approach to the provision of health evaluations as a part of personal preventive services within a health care program. If the program aims to provide such health evaluations, then the most efficient way to do so is by MHTS. (See Chapter Seventeen.) The primary goal is to help the physician provide economically to his patients a good quality of preventive health care.

Multiphasic health testing services function best when integrated into an organized health care delivery system, and they are rapidly evolving into an important subsystem.[1] MHTS, by its system approach utilizing automated instrumentation, computers, and allied health personnel, can serve as the basis for an efficient program for personal preventive health maintenance services;[2] it can identify individual patient needs and serve as the entry mode to a health care delivery system;[3] and it can be used as a cost-effective method of providing general or special health examinations to large numbers of people (public preventive medicine).[4]

As described in Chapter One, MHTS was born in the realm of public health and preventive medicine and is now growing up in the arena of health care delivery and personal health services. As a result, many of the general problems inherent in the field of personal vs. public preventive medicine are reflected in the controversy around many MHTS applications and programs.

At a recent National Conference on Preventive Medicine[5] it was stated that "action to prevent ill health and its consequences has been taken in one form or another from the earliest cultures up to the present. The operational expressions of such action have varied greatly, depending on the nature, organization and circumstances of the particular social group and on the values, knowledge and technical means available to it." The conference report emphasized that, more often than not, the application of preventive medicine has depended not only on the urgency and dimension of the health problem but also on political, economic, cultural, and ideological factors. The report suggested that the future of preventive medicine is bright if one sees it as having begun a new period only 25 to 30 years ago.

Breslow's Task Force at this conference made the following comments and recommendations:[6]

> A series of preventive services including primary and secondary measures tailored to each age-sex group has been developed and is available for incorporation into personal health services. The measures include prophylaxis, screening for early detection of disease, patient education and counseling toward specific behavior change. The specific measures have been shown by conclusive evaluation or strong scientific evidence to have value in health maintenance and disease prevention. The preventive services packages should be incorporated into the set of comprehensive personal health services aimed primarily at health maintenance.

Although the practice of preventive medicine has always been a worthy concept, it has been difficult to implement and even more difficult to evaluate. White[7] has prescribed four conditions as necessary for the adoption of prevention as a national health goal: (1) changes in the organization of health services; (2) changes in professional education, (3) changes in the financing of health services, and (4) changes in general education. Steenwyk[8] suggested that a system of prevention should provide periodic health examinations, early sickness consultation, and health education, and he called for the support of such a concept from health insurance plans (such as Blue Cross). Terris[9] has recently stated that epidemiologists have avoided the study of health, which may explain their generally negative attitudes toward health examinations and MHTS. Nevertheless, the early identification of medical problems by MHTS is a feasible method of moving toward satisfying White's conditions, including the education of both health professionals and patients, as several chapters in this book will discuss.

With the support of preventively oriented groups, with the evolution of HMOs under the Health Maintenance Act[10] of 1973, and with the evolving public concept of ''health care as a right,''[11] it is likely that health examinations will be increasingly demanded by the American people and that efficient methods of providing such examinations, as by MHTS, will be readily accepted.

Glazier[12] suggested that, while American medicine has traditionally been geared to respond to acute illness, its main task has now become the care of chronic disease and a more active intervention in its course. He argued that preventive medicine, once a wholly public concern, must now also become a private concern, and that screening for specific diseases according to an individual's risk factors will inevitably become a significant part of medical care. White[13] reported that in one year in a typical American population 72 percent of people visited a physician in an ambulatory setting at least once, whereas only 1 percent were admitted to a hospital at least once; this finding suggests the need to improve the delivery of ambulatory health care—which is where MHTS can have the greatest impact.[3,14]

Since each person desires health, we must be concerned with preserving it as well as restoring it by curing disease or rehabilitating disability. We cannot achieve ''total'' health without being concerned with ''total'' systems—so MHTS should consider evaluation of the total person. It should not only investigate the impact on the person of his specific disease but should also collect information on the social and environmental conditions in which he lives and works.

The ''human dock'' is a very apt metaphor used in Japan[15] to characterize the MHTS concept: the individual, as the captain of his ship of health, can periodically dock for general health evaluation and preventive maintenance. The analogy draws power from people's ideas of water, air, and space ships, where the concept of regular preventive maintenance is well established. Garfield[11] envisioned periodic health appraisal establishing health profiles that serve as milestones to guide each individual along his personal course through life.

MHTS is a keystone of primary care in that it can provide a systems approach to first-contact medicine and it can identify the need for, and arrange, subsequent primary or secondary care. It is a method of introducing technology into primary care, whereas in the past it has been applied mainly to secondary care in hospitals. Through telecommunication (the use of audio or video data communication channels) the technology can be moved out of specialized central facilities into satellite small health centers. Caceres[16] has advocated the term ''clinical engineering'' for the uses of technology in the development of systems in health care, and he considered MHTS an ideal model for the solution of problems in medicine that can apply clinical engineering principles and methods. White[13] advocated viewing health care needs as those of human populations in addition to those of random individuals. The health of each individual is affected not only by the health care services he utilizes but also by his genes, health habits, and social and environmental factors.

Health care expenditures in the United States are approaching 10 percent of the gross national product.[13] Health care costs are rising as fast as, if not faster than, any other item in the consumer's budget, and increased productivity is often cited as necessary to combat this. In all countries there is a growing concern with preventive medicine and health care as a means of improving health and decreasing the proportion of gross national product going to "sick" care. Preventive medicine lends itself very well to a systems engineering approach that will improve productivity, and it can be customized to specific population groups. In preventive medicine and health care, automated instrumentation for test processing and automated data processing by computer have brought major changes, and better systems technology can facilitate the greater use of personnel with less training than physicians. (See also B.5.) Technology can also provide low-cost health education and training to the individual, so that hopefully he can alter his health habits and behavior for the better, all within a systems approach to include medical, social, and environmental factors. The public can no longer afford to pay the physician at his costs for low-technology, routine diagnostic preventive care and low-technology curative and supportive care for chronic conditions. A greater variety of allied health personnel are becoming standard in our health care systems, and the physician then functions as the head of a team. For this reason physician practitioners often are not the strongest supporters of preventive medicine, since they cannot retain the one-to-one relationship they now enjoy with the sick patient.

There has been an increasing trend in the United States toward more centralization and specialization to make acute care at the secondary and tertiary levels more efficient; however, decentralization with less specialization tends to make preventive health care and primary care more efficient. We can make MHTS a bridge between central and satellite facilities by locating it in both types of facilities or by locating it only in a central facility and connecting it by telecommunication to local health centers or even to individual physician offices.

Health care, health maintenance, assessment of risk and degree of individual vulnerability to specific diseases, preventive care and preventive maintenance, continuing care for chronic conditions, and triage to acute care are all essential aspects of ambulatory primary care—and MHTS with adjunctive services is an efficient subsystem for all of these requirements.

A reorientation toward personal preventive services has been emerging within clinical medicine, particularly in the care of children and pregnant women, in that pediatricians and obstetricians have been directing their practices more and more toward health maintenance. This shift is currently spreading into other branches of primary care including general internal medicine and family medicine.

B. GENERAL PRINCIPLES

Many writers have advocated principles to guide multiphasic programs, and specific principles have been referred to in various relevant chapters of this book, especially as related to history (Chapter One), implementation and test selection (Chapter Three), and evaluation (Chapter Seventeen). General principles advocated for MHTS, as developed from our experience, are summarized below. These are not necessarily in order of priority, for each is important.

(1) The MHTS should be an integrated component of a health care program and closely related to its physician services. Such integration is most effective in a formal organized system of care, but it can also function in an informal cooperative relationship, in which case the linkages must be truly operational. Provision for diagnoses, followup, and treatment is essential, for without it MHTS will fall into disrepute. Thus there must be a group of primary care physicians who will support the MHTS by referring to it patients for examination and by accepting patients referred from MHTS for followup care.[17-20]

(2) A defined or target population of adequate size must agree to support the MHTS. Unless at least several thousand people are willing to travel periodically to the MHTS for examinations, it cannot support itself. A population exceeding 25,000 adults, with an average health examination rate of at least every three years, is advisable.

(3) Population health needs should be clearly defined; conditions sought for and tests selected should satisfy criteria and requirements detailed in Chapter Three. Preferably, user needs should be defined in terms of medical, psychosocial, occupational, and environmental factors as well as preventive health maintenance. Conditions selected should be important, prevalent, and susceptible to management. A comprehensive battery of appropriate, accurate tests is necessary. A high quality of testing is essential, and a control program of good quality must be maintained.

(4) MHTS should satisfy the specific objectives determined by its sponsoring organization (see D and Chapter Three), whether this be personal or public preventive medicine, industry or military.

(5) The user population should be kept informed as to the benefits and limits of MHTS, and health education should be an adjunct to MHTS. (See Chapter Twelve.)

(6) MHTS should have a computerized and/or manual record system adequate to maintain continuing files on each patient and permit comparison of each examination's findings with earlier data on the patient. The record system should satisfy the same requirements for confidentiality of patient data as any hospital record room.

(7) Since MHTS is a systems or "clinical engineering" approach,[16] it must be carefully planned and designed; and it must be operated with trained personnel to provide reliable, acceptable service and high-quality patient examinations at sufficient volume to be cost-effective. (See Chapter Three.)

(8) The program should be periodically evaluated regarding the extent to which its effectiveness and its efficiency in achieving its objectives can be improved. (See Chapters Seventeen and Eighteen.)

C. DEFINITIONS

Medicine is increasingly concerned with health and disease in the broadest sense, with all mechanisms and processes by which health is maintained and by which disease develops, at all levels including biochemical, cellular, organ-system, psychological, and social, including their interrelationships. MHTS therefore attempts to collect relevant information at all these levels. Often there is no clear dividing line between health and disease. Furthermore, a person may satisfy all the criteria of health at any point in time simply because the adaptive capacity of a defective system (be it biochemical, physiological, or psychological) has not been exceeded.[21] He may remain presymptomatic or asymptomatic until, eventually, the defect exceeds the adaptive capability and a breakdown occurs that produces discomfort in the patient, called a symptom or complaint. Or it may produce a swelling or behavioral alteration visible to others, called a sign; or develop a measurable biochemical test alteration, such as an elevated blood sugar, or a physiological test alteration, such as an elevated blood pressure.

1.   Health and Medical Care

Health can be defined as the state of well-being in which all body systems are functioning optimally for longevity, within the specified environment. Optimal for longevity means that those "normal" physiological ranges found in persons who live a long healthy life are the models that a well person would seek to emulate for longevity. Although it is difficult to quantitate health, a person is generally classified as being well (or healthy) when he has no symptoms or medical problems and when a physician after a general examination reports no clinically important significant finding or abnormality. Symptoms, medical problems, or complaints include those of a psychological and psychosocial nature, such as so-called "problems in living." The World Health Organization suggests that the state of health should include not only physical and mental but also social well-being. It is also necessary to specify the general environment since, e.g., the state of health in mile-high Denver requires a different normal range of hemoglobin than at sea level San Francisco.

Normal ranges for test values can best be established by measurements obtained from large numbers of well persons. They are most reliably determined from those who, having had repeated examinations over several years, continue in a state of health. (The establishment of normal values will be considered in Chapter Nineteen.) Borderline test values will always be found for continuous variables (e.g., blood pressure measurements), where the ranges for health and for disease may overlap.

Health status classification, an important function of an MHTS, is a method of categorizing individuals, primarily for purposes of "triage" and referral to appropriate care resources to match patient care needs.[14] It is also used to standardize examinees for comparative studies and analyses. One simple, validated, health status classification method for MHTS purposes involves only four categories of patients derived from establishing, at the completion of the MHTS examination, concurrence or nonconcurrence of the physician's judgments and patient's perceptions.[3,22] We determine as part of the multiphasic history whether the patient has any significant medical complaints or problems and determine after the MHTS physical examination whether the examining physician (or nurse practitioner) recorded any clinically significant abnormality or finding. These perceptions and judgments are opposed in a concurrence matrix, as shown in Figure 2-1. The patient is determined as perceiving himself "well" when the history shows no significant complaint or "sick" when there is a significant complaint. The physi-

		PATIENT'S PERCEPTION	
		WELL (NO SIGNIFICANT COMPLAINT)	SICK (SIGNIFICANT COMPLAINT)
PHYSICIAN'S	WELL (NO SIGNIFICANT ABNORMALITY)	"WELL"	"WORRIED-WELL"
FINDING	SICK (SIGNIFICANT ABNORMALITY)	"ASYMPTOMATIC-SICK"	"SICK"

Figure 2-1. Health status classification of MHTS patients useful for referral to appropriate resources to match patient needs.

cian is determined as perceiving the patient as "well" by his (or his nurse practitioner's) recording from the examination findings (physical examination and the multiphasic laboratory tests) no significant abnormality or as "sick" when there is a significant abnormality. The patient's health status at the time of the MHTS can then be readily classified by opposing the physician's findings with the patient's perception.

A patient is classified as "well" when both his own perception and the physician's findings concur that he is "well." Such a "well" patient may benefit by referral to health education and counseling. A "worried-well" patient perceives that he is "sick" (i.e., he has given a history containing some significant complaint such as headaches, always tired, etc.) although the physician (and/or nurse practitioner) has recorded that he is "well" (i.e., no significant abnormalities found). Such a "worried-well" patient may be referred to health or psychological counseling.

The "asymptomatic-sick" patient has no significant complaints but the examination has found a significant abnormality (e.g., high blood pressure, elevated blood sugar, etc.). Such a patient should be referred to his physician or to an appropriate preventive maintenance clinic. "Sick" are those whom both the patient and physician perceive as "sick"; i.e., the patients have significant complaints and the physicians have recorded significant findings. Such "sick" patients should, of course, be referred to their physicians for appropriate followup care. (See also Chapters Ten and Fifteen.)

Health status index is a measure of the health of an individual or a community. Such indices are usually constructed for purposes of comparing the health status of populations or evaluating the effect of alternative health services interventions on their health outcomes.[23]

Health care, or health maintenance, in its most limited sense is the evaluation and counseling of the well and worried-well. The term health care is sometimes used in the broadest sense to include both health care and medical care—that is, the overall care of both the well and the sick.

Medical care in its most limited sense is the diagnosis and treatment of the sick, the "sick" being defined as above—i.e., those patients, either symptomatic or asymptomatic who have significant complaints and in whom the physicians find a clinically important abnormality.

Medical care delivery system is a term that has evolved from newer organizational systems concepts, which developed to define the interrelationships of medical care, medical education, and medical research. A "system" is a coordinated group of interfacing components. Most medical care delivery systems integrate various organizational components for the primary purpose of providing direct patient care. Medical schools have as their primary mission medical education and medical research but also often have or collaborate with a medical care delivery system. A large medical care program (or system) may actively engage in all three of these activities. So as to distinguish the direct patient care components from the educational and research activities, it is meaningful to call those organizational components that provide primarily diagnostic and therapeutic services the "medical care delivery system."

A *health care delivery system,* in its limited meaning, provides health care services by an organization in a systemized manner. Many persons who see primary care physicians are not "sick," in the sense that they do not have physical or psychological abnormalities that require diagnosis and treatment, but they are uncertain or worried about their health status and want a survey examination to reassure them that they do not have some asymptomatic disease. To this group the physician provides (or delivers) "health" care, in that he furnishes a health evaluation and health maintenance counseling.

In the broadest sense, a health care delivery system is one that provides both health care and sick (i.e., medical) care. Although some have objected to the term "health care delivery system,"[24] it has a definite meaning for those programs that contract to provide both health care and medical care to a population that contains both well and sick people. When subscribers contract with a health plan for specified benefits (services), a medical group (doctors) contract with the health plan to provide (or deliver) those benefits (services). The health plan organizes a program (system) of integrated facilities (system components) including a hospital, offices, laboratory, pharmacy, x-ray, etc. to provide (deliver) these services (benefits). This health plan (system) includes a medical-educational system (house staff), medical care research system (health services research), and a medical care delivery system (professional staff and facilities) to provide (deliver) services to patients who have contracted for these benefits. When the medical group sign such a contract, they clearly know what services they are expected to deliver.

Personal health services are those in which the patient uses available health care resources primarily for his own benefit and in which an individual medical and legal relationship exists between the patient and the health professional. Personal health services are usually provided by solo or group practitioners financed by payments of fees-for-service, private or governmental health insurance, or prepaid health service plans.

Public health services are those in which a community or a population group is provided specified health programs, wherein every individual receives similar services, conducted for the benefit of the community or the group and generally provided and financed by governmental or public agencies.

2. Prevention and Preventive Care

Prevention is defined as intervention to attempt to prevent or postpone the natural course of diseases, illnesses, or medical problems, including physical, mental, and psychosocial. *Primary prevention* seeks to prevent disease by protecting the individual from acquiring it (e.g., by immunization). *Secondary prevention* seeks to prevent the continuation and progression of a disease by its early detection; this is one of the primary objectives of MHTS (e.g., detection of early cervical cancer by cytological examination of cervical smear). *Tertiary prevention* aims at minimizing or preventing the effects or complications of a disease that has been acquired (e.g., early sickness consultation is tertiary prevention).

Preventive health care was defined at the 1975 National Conference on Preventive Medicine[6] as preventive interventions that are not exclusively in the domain of the physician specialist in preventive medicine, and *preventive medicine* was defined as the physician specialty of preventive health care. This conference recommended that preventive services packages should be incorporated into a set of comprehensive personal health services aimed primarily at preventive health maintenance.

Personal preventive medical services therefore are those preventive measures directed to the individual and are generally governed by the individual health professional-patient relationships.

Public preventive medical services are preventive programs directed to groups of people. MHTS can be used for both personal or public preventive medical services.

The concept of preventable disease, in this context, includes not only the communicable diseases (such as syphilis and tuberculosis) but also the noncommunicable diseases and conditions (such as cancer, complications of hypertension, nutritional disorders, anxiety, etc.).

Predictive (prospective) medicine is a subspecialty of preventive medicine that focuses on identification and management of high-risk groups, individual health hazard appraisal, etc. (See Chapter Nineteen.)

Clinicians generally are trained primarily in sick care and have only secondary interest in preventive care. Terris[25] has suggested that medical schools might be administrated by schools of public health so as to be encouraged to educate physicians in preventive medicine.

3. Health, Medical and Multiphasic Examinations

A *health examination,* health evaluation, health appraisal, or health checkup is a survey examination of a presumably well person. It generally employs relatively simple, low-cost methods (usually including a history, a physical examination, and a battery of tests) for identifying abnormalities in an attempt to detect asymptomatic or previously unknown disease.

Periodic health examinations are health examinations performed at regularly prescribed intervals, such as annually, usually as a part of a preventive health maintenance program.

Health surveillance is a public preventive medicine program of repeated or periodic health examinations of a population to observe for changes in health status.

A *medical examination,* medical workup, or diagnostic study is an evaluation of a presumably sick person with one or more specific medical complaints or problems, which often employs specialized techniques and resources to provide a specific diagnosis to lead to appropriate treatment or to monitor the status of known existing disease.

A *physical examination* is the portion of a health or medical examination that involves gathering information as to signs or findings of bodily impairment by direct examination of the various parts of the body; it is the process of determining the patient's physical status.

Early disease detection is a general term that includes physical examination, screening, testing, or any other process for early identification of abnormalities. It is a form of "secondary prevention,"[19] since it aims at discovering conditions that have not yet reached a stage at which a patient would customarily seek medical aid.

Early sickness consultation is the prompt seeking of medical advice for symptoms. It is often advocated by physicians as preferable to individual periodic health examinations, since the clinician is primarily interested in "sick" care rather than in "health care" or "preventive health maintenance." Most persons who seek health examinations do have some medical concerns or problems that are elicited during the history. Accordingly, for an individual who arrives with a request for a checkup or for advice on a specific medical problem, the medical workup in either case should similarly include a comprehensive history, a physical examination, and a battery of commonly done laboratory tests so as to detect early asymptomatic, important disease.

4. Screening and Testing

Screening for a disease (or a condition) refers to the performance of a test (see Figure 2-2) that is usually simple and quick but has sufficient sensitivity and specificity for detecting the disease, if present, to permit the examiner to separate

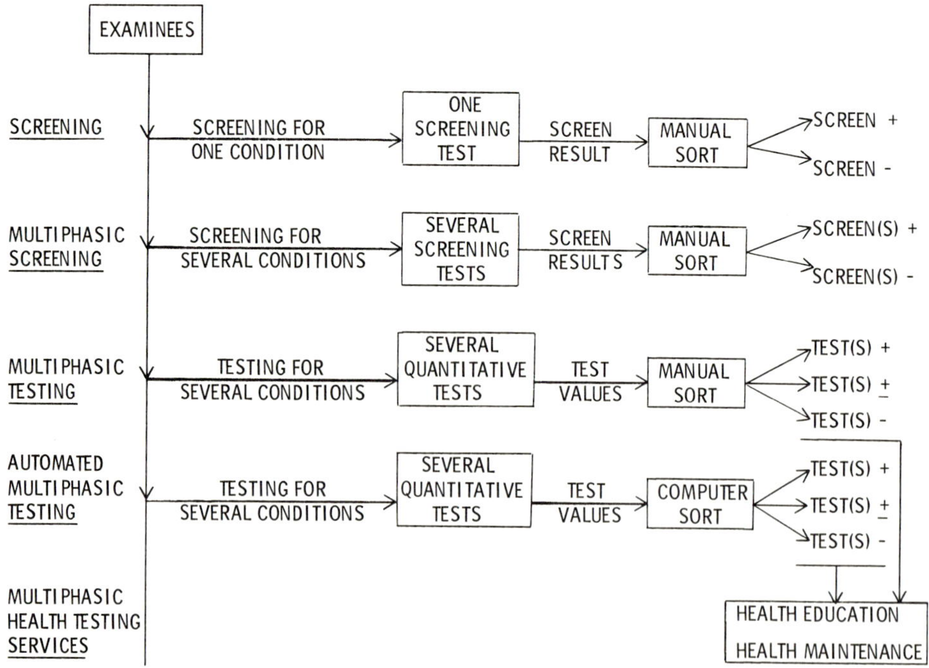

Figure 2-2. Diagrammatic representation of the progression of the screening process to multiphasic health testing services, with manual or computer sorting of patients with positive (+), negative (−), or borderline (±) results. The addition of adjunctive health education and maintenance completes the MHTS.

those persons who probably have the disease (i.e., have a positive screening test) from those who probably do not (i.e., have a negative test). Wilson and Jungner[19] emphasized that a screening test need not be diagnostic (e.g., urinalysis for protein) but may be so (as in some cancer screening tests). Screening tests include history questions for symptoms; physical examination for signs (e.g., cardiac auscultation and pelvic palpation); examination procedures, such as weight and blood pressure, x-ray, and electrocardiogram; and clinical laboratory testing of specimens, such as blood and urine analysis.

McKeown[33] interpreted screening to be "medical investigation which does not arise from a patient's request for advice for specific complaints." So considered, it comprises investigations of patients (a) who have not sought medical assistance (as in mass radiography), (b) who have sought medical assistance only for a screening test or examination (e.g., a health "checkup"), which they believe will be of value to them, and (c) who have sought assistance for a condition unrelated to the screening procedure (such as routine chest radiography of hospital patients). McKeown further identified screening for personal preventive medicine as *"prescriptive screening"*; although Wilson[4] defined prescriptive screening as *case finding*—examining subjects who have not sought medical advice for the condition for which they are examined, or searching for cases with a view of treating them.

Mass screening is the application of a test (or tests) to screen large populations for one or more specific diseases, generally as a part of a public preventive medicine program. (See Chapter One.) Mass screening is often used to conduct (a) *epidemiological surveys,* seeking information on the health status of a population, and (b) *disease surveillance,* seeking to assess changes in the health status of a population with reference to specific diseases.

Selective screening or *discriminate screening* involves the provision of selected screening tests only to preidentified high-risk individuals. Selective screening requires an adaptive design of the system to adjust the test panel for each patient. Holland[26] advocated selective rather than mass screening as a more effective and economical use of scarce resources. In this context he suggested that it may also be helpful to distinguish four different forms of screening: (1) screening for individuals with risk factors, such as obesity and cigarette smoking, that predispose to illness but are not themselves alerting symptoms; (2) screening for conditions, such as elevated blood pressure, that are the early signs of a disease; (3) identification of individuals with abnormalities in whom preventive action must be taken; and (4) identification of individuals who could benefit from surveillance and continuing care (e.g., those with visual or hearing loss where the disease process is irreversible but its effects can often be alleviated). Holland[26] pointed out the important need for development of effective methods of convincing these high-risk individuals to adhere to prescribed measures of prevention, such as antihypertensive medication, weight reduction, and ceasing to smoke. In this context, primary prevention in the form of identification and correction of the influences that encourage people to smoke, overeat, and lead sedentary lives may be more effective than identifying individuals in the early stages of disease. Holland summarized three discernible objectives: screening to prevent disease, screening to treat disease, and screening for conditions that are beyond prevention or curative treatment but that nevertheless can be alleviated or improved. In the middle-aged and elderly, for example, simple tests for vision and hearing, and tests to identify people in need of chiropody or walking aids, may be very effective in improving the quality of life. As discussed below, these latter objectives of Holland's can be better provided by testing than by screening programs.

Multiphasic screening (or multiple screening) is applied to the combining of several individual screening tests so as to provide an integrated test battery to screen for a number of diseases. (See Figure 2-2.) Multiple laboratory screening,[27] biochemical panels, and biochemical profiling are terms applied to a group of tests performed on a single blood specimen by an automated chemical analyzer, comprising a single phase in an MHTS.

Multiphasic testing has evolved from multiphasic screening by the employment of modern measurement technology. Semiautomated and automated instrumentation readily provides accurate quantitative test measurements. For example, instead of screening for a low hemoglobin by a copper sulfate falling-drop method, one can automatically and accurately measure the concentration of hemoglobin and print out the test value in grams. Accordingly, testing has replaced screening, and "multiphasic testing" is the term generally applied to current programs. (See Figures 2-2 and 2-3.)

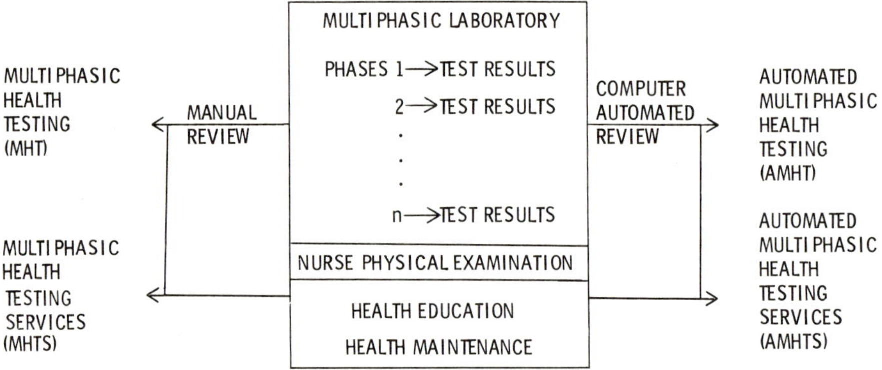

Figure 2-3. Diagrammatic representation of difference between MHTS and AMHTS.

Multiphasic health testing (MHT) is a systems engineering approach to providing the laboratory testing portion of a health evaluation. It employs automated laboratory procedures and specially trained allied health personnel to collect data on patients' medical histories, clinical laboratory, x-ray, and other physiological test measurements in a programmed sequence.

There is considerable confusion in the literature in distinguishing between screening and testing. The World Health Organization set forth the following definition of screening, whose aim is to discover latent and unrecognized disease:[4] "Screening, when used in the detection of either early or established disease, implies medical investigation that does not arise from a request for health care resulting from a specific complaint. In other words, screening is undertaken when tests or examinations are carried out on people who may be either well or ill; but who, if ill, are not suffering from the disease for which screening is being done. Screening aims at sorting out individuals who probably have a disease from those who probably do not."

Sackett and Holland[28] sought to clarify terminology thus: "Screening is the testing of apparently healthy volunteers from the general population for the purpose of separating them into groups with high and low probabilities for a given disorder. The objective of screening is unique: the early detection of those diseases whose treatment is either easier or more effective when undertaken at an earlier point in time. *Case finding* is the testing of patients who have sought health care for disorders which may be unrelated to their chief complaints. In contrast, *diagnostic testing* is the application of tests to patients who have actively sought health services in order to identify the exact cause of their chief complaints.'' Diagnostic testing is a part of a medical examination or diagnostic study.

Thus at least three issues differentiate testing from screening: (a) the accuracy of the test, (b) who requested the procedure, and (c) whether the examinee had a specific symptom or not. With reference to the first issue, screening does not require actual quantification of a test result; its consequence is a binary decision that the test result either is outside predefined screening limits (i.e., positive) and needs further study or is within the screening limits (i.e., negative) and does not need further testing. For example, the copper sulfate falling-drop method of screening for anemia can be adjusted to screen out all with a blood hemoglobin of less than 13 grams. Testing, as used in MHT, requires quantitative measurements, such as accurately measuring the blood hemoglobin to ascertain that the value is not only below 13 grams but is, for example, actually 10.2 grams.

The second issue—whether the patient, doctor, or public health officer initiated the request for the testing service—does have some ethical connotations, depending on whether the preventive medical services are of a personal or a public nature. (See E.) In mass screening programs the public health officer usually initiates the request for the testing. In most multiphasic programs currently operational in the United States the patient usually initiates the request for a health examination.

As to the third issue—whether the patient initiated the request for the test because of a specific complaint—in mass screening most screenees are unaware of any specific symptoms of the disease for which they are being screened. In MHTS, or for that matter in any good medical workup, owing to the comprehensiveness of the examination, it makes little difference whether the patient initiated the examination request because of a specific medical complaint or not. In MHTS this issue becomes a philosophical one of little practical consequence, since no person is physically perfect, and by the completion of the comprehensive history some symptoms can be elicited from everyone.

Automated multiphasic health testing (AMHT) is the expanded systems concept of utilizing automated equipment and a computer in an MHT to determine automatically whether there is sufficient likelihood of disease being present to warrant further specific diagnostic testing. (See Figures 2-2 and 2-3.) AMHT programs employ computerized decision (advice) rules that automatically sort out those patients whose test results exceed prescribed limits. The mere employment of automated equipment or a computer in a multiphasic testing program is not sufficient to satisfy the concept of *automated* multiphasic health testing.

The recent advent of electronics, computers, automation, and systems engineering into medicine offers the opportunity to improve and augment multiphasic testing so that not only more tests but more accurate and quantitative measurements can be performed in less time and at lower cost. Since diagnosis is defined as the identification of a specific disease, then as multiphasic testing becomes more comprehensive, precise, and quantitative, disease detection approximates disease diagnosis, and automated multiphasic health testing can approach *computer-aided diagnosis*. (See Chapter Nineteen.)

Multiphasic health checkup (MHC) is a health examination provided by using multiphasic health testing (manual or automated) followed by a physical examination. Figure 2-4 is a conceptual diagram in which multiphasic health checkups with physician or nurse practitioner physical examination are compared with the traditional health checkup.

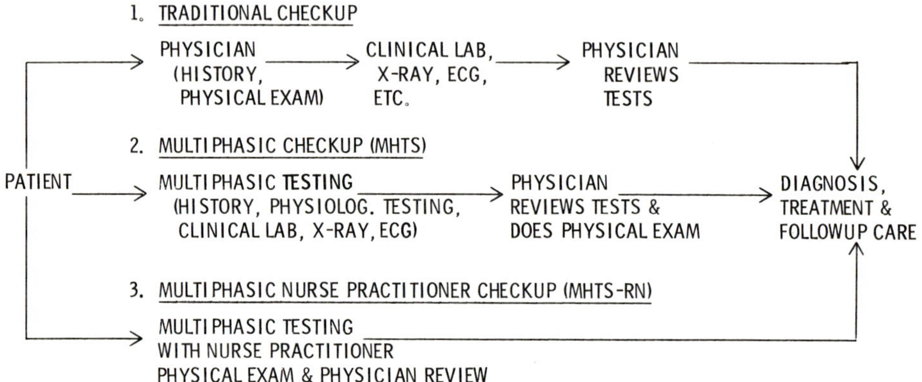

Figure 2-4. Conceptual diagram of systemized multiphasic approach to providing health examinations as compared to the traditional health checkup.

Multiphasic health testing services (MHTS) is the expanded use of multiphasic health testing programs (either manual or automated) within health care delivery systems to provide many adjunctive services such as entry triage, health counseling, health education, and preventive health maintenance. (See Figure 2-3.) Multiphasic testing for disease detection is thus only one of the uses of an MHTS.

MHTS can be provided with various levels of automation and computer processing. Smaller units may use entirely manual paper-and-pencil methods of recording and compiling test data onto a preprinted form for a report. Semiautomated MHTS use automated instrumentation and offline, batch processing of test data into a computer, which generates collated test reports.

Automated MHTS (AMHTS) is a total systems approach that combines automated testing procedures and computer data processing systems to automatically sort out patients with positive tests and advise followup and referral care.[29] History and test data are entered online into a computer, which, using programmed decision rules, automatically prints out in "realtime" (that is, before the patient leaves the multiphasic laboratory) advice on appropriate followup tests and care. In addition, AMHTS employs allied health personnel for adjunctive health and preventive maintenance services. (See Figures 2-2 and 2-3.)

5. Technology and Cybernetic Systems

Technology, as herein used, is the application of science to a practical task; it includes not only the instrument or machine but the procedures and personnel for using it. Technology, like science, is a cumulative process; each new development is an incremental addition to an existing level of capability.[30]

Automation is the use of devices to automatically perform sensing or motor tasks, replacing or improving on human capacities for performing these functions (e.g., the automated chemical analyzer).

Computers, or automated data processors, are devices that automatically perform logical or decision-making tasks by analyzing and interpreting data.

A combination of automation and computers, such as the use of automatic chemical analyzers with automatic data processing, provides a system with volume, precision, and rapidity unmatched by humans. The addition of data feedback to automatically arrange retesting or secondary (supplemental) testing based on preprogrammed decision rules or algorithms (such as in automated multiphasic health testing) is an example of *cybernetics* (communication and control in men and machines).

A cybernetic system usually not only improves the efficiency of people on a job by machines but results in a new way of thinking. For example, bringing automated chemical analyzers into the clinical laboratory reduced the number of technicians required, increasing their performance and productivity by increasing the number, variety, and accuracy of tests. It also greatly altered medical practice in the hospital and the way of thinking about the laboratory. For example, clinicians began to order routinely on every patient a whole profile of tests for asymptomatic disease rather than just the individual tests indicated by the patient's medical problems.

Automated multiphasic health testing is another example of a cybernetic system that has changed medical thinking. Rather than having physicians provide traditional examinations to a few patients on a one-to-one basis, the MHTS employs automated equipment and computers with allied health personnel to provide more comprehensive, better-quality examinations faster and at lower cost, permitting everyone, regardless of economic status, to receive periodic personal preventive health maintenance and referring them through a new entry mode to necessary medical care. Such cybernetic systems increase productivity and performance by increased volume and diversity at lower unit cost, improve precision and quality control, improve communication, decrease human and employee relations problems and errors, free up highly skilled professionals (e.g., physicians) for optimal utilization of their time, and upgrade the capability of lower-skilled personnel. On the other hand, such cybernetic systems tend to create unemployment for lower-skilled persons, require adjustment and extensive reorientation of higher-level professionals, require retraining of displaced personnel, require protection of confidentiality of privileged information, create socioeconomic pressures for more pay for same work period, can tend to depersonalize service (but patients soon seem to separate such service from their physicians and soon prefer it), and require creative planning to cope with these problems.

D. GOALS AND OBJECTIVES OF MHTS

Since an MHTS should always function as an integral part of some medical community, program, or system (e.g., a medical foundation, a health care delivery system, a public health program, an industry, a military program, etc.), its goals and objectives should support the mission and goals of the overall program. Goals are herein defined as long-term, while objectives are short-term aims. Each goal consists of one or more objectives. (See also Chapter Three for MHTS Objectives.)

1. Health Care Delivery MHTS

Within an organized health care delivery system, such as a fee-for-service group practice, a prepaid group practice health plan, or a health maintenance organization (HMO), the goals of an MHTS are, first, to provide effective personal preventive medical services, to determine the examinee's health status or physical fitness, identify any clinically important abnormalities, arrange for appropriate followup services, provide a high-quality service at a reasonable cost, and satisfy both the users and the providers of care. Second, the MHTS aims to improve the efficiency of the health care delivery system.

More specifically, the objectives of such an MHTS include:

a. Economically provide good-quality personal health evaluations. Since in a prepaid group practice health plan, or an HMO, the subscriber members of the program are eligible to receive periodic health checkups as a contractual benefit, the program will not readily be able to provide such health examinations in a cost-effective manner by using the traditional methods.

The traditional health checkup, as practiced in the United States, usually consists of the physician's taking a medical history from the patient, doing a physical examination, and then arranging for supplemental diagnostic tests and procedures that, in the physician's judgment, are essential to complete the health evaluation. The high costs of physician-provided examinations and the shortage of primary care physicians make such health checkups expensive, with long waiting periods.

The multiphasic health checkup is a systemized examination of a patient, including a self-administered questionnaire and a battery of physiological tests, the results of which, when completed, are printed in a report for the physician. When the physician sees the patient, he completes the physical examination, reviews the MHTS report, and arranges for followup care as indicated. Some MHTS centers provide physical examinations within the MHTS unit by certified nurse practitioners supervised by physicians. Such MHTS examinations are more economical and have shorter waiting times. (See Figure 2-4 and Chapter Ten.)

The subobjectives of MHTS in a health care delivery system are:

(1) *Health surveillance.* Multiphasic testing for the detection of asymptomatic or early disease is the oldest application of MHTS and still a very important function. Approximately one-third of all diseases found in an ongoing MHTS have been newly detected. (See Table 17-6, Chapter Seventeen.) Health surveillance also includes the application of predictive medicine to identify those with a higher-than-average risk of developing specific diseases.

(2) *Patient surveillance.* Chronic disease monitoring is an evolving application of any continuing MHTS. Usually about two-thirds of diseases found in an MHTS program that has been testing a defined population for several years will be known chronic conditions, which bring the patient back for an examination to evaluate and monitor the status of the condition and its impact on target organs and to detect any possible early complications.

(3) *Health maintenance.* Adjunctive services to patient care in an MHTS include health education, attempting to direct each patient into a positive program for continuing health, and also patient education, instructing a patient about a specific disease and about the care program prescribed by the physician. (See Chapters Eleven and Twelve.)

(4) *Maintain a high level of patient acceptability, compliance, and satisfaction.* An MHTS must satisfy its users, the patients. Since most persons have become accustomed to the traditional individual examinations by personal physicians, it is essential that an MHTS be very acceptable and satisfying in its conduct, or patients will not comply with its advice and referrals nor return for periodic reexaminations. Hopefully, MHTS will serve to improve patient understanding of health and disease.

(5) *Save patient time and costs and improve service and accessibility.* MHTS clearly can save examinee time, since many tests can be provided faster and in one location. The waiting time for appointments, especially when the physical examination is performed by nurse practitioners, should be much less than for the traditional examinations, since it is not necessary to wait for available physician time. MHTS examinations should cost much less than the traditional kind.

(6) *Improve the quality and comprehensiveness of health examinations.* Quality control of tests and procedures in an MHTS should be of a very high order. The establishment of normal limits should be more precise and can be more individualized, since they can be derived from the population tested and assigned age- and sex-specific values. The large battery of tests assures a highly comprehensive examination.

When MHTS is used as a part of a preadmission hospital workup or a routine ambulatory care office workup, it can serve as an adjunct to diagnosis by furnishing a comprehensive data base on the patient's overall health status.[29,31]

(7) *Be acceptable to physicians; conserve physician time and costs.* An MHTS must be acceptable to the physicians who participate in the health care delivery system. The increasing costs of medical care prohibit the use of large amounts of physician time for routine, repetitive health examinations that can be provided equally well by allied health professionals when supported by automation and protocols.

b. Provide an efficient entry mode to the health care delivery system. A serious problem in any health care delivery system is how the patient who needs medical care gets into the system. Traditionally, in nonurgent cases, the patient first telephones to book an appointment to see a physician. The doctor at this first (entry) visit will usually determine the patient's needs and arrange appropriate care to meet them. A more efficient method of entry is by the patient's booking an appointment for MHTS, where his needs can be determined and appropriate followup care arranged with much less cost and use of physician time. (See Chapters Fifteen and Seventeen.)

c. Improve patients' outcomes by decreasing disability, morbidity, and mortality. This objective is, of course, the overall primary objective of medical care. There would be little demand for health evaluations if they did not help the patient or his condition or at least decrease his anxiety. (MHTS effectiveness in these directions is evaluated in Chapter Eighteen.)

2. Specialized MHTS

MHTS also are used to provide a variety of special-purpose examinations to determine an individual's health status and physical fitness or capacity for specific environmental, organizational, or population group requirements. Such examinations may be designed to meet the objectives of the examiner rather than of the examinee; if so, the examinee should always be informed if an abnormality is detected and should be referred for appropriate followup care.

a. Public health screening programs. Historically, most multiphasic programs were established for mass screening or testing of a target population to detect disease and for referral of all who were found to have positive tests to physicians for secondary testing and followup care. Health surveillance of defined populations includes health assessment of persons who may or may not already be patients and surveys of populations to determine health care needs.

b. Preadmission testing of hospital patients. MHTS can very efficiently satisfy the laboratory test requirements for hospital admission for ambulatory (non-emergency) patients by arranging such examinations prior to admission.[31,32] Such an MHTS examination on or just prior to admission will generally require online data processing and more selective test selection. (See Chapter Ten, Figure 10-20.) Biochemical panel testing is already routine for many hospital admissions.

c. Prenatal examinations. Selective screening tests for conditions complicating pregnancy have been standard practice for many years, and such examinations can be readily incorporated into an MHTS with simple modifications, including protecting fetus from x-ray exposure, testing for congenital conditions, etc.

d. Preschool examinations. Preschool, precamping, and similar examinations can be provided very efficiently to large numbers of persons who must obtain a fitness examination to establish their physical capacities as an enrollment requirement.

e. Industrial and occupational examinations. Preemployment or periodic employee and executive examinations can be economically arranged, usually at hours suitable for employers. They often include special-purpose tests for high-risk safety hazards (e.g., spine x-rays for heavy lifting jobs) or environmental exposures (e.g., noise, dust, chemicals, etc.). MHTS can readily perform examinations to determine fitness for employment and additionally provide physical capacities analysis of employees to meet specific job requirements in industry. (See Chapter Sixteen.)

f. Other fitness examinations. MHTS is ideally suited to screen out persons unfit for military service (see Chapter Sixteen), for identifying high-risk applicants for life insurance, and the like.

E. INTEGRATION WITHIN A HEALTH CARE DELIVERY SYSTEM

In the developed countries of the world, technological innovations have so greatly affected the practice and costs of medicine that major legislation has been aimed at improving the financing, organization, and delivery of a higher scientific level of medicine to all people. A worldwide interest in health care delivery systems is evolving, within which MHTS or its equivalent is an important subsystem.

Forrester[34] defines a system as a grouping of parts that operate together for a common purpose. Man lives and works within social systems. His technology produces complex physical systems, which include people as well as physical parts. In industrial societies, social systems become very complex and evolve subsystems for health, politics, education, religion, economics, legislation, etc. The workings of the health care system are complicated by its interactions externally with the political, educational, economic, and other systems. An understanding of the health care system requires study of the internal interactions of its preventive, diagnostic, therapeutic, rehabilitative, public health, personal health, emergency, multiphasic, and other subsystems. Man is not an island in his social system, and neither can MHTS be treated as an island in a health care delivery system.

Systems principles provide guidelines for organizational structure and operational procedures for health care delivery, and they are essential for the efficient interaction of health care planners, administrators, physicians, and patients, so that each may efficiently achieve his individual objectives.

Social systems (such as health care systems) are much more complex than physical systems (such as electronic systems), but the fundamental principles apply, and appropriate input, output, and feedback relationships are essential for their successful functioning.

Health care delivery in the United States has generally functioned as a loose, "open" system, in which solo practitioners, as individual providers of care, deliver services (inputs) to patients. When such patients are acutely ill, information about their outcomes (outputs), whether death or recovery, usually is readily acquired by both provider and patient (feedback). When patients have chronic disease or long-term conditions, or are worried-well and wander from doctor to doctor, going in and out of the local medical community, feedback on their outcomes is not obtainable in any systemized manner.

With the emergence of prepaid group practice health plans that have a continuing contractual relationship to groups of people, organized health care delivery systems have come into existence. Feedback mechanisms built into these systems provide a closed-loop structure, bringing back information on the results of past actions of the health care system on its patients so as to influence and control future actions. In MHTS, for example, when the input of patient data indicates that a significant abnormality has been detected, it automatically triggers a feedback "advice" loop generating an output report to direct the patient to the clinical laboratory subsystem and/or the preventive maintenance subsystem and/or the sick care subsystem for further actions. From a management or planner's viewpoint the input and output data will feed back into a data base, providing essential information on the needs of appropriate allocation of resources for, and effectiveness of services delivered to the population for which the system is providing health care.

The operational integration of an MHTS into a health care delivery system is essential, so that patients can readily go from MHTS to physicians and ancillary services and also periodically go back to MHTS. Patient data also are transferred more readily and their confidentiality better maintained.

F. PROFESSIONAL RELATIONSHIP WITH MHTS

MHTS does require modification of the traditional fee-for-service relationship between patient and primary care physician, since a major objective is to save physician time. Traditionally, patients come to their doctors with medical problems; personal health care has been essentially a complaint-response type system. This system, however, is increasingly recognized to be insufficient for complete health care, the intent of which is to avoid premature death and unnecessary disability. As advocated by Breslow's Task Force,[6] "complaints need an appropriate response, but the presentation and handling of them can be more effective as a part of a larger health maintenance system of care. . . . The incorporation of preventive medicine into general health services . . . will obviously entail a change in orientation and a change in organization of personal health care services."

Many persons, moreover, come in allegedly for a "checkup," but the routine history elicits one or more medical problems or concerns. The physician then conducts a diagnostic workup for the specific complaints. Usually, as part of this medical workup, he also obtains a general history, including an inventory-by-systems; he then provides a general physical examination and finally arranges for several routine laboratory tests such as a blood count, urinalysis, electrocardiogram, etc. Most of the tests will probably be related to the specific complaints, but some will be of a screening nature to attempt to rule out common asymptomatic disease.

In MHTS, all examinees generally receive a similar battery of tests, with some variations by age (e.g., chest x-ray for adults only) or by sex (e.g., mammography), selected in accordance with the most common clinically important conditions in the target population. Some MHTS systems attempt to provide selective testing and furnish certain tests only to high-risk groups, e.g., mammography only to women over age 50. (See also Chapter Five.)

An important concept is that of the multiphasic laboratory as a patient data acquisition center for the physician. The primary care physician's activities can be divided into (1) collecting patient data and (2) making decisions on diagnosis and treatment. For a general health checkup, the physician goes through about the same history and physical examination and then orders a battery of tests; when all this information is gathered, the patient returns for diagnosis and treatment. The data gathering process is very routine and repetitive; in fact, the periodic health examination is probably the most routine and repetitive activity in the whole practice of medicine. That is why a systemized MHTS approach is most suited to this sort of practice.

McKeown[33] has identified what he terms an ethical issue in the screening of large groups, where essentially the doctor undertakes to identify the patient who needs his assistance. McKeown asserts that when the patient on his own initiative seeks medical advice, the doctor's position, ethically, is relatively simple: he undertakes to do his best with the knowledge and resources available to him. In traditional screening, however, when a doctor or public medical authority takes the initiative in looking for illness or disability in persons who have not complained of signs or symptoms, McKeown believes there is then a presumptive undertaking, not merely that an abnormality will be identified if it is present, but that those affected will derive benefit from subsequent treatment or care. The obligation exists, McKeown feels, even when the patient asks to be screened, for his request is then based upon the belief that the procedure is of value; if it is not, it is for medical people to make this known. McKeown cites the example that national screening for breast cancer would make heavy demands on medical resources; therefore it would clearly be essential to justify such diversion of resources and apply a validation procedure to such screening programs before they were put into use.

There can be little disagreement that the validation of cost-effectiveness of specific procedures is an important criterion for thc selection of tests both for public health mass screening and for an MHTS program providing personal preventive medical services (see Chapter Three, D, "Criteria for Test Selection").

Personal preventive medical services provided by an MHTS are arranged by and for the individual patient, so they do not incur McKeown's concern. The ethical issue he raises applies primarily to public preventive medicine such as mass screening programs (for which an MHTS may be used). In such an instance, where a population is screened for several diseases, and where those with positive screening tests are then referred to their physicians for validation and followup care, the patient comes to the doctor because of a positive test result. In some cases this may be a borderline, clinically unimportant finding (e.g., a blood sugar just above the normal screening limit) or even a "false positive" test (as proven by followup secondary testing). The effects of false positive and false negative tests on followup are also relevant to the relationship of the physician to the MHTS; this issue is considered in detail in Chapter Seventeen.

Ingelfinger,[35] commenting on the ethical issue raised by McKeown, pointed out that it was of practical consequence in testing populations at risk who are a sensitive minority group, such as in sickle cell screening programs for blacks. He advocated that when society initiates such public preventive medicine screening programs, not only the medical providers but the consumers should have an appropriate voice in the program.

An MHTS program is most commonly used (at least in the United States) as an efficient mode of providing personal health evaluations to individuals who desire them. McKeown's ethical issue does not apply when the physician uses the MHTS as a referral laboratory and sends the patient there for the testing phases of the health examination. In instances where the patient initiates the request for health examination and goes to the MHTS before making an appointment for followup, some physicians in fee-for-service practice find it an awkward situation when the patient appears after the MHTS. Strain may arise from divergence from the traditional method of the physician's first seeing the patient, taking a history, and establishing a doctor-patient relationship before referring the patient off to a laboratory for appropriate tests.

By designating a physician to whom his MHTS results are to be sent, the individual has requested the performance of professional services by that physician. The following recommendations for handling unsolicited Multiphasic Health Testing (MHT) reports have been developed by the American Medical Association:[36]

> 1. A physician who receives reports from an MHT organization involving persons who have made no prior arrangement with him for their evaluation may choose to accept such persons as his patients and communicate with them and provide such additional services as are necessary and usual in the physician-patient relationship.
>
> 2. If the physician elects not to accept the patient, he may return the reports to the MHT organization. If he does so, it is recommended that a covering letter be sent stating that he has not evaluated such reports and that the MHT organization take the necessary steps to inform the persons tested of the need

to make arrangements with a physician for their evaluation and followup care if required.

3. However, it is recommended that the physician evaluate any MHT reports involving patients whom he is actively treating or has treated in the past and that he communicate with such patients, especially if treatment or further testing is advisable. Failure to do so possibly may result in liability for malpractice if as a consequence the patient is not provided with prompt necessary treatment.

4. Even though the person involved is a stranger to the physician, if the testing results for a particular person indicate an urgent and immediate need for medical treatment suggesting a possible emergency situation, it is recommended that the physician communicate directly with the patient without delay for humanitarian reasons.

In a group practice prepaid health plan, which is essentially a form of contract medicine, the physician has a contractual obligation to provide health examinations to any plan member on request. A subscriber to the health plan who wishes to avail himself of this prepaid benefit, whether or not he has specific medical complaints, may elect one of two methods to obtain such: (1) he may first go to the physician in the traditional manner and be referred to the MHTS or clinical laboratory, or (2) he may first go to MHTS and be referred to the physician. The legality and ethics of these two modes of practice in a prepaid health plan are identical. The purpose of both types of health evaluations is to determine the health status of the individual, to screen for previously unknown or asymptomatic disease, and to arrange followup care in accordance with the patient's needs. Any differences are in the effects on the doctor-patient relationship caused by the patient's first contacting the physician before or after the laboratory testing—that is, at the beginning or at the end of the examination. These are not legal or ethical issues but rather are different styles of practice. In 25 years of providing multiphasic checkups to more than one-half million patients in the Kaiser-Permanente program, no medical cases occurred unique to the MHTS; the rare malpractice suits that did occur alleged missing early pulmonary tuberculosis by chest x-ray or breast cancer by mammography.

Bates[37] reported that physicians may react unfavorably to MHTS because they want to control access to the system through medical referral, because they want to oppose intervention by outside groups into medical practice, and because they want to be selective in choosing tests, often on the basis of clinical indication.

Physicians have similar variable reactions to their first exposure to panel or profile testing, wherein multiple blood chemistry tests are performed simultaneously on a single blood specimen. With the advent of automated chemical analyzers it is more economical to do 6, 12, or even 18 different tests routinely on a single blood sample than to do one or two individual blood chemistry tests on specific request. This issue is similar in MHTS programs as in those hospitals where routinely a panel of tests is performed on admission of the patients. Since most of the tests in the panel are unsolicited by the physician, he may be uncertain about his obligation to the patient when an abnormal test result is reported. The issue is no different when the physician finds an unsuspected abnormality by a routine hospital admission biochemical profile or MHTS test panel[27] than when he finds an unsuspected abnormality by a traditional routine inventory-by-systems history, by a "complete" routine physical examination, or by a "routine" blood count or a "routine" urinalysis. The difficulty lies merely in the current innovative status of the test panel. The medical professional will soon become accustomed to it, just as he became accustomed to the routine preadmission hospital workup. Friedman[38] has shown that providing more biochemical tests does indeed detect more clinically important abnormalities that warrant intervention.

The problem of false positive and false negative tests also affects the relationships of physicians to MHTS; this issue is discussed in Chapter Seventeen. Although MHTS clearly modifies the traditional role of the primary care physician, when the physician is satisfied that the patient can receive good-quality care at a lower cost and that the physician's time is saved without decreasing his income, he will support MHTS.

MHTS employs a variety of other health professionals (see Chapter Three), and their relationships with patients, physicians, and the MHTS are similar to those of other technologists in hospital clinical laboratories or x-ray departments. MHTS helps support new health careers, including those of nurse practitioners, various test-phase technologists, clinical engineers, medical application computer programmers, and health educators. An especially sensitive area is the need to indoctrinate all MHTS personnel as to the legal requirements for safeguarding patient data confidentiality.

G. PATIENT AND COMMUNITY RELATIONSHIP

Studies of social determinants of the use of preventive medical services,[39] which would include MHTS, suggest that people are less likely to use preventive services when they are poor, have little education, are isolated from community groups and social networks, have limited health knowledge and unfavorable attitudes toward preventive care, and have little confidence in the health care system. They are also less likely to use such services when their pattern of medical care is fragmented and episodic as compared with a more regular and continuous association with a medical provider.

The individual patient's relationships with an MHTS are, in one respect, similar to those of a patient to any clinical laboratory, x-ray department, or hospital when the MHTS serves as a referral or auxiliary service for the physician. MHTS provides services by examining the patient, his blood and urine specimens, his x-rays and ECG and reporting the results to his doctor for diagnosis and treatment. Any differences in MHTS-physician-patient relationships occur only when the patient, rather than the physician, initiates the MHTS; this issue was considered in the preceding section.

That the MHTS process significantly affects the traditional doctor-patient relationship has been acknowledged. Szasz and Hollender[40] consider the relationship between the patient and his doctor a "novel one" in which there is a joint participation of the two persons involved; it is an abstraction embodying the activities of the two interacting persons and can be represented by two basic models for ambulatory patients: (1) guidance-cooperation, in which the physician tells the patient what to do and the patient cooperates by obeying, by compliance; and (2) mutual participation, in which the physician helps the patient to help himself and the patient's role is one of the participant in a partnership who uses expert help. The model of mutual participation predominates in an MHTS program, since for the majority of MHTS patients (who are well, worried-well, or asymptomatic-sick) the physician does not profess to know what is best for the patient. The patient's own experiences furnish indispensable information for agreement as to what "well" might be for him. In the treatment of organic disease, such as cancer, a concurrence is readily obtained between doctor and patient as to whether the treatment is successful or not, but for most psychosocial conditions, such as "nervousness," "run-down," or "dizziness," it is more difficult to agree on a measure of successful outcome. MHTS introduces the additional factor of detecting variations from normal that were previously unknown to both doctor and patient, such as finding a uric acid of 10 in a middle-aged man who feels well and is seeing a physician who sees no agreement in the literature as to what is the proper management of asymptomatic hyperuricemia.

Patients' acceptance of and satisfaction with MHTS depends upon their prior orientation to the multiphasic process, how it works, and what it is expected to accomplish. Once patients understand the MHTS process, their acceptance of it is excellent.[41] Concern is often expressed that systems technology provides assembly-line medicine, and computers tend to dehumanize and depersonalize the medical care process. Hall,[42] a past president of the American Medical Association, cleverly coined the acronym "AMHTLC" to emphasize that Automated Multiphasic Health Testing (AMHT) must include Tender Loving Care (TLC). It is certainly essential that all MHTS personnel show concern, patience, understanding, and kindness to each patient, as all health care personnel should do in all medical care services. MHTS patients have no difficulty in separating the laboratory services (whether clinical laboratory, x-ray, or MHTS) from their primary care physician, so the extensive technology of the laboratory does not detract from the patient-physician relationship; on the contrary, the more modern the laboratory technology, the more confident is the patient with the physician's technical capabilities. Furthermore, the computer gives the physician a report that can furnish normal values that are age-sex specific and adjusted to time of day and hours since last food ingestion, thereby personalizing each report and individualizing the care for each patient in a way that is just not possible in the traditional care process. This not only increases the personalization of care but improves its quality.

With increasing numbers of organized medical groups providing medical care to consumer groups by contractual arrangements, MHTS will be used more and more to meet the growing public demand for *health* care (that is, health examinations and health maintenance) as a right. To be most effective, MHTS will need to provide health education to the public that will teach individuals how to better take care of their health. (See Chapter Twelve.) It appears that health care programs will need to become more responsive to what the people that it serves want in the form of medical care, including personal preventive services.[6] The increasing trend to organized arrangements for payments for health care will probably encourage preventive health maintenance services for improvement of personal health and stimulate MHTS development that is customized for the community it serves.

Consumer (cooperative) groups and unions are increasingly negotiating for periodic health examinations as a health welfare benefit. As the general public becomes more aware that company executives, political leaders, union groups, and health plan members are receiving periodic health examinations, it can be expected that the general public will increasingly want such health checkups.

The community's growing concern for its members can be fulfilled by MHTS in the early detection of communicable diseases such as tuberculosis and syphilis. Experience with sickle cell screening programs has alerted minority groups that, besides the potential benefits, there can be problems associated with identifying genetic or environmental high-risk groups. One should balance any possible medical benefits against potential societal harm, such as by having health status stigmatize an ethnic group.[35]

Elinson[43] believes that whether or not a person will use MHTS services or engage in any preventive health behavior is likely to depend on a wide variety of personal and social psychological factors and on factors characterizing the organization of health services. On the one hand, for example, preventive behavior depends on the person's orientation to health care, the perceived value of the service offered, and concern about health. On the other hand, the utilization of preventive opportunities depends on the physical proximity and convenience of the service offered, the response one expects from health personnel, and the monetary and psychological costs of using the service. Elinson further makes the following suggestions with respect to "customizing" the MHTS process: "Consideration might be given to use of mobile facilities, transportation services, baby-sitting services, hours of accessibility, friendliness of staff, allowing participants to bring someone with them, giving a description of the process while they are waiting, providing someone to talk with at convenient breaks in the process, using tour leaders from the community to bridge the gap between lay consumer and status-authority personnel, a final debriefing stage to give the consumer a chance to express his reactions to the process, and giving consumers small tangible gifts." Elinson contends that "as consumers more actively influence and interact with the services they receive, they are also more likely to value and support such services. Satisfaction will depend on how much personalization the system will allow and the consumers ultimately demand." He believes that personalized or customized systems of communication are not incompatible with effective use of highly standardized automated systems of technology. He suggests that customizing, for example, might include making staff resources available for reinterpretation of standardized information and arranging the ongoing accessibility of staff persons with this capability throughout the testing process.

Since the effectiveness of personal preventive services depends to a considerable extent upon the cooperation and compliance of patients with physicians' advice, this will be further discussed in Chapters Ten and Eighteen.

REFERENCES

1. *Detection and Prevention of Chronic Disease Utilizing Multiphasic Health Screening Techniques.* Hearings before the Subcommittee on Health of the Elderly of the Special Committee on Aging, U.S. Senate, Sept. 1966.

2. Thorner, R. M. "The Status of Activity in Automated Health Testing in the U.S.," in *Automated Multiphasic Health Testing.* Proceedings of Engineering Foundation Research Conferences. New York: Engineering Foundation, 1971.

3. Garfield, S., Collen, M., Richart, R., Feldman, R., Soghikian, K., Richart, R., and Duncan, J. "Evaluation of an Ambulatory Medical-Care Delivery System." *New Eng. J. Med.* 294(1976): 426–431.

4. Wilson, J. M. G., and Hilleboe, H. E. *Mass Health Examinations.* Pub. Health Paper No. 45. Geneva: W.H.O., 1971.

5. Rosen, G. "Preventive Medicine in the U.S., 1900–1975." Pages 716–809 in *Preventive Medicine USA.* New York: PRODIST, 1976.

6. Breslow, L., et al. "Theory, Practice and Application of Prevention in Personal Health Services." *Preventive Medicine USA.* New York: PRODIST, 1976.

7. White, K. L. "Prevention as a National Health Goal." *Preventive Medicine* 4(1975):247–251.

8. Steenwyk, J. V. *Implementing Programs for Preventive Health Care Services.* Blue Cross Repts. Res. Series 2, 1969.

9. Terris, M. "Approaches to an Epidemiology of Health." *Am. J. Pub. Health* 65 (1975).

10. Peacock, P. B., Gelman, A. C., and Lutins, T. A. "Preventive Health Care Strategies for Health Maintenance Organizations." *Prev. Med.* 4(1975):183–225.

11. Garfield, S. "Multiphasic Testing and Medical Care as a Right." *New Eng. J. Med.* 283(1970): 1087–1089.

12. Glazier, W. H. "The Task of Medicine." *Scientific American* 228(1973):13–17.

13. White, K. L. "Life and Death in Medicine." *Scientific American* 229(1973):23–33.

14. Garfield, S. "The Delivery of Medical Care." *Scientific American* 222(1970):15–23.

15. Yamaguchi, K. "The Toshiba Multiphasic Screening Centre." *Med. & Biol. Engng.* 9(1971):421–429.

16. Caceres, C. "AMHT in Perspective—Accomplishments and Problems," in *Automated Multiphasic Health Testing.* Proceedings of Engineering Foundation Research Conferences. New York: Engineering Foundation, 1971.

17. Warshaw, L. J., et al. "New York Heart Association Conference on Automated Multiphasic Health Screening." *Bulletin of the New York Academy of Medicine.* 2d Series. Vol. 45, No. 12 (Dec. 1969).

18. Creticos, A. P. "Some Thoughts on the Management of an Automated Multiphasic Health Screening Center." In *Proceedings of Symposia International Health Evaluation Association.* IHEA, 1974.

19. Wilson, J. M. G., and Jungner, G. *Principles and Practice of Screening for Disease.* Public Health Paper No. 34. Geneva: W.H.O., 1968.

20. Watts, M. S. "Some General Principles and Some General Guidelines." Section II in *Provisional Guidelines for Automated Multiphasic Health Testing Services,* Vol. 1. N.T.I.S. Report No. PB 195 654, 1970.

21. Engel, G. L. "A Unified Concept of Health and Disease." Chap. 16 in Millon, T. *Medical Behavioral Science.* Philadelphia: W. B. Saunders, 1975.

22. Richart, R. H., Duncan, J. H., Collen, M. F., and Garfield, S. R. "An Evaluation Model for Health Care System Change." *J. Med. Syst.* 1(1977)30–41.

23. Berg, R. L., et al. *Health Status Indexes.* Chicago: Health Research & Educational Trust, 1973.

24. Moser, R. H. "Jangled Semantics." *J.A.M.A.* 231(1975):1371.

25. Terris, M. "Evolution of Public Health and Preventive Medicine in the U.S." *Am. J. Pub. Health* 65(1975):161–169.

26. Holland, W. W. "Screening for Disease. Taking Stock." *The Lancet* 2(1974):1494–1497.

27. Benson, E. S., and Strandjord, P. E. *Multiple Laboratory Screening.* New York: Academic Press, 1969.

28. Sackett, D. L., and Holland, W. W. "Controversy in the Detection of Disease." *The Lancet* 2(1975):357–359.

29. Sanazaro, P. J. "AMHT. Definition of the Concept." *Hospitals, J.A.H.A.* 45(1971):41–43.

30. Flagle, C. D. "Technological Development in the Health Services." *Proc. I.E.E.E.* 11(1969): 1847–1852.

31. Pryor, T. A., and Warner, H. R. "Admitting Screening at Latter-Day Saints Hospital." In D. F.

Davies, Ed. *Health Evaluation, An Entry to the Health Care System.* New York: Intercontinental Medical Book Co., 1973.

32. Warner, H. R. "Routine vs. Priority Procedures: Challenging the Medical Checkup." Colloquium
8 in M. Schorow, Ed. *Hearings on Issues and Trends in Medical Care,* p. 135. Salt Lake City:
Intermountain Regional Medical Program, 1970.

33. McKeown, T. "Unvalidated Procedures Have No Place in Screening Programs." In F. J.
Ingelfinger et al. *Controversy in Internal Medicine II,* p. 92. Philadelphia: W. B. Saunders, 1974.
Also "Validation of Screening Procedures." Chap. 1 in *Screening in Medical Care.* Nuffield
Provincial Hospitals Trust. London: Oxford Univ. Press, 1968.

34. Forrester, J. W. *Principles of Systems.* Cambridge, Mass.: Wright-Allen Press, 1971.

35. Ingelfinger, F. J. "Comment on Multiphasic Screening." In F. J. Ingelfinger et al. *Controversy in
Internal Medicine II.* Philadelphia: W. B. Saunders Co., 1974, p. 29.

36. *Statement on Multiphasic Testing.* Chicago: American Medical Association, 1972.

37. Bates, B., and Mulinare, J. "Physicians' Use and Opinions of Screening Tests in Ambulatory
Practice." *J.A.M.A.* 214(1970):2173–2180.

38. Friedman, G., Goldberg, M., Ahuja, J., Siegelaub, A., Bassis, M., and Collen, M. F. "Biochemical Screening Tests: Effect of Panel Size on Medical Care." *Arch. Int. Med.* 129(1972):91–97.

39. Hinkle, L. E., et al. "Social Determinants of Human Health." Pages 617–675 in *Preventive
Medicine USA.* New York: PRODIST, 1976.
Bethesda, Md., 1975.

40. Szasz, T. S., and Hollender, M. H. "A Contribution to the Philosophy of Medicine: The Basic
Models of the Doctor-Patient Relationship." Chap. 35 in T. Millon, *Medical Behavioral Science.*
Philadelphia: W. B. Saunders, 1975.

41. Soghikian, K., and Collen, F. B. "Acceptance of Multiphasic Screening Examination by Patients." *Bull. N.Y. Acad. Med.* 45(1969):1366–1375.

42. Hall, W. "AMHTLC." In *Automated Multiphasic Health Testing.* Proceedings of Engineering
Foundation Research Conferences. New York: Engineering Foundation, 1971.

43. Elinson, J. "Subcommittee Report on Human Factors in AMHTS." Pages 211–220 in *Provisional
Guidelines for Automated Multiphasic Health Testing Services,* Vol. 3. DHEW Publication No.
72-3011, 1970.

CHAPTER THREE

MHTS Planning and Implementation

Morris F. Collen

A. **Sponsorship, Financing, and Organization**
B. **Personnel Selection and Functions**
C. **Defining Specific Objectives**
D. **Patient Processing Needs**
E. **Test Selection for Health Problems**
F. **Selection of Facility and Equipment**
G. **Systems Design**
H. **Implementation Scheduling**
 I. **Quality Control and Standard Operations**
J. **Guidelines for Successful Operation**

A. SPONSORSHIP, FINANCING, AND ORGANIZATION

MHTS programs have been sponsored and operated by a variety of agencies. They have been financed through government grants and public subsidy, through health insurance premiums that prepay their costs fully or in part, through fee-for-service where the examinee pays for all the costs, and through health and welfare benefits negotiated in collective bargaining between labor and management. Of approximately 200 MHTS programs reviewed in the United States,[1,2] private corporations operated about one-fifth and provided multiphasic testing services for personal health examinations on a fee-for-service basis or for employees at company expense. Governmental agencies (federal, state, county, and city health departments) operated about one-sixth of MHTS programs, including military personnel programs. Hospitals (both public and private) operated about one-tenth of the programs in the United States. Other MHTS program sponsors included individual and group practice physicians, health insurance companies, industrial corporations, health organizations, clinical laboratories, medical societies, and labor unions. In the past, health insurance plans generally have been, in fact, "sickness" insurance plans, and many have excluded health examinations and multiphasic checkups. With the advent of the "Health Maintenance Organization" (HMO) Act of 1973, more MHTS programs probably will be sponsored by prepaid group practice plans because of the orientation of HMOs to preventive medicine. Generally, the less the direct charges for health examinations, the greater is their utilization by the public.

In the 1960s most MHTS programs were financed totally or in part from governmental funds. In the 1970s most MHTS facilities were financially supported by their users, on either a prepaid insurance or fee-for-service basis, or by a company for its employees.

A MHTS is essentially a technological system, and its potential cost and profit will depend largely on technology considerations. Operational costs will depend upon the number of tests, the number of personnel employed in the program, the facility design, amortization rate of capitalized equipment, cost of supplies, plant maintenance, etc. Of all these factors, the most critical in determining the unit cost per examination (which primarily determines the charges to users) are the MHTS work load (that is, the number of examinees per day), the facility's design (which affects the efficiency of the program), and the degree of automation of equipment (which influences the number of personnel required).

The purpose of automation is usually to facilitate the handling of a work volume that exceeds reasonable manual capacity. The addition of automated equipment in MHTS improves the efficiency of operations by providing more tests at lower unit costs and maximizes the use of allied health personnel and technician aides. It also improves the accuracy of the testing, the quality of the data acquisition process, and the resultant report to the physician.

The majority of MHTS programs utilize some automated equipment—at least in the clinical laboratory phase for the serum chemistry and hematology tests. Many use automated self-administered histories, automated electrocardiogram interpretation, automated spirograms and/or audiograms, and automated data processing either by a dedicated computer or by sharing a large computer. A few MHTS programs use no automated equipment and perform all functions in a manual mode.

Generally, an MHTS program that examines less than 25 persons a day five work days a week, or 500 examinees a month, will not be able to support the large capital investment for automated equipment, will be almost entirely a manual operation, and for any minimally comprehensive number of tests will probably cost more than $50 an examination. An MHTS program that examines about 50 persons a day, or 1,000 a month, will probably be able to successfully finance some automated testing equipment and a small computer and should be able to provide a reasonably comprehensive battery of tests at a cost of less than $50 an examination. An MHTS program that examines 100 persons a day, or 2,000 a month, will be able to utilize primarily automated equipment with automated data processing and computer algorithms to triage patients (this being an automated MHTS) for a cost of about $25 per examination (exclusive of the physical examination). (See also Chapter Seventeen, Figure 17-1.)

MHTS charges to examinees are extremely varied and depend not only upon the operational costs but upon whether the program is part of a larger health care delivery system, whether it is operated on a for-profit or nonprofit basis, and whether it is fee-for-service or part of a prepaid insurance program. The usual charges in the mid 1970s for multiphasic testing (excluding physical examination) varied from $30 to $200; the usual range was $50 to $100 for a fee-for-service program.

Critical to financing is the sponsor's decision whether to develop its own MHTS or to acquire a turnkey commercial system. Whether to purchase or whether to lease the facility, the system, and/or the capital equipment also becomes a major decision. For a commercial turnkey system, under a lease contract, the advantages are that the longer the duration of the lease, the more favorable the program's terms and conditions can be, since no large initial investment is required for equipment, and an adequate load of examinees allows monthly payments to be budgeted and met. The disadvantages are that the MHTS system will have been designed to satisfy a large market rather than tailored to the individual needs of the individual MHTS program, and the MHTS program will be relatively fixed in its services during the period of the lease, since significant program changes will usually result in additional charges from the system vendor. Usually, the lessee has an option to purchase the system at the termination of the lease. Purchase of a turnkey system would be similar to a lease contract arrangement, except that full payment is due the vendor upon delivery of the system, and separate maintenance services must be arranged.

If the sponsoring organization is a large one and the MHTS will process 100 or more examinees a day, it will usually find it preferable to design and develop its own MHTS, which it can customize to suit its own objectives and more specifically meet the needs of its target population. The main disadvantages of developing a customized MHTS are its great expense and long development time.

Galbraith[3] was one of the first to point out just what is required for developing complex technological systems such as a large automated MHTS:

(1) Long-term investment—the more complex the technology the greater the lead time from planning to completion.

(2) Heavy investment of capital equipment and manpower.

(3) Need for accurate planning to inflexibly commit people and capital for long lead times—usually several years between planning and completion.

(4) Specialized technological manpower to design, develop, and implement most effectively.

(5) Organization—especially competent to coordinate mixed medical, systems, and engineering specialties.

For these reasons most MHTS sponsors prefer to buy or lease commercial turnkey systems rather than design and implement their own.

For sponsors who already have a medical center available and can project an MHTS program examining less than 50 patients a day, a special MHTS facility is not necessary. If existing radiology, electrocardiography, and clinical laboratory facilities and existing outpatient examination rooms are used each evening from 5:30 to 8:00 and all day Saturdays, 1,000 patients can be seen each month with no new investment in facilities or capital equipment.

The organization of an MHTS depends upon the sponsor's determining its objectives, arranging financing, selecting a physician-director, and appointing an advisory committee.[4,5]

An advisory committee is indispensable to advise the MHTS director on policies governing objectives and operations. It should represent professional users of MHTS, including referring physicians and hospitals. It may consider including consumer users of the MHTS when appropriate to its organizational structure and objectives. It should include the physician-specialists who are advisers to the medical-technical aspects of the various MHTS stations (for example, the consulting cardiologist for the ECG test station, the radiologist for the x-ray phase, and the clinical pathologist for the clinical laboratory phase).

It is essential that the advisory committee be only advisory and not controlling, since a subgroup within it may aggressively advocate its own interests and tend to suboptimize the overall program. Clinical specialists, since they are primarily trained in sick care, often do not appreciate or support preventive health care, and they often advocate terminating phases within MHTS that are primarily preventive or health care oriented.

After the physician-director is chosen, the remaining MHTS personnel can be selected as shown in Figure 3-1.

B. PERSONNEL SELECTION AND FUNCTIONS

The selection of qualified personnel to make up a multidisciplinary, closely functioning team is very important for an MHTS. Any large MHTS will do well to have an advisory committee and a group of key personnel including a physician-director (who may be part-time), a full-time nurse supervisor, an administrator or administrative assistant, and several supporting technical people in addition to the personnel who operate the test stations (see Figure 3-1).

1. MHTS Director

a. The MHTS director should be a physician who has great interest in preventive medicine, administrative experience, and some background in the physical sciences so as to understand the technological aspects.

b. He should be responsible for all administrative and medical aspects of the

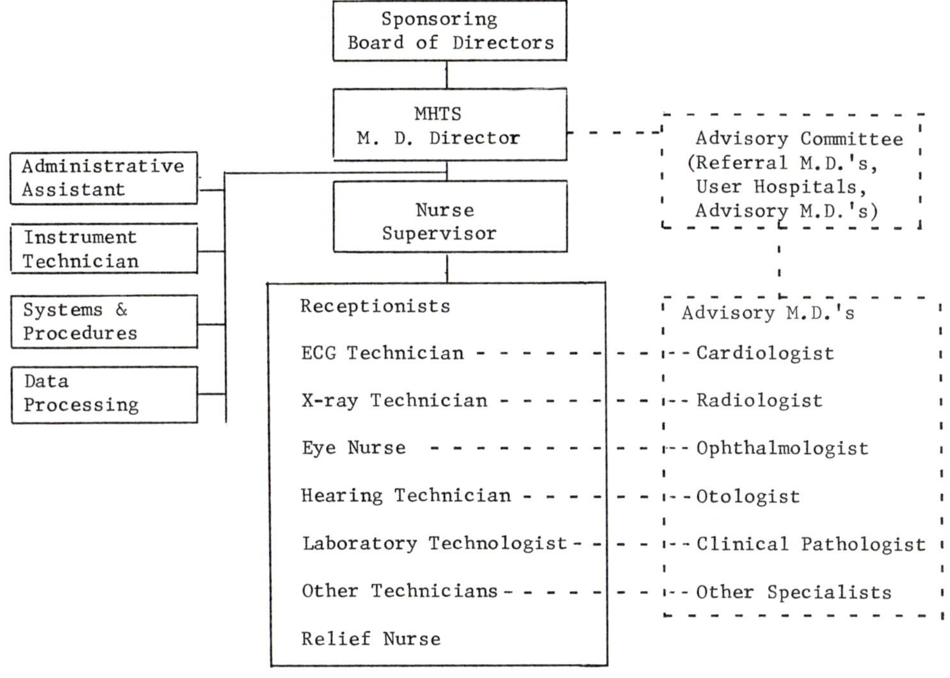

(Modified from Collen[4])

Figure 3-1. A suggested organizational chart for an MHTS.

MHTS and should authorize any changes and additions to standard operating procedures.

c. He reports to his board of directors or their designated administrative officer, and he consults with the advisory committee on all policy matters or major procedural problems.

d. He appoints the nurse supervisor, adminstrative assistant, instrumentation technician, and systems and procedures and data processing personnel.

e. He should be willing to spend at least half his time on the project. He makes regular rounds at least twice weekly to insure maintenance of quality control and performance of standard procedures.

f. He is available to supervise and assist the nurse supervisor in the performance of her functions.

g. He communicates and cooperates with specific medical and technical consultants (cardiologists, radiologists, etc.) in problem solving.

h. He functions as liaison between the MHTS and the patients' physicians, keeping them informed on problems and changes.

2. Nurse Supervisor

a. The nurse supervisor is the key person for day-to-day operations.

b. She supervises and coordinates the MHTS under the direct supervision of the director.

c. She is responsible for making decisions related to patient disposition, and:

(1) personally arranges disposition of any patient becoming ill or injured during the examination, following consultation with the physician director.

(2) personally arranges for patients whose test results indicate they require emergency medical care.

(3) releases patients when a station ceases to function owing to insufficient personnel or equipment breakdown (and notifies instrumentation and data processing personnel).

(4) authorizes (when necessary) the acceptance of unscheduled or excessively late patients.

(5) attends personally any patient involved in complaints or misunderstandings.

(6) answers patients' questions regarding tests and followup, insofar as nursing ethics and MHTS policies allow.

(7) reports in writing any unusual occurrence, to avoid future complications.

d. She is responsible for supervision and coordination of job performance of all phase technicians, and:

(1) supervises personnel performance and methods to assure maintenance of quality control and standard procedures.

(2) orients and trains new personnel concerning MHTS policies and objectives.

(3) is responsible for continuing orientation training of personnel for all new or revised procedures and policies.

(4) prepares staffing schedules adequate to the need.

(5) makes appropriate adjustments to personnel necessary to cover all testing phases for absences, illness, lateness, breaks, lunches.

(6) monitors flow of patient traffic, making adjustments in staffing of phases as necessary, to insure a smoothly operating unit.

(7) evaluates personnel for the director.

e. She functions as internal coordinator for MHTS operations, and:

(1) coordinates with advisory physicians in the absence of the director.

(2) reports to the director all operational problems involving patients.

(3) maintains close communication with data processing staff with regard to problems in processing data, missing data, etc.

f. She is responsible, with the administrator, for proper maintenance of the facility, equipment and supplies, and:

(1) is responsible for controlling use of supplies and medications; orders drugs, linens, forms, and other supplies, as necessary.

(2) assures proper functioning of equipment in the unit, instituting work orders and repair orders as necessary; notifies instrumentation technician promptly of equipment malfunction.

(3) observes the physical plant and suggests changes or improvements in maintenance.

3. Administrator or Administrative Assistant

a. An administrator for a large MHTS may take over many of the functions listed above for the nurse supervisor. An administrative assistant for a small MHTS can still be very helpful for proper planning and operation.

b. He is responsible to the director for administrative matters pertaining to the MHTS planning, implementation, and operation.

c. He supervises appointment scheduling and registration procedures.

d. He is responsible for supervising followup appointments and test reporting to physicians.

e. He arranges for plant maintenance.

f. He is responsible for proper processing of all purchase and personnel requisitions to be approved by the director, and for the maintenance of cost accounting data to permit suitable cost analyses as authorized.

4. Instrumentation Technician

a. An instrumentation technician is needed to maintain all MHTS equipment in proper working order, and he arranges repairs as necessary.

b. He establishes an adequate preventive maintenance program. He maintains a library of plans, specifications, and circuit diagrams for all equipment.

c. He monitors the quality control for equipment and provides regular reports as authorized.

d. He advises the director concerning desired modifications or replacement in equipment to improve reliability, accuracy, and efficiency.

e. He advises and assists in planning, designing, building, and/or selecting new equipment; and he interfaces equipment for data processing and for stand-by.

f. He cooperates with the director, nurse supervisor, and phase technicians to solve equipment problems.

5. Systems and Procedures (Supervisor)

a. A person trained in systems and procedures work is critical to the efficient functioning of an MHTS. In a large program he will be a supervisory-level person and be responsible for maintaining, preparing revisions, and distributing a Standard Operating Procedures Manual. (See Chapter Twenty.)

b. He advises on MHTS scheduling procedures for patient appointments. (See Chapter Five.)

c. He advises and assists with design and implementation of data acquisition forms.

d. He advises on modifications to improve patient flow through MHTS phases.

e. He carries out system analyses as authorized by the director.

6. Data Processing (Supervisor)

a. For a large automated MHTS a person capable of computer programming is essential and should be at supervisor level to handle the extensive data processing requirements.

b. He advises and assists with data processing planning and operation. (See Chapter Eight.)

c. He implements and maintains programs and procedures for MHTS computer requirements, including:

(1) computer preparation and processing of cards, forms, labels, appointments, etc.

(2) data output (test reports).

(3) data storage and retrieval.

(4) computer program library and documentation.

(5) writing computer programs for data quality control (such as for test validity limits), printout of normal values, etc.

(6) advising instrumentation technician on interfacing requirements between test equipment and data processing equipment.

d. He is responsible for control of the integrity and confidentiality of all patient data in magnetic storage and within the computer center.

e. He communicates with the nurse supervisor for all data processing problems.

f. He cooperates with the director for problems in data acquisition and data reporting.

7. Personnel Requirements for Individual Test Stations

The personnel for the various test stations must be selected in accordance with technology requirements. For x-ray tests a lesser trained technician than usually needed in a traditional radiology department can provide the one or two routine x-ray procedures performed; however, the quality of the films must still be supervised by and acceptable to the radiologist who will interpret them. The same quality of electrocardiography technician is advisable for screening ECGs as for routine clinic ECGs, since for nonautomated ECGs it is helpful if the technician can identify a serious variation from a normal ECG even though she may be unable to interpret the abnormality; thus, the seriously abnormal ECG can be shown to a physician before the patient leaves the MHTS site.

Tonometry testing is best done by a nurse who has been trained by an ophthalmologist as to the procedure and how to safely screen out patients for whom it is contraindicated.

At the history station it is advisable to have a nurse available to answer questions of a medical nature.

One technologist, who can receive supervision from a clinical pathologist, is necessary in the clinical laboratory. Since most of the automated procedures now provide digital readout, such equipment can be operated by laboratory aides.

Otherwise, for other MHTS phases, formally trained health professionals are not necessary, and high school graduates can be trained in a few weeks to be effective test personnel.[6]

Generally, to ease the monotony of doing the same repetitive test all the time, technicians appreciate being trained in two or three test stations and rotating tasks for variety. A relief nurse, trained to serve as a backup person for most test stations, is important.

To process 150 patients a day, the Kaiser-Permanente MHTS in Oakland staffs each test station as shown in Table 3-1. Staff are often trained in two test functions, so they can fill in for those out sick and vary their work. Multiphasic station personnel must be of a personality type who can follow protocols and standardized procedures repetitively without boredom; they must be able to do the same procedure exactly the same way a hundred or more times each day, day after day, to insure continuing uniform quality. It is therefore important to select

Table 3-1. Personnel Requirements for Individual Test Phases as Related to Work Load

Test Phase	Examinations Per Day			
	200	150	100	50
Registration	2	2	1	1
Referral	2	1	1	
Electrocardiogram	2	2	1	1
Blood pressure	2	1	1	
Chest x-ray	1	1	1	1
Mammography	2	1	1	
Height, weight, spirometry	1	1	1	1
Vision	1	1		
Tonometry	1	1	1	1
Hearing	1	1	1	
History	3	2	2	1
Clinical laboratory	5	4	3	2
Relief nurse/aide	2	2	1	1
Data processing	3	3	2	1
Total	28	23	17	10

people who like this type of work and then train them to do two or perhaps even three tasks to vary the job somewhat.

C. DEFINING SPECIFIC OBJECTIVES

Chapter Two discussed the various goals of MHTS. Obviously, no single program can suit all applications and satisfy all objectives. Each MHTS must define its own organization's objectives for the needs of the target population that it must satisfy. Each MHTS must be customized to meet its own specific objectives; the more objectives to satisfy, the more costly the program. An MHTS for patient care will need to be modified somewhat for research or for teaching. An MHTS for health care delivery will be very different from one for a large manufacturing industry or one for military inductees. An MHTS for adults will differ greatly from one for children.

Cost-effectiveness analysis is very useful in the planning of a health care system for an MHTS. Given a defined objective or benefit, it permits comparisons of alternative methods in terms of their effectiveness in achieving that objective. (See Chapter Seventeen, F.) If the objective or highest priority of a health care system is to prevent strokes, then a cost-effectiveness study would probably show that an MHTS blood pressure station for detection (and early treatment) of hypertension should receive very high priority. If the objective or highest priority of the health care system is the treatment and improvement of disability from strokes, then a cost-effectiveness study would give a low priority to an MHTS blood pressure station and a high priority to clinical remedial and rehabilitative services.

Proper planning will require defining both short- and long-term objectives.

1. Short-Term Objectives

An MHTS within a health care delivery system might have the following short-term objectives:

a. Provide reassurance. The majority of patients who come to MHTS in a health maintenance organization such as Kaiser-Permanente are well or worried-well; reassurance is therefore the most common immediate objective.

b. Define the health status of examinees and determine individual fitness *(health appraisal)*.

c. Monitor the status of continuing health of individuals by periodic examinations *(health surveillance)*.

d. Detect unknown abnormalities *(disease detection* or *case finding)*.

e. Monitor previously detected abnormalities by the periodic examination of patients with known diabetes, hypertension, etc. *(patient surveillance* and *disease monitoring)*.

f. Serve as a referral laboratory for physicians whose patients need early sickness or diagnostic surveys *(diagnostic adjunct)*.

g. Serve as an entry mode to the health care delivery system *(triage)*.

h. Provide admission hospital and pre-operative examinations. (See Figure 3-2.)

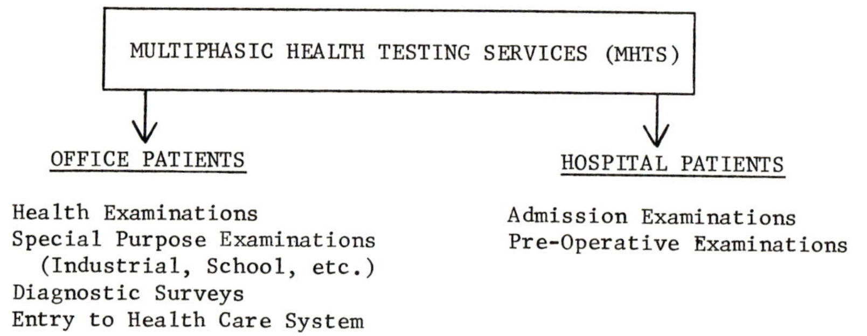

Figure 3-2. Typical objectives of an MHTS.

i. Provide health education and health maintenance to improve health habits and behavior.

j. Provide efficient, satisfying, and quality testing service to patients.

k. Improve accessibility of health care delivery by making health status evaluation more readily available.

l. Provide efficient, satisfying, and quality service to physicians; save physician time by providing a high-utility report, comprehensive in content and readable in format.

m. Provide a comprehensive, quality, patient health profile to furnish baseline measurements for continuing or future care.

n. Operate a cost-effective program.

o. Contain the cost of the process of providing medical care by decreasing use of hospital beds and costs of ancillary (clinical laboratory and x-ray) services, in addition to conserving physician time.

p. Secondary objectives may involve using the MHTS data for clinical, epidemiological, or health services types of research, which may require supplemental data collection and processing procedures and may increase accuracy requirements for testing. An additional objective of the MHTS may be to serve as an adjunct for professional education and allied health personnel training; this will require some adjustment of space and personnel time.

2. Long-Term Objectives

The long-term objectives of an MHTS might be to:

(1) decrease morbidity, disability, and mortality (outcome) of patients; and thereby
(2) decrease long-term utilization of hospital services and costs of care.

3. Specific Functional Objectives for Each Test Phase

Each MHTS must define specific objectives for each test customized for its examinees, depending upon their racial, ethnic, and socioeconomic characteristics. It is essential to define precisely the short-term functional objectives for each test phase, after choosing tests that satisfy the criteria for selection (see E). Objectives should include:

(1) A desired sensitivity and specificity for each test. The determination of the accuracy required for each test and the setting of boundary limits for "normal" and "abnormal" will define the percentage of true positives and true negatives, false positives and false negatives. If MHTS is used for preadmission hospital patients, inpatients usually have more numerous and severe abnormalities, and normal limits for certain tests are different for ambulatory than for bed patients.
(2) A projected prevalence of true positives for each phase. The estimated prevalence of targeted diseases in the population to be tested is essential.
(3) An expected cost effectiveness for each phase. The usual objective is to detect a significant number of specified conditions at a reasonable cost.

It cannot be emphasized too strongly that the more precisely the sponsor can define the objectives of the MHTS and of its testing phases, the greater the likelihood that it can successfully achieve them. In a health care program or medical center, if the director is a preventive medical specialist, its objectives will probably include and emphasize preventive and predictive medical tests. On the other hand, if the control of the MHTS lies with a specialist in internal medicine, the objectives will emphasize disease detection and disease monitoring and may very well eliminate many early preventive and predictive tests, since the traditional practicing internist is oriented to sick care rather than health care.

D. PATIENT PROCESSING NEEDS

1. Identifying User Population Needs

A cost-effective MHTS depends on data that can identify the user population needs. Demographic and cultural characteristics and environmental and industrial health hazards of the target population together with available disease prevalence data are a necessary basis for estimating specific disease rates. For example, if pulmonary tuberculosis or exposure to environmental or occupational dusts is a significant problem in the community, then obviously chest x-rays should be included in every examination; if not, then chest x-rays could be omitted from examinations after the first one.

The prevalence of the specific conditions in the target population is important in influencing yield rates, cost per positive case, and cost effectiveness of the MHTS program. (See Chapter Seventeen.) Mammography is indicated for postmenopausal women but certainly not justified for young women. The identification of genetically high-risk groups (testing blacks for sickle cell anemia) or environmental high-risk groups (pulmonary disease in high-dust occupations) is very important.

2.   Patient Safety, Acceptability, and Comfort

An MHTS must be designed and operated to meet patient needs for safety, acceptability, satisfaction, and comfort. Tests must be harmless. Exposure to x-ray and isotope radiations should be minimized and carefully evaluated for a given population with regard to yield of information for the hazards involved.

Tests should cause no unreasonable discomfort. Putting drops in the eyes and using needles to draw blood, although uncomfortable, are standard procedures accepted by patients; but gastric intubation for acid analysis, for example, is usually not warranted. Significant discomfort is unacceptable, since it can alter patients' responses to questions and may affect test results.

MHTS should provide comfortable waiting areas between test phases. MHTS personnel should be sensitive to opportunities to reassure examinees regarding the test procedures.

3.   Patient Processing Time

The time for MHTS processing for individual tests should not be so prolonged as to cause undue fatigue, which could significantly alter patients' responses and test results. The accuracy of testing is benefited by the high standardization of timing and procedure that can be maintained within an MHTS laboratory, and gross exceptions may significantly alter test results. It may, however, be necessary to permit flexible scheduling and processing for special population groups or patient abnormalities.

4.   Patient Identification and Codification

Planning must provide the means for identification of each patient at the time of registration and for verification at each subsequent individual station. Positive identification requires agreement on four identifiers:

(1) Encoding each patient by a unique number (which may be the laboratory accession number, social security number or some other externally assigned patient medical record number, which should never be reassigned by the MHTS).

(2) Patient's name.

(3) Sex.

(4) Birth date (at least by month and year).

Any identification procedure using less than all four of the above identifiers will probably have a significant error rate in reporting tests for incorrectly identified patients.

Planning for encoding of patients' identifying data by use of embossed or punched paper, plastic, or metal cards is important, since the use of such cards minimizes errors due to reporting tests for wrong patients within the laboratory. However, since family members in haste may exchange identification cards, it is mandatory at registration to check all four identifiers to validate that the encoded card being used does in truth identify the person being tested.

5. Patient Followup

It is essential that medical decisions based upon MHTS test results be made by a physician who assumes responsibility for the patient's care. Accordingly, it is necessary to plan for the MHTS to return every patient to the referring physician and to arrange to refer nonreferred examinees to a followup physician who will agree to receive the MHTS results and accept the patient.

It is advisable to arrange a procedure so that the physician reports back to MHTS as to the followup diagnosis, therapy, and outcome.

E. TEST SELECTION FOR HEALTH PROBLEMS

It is important to identify a set of health problems, tests, and preventive procedures for each MHTS, customized to fit the needs of its target population. A different package needs to be designed for children, as compared to adults. It is advisable to have a somewhat different battery of tests for young, middle-aged, and older adults. Certainly different tests will be selected for personal (individual) vs. public health (mass), industry vs. military, etc. The program should be designed to be flexible, so that tests can be added and removed to meet changing health problems and technological innovations.

For common chronic diseases, such as heart disease and cancer, it is necessary first to identify the specific factors that increase the risk to health. For example, identifying high-risk patients for coronary disease (to prevent or postpone myocardial infarction) involves including questions on diet, smoking, and exercise; family history; blood chemistry tests (glucose, cholesterol, and triglycerides); electrocardiography, weight, blood pressure, etc. Adjunctive services would then include health education and counseling and preventive health measures to decrease these risk factors.

1. Criteria for Selecting Conditions for Testing

A critical decision for every MHTS is the conditions for which to implement test stations. Many writers have propounded selection criteria. Some who are epidemiologically oriented insist on selecting only conditions for which the natural history is adequately understood and for which treatment is available that effectively alters it.[7-11] However, as emphasized in Chapter Two, in personal health care many patients come to physicians with complaints, problems, and conditions for which the natural history is not understood and/or for which effective treatment is not available. These include nondisabling conditions such as visual and hearing defects, for which corrective devices are of benefit; and overweight, smoking, problems-in-living, and psychosocial problems, for which health and psychosocial counseling may be of benefit. These also include fatal conditions such as those cancers the natural course of which cannot be altered, where earlier detection at least provides more lead time for planning estate and family matters as well as general supportive care and palliation to the patient.

A controversial issue is whether anxiety and concern about one's health is an important health problem. Certainly to the individual it is important, and providing a health evaluation to reassure a person that he is well is the most effective method of removing this particular problem. Holland[7] has pointed out that it is also important to detect conditions that alter the "quality of life"; for example, in the middle-aged and elderly, tests for vision and hearing acuity are very effective in improving the quality of living.

From our experience, a MHTS for personal health services in a health care program should select conditions for testing that fulfill the following criteria:

(1) It is an important health problem for the individual and/or the community. Such problems include not only conditions that are potentially disabling or life threatening (e.g., hypertension, breast cancer, etc.) but also those that impair the quality of life (e.g., hearing acuity, anxiety, etc.).

(2) (a) The condition should be prevalent in the population tested with sufficient frequency and (b) a test should be available to detect the condition with sufficient sensitivity and specificity so that (c) the cost per positive test is acceptable to both provider and user of services.

(3) Appropriate health care services should be available for the condition, whether these be further diagnostic services, curative or rehabilitative services, health and psychosocial counseling, or terminal care—as may be indicated for each patient's problem. It is ideal (but not always achievable in reality) if the test can detect the disease early enough and if effective therapy is available such that the entire process of detection, diagnosis, and treatment can be demonstrated to be cost-effective. (See Chapter Seventeen.)

2.   Criteria for Test Selection

Determining which tests should be included in an MHTS depends upon decisions as to which conditions can and should be detected early, and whether the test is accurate, economical, and acceptable.[7-10] Criteria for the selection of specific tests for MHTS include:

(1) Predicted yield rate of the target population. Yield rates must be significant; if the condition is very rare, it will probably be too expensive to identify.

(2) Cost per test. If the test is too expensive, it will probably exceed what the users will accept as a reasonable charge. For example, although often included in MHTS in Japan owing to the high incidence of gastric cancer, gastrointestinal x-rays are rarely included in the United States because they are relatively costly in dollars and resources, and there are not enough physicians available to perform these tests. Generally, an MHTS does not have a physician present in its laboratory, since one of the usual MHTS requirements is that a test must be capable of being entirely performed by allied health personnel.

(3) Cost per positive test. This criterion follows from items (1) and (2) and is generally decisive in test selection.

(4) Cost per true positive test. This criterion introduces the essential requirements of sensitivity and specificity of tests, which affect followup costs. (See Chapter Seventeen.) The physician (after patients have been referred to him) primarily addresses himself to improving the specificity of the procedure, in order to determine whether the patient in fact has the given disease or condition or whether the test gave a false positive report. The followup costs addressed to ruling out conditions are troublesome to the doctor and costly to the patient.

(5) Cost effectiveness. This criterion attempts to measure the costs of early detection. A test should detect a condition sufficiently early to identify it before irreparable pathological changes have become disabling. Cost effectiveness is sometimes defined in terms of possible therapy—i.e., the ability to alter the course of the condition or disease. (See Chapter Seventeen.)

(6) Acceptability to patient. The test must be harmless, cause no unreasonable discomfort, and take a reasonable time. Gastric intubation is an example of a test that is unacceptable to patients.

(7) Usefulness. If not useful for patient care, it may be useful for research or for other specific objectives of the MHTS sponsor.

From a pragmatic viewpoint, the most important criterion for test selection is usually the projected cost to detect a patient with a positive test.[12] For example, if one has the projected cost for a chest x-ray ($1.45) and the estimated prevalence of clinically important abnormalities reported from a chest roentgenography (e.g., see Chapter Seventeen, Table 17–5), then unit costs can be projected for the following age groups as shown:

Ages	Prevalence	Cost per Positive Test
20–39	2.1%	$70
40–59	7.4%	$20
60+	19.2%	$8

For persons of age 60 or more, almost one in every five (19.2%) is reported to have an important abnormality in his chest x-ray, so the cost to detect one elderly patient with an abnormal chest x-ray is less than $8. An MHTS could readily justify doing chest roentgenography on all examinees of age 60 or more. For examinees of age 20 to 39 the prevalence of clinically important abnormalities reported by chest x-ray is much lower (only about one in 50, or 2.1%), and the cost per positive is $70. As a result, for young adults many MHTS provide a chest x-ray only for the first examination; if it is normal, they do not do repeat chest x-rays on subsequent routine checkups.

3. Recommended MHTS Tests

Lists have been published of recommended screening tests, but each MHTS should select its own in accordance with its objectives, the populations it serves, and the above criteria.

Frame and Carlson[13] provided a critical review of tests suitable for periodic health checkups. Breslow et al.[14] developed lists of recommended conditions and tests for personal preventive health services for adults, as shown in Tables 3-2, 3-3, and 3-4, which include those tests recommended on the basis of the Kaiser-Permanente experience. Table 3-2 lists the recommended tests that should be provided to young adults by an MHTS. Breslow advised that these batteries of tests should be given three times between ages 17 and 35: once between 17 and 20, once in the mid-20s, and again in the mid-30s. Kaiser-Permanente's recommendation is that, after an initial examination to provide a baseline health status, if the individual is found to be well, then checkups might be repeated every 3 to 4 years in the twenties or thirties.

Table 3-3 lists the tests that are recommended for the age group 36 to 64. Breslow[14] recommends these tests be given at least once every five years beginning at age 40 and ending at age 60. Kaiser-Permanente's studies indicate that

Table 3-2.   Recommended Tests for Young Adults (Ages 17–35)*

Test	FIC	ASPH, ATPM	APHA	TF	CKP
History	X		X	X	X
Height and weight	X	X	X	X	X
Blood pressure	X	X		X	X
EKG	X				X
Hearing and vision				X	X
Chest x-ray			X		X
Laboratory examinations					
Serum cholesterol	X	X		X	X
Serum triglycerides	X				X
Serum glucose	X			X	X
Serum uric acid	X				X
Serum SGOT	X				X
Hemoglobin/hematocrit	X			X	
Blood count, complete (exclude differential smear)			X		X
VDRL			X	X	X
Urinalysis	X	X	X		X
Gonococcal culture (females)		X	X	X	X
Pap smear (females)	X	X	X	X	X
Physical examination, general	X	X	X	X	X
Breast examination (females)			X	X	X
Rectal examination			X		X
Pelvic examination (females)			X		X

*Modified from Breslow et al.[14]
  FIC   = Fogarty International Center Task Force, 1974
  ASPH = Association of Schools of Public Health, 1973
  ATPM = Association of Teachers of Preventive Medicine, 1973
  APHA = American Public Health Association, 1974
  TF   = Breslow's Task Force, 1975
  CKP   = Collen, Kaiser-Permanente, 1976

Table 3-3. Recommended Tests for Middle-Aged Adults (Ages 36–64)*

Test	FIC	ASPH, ATPM	APHA	TF	CKP
History	X		X	X	X
Height and weight	X	X	X	X	X
Blood pressure	X	X	X	X	X
EKG	X	X	X		X
Vision		X		X	X
Tonometry	X	X	X		X
Spirometry			X		X
Mammography (females)	X	X		X	X‡
Chest x-ray			X		X
Laboratory examinations					
Serum cholesterol	X	X	X	X	X
Serum triglycerides	X		X		X
Serum glucose	X	X		X	X
Serum uric acid	X				X
Serum SGOT	X				X
Serum BUN			X		
Serum creatinine			X		X
Serum calcium					X
Hemoglobin/hematocrit	X			X	
Blood count, complete (exclude differential smear)			X		X
VDRL			X	X	X
Urinalysis	X		X		X
Gonococcal culture (females)			X		
Pap smear (females)	X	X	X	X	X
Stool guaiac	X	X	X	X	
Tuberculin			X	X	
Physical examination, general	X	X	X	X	X
Breast examination (females)		X	X	X	X
Rectal examination		X	X		X
Pelvic examination (females)			X		X
Sigmoidoscopy			X		X

*Modified from Breslow et al.[14]
FIC   = Fogarty International Center Task Force, 1974
ASPH = Association of Schools of Public Health, 1973
ATPM = Association of Teachers of Preventive Medicine, 1973
APHA = American Public Health Association, 1974
TF   = Breslow's Task Force, 1975
CKP = Collen, Kaiser-Permanente, 1976
‡For females over age 50 only.

periodic multiphasic health checkups do favorably decrease mortality after age 35 (see Chapter Eighteen), so it would appear advisable to recommend health examinations at least every 2 to 3 years from ages 36 to 44 and every 1 to 2 years after age 45.

Table 3-4 lists the recommended tests for the examinees aged 65 or greater. The Kaiser-Permanente experience indicates it is advisable for this age group to have

Table 3-4.   Recommended Tests for Older Adults (Ages 65 or More)*

Test	FIC	ASPH, ATPM	APHA	TF	CKP
History	X		X	X	X
Height and weight	X	X	X	X	X
Blood pressure	X	X	X	X	X
EKG	X	X	X	X	X
Vision	X	X	X		X
Tonometry		X	X		X
Hearing	X	X		X	X
Spirometry			X		X
Mammography (females)		X		X	X
Chest x-ray			X		X
Podiatric examination	X				
Dental examination	X				
Laboratory examinations					
Serum cholesterol	X		X		X
Serum triglycerides	X		X		X
Serum glucose	X	X		X	X
Serum uric acid	X				X
Serum SGOT	X				X
Serum BUN			X		
Serum creatinine			X		X
Serum calcium					X
Serum triiodothyronine (T_3)					X
Serum thyroxine (T_4)					X
Hemoglobin/hematocrit	X			X	
Blood count, complete (exclude differential smear)			X		X
Urinalysis	X		X		X
VDRL			X		X
Tuberculin			X		
Pap smear (females)	X	X		X	X
Stool guaiac	X	X	X	X	
Physical examination, general	X	X	X	X	X
Breast examination (females)	X			X	X
Rectal examination	X	X	X		X
Pelvic examination (females)					X
Sigmoidoscopy			X		X

*Modified from Breslow et al.[14]
FIC   = Fogarty International Center Task Force, 1974
ASPH = Association of Schools of Public Health, 1973
ATPM = Association of Teachers of Preventive Medicine, 1973
APHA = American Public Health Association, 1974
TF   = Breslow's Task Force, 1975
CKP = Collen, Kaiser-Permanente, 1976

such a test battery every year, and perhaps even more often, owing to the increasing rate of change of abnormalities with age. (See also Chapter Seventeen, F.)

The selection of tests for specialized MHTS will vary, of course, to suit specific objectives. For example, if one were to design an MHTS specifically for cancer screening, the various test stations might include: (1) self-administered questionnaires (present and past history, family and environmental history); (2) x-rays (chest, breast for women older than 47; in Japan, gastrointestinal); (3) clinical lab tests (blood and urine, stool for blood); (4) physical examination (skin, breasts and abdomen, thyroid and lymph nodes, rectum and prostate, pelvis and cervical smear); and (5) sigmoidoscopy.

The implementation of specific test phases is discussed in Chapter Six.

F. SELECTION OF FACILITY AND EQUIPMENT

1. Facilities Selection

The design of MHTS facilities is discussed in detail in Chapter Four. The program's objectives, its financing, and the patient load will generally determine the facility it selects.

A small patient load (less than 50 examinees a day) in an MHTS associated with an existing medical center will probably do best to use its facilities evenings or weekends to avoid investing in a new facility and new capital equipment.

A patient load in excess of 50 per day will be processed more efficiently in a specially designed dedicated facility. Careful consideration of alternative designs becomes paramount; these are considered in Chapter Four. A poorly designed facility can cause inefficiency and cripple a program; a well-designed, flexible facility can support many years of cost-effective operations.

2. Equipment Selection

The selection of complex mechanized or automated equipment to provide quality test results requires consideration of the following general guidelines:

(1) Accuracy should be sufficient to achieve functional objectives. (For example, clinical service functions may accept a 5 percent instrumental coefficient of error, whereas epidemiological research may tolerate only 2 percent.)

(2) Equipment cost is critical, since the initial capital investment may be sizable. Equally important is the amortization schedule (which is related to instrument life and rate of obsolescence). The actual capital costs for equipment will vary with the size of the MHTS program but for the test stations will be $100,000 to $200,000. The computer costs will vary with the requirements for online vs. offline; leased equipment will probably cost $1.50 to $3 per patient.

(3) Operational personnel requirements must be considered, since within a few years cumulative personnel costs almost always exceed initial equipment costs.

(4) Equipment reliability is very important. All equipment integral to patient processing should generally perform with a reliability of at least 95 percent (i.e., it must operate 19 out of 20 work days) and preferably 98 percent (or a down time of only one day in 50). For automated online MHTS programs that require the test results to be available before the patient leaves the MHTS, an even higher degree

of reliability may be necessary. If, for example, 20 pieces of equipment were essential to the processing of MHTS patients at a planned scheduling rate, and if none of them were backed up with alternative systems that could process their functions at the planned rate, a reliability of 99 percent for each phase would still mean program breakdown, delays, and rescheduling on the average of every fifth operating day. It is therefore essential to plan for a proper mix of backup equipment, modules, parts, and maintenance capability to maintain operations despite failure and breakdown.

(5) Calibration procedures and reference standards should be available and capable of being applied at necessary intervals for proper test quality control. (See Chapter Nine.)

(6) The environmental requirements for each piece of equipment (space, heat, light, noise suppression, etc.) should be achievable within the allocated investment.

(7) Digital readout and/or interfacing capabilities should be available when necessary for direct coupling to data input equipment and for integration with other subsystems components.

(8) Data processing equipment has special functional requirements[20] for:

(A) Data acquisition. Computer resources may be required with abilities for handling marksense cards, keypunched cards, punched paper tape, optically scannable marked forms, digital and analog magnetic tape, and keyboard and visual display terminals.

(b) Data storage and retrieval. Magnetic tape storage generally fulfills requirements for offline batch processing of data. Direct-access magnetic disk storage will permit online processing of data before the patient leaves the MHTS laboratory. This will permit providing advice as to additional secondary or confirmatory tests the patient should receive before his next visit to a physician, so as to conserve patient and doctor time. Online processing will also permit data quality to be monitored at the time of data input, while the specimen or patient and source information are still available, since correcting errors offline at a later time is much more expensive. A machine-retrievable file should be maintained on each patient. Error-checking programs are essential. (See Chapter Eight.)

(c) Data output. Printout of test reports provided to the physician should be planned to include:

(i)   Patient identifying data and date of examination.

(ii) All test results, with normal values reported for each patient as applicable for his age and sex.

(iii) Flagging of clinically important abnormalities (such as by an asterisk or by prominent grouping in a summary abstract).

(iv) Acceptable format to user physicians, permitting easy reading.

(d) Data security. All patient data within an MHTS or its computer center (whether on punched cards, magnetic storage, or computer printouts) should be subject to the same security measures governing privacy and confidentiality as those in a hospital medical record room.

G. SYSTEMS DESIGN

Prior chapters have emphasized that the systems approach involves careful problem definition. For an MHTS this involves identifying the prevalence of the

medical problems in the target population. Then one can begin a systems design.
Churchman[15] summarized the basic factors in systems design as:

(1) Exterior design: relationship of the system to its environment
    (a) Functional objectives and performance measures
    (b) System environment, including constraints
    (c) Resources used in the system
(2) Interior design: details of the system itself and of its components
    (a) Components of the system
    (b) Overall configuration of the system and its interfaces
    (c) Operating characteristics of the system

Systems component analysis models deal with various parts of the health
service system, such as for MHTS. Systems design models tend to be descriptive
and are used in planning health care delivery systems. Detailed analyses and flow
charting of each phase (see Chapter Twenty) and the integration of all the phases
into a smoothly operational MHTS (see Chapter Five) are very critical. Systems
design must consider in minute detail the patient flow, specimen flow, data flow,
and personnel activities; it must carefully specify system requirements (what it
must do), systems design (how it will do it), and systems evaluation (how well it does it).

An ideal systems design would permit a basic test battery plus flexible selective
testing for each individual in accordance with his identified risk factors, with
immediate (online) feedback to permit indicated secondary (supplemental) testing
to improve the sensitivity and specificity of the testing process before referral to
the physician. (See Chapter Two.)

H. IMPLEMENTATION SCHEDULING

The implementation of a MHTS will require detailed planning and scheduling of
many procedural steps,[45] including:

(1) Determination of the basic demographic characteristics and medical needs
of the community that will use the MHTS.

(2) Definition of the objectives of the MHTS to meet its community's needs.

(3) Establishment of liaison and advisory committees with user physicians
and hospitals.

(4) Determination of needs of the physician and hospital users of MHTS.

(5) Selection of the tests to be included. (If the hospital will use MHTS for
preadmission and preoperative examinations, tests in addition to those selected
for physician-referred periodic health examinations may be necessary.)

(6) Selection of the testing equipment. Adequate backup equipment should be
included in the event of failure.

(7) Determination of patient scheduling requirements. The selected hours of
operation and the number of patients examined per hour will influence system
design and operational characteristics.

(8) Design of each of the individual test phases for the MHTS system. This
will require a multidisciplinary team, including medical, systems, automation, and
data processing personnel.

(9) Design of the total system by efficient integration of the phase components. (Requirements for online vs. offline data processing are different.)

(10) Preparation of implementation progress schedules and cost forecasts. Rational planning and efficient implementation require very detailed projections.

(11) Development of program evaluation procedures. To permit appraisal of the extent to which MHTS achieves desired objectives, a protocol for short-term and long-term evaluation should be developed.

(12) Preparation of the facility's structural design. An architect with experience in the design of medical facilities will be very helpful. Special requirements for noise, heat, light, and laboratory toilet facilities must be met.

(13) Construction of the facility. Construction of a new facility will involve considerably more time and cost than reconstruction or alteration of an existing structure.

(14) Installation and testing of equipment. It is critical that equipment be adequately tested prior to implementation of the program, because it is rare to have equipment operate with complete satisfaction directly after installation.

(15) Development of a manual of quality control and standard operating procedures. The maintenance of a good quality of testing is the most difficult part of operating an MHTS, so it is of the highest priority to establish a high-quality control program with standardized operating procedures for every test phase.

(16) Development of a personnel training program. The help of affiliated medical center personnel is indispensable for training personnel for the ECG, x-ray, and clinical laboratory phases.

(17) Selection and training of personnel. The quality of the initial personnel will greatly influence the success of implementation.

(18) Development of the format of test reporting to physician users of MHTS. Because MHTS is clearly a service to clinicians, it should provide a summary report of maximum utility to physicians.

(19) Development of procedures for physician followup of patients. MHTS is a referral service, an adjunct to medical care, so it must coordinate its scheduling and followup with the needs of the community physicians.

(20) Conducting of pilot testing. A few days of pilot testing will usually be adequate if each of the above has been completed satisfactorily.

(21) Implementation of the fully operational MHTS. (Steps 1 through 20 usually will take 12 to 24 months, depending upon the availability of equipment and facilities).

(22) Conducting of periodic reevaluations and cost analyses, and revision and improvement of the MHTS and of the individual test phases as needed.

It is very useful in planning, implementing, and monitoring the progress of implementation of an MHTS to draw up a Gantt type progress planning chart. Figure 3-3 shows an overall projected schedule for implementing an MHTS over a one-year period, after objectives have been defined and authorization to proceed has been obtained. In addition to a general macro chart, as shown in Figure 3-3, a detailed micro chart for each phase should also be prepared so that no important item is omitted.

For large MHTS, other techniques to insure accurate planning, scheduling, and implementation of the project are the *program evaluation review technique (PERT)* and *critical path method (CPM)*.[18] PERT is an arrow diagram representing all tasks and activities by arrows in sequential or parallel relationships. The network of arrows shows all the relationships and interdependencies of all the

	First Year				Second Year
	1st Qtr.	2nd Qtr.	3rd Qtr.	4th Qtr.	
Registration & referral	Design and develop forms and procedures		Test forms and procedures		Implement and operate MHTS phases
History	Develop and design questionnaire		Pilot test, revise and retest		
EKG and B.P. Height & Weight Spirometry Chest x-ray Mammography Vision Tonometry Hearing Laboratory	Select and order equipment Develop standard operating procedures Develop quality control programs		Pilot test		
Data processing	Develop require-ments	Design system	Purchase or lease system Program or lease software		
Evaluation	Document objectives	Develop study design Conduct pilot study			Conduct evaluation

Figure 3-3. An overall progress planning chart for implementation of an MHTS.

activities to be completed. The time required for each activity is noted for each arrow. Study of the diagram will usually show several alternative paths for completing activities, and one can calculate the total time required to complete the MHTS by each of these paths. The path that takes longest from beginning to end is usually called the critical path or the most "pessimistic." The shortest path is the most "optimistic," and one can select a mid-time as the "normal" path. PERT can thus identify "slack" time for those activities that can be completed earlier than the critical path time; such tasks can be permitted to slip for this amount of time without delaying the overall project.

I. QUALITY CONTROL AND STANDARD OPERATIONS

1. General Quality Control Requirements

A most important requirement for a high-quality MHTS is to establish and maintain a good quality control program. (See Chapter Nine.) It generally requires greater accuracy to detect the slight abnormalities of early disease than the gross changes of overt disease. It is more difficult to plan effective quality control monitoring for personnel than for instruments.

Proper control and maintenance of quality testing requires: (a) explicit definitions of methods and procedures, (b) precise setting of limits of performance, and (c) regular monitoring to detect any variations.

Definition of quality control procedures includes: (a) standard operating test procedures for (1) personnel supervision, and (2) instrumental accuracy; (b) reference standards for (1) specimens, and (2) patients (recommended are specific normal limits by age and sex); and (c) interlaboratory comparisons for measurements of variations in (1) instruments, (2) standards, and (3) populations.

2. Standard Operating Procedures

a. Standard procedures manual for personnel.   It is essential that a Standard Operating Procedures Manual be prepared that includes detailed, explicit instructions on methods and procedures for each technician for each phase of each task. (See Chapter Twenty.) Those pages of the Procedures Manual that pertain to each testing phase should be prominently posted at that station for continual reference by technicians.

b. Standard procedures supervision.   At least once each day, preferably at unscheduled times, the nurse supervisor should make rounds and inspect each testing phase, observing the complete testing for at least one patient. Periodically the MHTS director should also make rounds to see that standard procedures are being precisely followed.

Any observed significant variation should be immediately noted and corrected. It is possible that technicians may develop improvements in procedures. Such changes from the Procedures Manual should be evaluated by the director and appropriate advisory specialists. Valid improvements should then be incorporated into the Procedures Manual. Deviations from standard procedures that diminish quality of testing should be immediately corrected by intensive retraining of the technician at fault.

3. Standard Operating Procedures for Equipment

Standard procedures and corresponding manuals should be developed for both equipment and analytic methods as to:

(1) Standard operating procedure, including calibrations and accuracy testing.

(2) Performance characteristics, reliability, failure backup, preventive and corrective maintenance.

(3) Reference standards and controls.

(4) Monitoring of quality control, which should include reports of errors, missing data, and percentage of unsatisfactory tests.

J. GUIDELINES FOR SUCCESSFUL OPERATION

1. Factors Leading to Success

An MHTS program can be considered successful if it accomplishes its objectives. These objectives usually include providing good-quality examinations and acceptable service to both providers and users at an acceptable cost (or profit). Sanazaro[16] identified the most important factors to be observed in any MHTS program as:

a. Planning. The purpose of a MHTS must be clear. The population to be reached must be defined, the aides and technicians must be trained, the instrumentation to be used must be reliable and dependable, the space must be properly designed, optimum patient flow must be established, and the entire process must be set up to function more or less automatically.

b. Economy of scale. Because personnel are trained and instrumentation is programmed to repeat a predetermined sequence of tasks many times, the scale of utilization must be great enough to make the MHTS program economical. Unless sufficient patient volume can be achieved, a program will be unjustifiably costly and wasteful of both trained personnel and expensive instrumentation.

c. Integration into a delivery system. The relationship between the MHTS program and the health care delivery system must be operational. The means must exist for patients and examinees to move easily from MHTS to the health care system. Data and information must be readily transferrable within the MHTS system, with attention to patient privacy when this is indicated.

The most important principle to be observed is that MHTS cannot be a free-standing entity independent of the health care system. Rather it is to be linked closely to that system for the purpose of increasing its reach, its productivity, its economic efficiency, and the quality and effectiveness of its services.

d. Acceptability to physicians. MHTS must be acceptable to the physicians who participate in the program and in the health care delivery system with which it is linked. Physician participation and satisfaction are essential corollaries of the requirement that MHTS always be integrated within the health care delivery system.

e. Acceptability to examinees, patients, and the community. The program should be acceptable to the persons who are processed through it. This acceptance will depend on an adequate explanation of the purpose to be served, the manner in which the testing is carried out, and the liaison between the sponsors of the program and the community.

f. Financial soundness. The program must meet the ultimate financial test of whether the intended benefits are realized; that is, it must become self-supporting or worth subsidizing.

2. Pitfalls Leading to Failure

The following will almost assure failure for an MHTS:

(1) Assuming that an MHTS can be transferred from one program to another with equal success.

(2) Ignoring the patients' physicians in organizing the MHTS and failing to obtain physician support.

(3) Assuming that the MHTS can operate separately from a health care delivery system and that health checkups are simply case detection, not requiring physical examinations or physician followup.

(4) Failing to orient the physicians as to the service role that MHTS can provide to them and their patients.

(5) Assuming that operating an MHTS is easy.

(6) Attempting to implement an MHTS in too short a time.

(7) Failing to analyze population needs and to reassess those needs periodically. Failing to alter the system when new needs develop and old needs disappear. Failing to obtain continuing patient support.

(8) Assuming the MHTS will produce rapid and/or obvious beneficial results in the target population.

3.   Criteria for Success

A review of our own 25 years of experience in this field suggests some guidelines for a successful MHTS program.[17] The minimum criteria for success appear to be three: good quality, service, and economy.

a.   *Good quality* for an MHTS means:

(1) Accurate testing procedures so as to achieve acceptable reproducibility and validity of test measurements. This requires expensive, continuing quality control monitoring of personnel and equipment.

(2) High utility, so as to provide good sensitivity and specificity for detection of important diseases for which effective therapy is available.

(3) Completeness of testing, so as to screen for many common conditions. A chemistry profile alone will not satisfy patients who expect a relatively comprehensive battery of tests.

A reputation for poor quality will irrevocably lose the confidence of referral physicians; serious errors will result in malpractice suits by patients.

b.   *Good service* for an MHTS means:

(1) Integrating the MHTS program into the community of patients and physicians. All patients should be referred to their physicians, and MHTS laboratory reports should be provided only to the patient's physician.

(2) Conserving the physician's time. MHTS reports should be provided quickly enough and be of such format and content so as to reduce significantly the time the physician spends on a periodic health examination.

(3) Reliability of service. Patients will be dissatisfied if equipment or personnel failures too often result in "test not done" or "unsatisfactory test," requiring the patient's return for repeat testing.

(4) Acceptability to patients. Prompt and pleasant service to examinees at each test station and efficient scheduling, organization, and followup procedures are essential for patient satisfaction.

(5) Maintaining continuing patient records. The occasional checkup is of lesser value than periodic health examinations. Providing the physician with test results of prior examinations for comparison permits trend analysis for borderline abnormalities and aids in better diagnoses.

An MHTS laboratory that lacks the support of the physicians who provide care to the patients is doomed to failure.

c.   *Good economy* means:

(1) Processing enough patients each day (e.g., 100 or more) so that the MHTS unit cost per patient will be much less (25 to 50 percent) than that of traditional methods.

(2) Selecting tests with an acceptable cost per positive case. This requires "tailoring" the MHTS test phases to the specific needs of the community of patients and physicians served (e.g., providing chest x-ray to adult groups but not to children; modifying medical questionnaires for different socioeconomic and ethnic groups, etc.).

Good quality and good service are measures of effectiveness of a program; good economy is a measure of its efficiency. As Drucker[19] has so well stated: "Effectiveness is the foundation of success—efficiency is a minimum condition for survival after success has been achieved. Efficiency is concerned with doing things right. Effectiveness is doing the right things."

History shows that whenever one of these basic requirements of quality, service, or economy has not been met, the MHTS program has failed. Where all three requirements are fulfilled, the program should be successful and profitable for the MHTS, the patients, the physicians, and the community.

REFERENCES

1. Schoen, A. W. *AMHT Programs Directory*. 3d ed. Burbank: Bioscience Pub., Inc., 1973.

2. *Statement on Multiphasic Health Testing*. Chicago: American Medical Association, 1972.

3. Galbraith, J. K. "The Imperatives of Technology." In *The New Industrial State*. Boston: Houghton Mifflin, 1967.

4. Collen, M. F. "A.M.H.T. Implementation of a System." *Hospitals, J.A.H.A.* 45(1971):49–53.

5. Collen, M. F., et al. *Provisional Guidelines for Automated Multiphasic Health Testing and Services*. Vol. 2. N.T.I.S. PB 196 000, 1970.

6. McCormick, J. B., and Kopp, J. B. "AMHT Manpower Considerations." *Hospitals, J.A.H.A.* 45(1971):56–57.

7. Holland, W. W. "Screening for Disease. Taking Stock." *The Lancet* 2 (1974):1494–1496.

8. McKeown, T. "Validation of Screening Procedures." In *Screening in Medical Care*. Nuffield Trust. London: Oxford Univ. Press, 1968.

9. Wilson, J. M. G., and Jungner, G. *Principles and Practice of Screening for Disease*. Public Health Paper No. 34. Geneva: W.H.O., 1968.

10. *Mass Health Examinations*. Public Health Paper No. 45. Geneva: W.H.O., 1971.

11. Sharp, C. L., and Keen, H. Chaps. 6 and 16 in *Presymptomatic Detection and Early Diagnosis*. Baltimore: Williams & Wilkins Co., 1968.

12. Collen, M. F. "Diseases Which Can and Should Be Detected Early." *Industrial Med.* 39(1970): 27–29.

13. Frame, P. S., and Carlson, S. J.. "A Critical Review of Periodic Health Screening Using Specific Screening Criteria." *J. Family Practice* 2(1975):29–36, 123–129, 189–194, 283–288.

14. Breslow, L., et al. "Theory, Practice and Application of Prevention in Personal Health Services." Pages 257–359 in *Preventive Medicine USA*. New York: PRODIST, 1976.

15. Churchman, C. W.: *The Systems Approach*. New York: Dell Pub. Co., 1968.

16. Sanazaro, P. J. "AMHT. Definition of the Concept." *Hospitals, J.A.H.A.* 45(1971):41–43.

17. Collen, M. F. "Guidelines for Multiphasic Checkups." *Arch. Int. Med.* 127(1971):99–100.

18. Malcolm, D. G., and Hill, L. S. Chap. 3 in H. B. Maynard, *Industrial Engineering Handbook*, 3d ed. New York: Harper & Row, 1971.

19. Drucker, P. F. *Management*. New York: Harper & Row, 1974.

20. Collen, M. F. "Automated Multiphasic Health Testing." Chapter 11 in M. F. Collen, ed. *Hospital Computer Systems*. New York: John Wiley & Sons, 1974.

CHAPTER FOUR

Facilities Design and Construction

Sidney R. Garfield

A. INTRODUCTION

The relatively recent evolution of MHTS as an important new subsystem of medical care in the United States has focused attention on the planning and design of facilities to efficiently house its specific services. Aside from the commonly accepted standards pertaining to building components, such as foundations, structure, electrical, heating, ventilating, and plumbing systems, MHTS facilities must meet the fairly rigid codes for medical facilities, which require special attention to safety and fire protection, easily cleaned interior finishes, and adequate utility services. Electrical systems may need extra capacity for equipment loads such as x-ray, laboratory, and other diagnostic and testing equipment. Heating, ventilating, and air conditioning systems must be carefully designed to assure comfort and proper temperature and humidity ranges in the testing and computer areas. In addition, an MHTS unit requires a design that suits the variety of services provided in its test stations and supports the interrelations that permit a smooth flow of patients, data, and material for optimum patient throughput and cost effectiveness.

There is no single best way today to design MHTS facilities. The system is relatively too new, too varied in operational concepts and goals, and too diverse in its organizational settings to be standardized at this time. Many existing MHTS units have been constructed in renovated spaces and may be limited by those space constraints to less than optimal design. On the other hand, newly constructed designs have been constrained by lack of standards and often by funding restrictions.

This chapter will attempt to acquaint the reader with the present state of the art and provide guidelines that may be generally applicable in a variety of MHTS designs. The information presented is based in large part upon our own experience in designing and operating such facilities, a prior excellent review of MHTS facilities,[1] and inspection of a number of operating centers in the United States.

B. ORGANIZATION FOR DESIGN AND CONSTRUCTION

The designing of a functional program that will integrate goals, conceptual objectives, and operations into an effective building plan requires a clearly defined chain of authority, which will vary with the specific organizational setting of each MHTS. As described in prior chapters, the setting may be a prepaid group practice, a hospital, a medical and hospital center, a medical society foundation, or simply a solo practitioner's office. The chain of authority for planning should include the MHTS medical director and administrator, who should work very closely with the design consultant and architect.

The functional program specifies the operational requirements and details of the services to be provided and tests to be performed at each station, the interrelation of stations, auxiliary nontesting areas, the equipment and staffing for each station, utilities essential for each unit, the space needed, the preferred arrangement of space and equipment for each station, and any other special requirements.

The functional program will vary with the various operational concepts, organizational settings, and the desired throughput capacity of the proposed center. Figure 4-1 is a flow diagram of a functional MHTS developed for a large-volume,

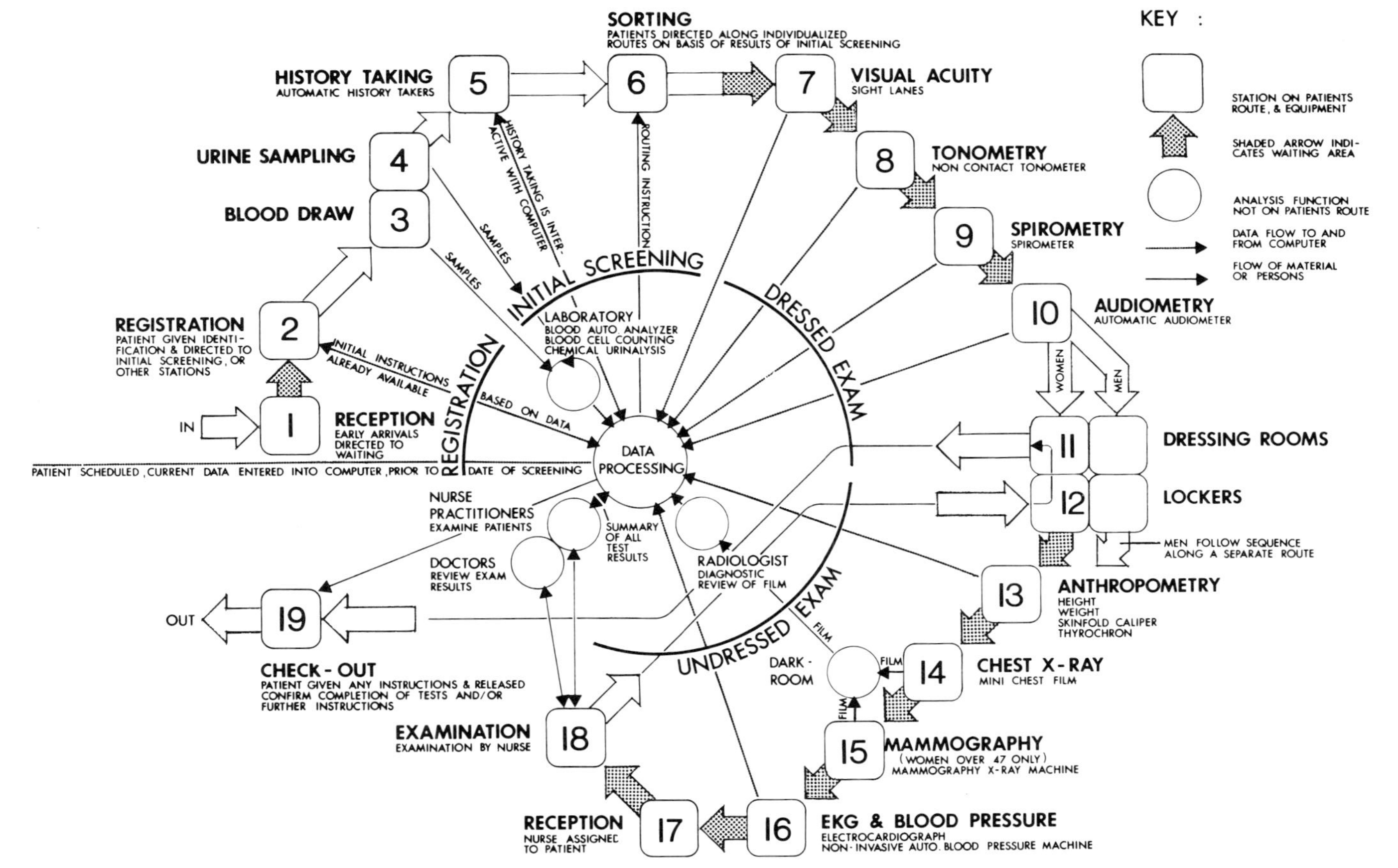

FLOW DIAGRAM OF THE HEALTH APPRAISAL PROCESS

Figure 4-1. Flow diagram representing the MHTS functional process in Kaiser Permanente Oakland.

105

comprehensive self-contained MHTS center (Kaiser-Permanente, Oakland). It demonstrates the usual test stations, station interrelations, and patient and data processing flow, and it includes the physical examination space required to complete the entire MHTS process in a single (online) visit. (See also Chapter Five.)

This comprehensive program is still operating at the Oakland Kaiser-Permanente Medical Center (which in 1976 processed an average of 200 patients per day) and has served as the demonstration model for many MHTS in the United States and other countries. It still reflects our present thinking on requirements for optimal function of an MHTS.

Functional program design should include:

(1) Modular flow requirements to permit processing of desired number of examinees per hour.

(2) Registration and appointment functions.

(3) Controlled time functions (for example, glucose challenge dose ingestion to blood drawing equals 60 minutes).

(4) Patient control centers (for example, the questionnaire phase may control the location of patient for time of blood drawing).

(5) Undressed functions (for example, electrocardiograms, chest x-ray, etc.).

(6) Environmental control (for example, for temperature, irradiation, noise, light, etc.).

(7) Patient waiting areas.

(8) Requirements for each test station.

After the goals and concepts for the MHTS center have been established and the functional specifications generated, the MHTS physician and administrator and the architect cooperate in translating the functional program into a design that will fulfill the program's objectives in an efficient and esthetically pleasing facility—form must follow function. The architect designs floor layouts and building configuration and coordinates the work of the various consultants responsible for design of the building components—the structural engineer, the mechanical and electrical engineers, the interior decorating expert, etc. He also arranges for bids, supervises construction, certifies requests for progress payments, and initiates change orders after the builder has been selected and the contract awarded.

C. OVERALL SEQUENCE OF PLANNING, DESIGN, AND CONSTRUCTION

Four stages in the planning, design, and construction of multiphasic health testing facilities are identified in Figure 4-2. The first is Specifications Development. In this stage, after the mission, affiliation, and other administrative aspects of the MHTS center are defined, the detailed functional and physical requirements of the center are developed. The remaining activities may be grouped under three headings: Preliminary Design, Final Design, and Construction. (See Figure 4-2 for details of the four stages.)

D. OPTIONS IN MHTS FACILITY DESIGN AND CONSTRUCTION

A considerable number of options are available for the design of an MHTS. An MHTS unit may be mobile or stationary; it may be fitted into existing medical

1. <u>Specification and Program Development</u>

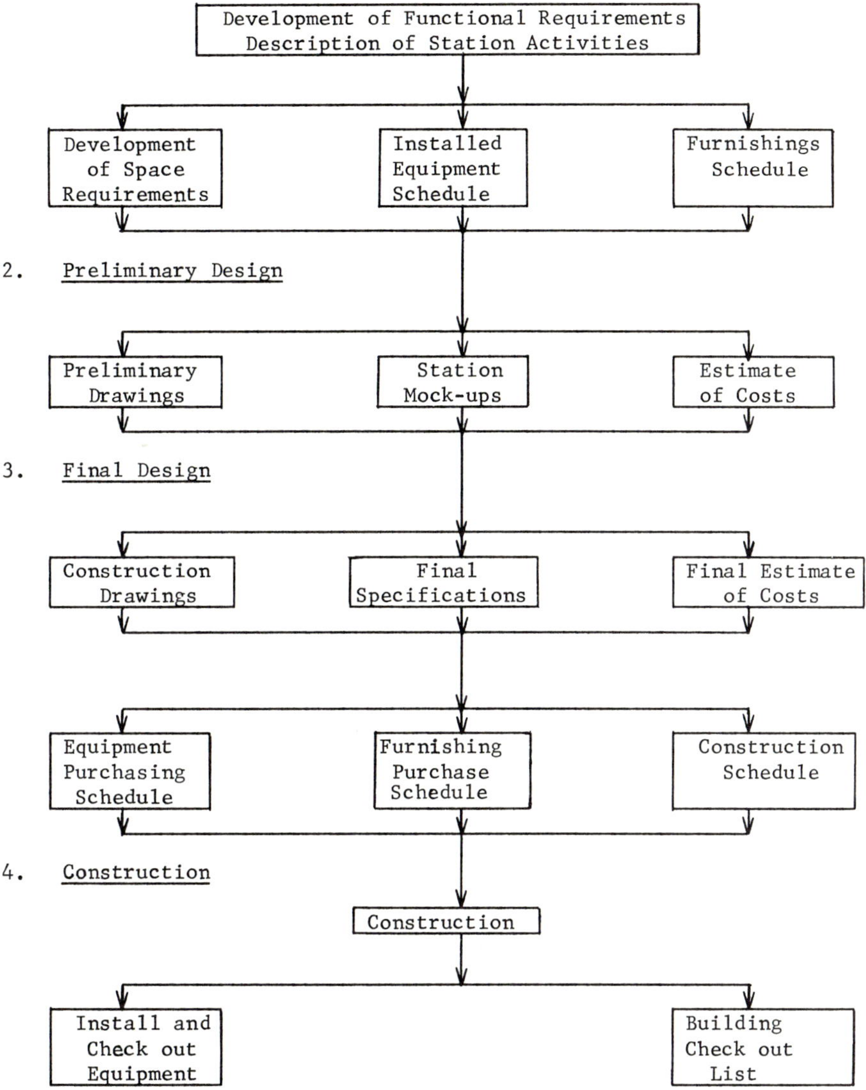

2. <u>Preliminary Design</u>

3. <u>Final Design</u>

4. <u>Construction</u>

Figure 4-2. Sequence for planning, designing and constructing an MHTS. (Modified from De Cicco.[1])

center space "as is"; it may be designed into renovated space, entirely new space, or combinations of both. It can vary in the number of tests as well as in the throughput capacity desired, and the testing stations can be arranged in sequential or carrel type configurations.

Factors influencing the choice of these options will depend mainly on the mission of the system, the organizational setting, throughput capacity desired, and funds available.

1. Mobile MHTS Units

Multiphasic screening units often originated historically as mobile units used to survey defined populations for a few specific illnesses, such as pulmonary tuberculosis and diabetes mellitus. (See Chapter One.) Specially designed vans containing a limited amount of equipment would move into a town or city, and their accessibility and publicity would influence public acceptance of the tests.

The mobile-unit principle has been expanded through a variety of well-designed units to (1) bring a modest variety of testing to sparsely settled rural areas (Figures 4-3, 4-4, and 4-5); or (2) bring a comprehensive variety of testing to larger

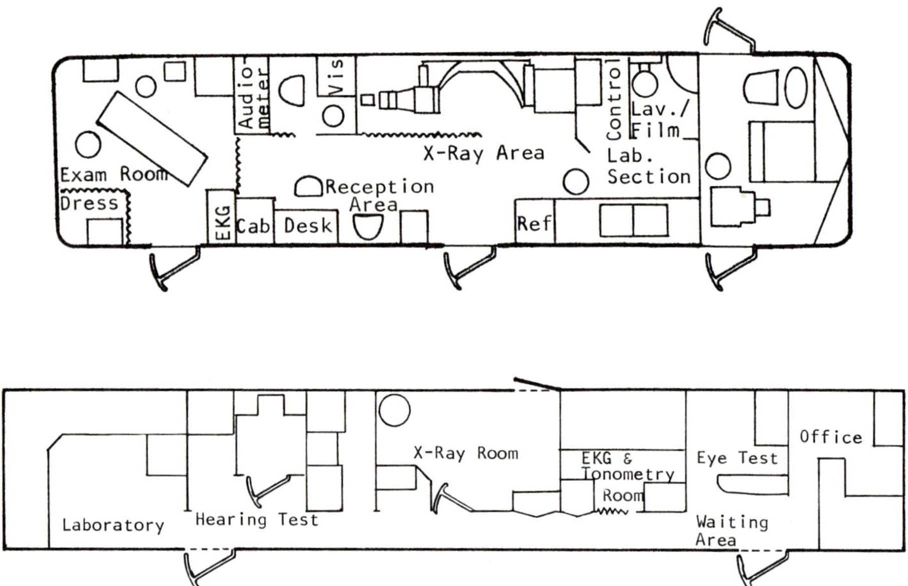

Figure 4-4. Floor plan for the TVA mobile unit.

populations as shown in the TVA unit design (Figure 4-4) and the California Cannery Workers multiple-van design (Figure 4-5). Mobile units require special functional considerations for patient flow, handling of blood specimens not done locally, batch data processing, utilities (electricity, water, waste disposal), and others. (See also Chapter Sixteen, E.)

2. Stationary MHTS Units

Many of today's stationary MHTS facilities have evolved as subsystems within defined medical care programs and therefore have been constrained in area and relationships by those existing organizational settings. The resulting variety of optional MHTS configurations can be generally classified as follows:

(1) *Total sharing of facilities and equipment* in an existing medical center during off-use hours. A very creditable MHTS can be operated after regular clinic hours, using existing laboratory and x-ray departments. This is obviously the easiest and speediest way to initiate an MHTS and offers the lowest possible starting costs. However, there are inherent inefficiencies in adapting regular clinic

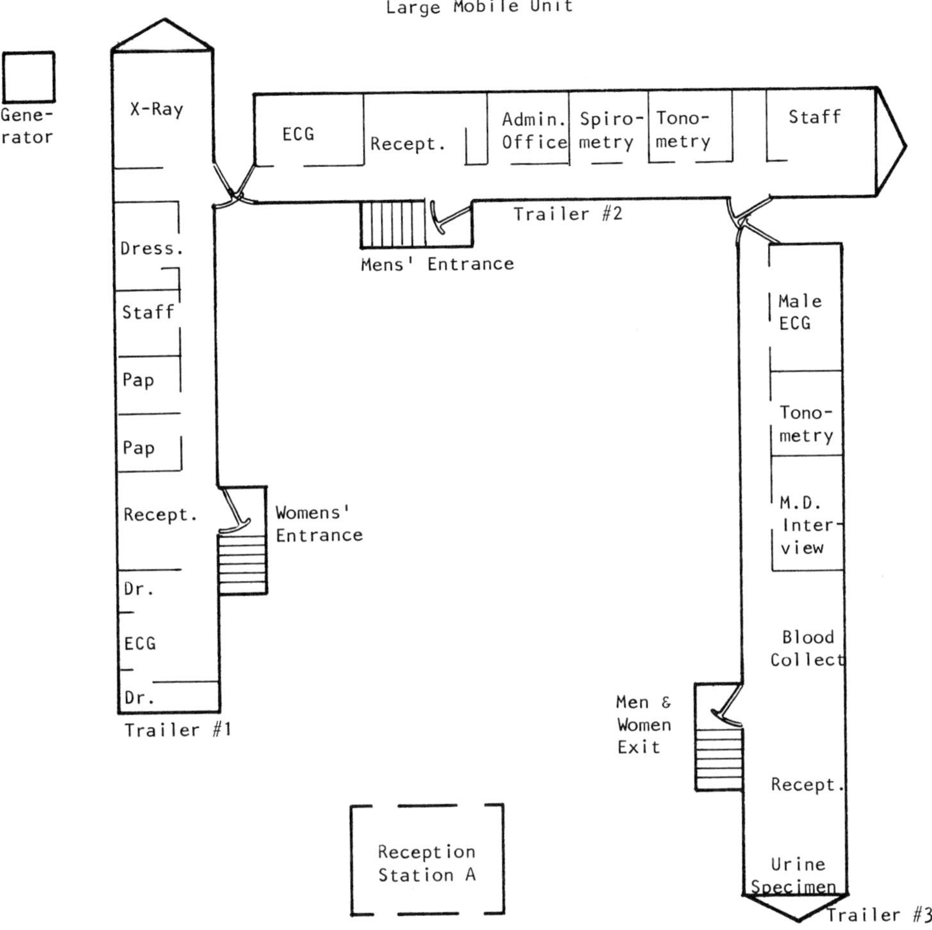

Figure 4-5.   Floor plan for the large mobile unit for the California Cannery Workers.

examination rooms to MHTS testing stations, and the patient traffic routes to laboratory and x-ray may be quite long. Such an adaptation is rarely suited to large-volume operations and is usually incompatible with online completion of the multiphasic examination in one patient visit.

(2) *Partial sharing of facilities and equipment* in an existing setting. A new MHTS facility can be added to an existing medical center either by new construction or by renovation in a fashion that permits sharing the most expensive testing phases—i.e., clinical laboratory and x-ray departments. This can be more efficient than total sharing and permits greater volume, but the x-ray and laboratory services may be so inconveniently far away that patients must return another day for completion of these tests.

(3) *Renovation of existing clinic space* into a completely self-contained MHTS unit. This was accomplished at San Francisco Kaiser-Permanente's MHTS center (see Figure 4-6), which was redesigned from an orthopedics outpatient clinic and which for 10 years has processed about 100 patients a day. The constraints imposed by renovated areas usually result in a less-than-optimum design.

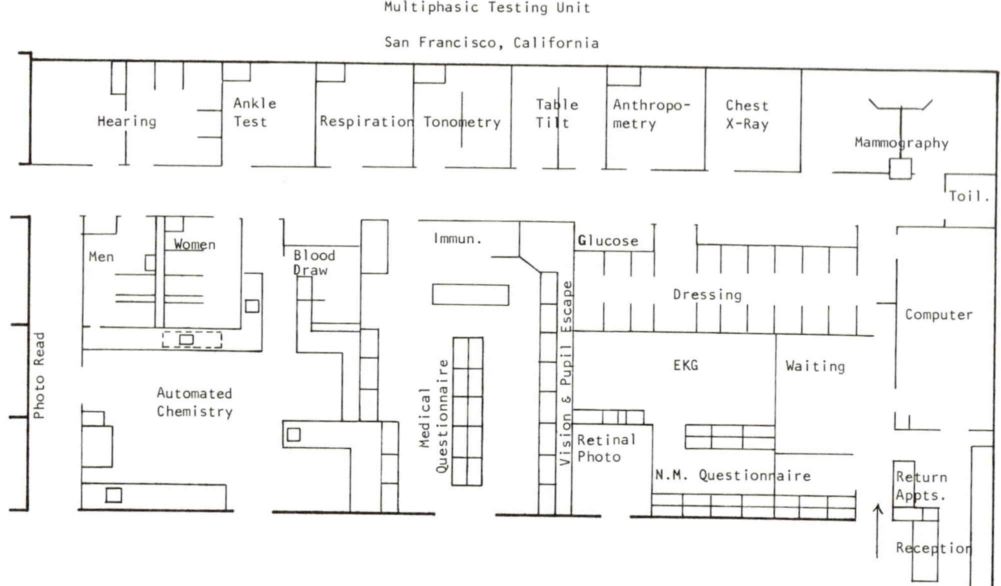

Figure 4-6. Floor plan for an MHTS redesigned from an existing orthopedic clinic in Kaiser-Permanente, San Francisco.

(4) *Completely new construction* provides the greatest opportunity for ideal design, permitting optimum location and interrelation of testing stations, shortest patient flow routes without backtracking, proper separation of traffic, and expansion flexibility. Oakland's Kaiser-Permanente MHTS was thus designed and constructed; in 1975 it processed an average of 185 patients daily, and in 1976 200 patients a day (see Figure 4-7). Large-volume MHTS definitely favors new construction and completely self-contained units. It is likely that newly constructed MHTS units will have the lowest life-cycle costs, operate more efficiently, and be more satisfactory to staff and patients than any of the other modes of shared or renovated installations. Because the initial cost is highest, enlightened high-level policy decisions are required that take account of the real values of the MHTS in the future of medical care.

(5) *Need for flexibility.* Through time, new tests will be introduced into an MHTS and others discarded. For this reason partitions, pipe runs, etc. should be designed to permit greatest flexibility for change. The design of the whole facility should be open-ended for future unobstructed expansion.

3. MHTS Sequential Testing vs. Carrel Testing

In *sequential testing* the patient travels from one testing station to the next in a timed, relatively fixed sequence within two general operational phases: (1) a "dressed" phase, which permits the mingling of men and women for such tests as visual acuity, tonometry, audiometry, spirometry, etc.; and (2) an "undressed" (gowned) phase, which for nicety of operation requires separation of sexes for such tests as require exposure of the trunk (e.g., EKG, anthropometry, chest x-ray, mammography, etc.).

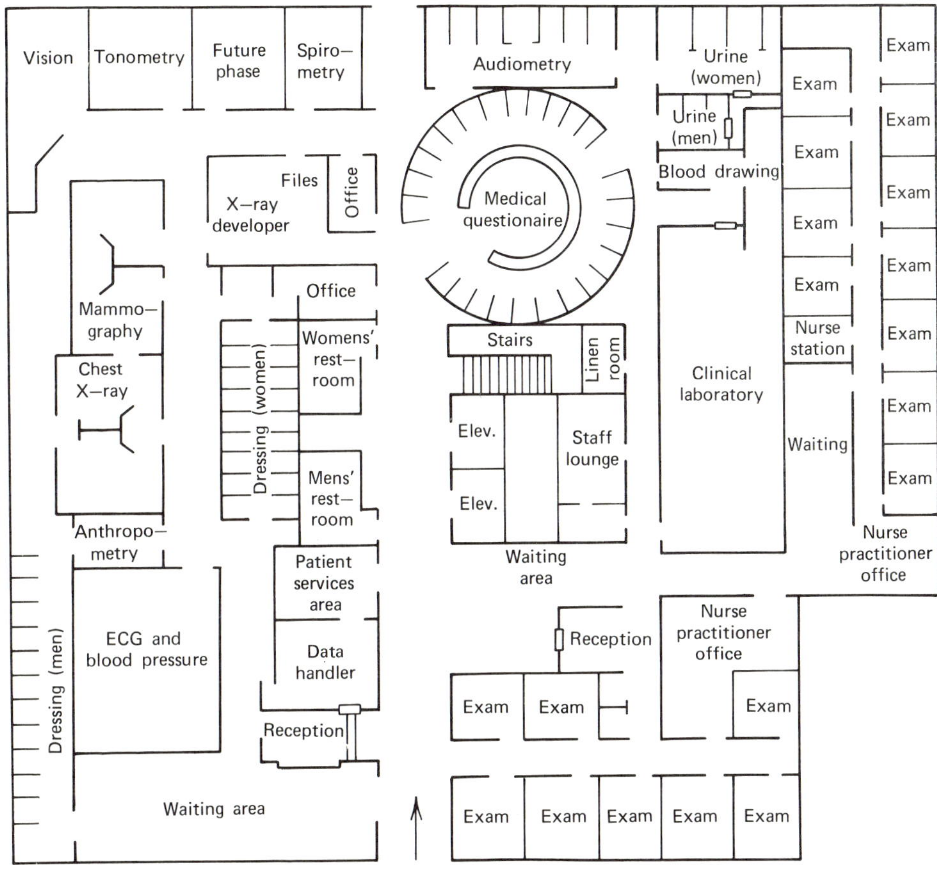

Figure 4-7. Floor plan for the Oakland Kaiser-Permanente MHTS, a large sequential flow program.

It is generally believed that a large-volume MHTS requires sequential testing for best cost effectiveness. The sequential mode, however, creates some inefficiencies, such as patient flow surges and occasional queuing between stations. It also is relatively inflexible and does not lend itself to variation of the tests according to selective patient needs. Skipping tests that may not be essential at every return visit, for example, may cause overloading at some stations and underloading at others.

In *carrel testing* (pioneered by Gilbert[2,3] at the Straub Clinic, Honolulu), a group of tests are combined in one room staffed by one technician. These grouped tests may include visual acuity, tonometry, audiometry, height, weight, and skinfold testing, blood pressure, ankle reflex test, and, if desired, a screening EKG. The same technician draws a blood sample for hematology and chemistry tests and can take a mini-chest film in a unit conveniently located to serve a group of carrels. Each carrel technician can handle approximately 20 to 25 patients per day.

The advantages of the carrel type operation are: (a) a seemingly more personalized service; (b) freedom from the delicate timing constraints of sequential testing, with its occasional test-to-test queuing; (c) greater flexibility in selection of tests for each patient without affecting a sequential line; (d) greater adaptability to volume; e.g., one carrel can handle 20 patients per day, two carrels, 40 patients, etc. Its disadvantages are: (a) there is duplication of equipment in each carrel (though Gilbert points out that the equipment within a carrel is of relatively minor cost); and (b) some experts believe this type of MHTS cannot handle large volume (over 80 patients per day) at the low unit cost of the sequential MHTS, though until recently no large-volume (100 to 200 patients per day) carrel type operation existed to provide comparative data. The Kaiser-Permanente new MHTS at San Jose pictured in Figure 4-8 is a combined sequential and carrel type, large-volume unit which may assist such evaluation.

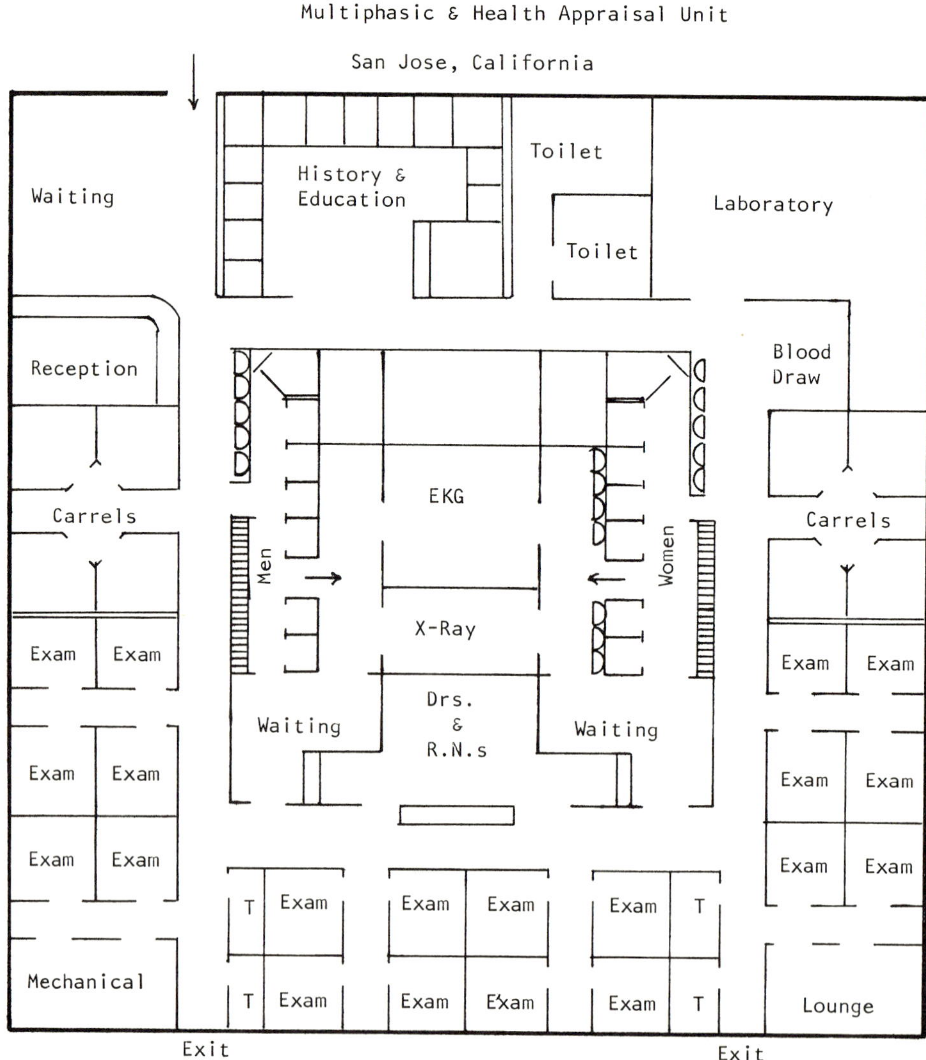

Figure 4-8.   Floor plan for San Jose Kaiser-Permanente MHTS which employs carrels.

E. GUIDELINES FOR PLANNING

1. Testing Stations

A review of multiphasic health testing systems reveals a wide degree of variation in tests and measurements. Figure 4-1 includes the majority of tests now being used. Tests will be added in the future and some discontinued. For flexibility, extra space should be made available for changes, or a new building be constructed open-ended to permit expansion.

Most MHTS installations for adults include stations for:

(1) History taking.
(2) Height and weight.
(3) Chest x-ray.
(4) EKG and blood pressure.
(5) Visual acuity.
(6) Tonometry.
(7) Spirometry.
(8) Blood drawing (for hematology and blood chemistry).
(9) Urine collection.

In addition some installations include:

(10) Skinfold measurements.
(11) Achilles reflex test for thyroid function.
(12) Mammography.
(13) Thermography.
(14) Other x-rays (sometimes for gastrointestinal or back examinations).
(15) Dental x-rays and oral examinations.
(16) Health education.
(17) Immunizations.
(18) Physical examinations.
(19) Pelvic examinations and cervical smears (Pap test).
(20) Proctosigmoidoscopy.

It is important that these stations be planned carefully so as to permit optimum traffic flow without backtracking. Privacy should be planned for men and women in the undressed phase. This sex problem can be avoided by alternating female and male MHTS days, although a problem then arises for families wishing to be examined the same day.

2. Supporting Facilities

Depending on the size and capacity of the unit and whether it is attached to existing facilities or self-contained, the following auxiliary areas may be needed:

(1) Waiting areas, both at the entry point for registration and strategically situated between testing stations.

(2) Reception, registration check-in, and referral followup check-out windows.

(3) Nurse supervisor's office.

(4) Toilet areas for patients with pass-through windows to clinical laboratory station for urine specimens.

(5) Lounge and toilet areas for staff.

(6) Data processing areas for the computer and associated equipment and for remotely located terminals (e.g., for online reports to the physical examination area).

(7) Secretarial space.

(8) Vending machine space for refreshments.

(9) Instrument repair shop.

(10) Janitor and housekeeping closets.

F. SOME ARCHITECTURAL DETAILS FOR STATIONARY MHTS

(1) Tables 4-1 to 4-4 show some alternative uses of space and staff for six stationary sequential-flow MHTS. Tables 4-1 and 4-2 show allocated space for major functional areas, and Tables 4-3 and 4-4 show space and staffing for individual testing stations.

(2) Floor areas will vary with the size of the MHTS and the number of tests provided and may occupy 5,000 to 10,000 square feet. The latter figure would include a sizable area for physical examinations and health education and would accommodate approximately 200 patients per day in a self-contained unit.

(3) Where the MHTS unit includes a physical examination area to provide complete "one-visit" health appraisal, it is important to have the dressing areas central to both the undressed phases (EKG, chest x-ray, mammography, thermography, etc.) and the physical examination areas so as to avoid repeated undressing during the examination (see Figures 4-8, 4-9 and 4-10).

Table 4-1. Major Components of Allocated Space in Square Feet in Various MHTS Centers

Components	MHTS Center*					
	A	B	C	D	E	F
1. Reception, registration, and waiting	420	899	1,016	600	700	1,000
2. History acquisition area	594	224	500	200	480	825
3. Laboratory space	476	152	1,320	345	700	700
4. Testing stations	1,160	1,381	4,980	3,201	5,185	6,810
5. Office and secretary space	977	694	338	500	100	200
6. Patient lockers and dressing cubicles	390	214	868	150	720	1,200
7. Data processing area	270†	0	208†	150†	0‡	240†
8. Staff lounge and toilets	530	312	400	300	300	300
9. Conference area	128	0	160	500	120	200
10. Circulation	1,570	1,420	2,660	1,600	1,700	2,600

*A = Rhode Island[1]   D = Kaiser-Permanente Sacramento
 B = U.S.P.H.S.-Baltimore[1]   E = Kaiser-Permanente San Jose
 C = Kaiser-Permanente Oakland   F = Kaiser-Permanente Santa Clara
†Peripheral terminals only.
‡Pneumatic tubes to computer area.

Table 4-2. Major Components of Space by Percent Distribution in Described MHTS Centers

Components	MHTS Center*					
	A	B	C	D	E	F
1. Reception, registration, and waiting	6	16	8	8	7	7
2. History acquisition area	9	4	4	3	4	6
3. Laboratory space	7	3	10	4	7	5
4. Testing stations	17	25	39	42	53	49
5. Office and secretary space	15	13	3	7	1	2
6. Patient lockers and dressing cubicles	6	4	7	2	7	7
7. Data processing area	4	0	2	2	0	2
8. Staff lounge and toilets	8	6	4	4	3	2
9. Conference area	2	0	2	7	1	1.5
10. Circulation	24	26	21	21	17	18

*A = Rhode Island[1]
B = U.S.P.H.S.-Baltimore[1]
C = Kaiser-Permanente Oakland
D = Kaiser-Permanente Sacramento
E = Kaiser-Permanente San Jose
F = Kaiser-Permanente Santa Clara
Note: The large difference in testing space is due to the large amount of physical examination space in Kaiser-Permanente MHTS Centers.

Table 4-3. Some Variations of Square Feet Allocation for MHTS Testing Stations

Tests	MHTS Center*					
	A	B	C	D	E	F
1. Visual acuity	128	0	120	84	750	100
2. Tonometry		0	105	190		100
3. Audiometry	135	144	200	402		300
4. Spirometry	105	180	100	120		100
5. Achilles reflex test	95	0	100	0		100
6. Retinal photo	72	135	0	0	0	0
7. Anthropometry	45	0	100	150		190
8. Dental x-ray	50	50	0	0	0	0
9. Blood pressure	122	0				
10. Electrocardiography	117		408	225	265	540
11. Chest x-ray	135	260	200	240	172	230
12. Mammography	64	0	230	0	0	240
13. Cervical smear Pap test	143	0				
14. Physical examination	0	612	2,536	1,800	4,000	5,000

*A = Rhode Island[1]
B = U.S.P.H.S.-Baltimore[1]
C = Kaiser-Permanente Oakland
D = Kaiser-Permanente Sacramento
E = Kaiser-Permanente San Jose (carrel type)
F = Kaiser-Permanente Santa Clara
†Brackets indicate tests performed at common station.
Note: Large physical examination spaces in Kaiser-Permanente MHTS allow for nurse practitioner completion of examinations under MD supervision.

Table 4-4. Space and Staffing for Various MHTS Throughput Capacity

Tests	200/day	150/day	100/day	50/day	25/day
1. Visual acuity	1T	1T			
2. Tonometry	1T				
3. Audiometry	2T	1T	3T	2T	1T
4. Achilles reflex test	1T				
5. Spirometry	1T	1T			
6. Anthropometry	1T	1T			
7. Blood pressure	3T	2T	2T	1T	$\frac{1}{2}$T
8. EKG					
9. Chest x-ray	3T	2T	1.5T	1T	$\frac{1}{2}$T
10. Mammography					
11. Physical examination	16NPs	12NPs	8NPs	4NPs	2NPs
	2MDs	1MD	1MD	$\frac{1}{2}$MD	$\frac{1}{5}$MD
Space Required (square feet)					
Estimated space	17,000	14,000	12,000	8,000	3,000
Without physical examination	8,000	7,000	6,000	3,000	1,500
Flow					
Type of flow	S	S	S or C	C	C

T = technician; NP = nurse practitioner; MD = medical doctor.
S = sequential; C = carrel.

(4) Computer installations may require special construction such as raised floors, environmental control systems, special power lines, and noninterruptible power supply (for online programs).

(5) MHTS systems of any considerable size generate a large amount of records, and adequate record room space is important. Consideration should be given to the use of pneumatic tubes or alternate paper transportation systems between stations, computer room, and medical record storage and clerical areas.

(6) Space allocation for the clinical laboratory phase will depend on whether the unit is self-contained or merely collects specimens to be processed elsewhere. The Oakland floor plan shown in Figure 4-7 included automated clinical laboratory equipment (Technicon SMA 12 and Coulter-S blood counter). Toilets adjacent to the laboratory permit pass-through specimen collection.

(7) An isolated self-contained MHTS will require a moderate sized storage area to permit purchasing and storing of supplies in cost-efficient quantities. Some testing areas (such as EKG, x-ray, and lab) will require special storage areas for supplies, solutions, films, and records.

(8) Depending upon available service, backup equipment may be needed. A small instrument repair shop may be desirable for maintenance of large-volume equipment.

(9) Patients in the medical history areas require supervision and assistance. Booths preferably should be dispersed around a central supervision desk, so the supervisor can see the patients and know when they need assistance.

(10) Dressing areas should be as pleasant as possible, and lockers with locks and keys should be provided for clothing. To conserve space a limited number of dressing rooms can be provided with a bank of keyed lockers for storing clothes during the examination, as shown in the San Jose and Santa Clara floor plans (Figures 4-8 and 4-9).

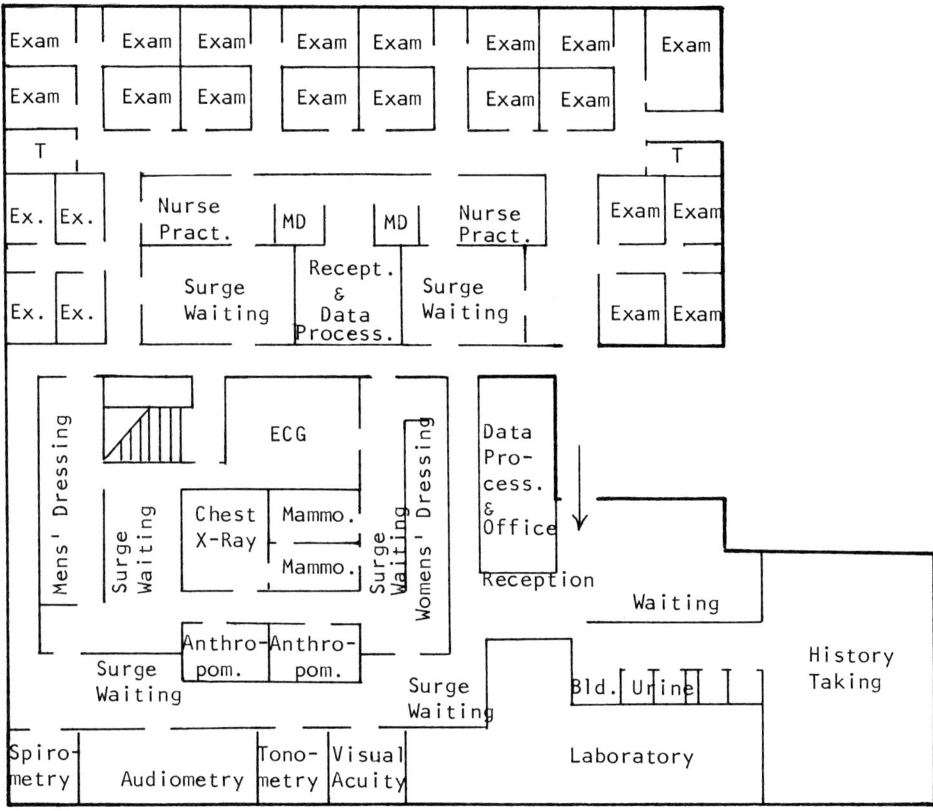

Figure 4-9. Floor plan for Kaiser-Permanente MHTS in Santa Clara.

(11) Since MHTS test rooms may be small, it is well to anticipate the necessary equipment and furniture locations. Writing shelves or tables may be required for personnel use.

(12) Doors to test rooms and examination rooms should open so as to screen the interior of the room from outside vision.

(13) Signal lights or "flip" signs showing that a room is in use and naming the professional users are useful in achieving effective operations and retaining patient privacy.

(14) Built-in furniture and cabinets should be minimized so as to permit flexibility for change. Prefabricated audiometry cabinets are preferable to built-in-place units for the same reason.

(15) Educational signs and models should be placed on walls opposite waiting-area seats so patients can learn while waiting. At each testing station attractive, readable signs should explain the next tests to be done.

(16) Rooms and special areas should be lockable to provide security for expensive equipment.

(17) A lounge chair or stretcher area should be close to blood drawing for

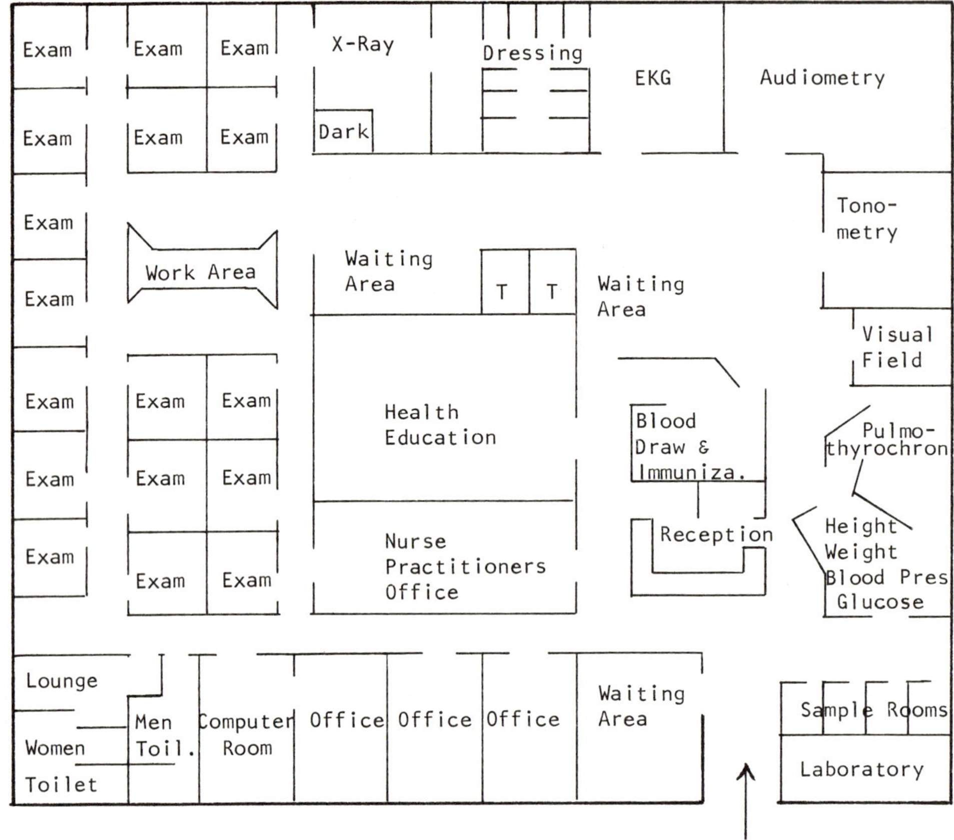

Kaiser-Permanente
Multiphasic & Health Appraisal Unit

Sacramento, California

Figure 4-10.   Floor plan for Kaiser-Permanente MHTS in Sacramento.

occasional fainting patients, or for one who might have to be moved to adjacent facilities.

(18) Proper ventilation and air conditioning need special consideration in areas such as waiting rooms, clinical laboratory, and history-taking area if automated history terminals with film-slide projection are used (these generate a great deal of heat). Dressing areas should be warm enough, and the heating-air conditioning system should be well balanced.

(19) Sufficient power capacity and electrical outlets should be provided in each testing station. Some provision should exist for unanticipated power load.

(20) Communications both within the MHTS and with the exterior should be carefully planned to optimize receiving and transmitting of essential telephone calls.

G.   ENVIRONMENTAL FEATURES

The center should be made as attractive as possible by the use of color, interior finishes, and pleasing graphics. Illumination should not be glaring but adequate where needed. Sound control is essential where patients will be questioned or must discuss personal intimate matters. Ventilation drafts should be avoided.

Often an in-house lunch and coffee-break room for the MHTS staff is included; it should be designed attractively for staff morale.

Interior finishes, walls, ceilings, and floors should be planned for easy cleaning and minimum maintenance costs.

Waste disposal should entail no serious problems—less, certainly, than in a regular medical clinic, since few MHTS patients are acutely sick.

H. FUTURE SCREENING CENTERS

The advent of Health Maintenance Organization (HMO) legislation and the spread of health insurance will no doubt mean more and bigger MHTS. One can anticipate that the demand for MHTS and for periodic updating of patient profiles will markedly increase in the near future. It is likely that these MHTS centers will become the admitting departments for ambulatory care and that they will monitor and provide surveillance for both the well and the chronic sick. Pediatric and mental health are important new components that will probably be added to MHTS (see Chapters Thirteen and Fourteen). There will be a higher level of automation, new technology in instrumentation, and improved data processing. These changes will require a flexibility for expansion that can best be provided for by open-ending the MHTS facility of the future.

REFERENCES

1. De Cicco, P. R. *Physical Facilities in Provisional Guidelines for AMHTS*, Vol. 3, 135–165. H.E.W. Publication No. (HSM) 72-3011, N.T.I.S., 1970.
2. Gilbert, F. "Multiphasic Screening Cut Down to Size." *Med. World News* 9(1968):60–61.
3. Gilbert, F., and Nordyke, R. "Automated Multiphasic Health Testing in Multispecialty Group Practice." *Prev. Med.* 1(1973):261–265.

CHAPTER FIVE

MHTS Systems Engineering

James H. Duncan

A. INTRODUCTION

The *Oxford English Dictionary* defines a system as a group, set, or aggregate of things, natural or artificial, forming a connected or complex whole.[1] In terms of an engineered system, however, this definition is not complete. A system does not exist in a vacuum; therefore it must exist for a specific goal or objective.[2] It follows, then, that specific systems can incorporate skills, procedures, equipment, and physical facilities to accomplish defined objectives.

The objectives for which a system is engineered should dictate its design. Two basic principles must be considered. The first is planning: planning is the methodologies engineered into the system to attain the objectives. The second is control: control is the device(s) engineered into the system to provide decision makers with current and meaningful data with which they can evaluate the system vis-à-vis the objectives.[3]

Multiphasic Health Testing Services (MHTS) is a system designed to use information provided by the patient (i.e., history) and by specific tests to provide first-level health status information to the medical decision maker (physician or nurse practitioner). Defined from a somewhat different frame of reference: MHTS is basically a system wherein patients who may have a particular identifiable disease can be readily detected.[4] In effect, MHTS is a series of subsystems, each having a specific objective, integrated into the planned system. This integration, with controls for continuous evaluation of the performance of these subsystems, is necessary for the system to attain its overall objective; therefore, it defines the system as a whole.

B. GENERAL SYSTEM REQUIREMENTS

1. Objectives

The most important primary system requirement is a clear and concise statement of objectives. (See Chapter Two, B.) From a system standpoint, the objectives ultimately have to be stated in terms of specifications. How many, when, with what, who, where, and how—these questions must be answered with numbers and/or specifications.[5]

Each component or subsystem has a precise goal or objective, and these must be developed from, and be a part of, the whole system's set of objectives. Since MHTS is a probabilistic system,[6] i.e., its outcomes are not fully predictable, the objectives must be stated to cover this contingency. The following objectives are primarily systems oriented:

(1) Provide a fast, courteous, and comprehensive health testing service.

(2) Provide a health testing service that is cost-effective and optimizes the use of resources.

(3) Provide appointment times, at convenient hours, to as many patients as possible.

(4) Utilize automation (where economically feasible) to quickly and accurately collect and collate patient history and test data.

(5) Utilize data processing (when economically feasible) to disseminate the data generated, evaluate test results, flag abnormal values, and produce advice rules.

Each subsystem, or component, must have as its goal one or more of these objectives, in addition to its own specific goal. For example, the appointment-making function or subsystem has as its primary objective: "Make patient appointments in a cost-effective manner." This objective, however, must be in consonance with other objectives of MHTS. In this example the subsystem objectives must complement or augment items (1) through (4) above.

2. Systems Analysis

When the systems approach is used, the first logical step is a systems analysis. For an MHTS system there are several critical factors to be analyzed, including:

(1) The objectives of the system, especially those objectives that impact most heavily on the system—such as those listed above in B.1.

(2) The ratio of males to females in the population to be served.

(3) Median age of the population to be served and other demographic data such as size, density, and distribution.

(4) Physical constraints of an existing building or building-code requirements of a new building.

(5) The specific tests to be performed on various classifications of patients (e.g., mammography on females over 50 years of age) and the quality control requirements for the testing equipment.

(6) Number and classification of personnel to be budgeted for the operation of the MHTS (e.g., number of receptionists, clerks, technicians, etc.).

(7) The location of the MHTS (e..g, the area, proximity of public transportation, etc.).

(8) Patient volume anticipated by age and sex.

(9) Personnel training—how much, when, initial and ongoing programs.

(10) Administrative policies (e.g., how will late cancellations and no-shows be handled?).

3. Systems Design

The basic methodology for MHTS systems design is to use the data from the analysis for the following procedural steps (see also Chapter Two, F):

(1) Study the objectives of the proposed MHTS program and understand the scope of the project.

(2) Develop a tentative set of design specifications.

(3) Match the tentative design specifications against the overall objectives and determine the objectives of each subsystem. The subsystem objectives must complement and be in consonance with the overall objectives.

(4) Develop design specifications for each subsystem.

(5) Develop tentative testing sequence.

(6) Match the design specifications against the testing sequence, then match both against the individual and overall objectives.

(7) Redesign specifications as dictated by step (6).

(8) Synthesize the information produced in the seven steps above and design the MHTS system.

(9) Test the system design. Use whatever type of simulation model that best tests the design. The simulation model should use "real" data.

(10) Redesign the system to correct design problems uncovered by the simulation.

(11) Provide information to management with respect to the following:

(a) Specific requirements for testing equipment (e.g., a tonometer that meets requirements for testing times, quality of results, costs, and maintenance).

(b) Specific manpower staffing requirements for each test station as well as for administrative functions.

(c) Type, duration, and costs of training program for all personnel by classification.

(d) The standard operating procedures for each test station.

(e) Optimum building configuration and site requirements.

(f) Staff, equipment, training, and operating costs.

(g) Time parameters for patient flow.

(h) Communication requirements including equipment and personnel (e.g., what will be required for making appointments and the subsequent scheduling of patients for the MHTS?).

(i) Data handling (e.g., how will test results be accumulated, collated, and sent to the appropriate physician and/or clinic?).

(12) When requirements listed in step (11) have been satisfied, install the MHTS system.

(13) Establish control parameters for the whole system and for each station (subsystem). These should include:

(a) Time parameters on patient flow through the system, station by station.

(b) Upper and lower limits on the test times at each testing station.

(c) Number of man-hours allocated for each testing station based on number of patients tested.

(d) Patient queuing times at each station—upper and lower limits.

(e) Number of late cancellations and no-shows or a percentage of the total number scheduled.

(f) The flow of data (test results) from each station and the compilation of these results into a standard printout with appropriate "advice" rules.

(14) Install system monitor to measure performance against control parameters and report results to those responsible for the operation and management of the system.

(15) Set up procedures (such as a System Modification Request—see Figure 5-1) to implement any required changes to the system. This should include an information loop, then an approval process loop. This procedure should help insure that any system change will be known to both operations and management decision makers prior to the change.

C. NONSELECTIVE VS. SELECTIVE MHTS

The objectives and resources available will probably dictate the type of MHTS program to be installed. System requirements will be different for each type, but the basic system principles will still apply. A "selective" MHTS is one in which each patient is scheduled for specific tests in advance and only those scheduled tests are done. A "nonselective" MHTS provides the same tests (usually) in the same sequence for all patients; few provisions are made for selectivity.

1. Nonselective MHTS

The system requirements for nonselective MHTS impact most heavily on scheduling, patient flow, communications, equipment, and manpower. The most complex interrelationships, however, involve patient flow, queuing, equipment, and manpower. There are two basic types of nonselective MHTS: the carrel[7] type and the sequential type. System requirements for each are significantly different. (See also Chapter Four, B.)

a. Carrel type.

The carrel type of nonselective MHTS utilizes individual testing rooms (see Figure 5-2); all tests except history, x-ray, and clinical laboratory are accomplished in the same testing room by one technician. System requirements for this type are less complex, since queuing and flow problems are minimized. Equipment costs, however, would be proportionately higher, depending on the number of testing rooms required.

Scheduling, patient flow, and queuing can be systemized rather easily, since the time required to perform all tests in the testing rooms can be measured and future scheduling adjusted accordingly. For example, if the testing phase per patient is timed at 15 to 18 minutes and the clean-up, data entry function, etc., can be completed in seven minutes or less, one patient can be scheduled for each technician every 25 minutes.

b. Sequential type.
The sequential type of nonselective MHTS system presents more complex problems in optimizing scheduling, patient flow, and queuing. If 150 patients are to be tested in one eight-hour day (480 minutes), one patient has to be entered into each test phase approximately every three minutes. Since not all test phases will fall into this convenient time frame, extensive studies must be done to determine what and how much pretest, test, and posttest work is involved in each test phase; the sequencing must then be synchronized for a uniform patient flow pattern. If, for example, all the work involved in test A takes two minutes and in test B six minutes, it may be that the technician in test A can do a significant portion of the pretest or posttest work (such as instructions) for test B; these stations, then, should be adjacent and sequenced accordingly. If this is not feasible, then two testing devices will be required at station B if all 150 patients are to receive test B; in this instance, simultaneous testing on two patients will have to be accomplished. The objective, in either case, is to sustain the three-minute patient flow module.

2. Selective MHTS

a. Carrel type.
System requirements for selective testing would be more complex in a sequential type of MHTS but relatively simple in the carrel type. Sequencing and queuing problems inherent in a sequential-selective MHTS would require an inordinate amount of system work. This would not be true, however, for a carrel-selective MHTS, where the primary systems work (over and above

TASK/PROJECT CONTROL

ACCOUNT #: ______________________

BY: ______________________

DATE OF REQUEST: ______________________

REQUESTER: ______________________

LOCATION/DEPT: ______________________

EXT: ______________________

APPLICATION ______________________

____

DOCUMENT ______________________

____

TYPE OF REQUEST:

☐ NEW

☐ MALFUNCTION CORRECTION

☐ CHANGE TO EXISTING FEATURE

☐ ______________________

INITIAL APPROVAL

☐ APPROVED
☐ DISAPPROVED

TASK/PROJECT AUTHORIZATION   DATE   1

☐ FINAL MEDICAL APPROVAL IS REQUIRED, WITH SIGNATURE IN ITEM 9 BELOW, BEFORE IMPLEMENTATION.

PROGRAMMING APPROVAL

☐ APPROVED
☐ DISAPPROVED
☐ N/A

PROGRAMMING SUPERVISOR   2

RESOURCE ESTIMATE

(NAME)   (TITLE)   DATE   3

EST: ______   BY: ______________________   4
MAN-DAYS   (NAME)   (TITLE)

FINAL AUTHORIZATION

☐ PROCEED — PRIORITY: L   1   2   3   4   5   6   7   8   H 9
☐ HOLD   ______ WEEKS
☐ ARCHIVE

DIRECTOR   DATE   5

DESCRIPTION OF REQUEST ______

☐ ADDITIONAL DESCRIPTION ATTACHED

NOTES:

WORK ASSIGNED	TO: ______ (NAME) ______ (TITLE) ON: ______ DATE 6 FOR IMPLEMENTATION BY: ______ DATE
ACTUAL TIME REQUIRED TO COMPLETE	ACTUAL: ______ MAN-DAYS COMPLETE: ______ (NAME) ______ (TITLE) ______ DATE 7
FINAL ACCEPTANCE AND APPROVAL FOR IMPLEMENTATION	______ PROGRAMMING SUPERVISOR ______ DATE 8 ______ TASK/PROJECT AUTHORIZATION ______ DATE 9 ______ DIRECTOR ______ DATE 10
CLOSING DISTRIB.	______ SYSTEMS SUPERVISOR ______ DATE 11

Figure 5-1. System modification request (SMR) form.

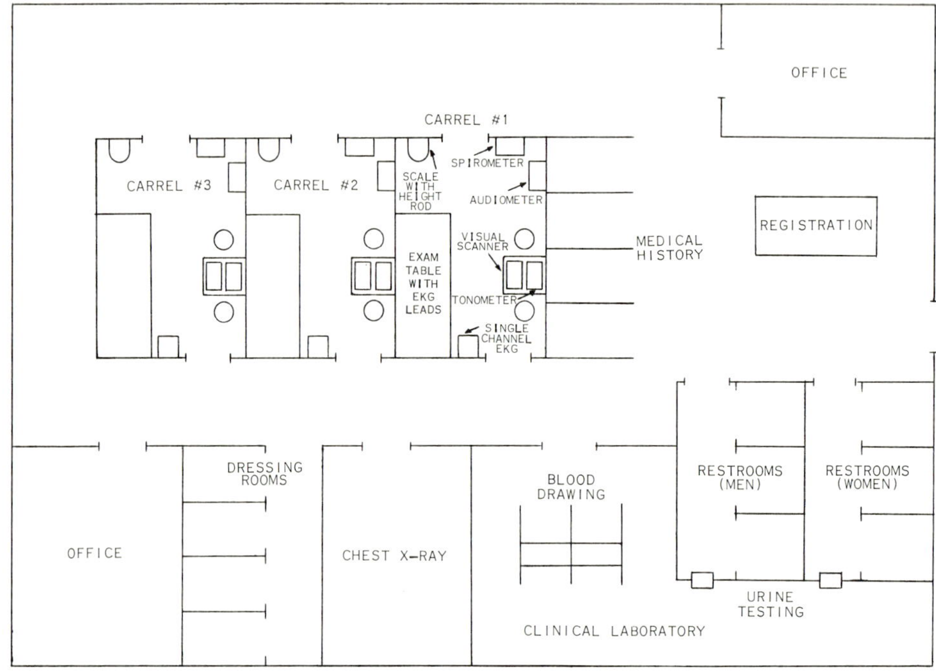

Figure 5-2.   One version of a carrel type MHTS floor plan.

usual) would be scheduling, assuming two or more testing rooms. The system would have to provide for variable-length scheduling based on the various total testing times. The next section on scheduling alternatives will detail some of the systems work required.

   b. Sequential type.   Sequential types of MHTS are almost always nonselective. The systems aspect of a sequential MHTS is the most complex. The system logic set forth earlier in this chapter must be rigorously applied. Obviously, the first objectives that must be known are (1) the number of people to be tested and (2) the specific tests to be performed. From these data, specific design specifications can be established. For example, if an objective were to test 120 people per eight-hour day, the average time per test station would have to approximate four minutes per test. This time should then be used to help determine the equipment specifications. In cases where the technician's skill is more important than equipment in determining test times, time studies can be used to establish average times. This type of study can be performed in other clinics where similar or identical equipment is being used.

D. APPOINTMENT SCHEDULING ALTERNATIVES

1. Selective—Carrel Type

A major systems consideration is patient scheduling. In a selective-carrel MHTS the scheduling work would be a function of the number of testing rooms and the number of different series (selective groups) of tests offered. If four different test series were offered, the systems analyst would have to take into account their different durations as well as other factors. The following are some procedures that could be used to establish a schedule for a selective-carrel MHTS.

Test Series	Tests Included	Duration (Minutes)
No. 1	EKG	5.2
	Anthropometry	2.5
	Respirometry	2.1
	Visual acuity	1.2
	Tonometry	2.6
	Chest x-ray	2.0
	Total	15.6
No. 2	EKG	5.2
	Respirometry	2.1
	Visual acuity	1.2
	Tonometry	2.6
	Urinalysis	5.0
	Blood Tests	2.0
	Total	18.1
No. 3	EKG	5.2
	Tonometry	2.6
	Chest x-ray	2.0
	Urinalysis	5.0
	Blood Tests	2.0
	Total	16.8
No. 4	EKG	5.2
	Respirometry	2.1
	Visual acuity	1.2
	Tonometry	2.6
	Chest x-ray	2.0
	Total	13.1

Systems requirements for scheduling will have to take account of variations in tests requested such as those shown above. In addition to the testing time per se there will be other times to factor into the equation—times for clean-up, clerical work, patient undressing, and integration (time spent with patient, over and above test times). These other times can be averaged, but they will vary with the number of tests performed. If more tests are done, more equipment has been used and hence must be cleaned and/or prepared for the next patient. For purpose of this example, assume 15 seconds is required (for the above) for each minute of testing. The times for the four selective test series will now be:

Test Series	Minutes
No. 1	19.5
No. 2	22.6
No. 3	21.0
No. 4	16.4

Finally, assume 15% percent for technician personal time per patient. The times would then be (rounded to the nearest minute):

Test Series	Minutes
No. 1	22
No. 2	26
No. 3	24
No. 4	19

Figure 5-3 illustrates a schedule based on four variable-length test series. The appointment clerk can assign patients to any unfilled appointment slot so long as the test series number is listed in that slot. The *desired* test series number for that time slot is the first number indicated. As an example of the use of the schedule, suppose a patient requested test series number 3, as specified by his physician, and preferably a morning appointment. The clerk could offer 0850, 0955, 1040 in room 1; 0825, 0855, 0940, 1045 in room 2; and 0910, 0950, 1020, 1105 in room 3. For maximum efficiency, however, the clerk would attempt not to use 0850 and 1040 in room 1, 0825 and 0940 in room 2, or 0950 and 1020 in room 3.

Registration in the variable-length test series schedule sheet is approximately 30 minutes prior to test time. In this example the registration time would range from two to four minutes. The medical history questionnaire would average from 12 to 21 minutes. The questionnaire would be taken back to the receptionist, who would check it for completeness. The patient would be called to the room by the technician and tested. The EKG would be the last test performed in the room, and since this test requires some undressing, the patient would remain partially undressed, but covered by a disposable gown, and taken to the x-ray room for the final test. After the x-ray the patient would dress in an adjacent dressing room.

2. Nonselective—Sequential Type

In a sequential type MHTS it is essential that patients be appropriately scheduled to insure an even, steady flow. One method is to book patients for an exact time (e.g., 0942, 1117, 1242, etc.) and specify that the patient arrive at least 15 minutes earlier for registration, prior completion of medical history, etc. The general experience, however, is that despite precise scheduling, precise instructions, and asking the patient to repeat appointment times and places, patients arrive late as well as early. Schedules, therefore, are probably better if they can accommodate this aspect of human nature. A system that attempts to do this is called block scheduling.

a. Block scheduling. The concept of block scheduling is based on overbooking and concurrent scheduling. The overbooking is to compensate (at a projected rate) for those who fail to show up and for those who cancel their appointment too late to fill it with another patient. Concurrent scheduling provides for a specific number of patients to be given the same appointment time in increments or blocks of time. For this example the increments or blocks are specified as 15 minutes in Figure 5-4. Note that ten appointment slots are scheduled for some blocks, while

	Testing Room 1	Testing Room 2	Testing Room 3
1	REG. TIME 0820 TEST TIME 0900 TEST #: 1 4 LAST NAME FIRST	REG. TIME 0825 TEST TIME 0900 TEST #: 2 3 1 4 LAST NAME FIRST	REG. TIME 0830 TEST TIME 0900 TEST #: 4 LAST NAME FIRST
2	REG. TIME 0850 TEST TIME 0922 TEST #: 2 3 1 4 LAST NAME FIRST	REG. TIME 0855 TEST TIME 0926 TEST #: 3 1 4 LAST NAME FIRST	REG. TIME 0845 TEST TIME 0919 TEST #: 1 4 LAST NAME FIRST
3	REG. TIME 0915 TEST TIME 0948 TEST #: 1 4 LAST NAME FIRST	REG. TIME 0920 TEST TIME 0950 TEST #: 1 4 LAST NAME FIRST	REG. TIME 0910 TEST TIME 0942 TEST #: 3 1 4 LAST NAME FIRST
4	REG. TIME 0935 TEST TIME 1010 TEST #: 4 LAST NAME FIRST	REG. TIME 0940 TEST TIME 1012 TEST #: 2 3 4 1 LAST NAME FIRST	REG. TIME 0930 TEST TIME 1006 TEST #: 1 4 LAST NAME FIRST
5	REG. TIME 0955 TEST TIME 1029 TEST #: 3 1 4 LAST NAME FIRST	REG. TIME 1005 TEST TIME 1038 TEST #: 4 LAST NAME FIRST	REG. TIME 0950 TEST TIME 1028 TEST #: 2 3 1 4 LAST NAME FIRST
6	REG. TIME 1015 TEST TIME 1053 TEST #: 4 LAST NAME FIRST	REG. TIME 1025 TEST TIME 1057 TEST #: 1 4 LAST NAME FIRST	REG. TIME 1020 TEST TIME 1054 TEST #: 2 3 1 4 LAST NAME FIRST
7	REG. TIME 1040 TEST TIME 1112 TEST #: 2 3 1 4 LAST NAME FIRST	REG. TIME 1045 TEST TIME 1119 TEST #: 3 1 4 LAST NAME FIRST	REG. TIME 1050 TEST TIME 1120 TEST #: 4 LAST NAME FIRST
8	REG. TIME 1100 TEST TIME 1138 TEST #: 1 4 LAST NAME FIRST	REG. TIME 1110 TEST TIME 1143 TEST #: 4 LAST NAME FIRST	REG. TIME 1105 TEST TIME 1139 TEST #: 3 1 4 LAST NAME FIRST

Figure 5-3. Variable-length test series schedule for three carrels.

BLOCK TIME	PT. CODE*	APPT TIME	BLOCK TIME	PT. CODE*	APPT TIME	BLOCK TIME	PT. CODE*	APPT TIME	BLOCK TIME	PT. CODE*	APPT TIME
0745-1	2	0745	0930-1	5X	0931	1145-1	2	1146	145-1	2X	1346
-2	2	0746	-2	2	0932	-2	2	1147	-2	2	1347
-3	3X	0747	-3	3	0933	-3	3	1148	-3	2	1348
-4	1	0748	-4	3	0934	-4	2	1149	-4	5	1350
-5	2	0749	-5	2	0938	-5	2	1155	-5	2	1352
-6	2	0751	-6	SX	0940	-6	2X	1156	-6	2X	1353
-7	3	0752	-7	2	0942	-7	3	1157	-7	3	1355
-8	1X	0753	0945-1	3	0947	1200-1	3	1201	200-1	3	1401
-9	3	0754	-2	3	0948	-2	3	1202	-2	3	1402
-10	2	0755	-3	5	0950	-3	2X	1203	-3	5X	1403
0800-1	2	0801	-4	3	0952	-4	3	1205	-4	3	1405
-2	2	0803	-5	S	0954	-5	S	1207	-5	S	1407
-3	3	0805	1000-1	5X	1001	-6	3	1208	-6	3	1409
-4	3	0807	-2	5X	1002	-7	2	1210	-7	3	1411
-5	S	0808	-3	5	1006	1215-1	2X	1216	215-1	2X	1416
-6	SX	0809	-4	5	1008	-2	2	1218	-2	3	1417
-7	3	0810	-5	5	1010	-3	2	1219	03	3	1418
-8	2X	0811	-6	5	1012	-4	2	1220	-4	5	1420
-9	2	0812	-7	5	1013	-5	2	1223	-5	3	1422
-10	3	0813	1015-1	5X	1018	-6	1X	1225	-6	5	1425
0815-1	2	0815	-2	5	1020	-7	3	1227	-7	3	1427
-2	1	0816	-3	5	1021	1230-1	2	1231	230-1	3	1431
-3	5X	0817	-4	5	1023	-2	3	1232	-2	3	1433
-4	1	0818	-5	5	1025	-3	2X	1233	-3	5X	1435
-5	2	0820	-6	5	1026	-4	3	1235	-4	3	1436
-6	1	0821	1030-1	5	1032	-5	5	1237	-5	5	1437
-7	1	0822	-2	5	1035	-6	5X	1240	-6	SX	1439
-8	2X	0823	-3	5	1038	-7	3	1243	-7	5	1441
-9	3	0824	-4	SX	1040						
-10	3	0825	-5	5	1041						

Block	Code	Time	Block	Code	Time	Block	Code	Time	Block	Code	Time
0830-1	5	0830	1045-1	5X	1047	1245-1	2	1246	245-1	3	1446
-2	3	0831	-2	2	1048	-2	2X	1247	-2	3	1447
-3	1X	0832	-3	5	1049	-3	1	1249	-3	3	1450
-4	2	0833	-4	5	1051	-4	2	1250	-4	5	1452
-5	1	0834	-5	5X	1052	-5	5X	1251	-5	5	1455
-6	2X	0835	-6	5	1053	-6	2	1253	-6	5	1456
-7	1	0836	-7	2	1055	-7	3	1255	-7	5	1457
0845-1	2X	0845	1100-1	2	1102	100-1	3	1301	300-1	5	1501
-2	1	0847	-2	3X	1103	-2	2X	1303	-2	5X	1502
-3	3	0848	-3	5X	1104	-3	5	1305	-3	5	1505
-4	5X	0849	-4	2	1105	-4	5	1307	-4	5	1507
-5	5	0850	-5	S	1108	-5	3	1310	-5	S	1509
-6	2	0852	-6	2	1110	-6	SX	1312	-6	5X	1510
-7	1	0855	-7	2	1112	-7	3	1313	-7	5	1511
0900-1	3X	0901	1115-1	2	1116	115-1	2X	1316	315-1	5	1516
-2	5X	0902	-2	2	1117	-2	2	1317	-2	5	1517
-3	2	0903	-3	3	1118	-3	5	1320	-3	5	1520
-4	5X	0904	-4	2	1120	-4	2	1322	-4	5	1522
-5	S	0905	-5	2	1122	-5	5	1324	-5	S	1525
-6	2	0906	-6	2X	1124	-6	2X	1325	-6	SX	1526
-7	2	0908	-7	2	1125	-7	3	1326	-7	5	1527
0915-1	3	0916	1130-1	2	1131	130-1	3	1332			
-2	3X	0918	-2	5X	1132	-2	3X	1333			
-3	5	0920	-3	5	1134	-3	3	1335			
-4	3	0922	-4	5	1136	-4	3	1338			
-5	3	0923	-5	2	1138	-5	3	1340			
-6	3	0924	-6	3	1140	-6	1	1342			
-7	5X	0925	-7	3	1141	-7	2	1343			

STUDY GROUP	- 14
CODE #1*	- 14
CODE #2*	- 66
CODE #3*	- 62
CODE #5	- 65
POSSIBLE	- 221
HES*	- 142
MAMMOGRAPHY	- 49

Effective: 4/1/76

Figure 5-4. Block/appointment time schedule. (Explanation of codes: Codes 1, 2, and 3—Time slots available for patients scheduled for HES after MHTS. Code 1: patients with significant complaints; code 2: patients with minor complaints; code 3: patients with no complaints. Code 5—Patients scheduled only for MHTS. X = time slots available for patients scheduled for a mammogram; S = time slots available for study-group patients.)

other blocks have five, six, or seven slots; most blocks have seven slots. When the patient makes an appointment, he will be given the block time nearest his requested time (which will usually be in increments of one hour). Note that all patients scheduled in the 0745 block have different actual times but are told they have a 0745 appointment and are asked to arrive 15 minutes earlier (i.e., at 0730). Patients are usually processed through in their order of arrival, not their actual time slot. Several advantages accrue from this approach. If a patient scheduled for the 0800 block arrives earlier than the requested 0745 (15 minutes before appointment time), he can be processed through in place of a late 0745 block patient. The late 0745 block patient can then be scheduled into the 0800 block.

Another feature of this scheduling procedure is that different types of patients can be programmed into the flow at whatever rate is required. For example, patients requiring a mammography (suffix X in Figure 5-4) are placed into the schedule at the rate dictated by the time to process patients through this procedure. The schedule illustrated in Figure 5–4 was designed not only to schedule MHTS patients but also to provide the proper flow of patients to a Health Evaluation Section (HES), which provides medical nurse practitioner physical examinations (under physician supervision) to patients coded 1, 2, and 3. (See Chapter Ten.)

b. Specific time schedules. The Block/Appointment Time Schedule Sheet could, with minor changes, be used for specific time scheduling; the major change would be to eliminate the block times. It would then be a matter of giving the patient an exact appointment time—8:35, 11:20, or whatever. As discussed earlier, it would be advantageous to ask the patient to arrive 15 minutes early.

E. PATIENT FLOW ALTERNATIVES

With some exceptions the type of MHTS, whether carrel or sequential, will dictate patient flow possibilities. In a sequential system the patients move through the testing stations starting with the first test and ending with the last. A basic consideration in the flow is the separation of male and female patients during the tests that require partial disrobing, such as EKG and chest x-ray. Additionally, the female patients who require mammography will have to be routed through that station, usually immediately after chest x-ray. Therefore, to expedite the flow, the physical layout must provide for this basic separation.

If, however, the separation is done by scheduling male and female patients on alternate days, the physical layout and the flow patterns can be less complex. Of course, this scheduling procedure introduces other problems of balance, especially with respect to the staff and patient load.

On days when only men were scheduled, the mammography technician(s) would not be needed. Conversely, for days when only women were scheduled, the appointment center would have to schedule a specific number of women requiring the mammography, and the balance not requiring this test. This might cause the schedule to become excessively long for women requiring mammograms.

Patient flow must take account of tests that are time dependent. For example, results of glucose determination (fasting, postprandial, or challenge) are dependent upon when the specimens are collected. Figure 5-5 illustrates the sequential time requirements for glucose challenge and for the two-hour postprandial tests.

1. For Glucose Challenge Dose

Test Time		Cumulative Time
8	Reception	8
4	Glucose ingestion	12
5	Dressing room	17
8	EKG/blood pressure	25
3	Anthropometry/spirometry	28
3	Chest x-ray	31
5	Dressing room	36
32*	Medical history	68
4	Venipuncture	72
3	Urine specimen (Lab)	75
3	Visual acuity	78
3	Tonometry	81
9	Audiometry	90
6	Discharge/registration for HES	96
35	Physical exam	131
4	Discharge	135

(60-minute interval between Anthropometry/spirometry and Chest x-ray)

2. For Two-Hour Postprandial Glucose

Test Time		Cumulative Time
8	Reception	8
4	Venipucture	12†
3	Urine specimen (Lab)	15
5	Dressing room	20
8	EKG/blood pressure	28
3	Anthropometry/spirometry	31
3	Chest x-ray	34
5	Dressing room	39
3	Visual acuity	42
3	Tonometry	45
9	Audiometry	54
25	Medical history	79
6	Discharge/registration for HES	85
35	Physical exam	120
4	Discharge	124

*Test time for the medical history phase is flexible and adjusts to meet the 60-minute interval required between glucose ingestion and venipuncture.
†Patient arrives at venipuncture phase two hours after eating a standard meal.

Figure 5-5.   Patient test sequential time requirements.

Note that for the challenge dose the MHTS laboratory functions occur immediately (or possibly during) the medical history function. In designing the system and the patient flow it would be advisable to have the MHTS laboratory located adjacent to a station, such as medical history, so that the time could be easily monitored. For the two-hour postprandial the receptionist would query the patient upon registration as to when the prescribed meal was taken. Two hours from that time the receptionist would direct the patient to the MHTS laboratory for blood and urine specimen collection. In this case the appointment clerk must advise the patient to take the prescribed meal two hours prior to the appointment time.

For the carrel type MHTS the flow would be less complex, since patients are basically taken by one technician through all tests, which with few exceptions (chest x-ray and mammography) are done in the same testing room. For the selective-carrel MHTS the patient flow would have to conform to the schedule, but otherwise no special system work should be required.

Another important consideration in planning patient flow is any patient service rendered immediately after the MHTS. For example, patients who had previously asked for a health appraisal might be scheduled for a physical examination by nurse practitioners in the Health Evaluation Service (HES) after the multiphasic laboratory tests; these patients would have to flow through MHTS at a rate equal to the predetermined HES schedule. This online patient flow and schedule requires not only preplanning but also intermittent monitoring of flow through MHTS.

If the health appraisal is not done immediately after MHTS but is done offline (e.g., two to three weeks later), the patient flow through MHTS will not be affected. However, both online and offline procedures affect data flow, as discussed at the end of F, below.

F. DATA FLOW ALTERNATIVES

An MHTS data processing system must provide for data generation and flow for the following functions: appointment scheduling, patient history, test results, advice rules, and summary reports. The system may also have to provide for computer storage and retrieval of data.

The system to be used for data flow depends primarily on the type and objectives of the MHTS clinic under consideration. If, for example, a small carrel type is being planned, and the objectives do not include computer storage and retrieval of data, a manual system could be the most cost-effective. Figure 5-6 is an example of a manual MHTS summary report on which test results would be written by the technicians. Subsequently, the results from the cardiologist, radiologist, and the clinical laboratory could be transcribed to this form by a clerk. When the form had been completed, it would be sent (mailed if required) along with the medical history to the patient's physician. If any serious gross abnormalities were noted, the patient's physician could be telephoned with these results immediately. The physician then could specify additional followup testing or arrange for an immediate examination.

The manual system described above could be semiautmoated if the size of the MHTS clinic increased sufficiently to warrant the cost. The data on the test report, along with the medical history, could be keypunched into cards and read into a computer processor. The computer printout summary report, along with other programmed data, would then be sent to the patient's physician.

A heavy-volume, sequential MHTS would probably require, at the very least, a semiautomated data flow system. Such a system might incorporate test results recorded directly on punch cards for batch processing when the patient completed the last phase of MHTS or might use a variety of methods for computer entry, online or offline.

The previous section discussed online and offline procedures for reporting. Obviously, the data flow system through MHTS must be designed to facilitate either online, offline, or a combination of both. In other words, test data on the patient going through MHTS and scheduled for online physical examination would have to be available when the patient arrived for the physical examination. Test data on those not so scheduled would not have to be available; hence the system for accumulating and handling these data would be different. (See Chapter Eight, Data Processing.)

MULTIPHASIC TEST REPORT

Name _________________________ _________________   Date ___________
           (last)   (first)

Address _____________________________________   Phone ___________

City _________________   State ___________   Zip ___________

Birthdate ___ ___ ___   Sex ________   MR# _ _ _ _ _ _ _ _
         mo day yr

1. |Height| ________ in/cm   Weight ________ lbs/kgs

2. |Spirometry| PRT   TNI   TND
                                                        Vital
                 Peak flow   FEVB-1s   FEVA-2s   Capacity

       Test 1   _____   _____   _____   _____

       Test 2   _____   _____   _____   _____

       Test 3   _____   _____   _____   _____

3. |Visual Acuity| PRT   TNI   TND   LABORATORY

       Right eye ______   Left eye ______ |Blood   PRT   TNI   TND
                                                                    am
4. |Tonometry| PRT   TNI   TND   Time blood drawn ________ pm

       Right eye _____mm Left eye _____mm   Hematology
                                               WBC________   RBC ________
5. |Hearing| PRT   TNI   TND   HCT________   MCHC________
                                               HGB________   MCV ________
       Right ___________________
                                             Chemistry
       Left ___________________   Na ________   BUN ________
                                               K   ________   T Bili_______
6. |Blood Pressure| ___________________   Ca ________   SGOT ________
                                               Gluc ________   Creat ________
7. |EKG| PRT   TNI   TND   Alk Phos_______ LDH ________
                                               Chol ________   Uric acid___
       ____
                                             |Urine
       ____
                                               pH ________   Gluc________
       ___________________________   Clin________   Acet ________
                                               Prot________   Hgb ________
       ____

8. |Chest X-Ray| PRT   TNI   TND
                                                     REMARKS
       ____

       ____

       ____

       ____

   PRT = Patient Referral Test   TNI = Test Not Indicated   TND = Test Not Done

Figure 5-6. Manual multiphasic test report form.

137

G. MHTS FLOW DIAGRAM

One of the keys to designing a system is to create a methodology to analyze the components as they relate to the system and to each other. Flow diagramming provides a methodology for building a system (if only on paper) to do this analysis. If the analysis suggests changes, these changes can then be incorporated and tested again in the analysis.

Building the system by testing and assembling the components—all in a flow diagram—is critical to the success of the system design. The method of flow diagramming must, therefore, be unique to the system design requirements. The flow diagrams depicted in Figure 5-7 are unique to the design requirements of an MHTS system.

The MHTS flow diagrams (Figure 5-7, a–n) begin with the appointment-making process and continue through all phases to patient discharge. The interrelationship of data generation and flow with patient testing and flow is shown functionally. Procedures are shown in sufficient detail to depict the functions, but they are not to be used as standard operating procedures. (See Chapter Twenty for standard operating procedures.)

As shown in Figure 5-7, flow diagramming is also necessary to insure due consideration to such items as physical location, facilities planning, patient and staff accommodations, reception, patient flow, test sequence, type of data generated, and data flow. The technique or convention used to flow-diagram is not as important as the accurate and logical inclusion of all facets of the system.

H. CONCLUSION

A number of different methodologies might be used to engineer an MHTS system. All, however, should be the result of systems analysis. As developed in this chapter, the steps used for the analysis are iterative, so that identifiable improvements can be incorporated in the design.

Finally, the system incorporates a continuing evaluation of its effectiveness and permits controls on modifications. This ability to monitor is essential in a system as dynamic as health testing.

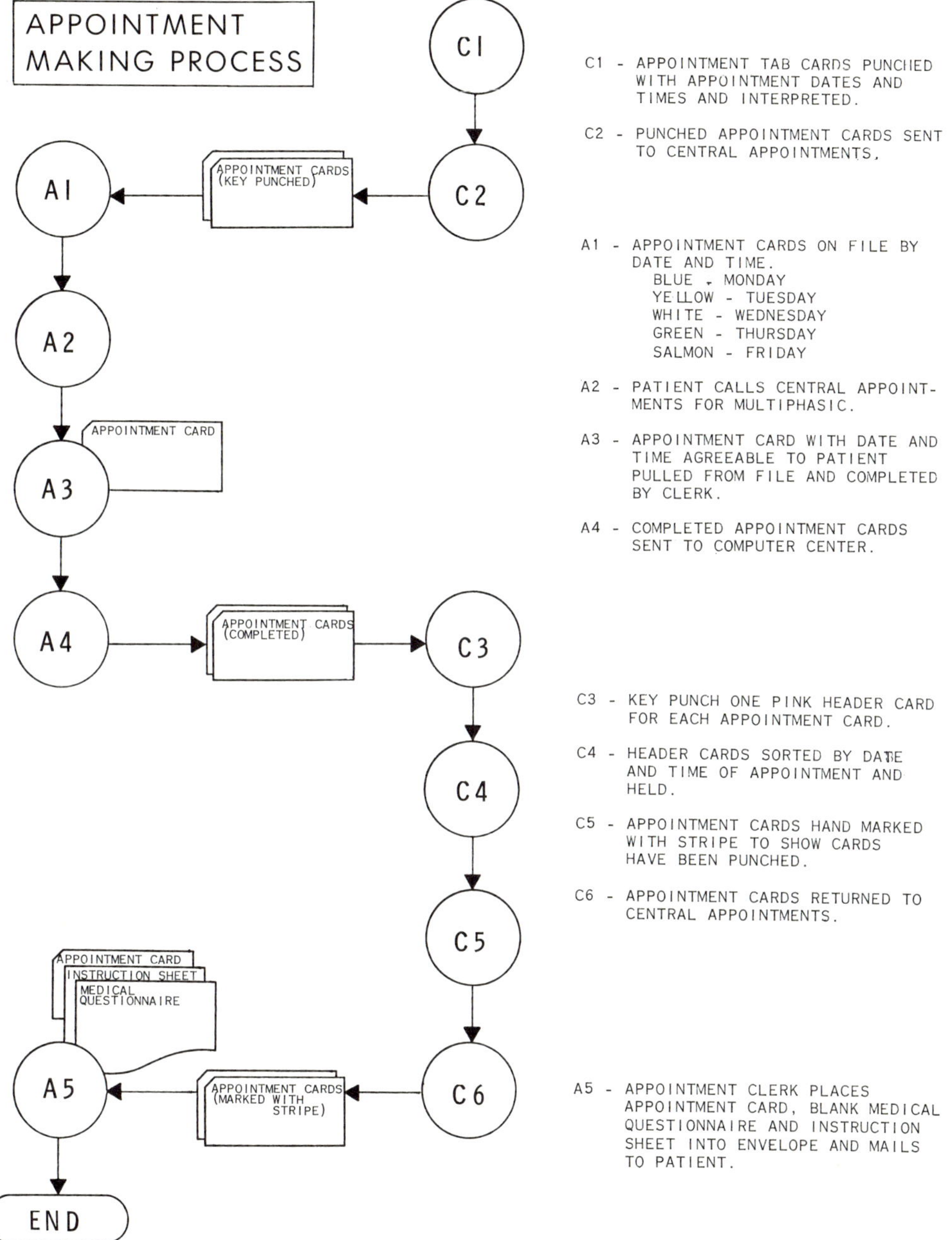

Figure 5-7a. Flow diagram for the current Oakland MHTS.

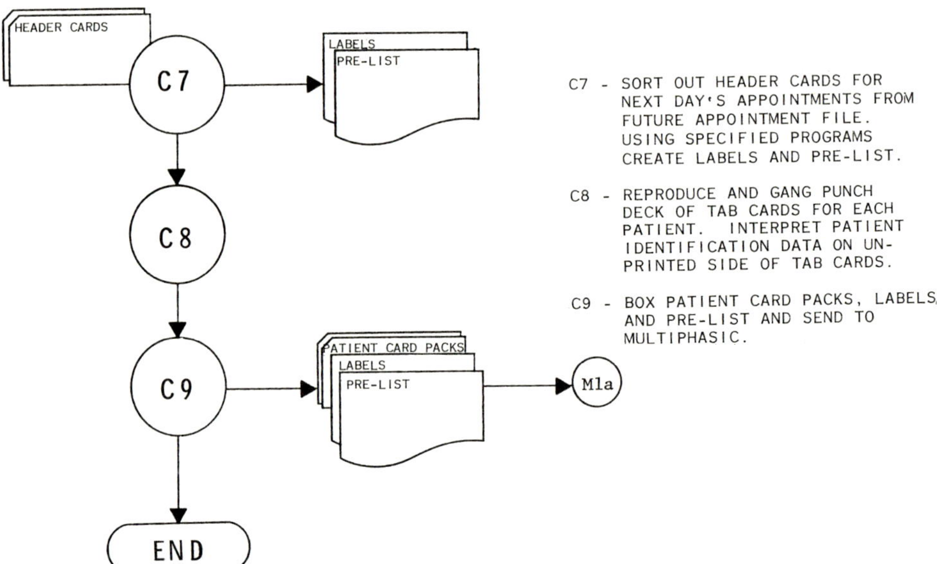

C7 - SORT OUT HEADER CARDS FOR NEXT DAY'S APPOINTMENTS FROM FUTURE APPOINTMENT FILE. USING SPECIFIED PROGRAMS CREATE LABELS AND PRE-LIST.

C8 - REPRODUCE AND GANG PUNCH DECK OF TAB CARDS FOR EACH PATIENT. INTERPRET PATIENT IDENTIFICATION DATA ON UN-PRINTED SIDE OF TAB CARDS.

C9 - BOX PATIENT CARD PACKS, LABELS, AND PRE-LIST AND SEND TO MULTIPHASIC.

Figure 5-7b.

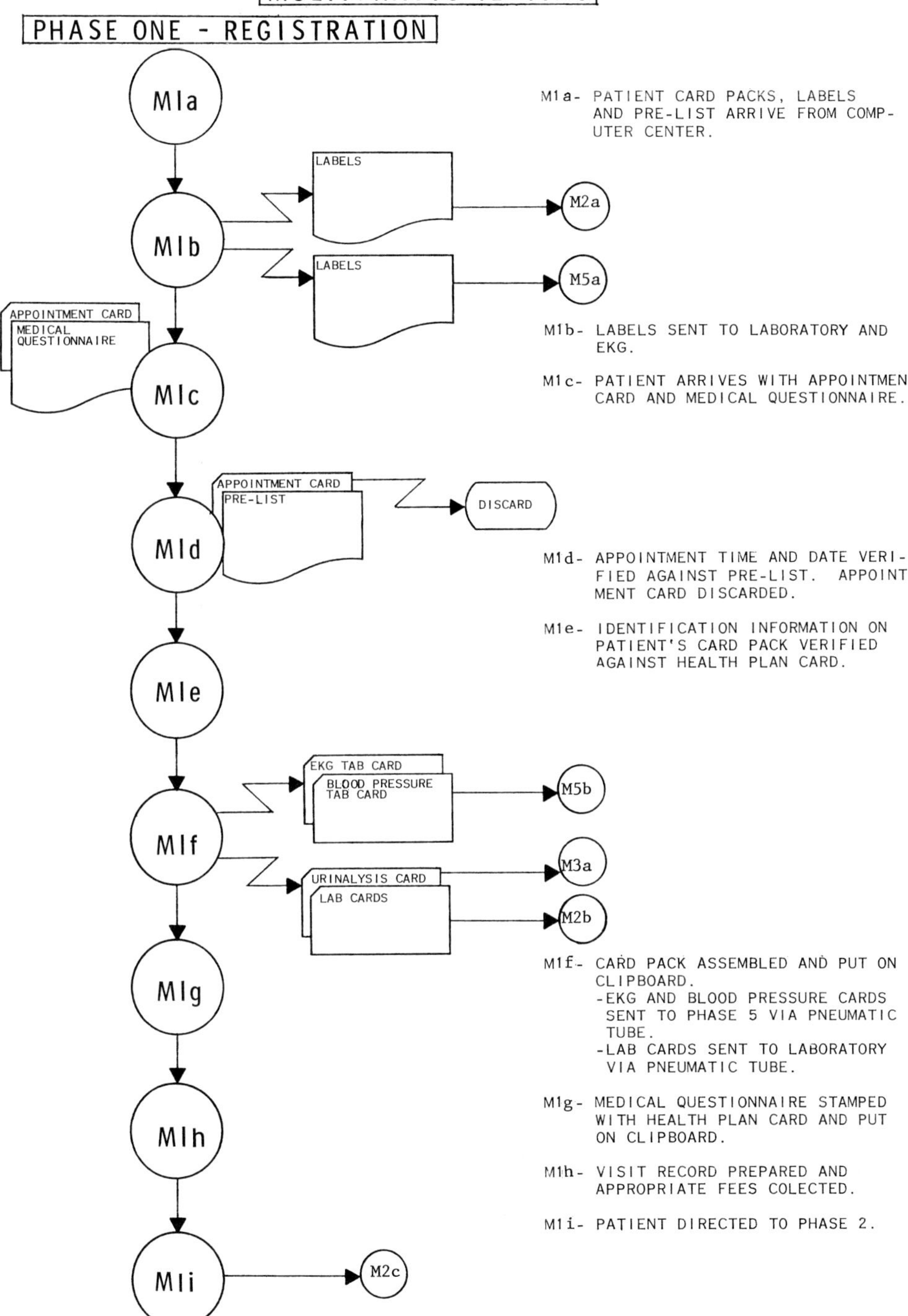

MULTIPHASIC TESTING
PHASE ONE - REGISTRATION
M1a
M1b
LABELS
LABELS
M2a
M5a
APPOINTMENT CARD
MEDICAL QUESTIONNAIRE
M1c
APPOINTMENT CARD
PRE-LIST
DISCARD
M1d
M1e
EKG TAB CARD
BLOOD PRESSURE TAB CARD
M5b
URINALYSIS CARD
LAB CARDS
M3a
M2b
M1f
M1g
M1h
M1i
M2c
M1a- PATIENT CARD PACKS, LABELS AND PRE-LIST ARRIVE FROM COMPUTER CENTER.
M1b- LABELS SENT TO LABORATORY AND EKG.
M1c- PATIENT ARRIVES WITH APPOINTMENT CARD AND MEDICAL QUESTIONNAIRE.
M1d- APPOINTMENT TIME AND DATE VERIFIED AGAINST PRE-LIST. APPOINTMENT CARD DISCARDED.
M1e- IDENTIFICATION INFORMATION ON PATIENT'S CARD PACK VERIFIED AGAINST HEALTH PLAN CARD.
M1f- CARD PACK ASSEMBLED AND PUT ON CLIPBOARD.
-EKG AND BLOOD PRESSURE CARDS SENT TO PHASE 5 VIA PNEUMATIC TUBE.
-LAB CARDS SENT TO LABORATORY VIA PNEUMATIC TUBE.
M1g- MEDICAL QUESTIONNAIRE STAMPED WITH HEALTH PLAN CARD AND PUT ON CLIPBOARD.
M1h- VISIT RECORD PREPARED AND APPROPRIATE FEES COLECTED.
M1i- PATIENT DIRECTED TO PHASE 2.

Figure 5-7c.

PHASE TWO - VENIPUNCTURE

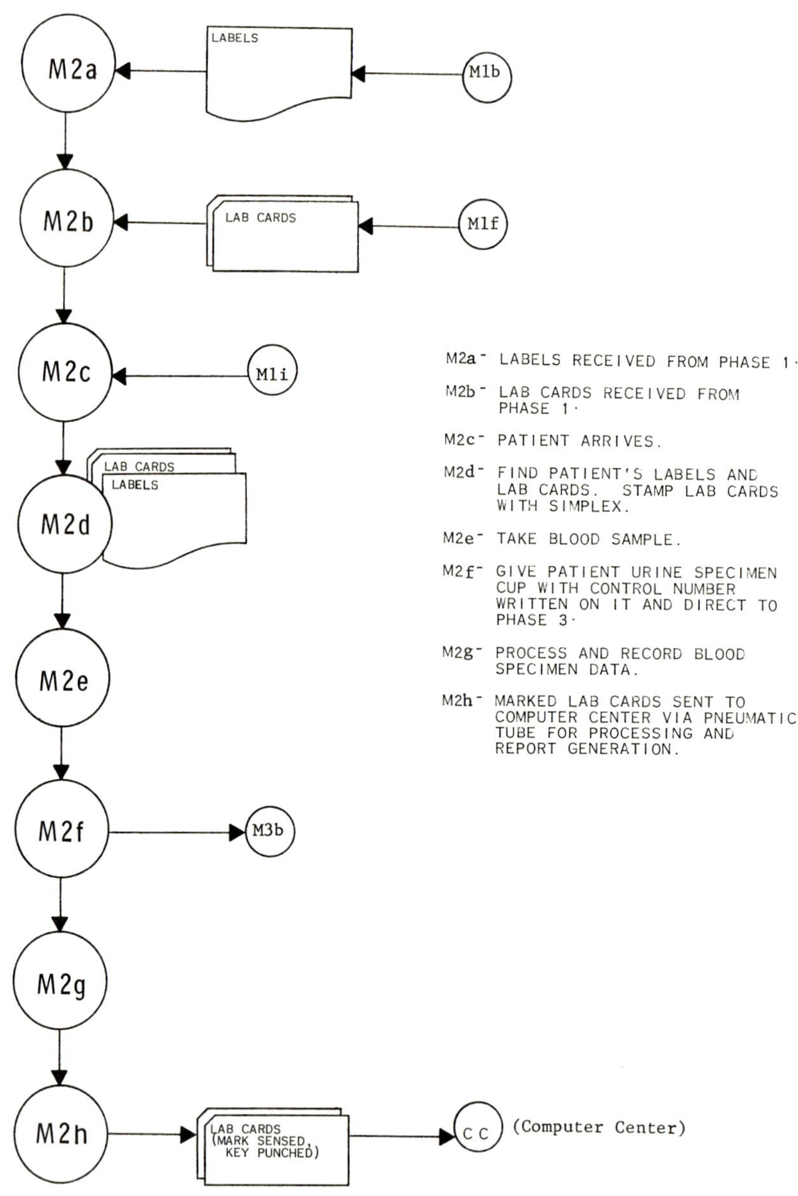
LABELS
M2a
M1b
LAB CARDS
M2b
M1f
M2c
M1i
LAB CARDS
LABELS
M2d
M2e
M2f
M3b
M2g
M2h
LAB CARDS
(MARK SENSED,
KEY PUNCHED)
C C
(Computer Center)

M2a - LABELS RECEIVED FROM PHASE 1.
M2b - LAB CARDS RECEIVED FROM PHASE 1.
M2c - PATIENT ARRIVES.
M2d - FIND PATIENT'S LABELS AND LAB CARDS. STAMP LAB CARDS WITH SIMPLEX.
M2e - TAKE BLOOD SAMPLE.
M2f - GIVE PATIENT URINE SPECIMEN CUP WITH CONTROL NUMBER WRITTEN ON IT AND DIRECT TO PHASE 3.
M2g - PROCESS AND RECORD BLOOD SPECIMEN DATA.
M2h - MARKED LAB CARDS SENT TO COMPUTER CENTER VIA PNEUMATIC TUBE FOR PROCESSING AND REPORT GENERATION.

Figure 5-7d.

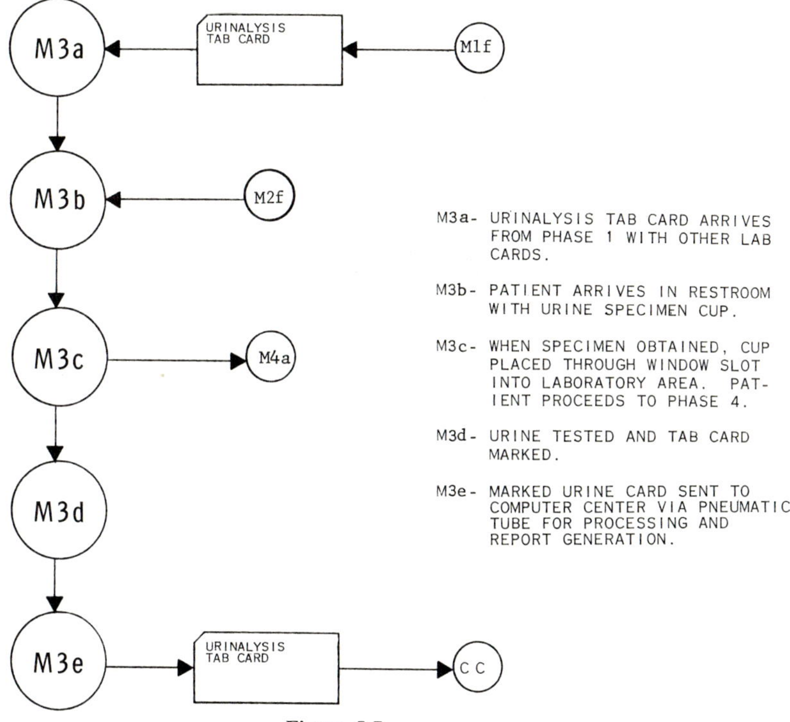

Figure 5-7e.

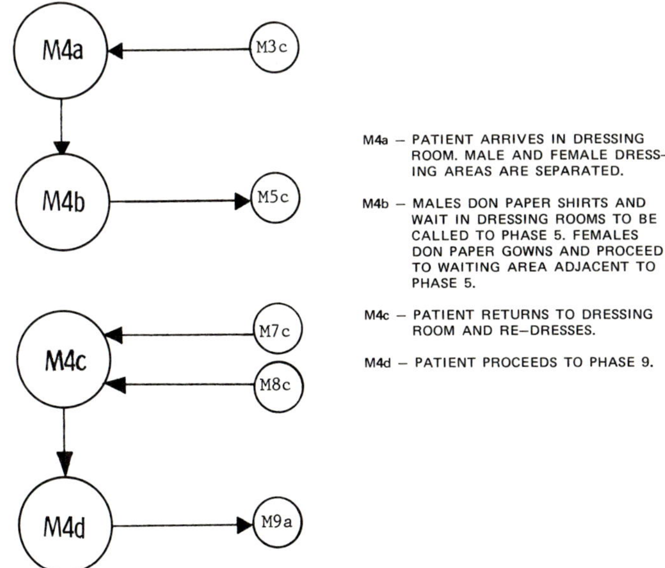

Figure 5-7f.

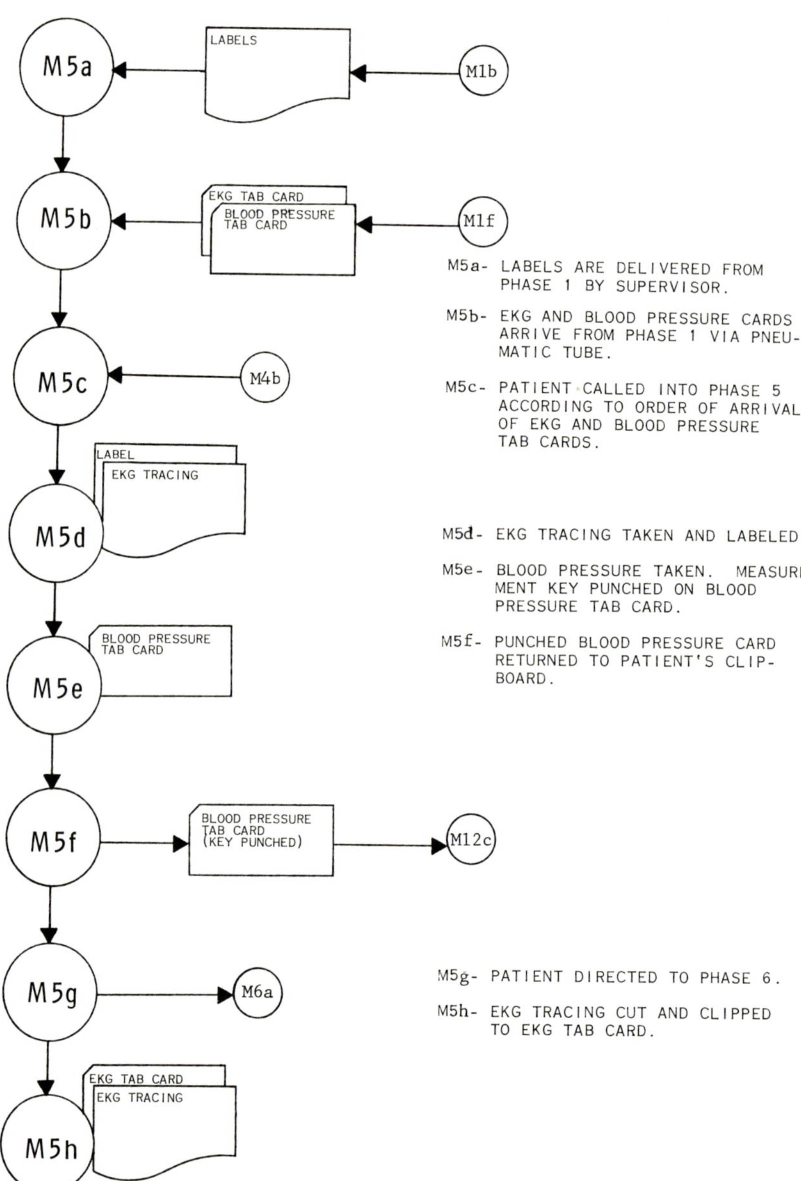

PHASE FIVE - EKG AND BLOOD PRESSURE
M5a
LABELS
M1b
M5b
EKG TAB CARD
BLOOD PRESSURE TAB CARD
M1f
M5a- LABELS ARE DELIVERED FROM PHASE 1 BY SUPERVISOR.
M5b- EKG AND BLOOD PRESSURE CARDS ARRIVE FROM PHASE 1 VIA PNEUMATIC TUBE.
M5c
M4b
M5c- PATIENT CALLED INTO PHASE 5 ACCORDING TO ORDER OF ARRIVAL OF EKG AND BLOOD PRESSURE TAB CARDS.
LABEL
EKG TRACING
M5d
M5d- EKG TRACING TAKEN AND LABELED.
M5e- BLOOD PRESSURE TAKEN. MEASUREMENT KEY PUNCHED ON BLOOD PRESSURE TAB CARD.
BLOOD PRESSURE TAB CARD
M5e
M5f- PUNCHED BLOOD PRESSURE CARD RETURNED TO PATIENT'S CLIPBOARD.
M5f
BLOOD PRESSURE TAB CARD (KEY PUNCHED)
M12c
M5g
M6a
M5g- PATIENT DIRECTED TO PHASE 6.
M5h- EKG TRACING CUT AND CLIPPED TO EKG TAB CARD.
EKG TAB CARD
EKG TRACING
M5h

Figure 5-7g.

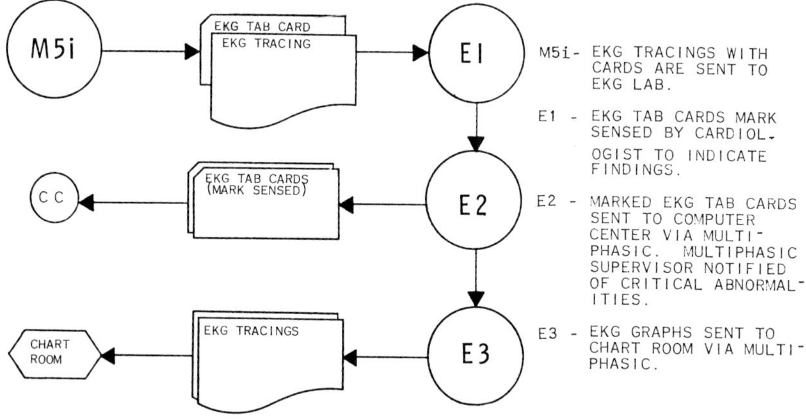

PHASE SIX - SPIROMETRY AND ANTHROPOMETRY

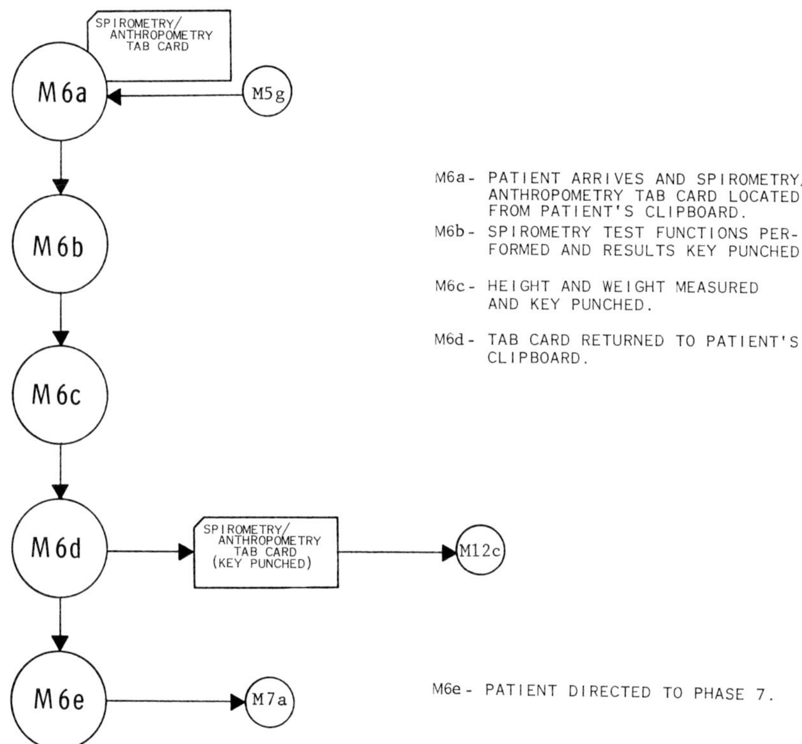

Figure 5-7h.

PHASE SEVEN - CHEST X-RAY

CHEST X-RAY
TAB CARD
M7a
M6e
M7b
M7c
MALES
M4c
FEMALES UNDER
48 YEARS OF AGE
M4c
FEMALES
OVER 48
M8a
M7d
M7e
CHEST X-RAY
TAB CARD
CHEST FILM
R1
CHEST X-RAY
TAB CARDS
(MARK SENSED)
CC
R2
R3
CHEST X-RAY
TAB CARDS
(PROCESSED)
CC
R4
R5

M7a- PATIENT ARRIVES AND CHEST
X-RAY TAB CARD LOCATED.

M7b- CHEST X-RAY TAKEN.

M7c- MALES AND WOMEN UNDER 48 WITH
NO PRIOR MASTECTOMIES DIRECTED
TO DRESSING ROOMS.
WOMEN OVER 48 OR WITH PRIOR
MASTECTOMIES DIRECTED TO PHASE 8.

M7d- FILM DEVELOPED.

M7e- FILM AND CHEST X-RAY TAB CARDS
SENT TO RADIOLOGIST FOR INTER-
PRETATION VIA MULTIPHASIC RUNNER.

R1 - CHEST X-RAY TAB CARD MARK
SENSED BY RADIOLOGIST TO
INDICATE FINDINGS.

R2 - CHEST X-RAY TAB CARDS TO
COMPUTER CENTER VIA MULTIPHASIC
PNEUMATIC TUBE.

R3 - FILM RETAINED UNTIL PROCESSED
TAB CARDS RETURNED FROM
COMPUTER CENTER.

R4 - PROCESSED CHEST X-RAY TAB
CARDS RETURNED FROM
COMPUTER CENTER VIA MULTI-
PHASIC RUNNER.

R5 - INDIVIDUAL FILM ATTACHED
TO EACH TAB CARD.

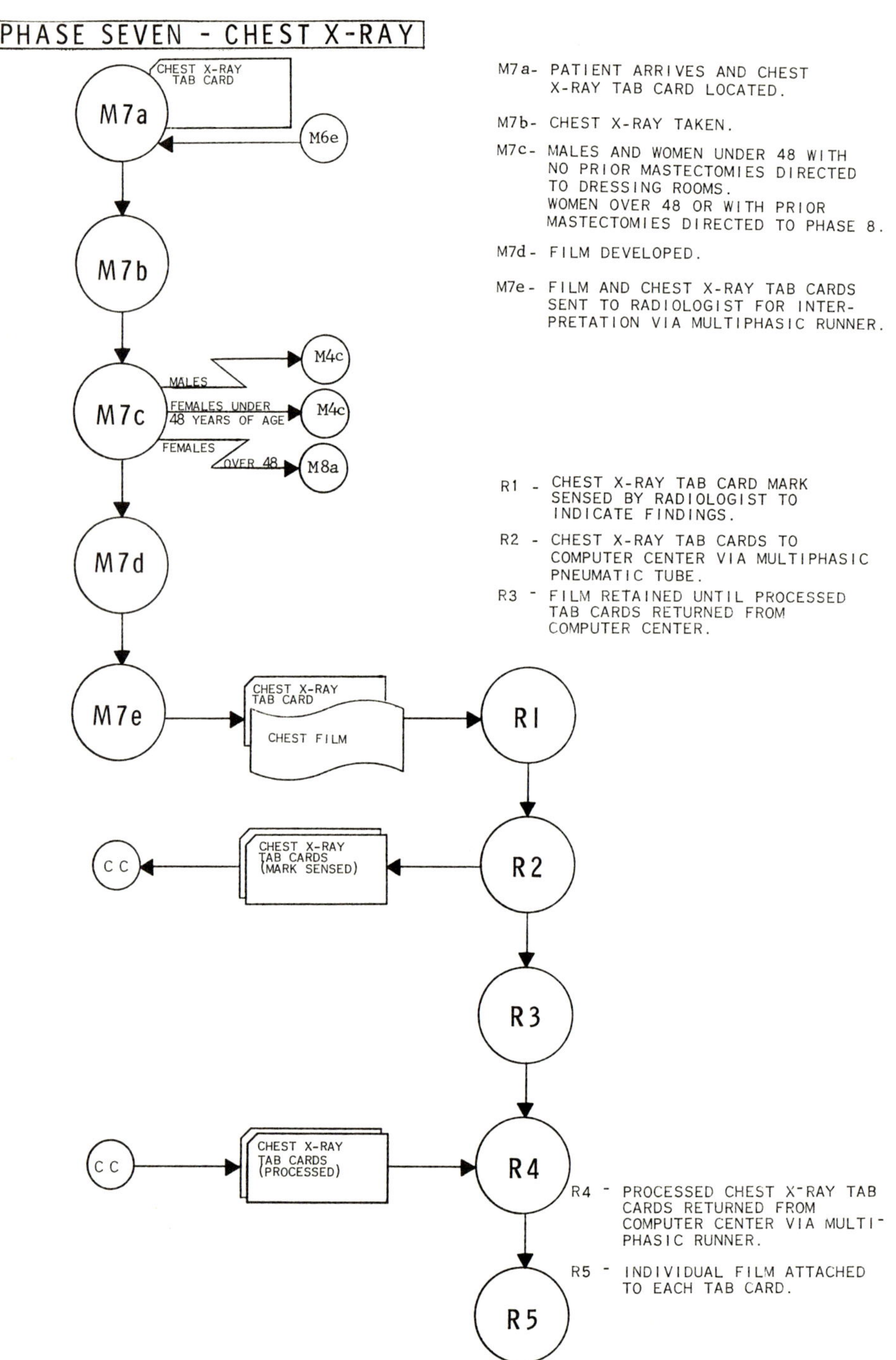

Figure 5-7i.

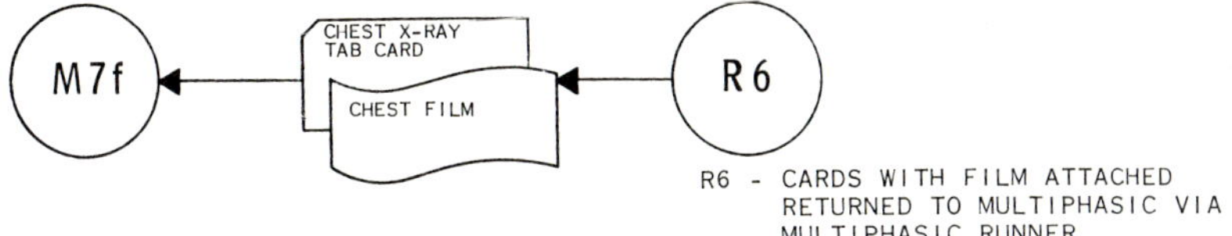

R6 - CARDS WITH FILM ATTACHED
RETURNED TO MULTIPHASIC VIA
MULTIPHASIC RUNNER.

M7f- CHEST X-RAY TAB CARDS (WITH
FILM ATTACHED) FILED BY MED-
ICAL RECORD NUMBER.

PHASE EIGHT - MAMMOGRAPHY

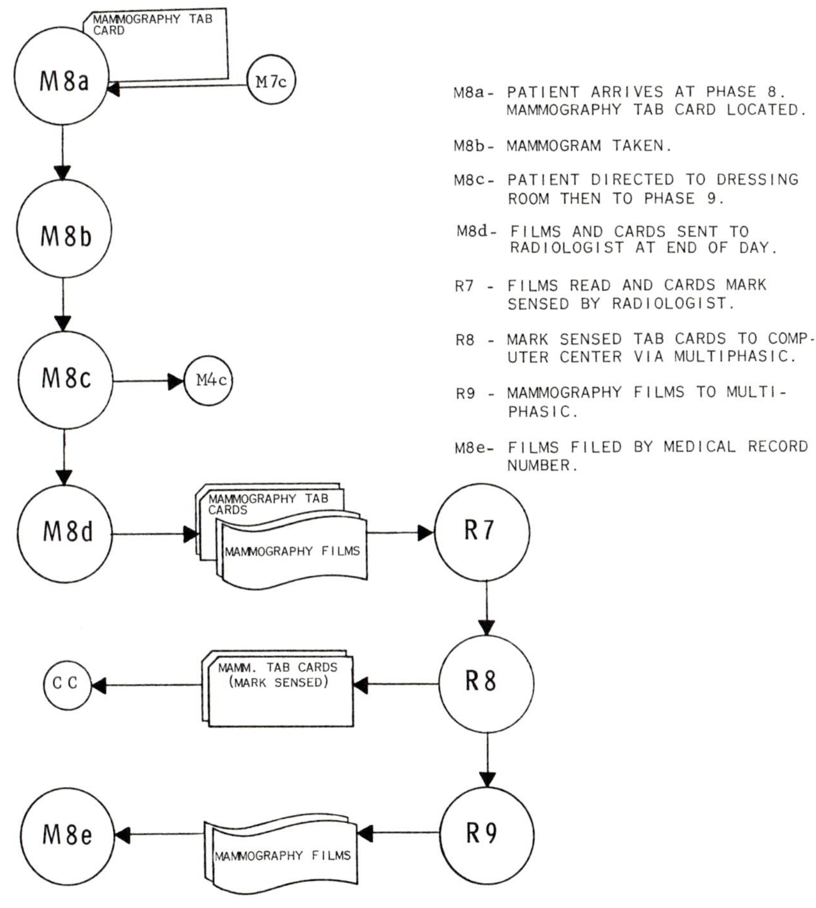

M8a- PATIENT ARRIVES AT PHASE 8.
MAMMOGRAPHY TAB CARD LOCATED.

M8b- MAMMOGRAM TAKEN.

M8c- PATIENT DIRECTED TO DRESSING
ROOM THEN TO PHASE 9.

M8d- FILMS AND CARDS SENT TO
RADIOLOGIST AT END OF DAY.

R7 - FILMS READ AND CARDS MARK
SENSED BY RADIOLOGIST.

R8 - MARK SENSED TAB CARDS TO COMP-
UTER CENTER VIA MULTIPHASIC.

R9 - MAMMOGRAPHY FILMS TO MULTI-
PHASIC.

M8e- FILMS FILED BY MEDICAL RECORD
NUMBER.

Figure 5-7j.

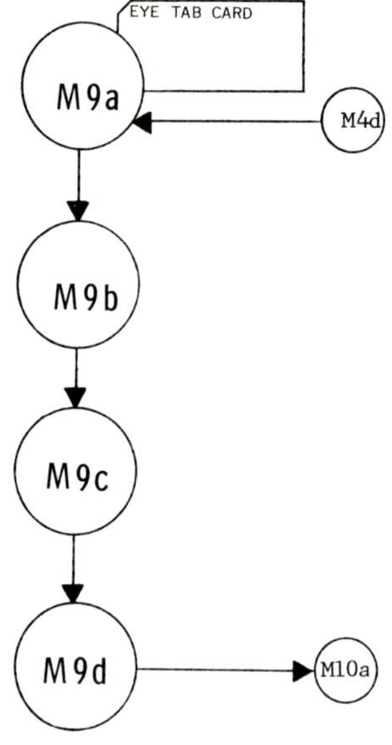

M9a- PATIENT ARRIVES FROM DRESSING ROOM AND EYE CARD LOCATED.

M9b- VISUAL ACUITY CHECKED AND MARK SENSED.

M9c- EYE CARD RETURNED TO CLIPBOARD.

M9d- PATIENT DIRECTED TO PHASE 10.

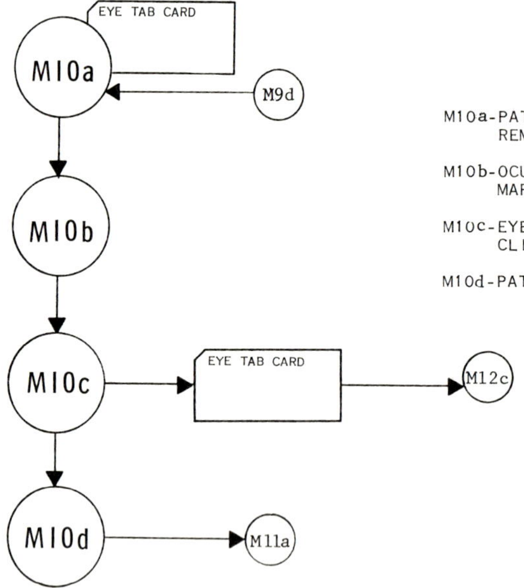

M10a-PATIENT ARRIVES AND EYE CARD REMOVED FROM CLIPBOARD.

M10b-OCULAR TENSION MEASURED AND MARK SENSED ON EYE CARD.

M10c-EYE CARD RETURNED TO PATIENT'S CLIPBOARD.

M10d-PATIENT DIRECTED TO PHASE 11.

Figure 5-7k.

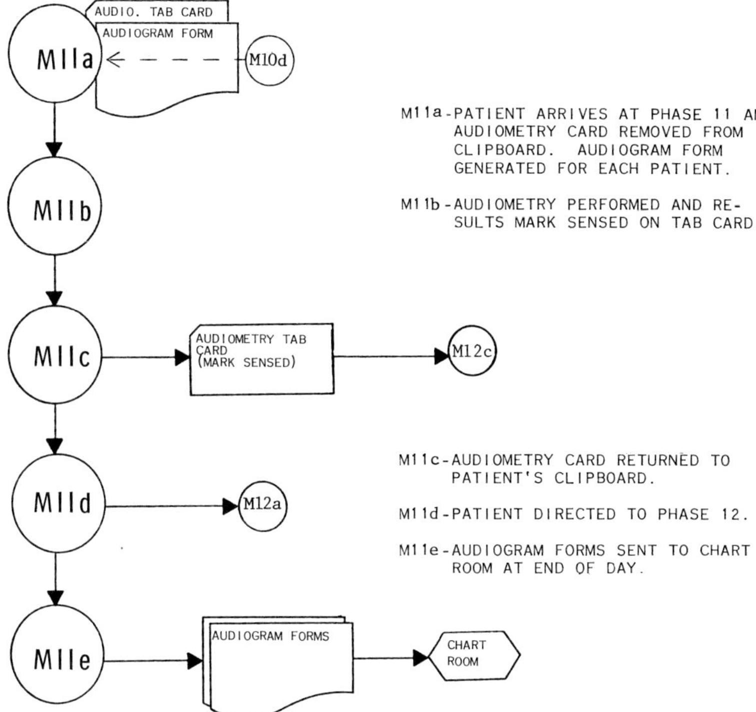
AUDIO. TAB CARD
AUDIOGRAM FORM
M11a
M10d
M11b
AUDIOMETRY TAB CARD
(MARK SENSED)
M11c
M12c
M11d
M12a
M11e
AUDIOGRAM FORMS
CHART ROOM
M11a-PATIENT ARRIVES AT PHASE 11 AND AUDIOMETRY CARD REMOVED FROM CLIPBOARD. AUDIOGRAM FORM GENERATED FOR EACH PATIENT.
M11b-AUDIOMETRY PERFORMED AND RE- SULTS MARK SENSED ON TAB CARD.
M11c-AUDIOMETRY CARD RETURNED TO PATIENT'S CLIPBOARD.
M11d-PATIENT DIRECTED TO PHASE 12.
M11e-AUDIOGRAM FORMS SENT TO CHART ROOM AT END OF DAY.

Figure 5-71.

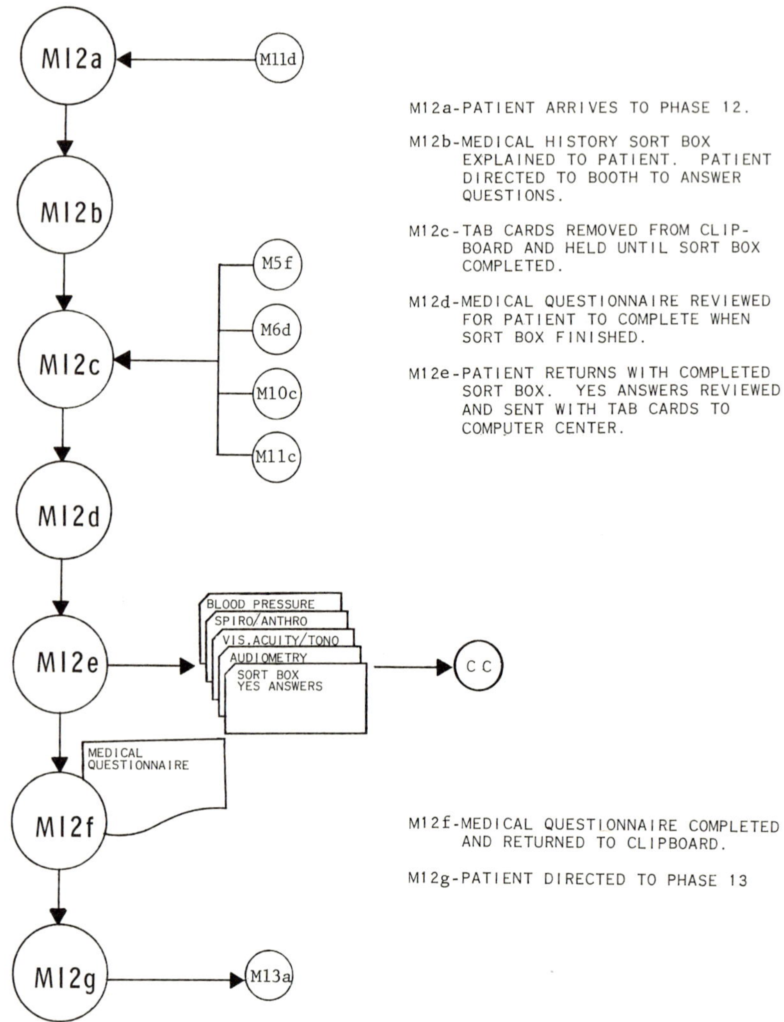

M12a-PATIENT ARRIVES TO PHASE 12.

M12b-MEDICAL HISTORY SORT BOX
EXPLAINED TO PATIENT. PATIENT
DIRECTED TO BOOTH TO ANSWER
QUESTIONS.

M12c-TAB CARDS REMOVED FROM CLIP-
BOARD AND HELD UNTIL SORT BOX
COMPLETED.

M12d-MEDICAL QUESTIONNAIRE REVIEWED
FOR PATIENT TO COMPLETE WHEN
SORT BOX FINISHED.

M12e-PATIENT RETURNS WITH COMPLETED
SORT BOX. YES ANSWERS REVIEWED
AND SENT WITH TAB CARDS TO
COMPUTER CENTER.

M12f-MEDICAL QUESTIONNAIRE COMPLETED
AND RETURNED TO CLIPBOARD.

M12g-PATIENT DIRECTED TO PHASE 13

Figure 5-7m.

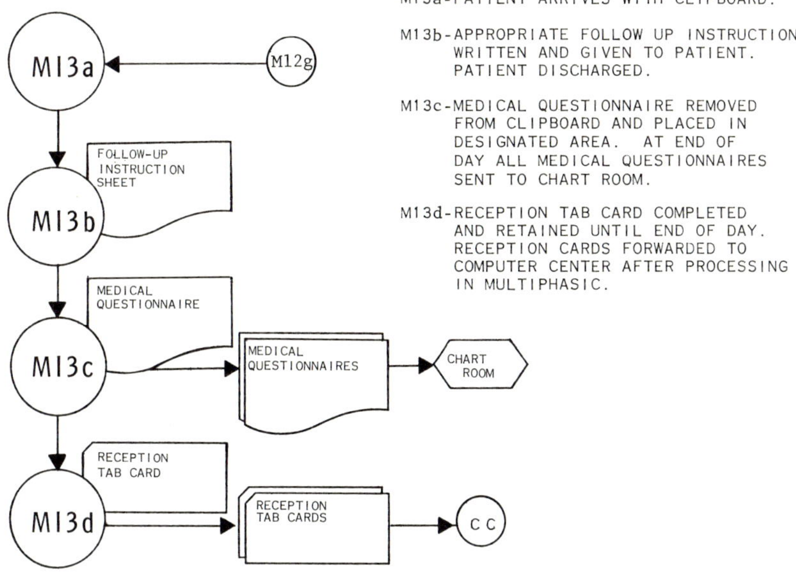

Figure 5-7n.

REFERENCES

1. Onions, C. T., ed. *Oxford English Dictionary*. New York: Oxford Univ. Press, 1955.

2. Maynard, H. B., ed. *Industrial Engineering Handbook*. 2d ed. New York: McGraw-Hill, 1963, Chap. 7, p. 3.

3. *Ibid.*, p. 4.

4. Collen, M. F. "Introduction to Multiphasic Health Testing Forum." *Prev. Med.* 2(1973):175–176.

5. Churchman, C. *The Systems Approach*. New York: Dell Pub. Co., 1968, pp. 41–43.

6. Beers, S. *Cybernetics and Management*. 2d ed. London: The English University Press, 1967, pp. 9–19.

7. Gilbert, F. "Multiphasic Screening Cut Down to Size." *Med. World News* 9(1968):60–61.

CHAPTER SIX

Specific Phases: Selection and Implementation

Edmund E. Van Brunt

A.   INTRODUCTION

Implementation of specific phases in a given multiphasic health testing service (MHTS) program logically follows their selection for inclusion in the MHTS. A test phase is defined as a set of one or more tests conducted at a single station or location (e.g., a room or part of a room). The test(s) at a given phase usually, but not necessarily, relate to a single organ system or function (e.g., blood pressure and electrocardiogram) or procedure (e.g., phlebotomy and clinical laboratory).

Selection and implementation of tests are inseparably related to the objective(s) of the multiphasic testing program, to the environment in which it is to operate, and to the available resources. This complex interdependent relationship is diagrammed in Figure 6-1, and elements of it are discussed in Chapters Two and Three. Once the precise mix of elements has been specified, implementation follows a number of dependent considerations, which are presented separately: systems analysis and facility design (Chapters Four and Five); data processing, instrumentation, and quality control (Chapters Seven, Eight, Nine).

Both the degree of comprehensiveness of any set of tests and the complexity of a given test will vary greatly depending upon their relation to the above factors. This is readily illustrated by considering the specific tests one might employ, for example, to monitor a single disease process (such as hypertension) for minimum adequate blood pressure control, for any known complications, or for research-oriented associated changes in physiology. Contrast the implied effects of such differing objectives on numbers and capabilities of personnel, choice of instrumentation, documentation (all aspects of data handling), quality control and cost, and expand these considerations to multisystem/multidisease orientation in different environments.

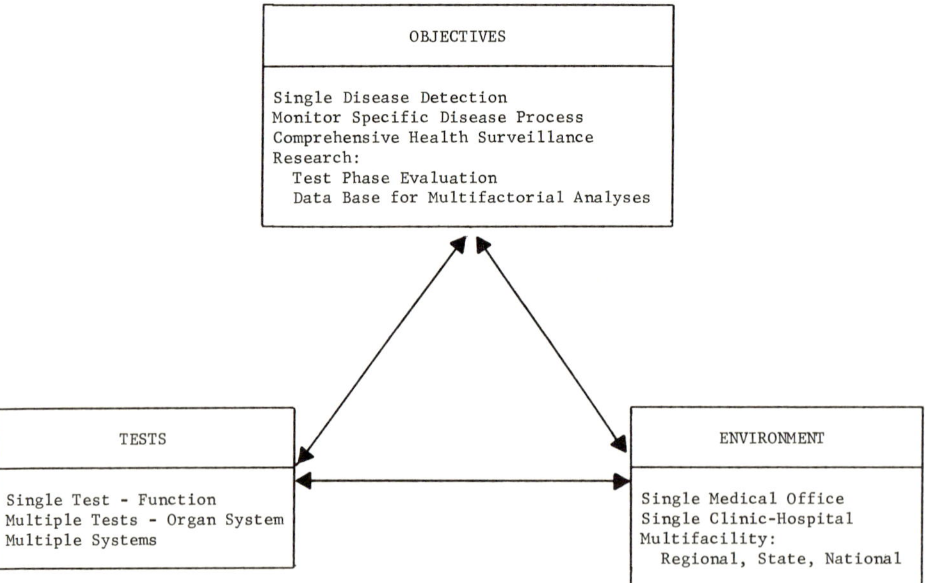

Figure 6-1.   Schematic presentation of the interrelation of program objectives, program environment, and tests.

Specific tests to be implemented will have been selected in accord with the considerations noted above and the criteria outlined in Chapter Three.

In 1970 the U.S. Department of Health, Education and Welfare published a set of *Provisional Guidelines for Automated Multiphasic Health Testing and Services* (AMHTS).[1-3] Taken as a whole, this three-volume set comprises one of the most thorough outlines extant of MHTS. The remainder of this chapter will follow, approximately, the organization of Volume 2, Sections IV through VIII: Scheduling and Registration, Medical and Psychosocial History, Organ and System Testing, Clinical Laboratory Testing, and Test Phases Using X-Ray and Other Radiations. Emphasis will be on selected medical aspects of screening. Allied topics of bioengineering, instrumentation, and quality control are discussed in Chapters Seven and Nine. There is no intent, in this chapter, to recommend one set of tests, or a method, over another; as indicated above, each must be selected in the light of program objectives and available resources.

In the planning, design, implementation, operation, and evaluation of any test phase, attention must be paid to the fact that a MHTS system of testing procedures, especially those used for large numbers of people, should not be allowed to create an impersonal or "cold" environment. Patients must be informed about the testing process in order to make appropriate arrangements for the required time, dress, and what to expect upon arrival at the MHTS center. Efforts should be made to maintain the highest possible degree of personal attention and individual dignity. This involves both the physical design and decoration of test stations and, more importantly, the appearance and behavior of the working personnel. Above all, frequent verbal communication with the individual patient, using his name correctly, will establish a sense of security and confidence. Conversely, little can be more dismaying to a patient than to be addressed by a number or an incorrect name. (See Chapter Three.)

Physiological measurements are notoriously variable. (See Chapter Nine.) Reproducibility, even among the same patients and under "basal" conditions, is difficult to achieve. The technical and professional personnel of the MHTS laboratory can contribute importantly to the validity of the test data by their competence, behavior, and appearance. Efforts must be made at all phases to maintain an atmosphere of calm, with attention to and understanding of individual patient needs. Time must be taken to assure that patients, who are usually cooperative, willing to please, but nonetheless apprehensive, understand fully what is expected of them. Their level of understanding and cooperation will materially influence the outcomes of most tests.

In addition to careful training of personnel in the operation of the phase(s) for which they will be responsible, their performance must be checked periodically by the supervisory staff in order to maintain good quality control.

Most testing phases can be operated very well by trained nonprofessional technicians. Exceptions would seem to be those phases where there is direct manipulation or instrumentation of the patient, as in glaucoma testing (tonometry), Papanicolaou smear (pelvic examination), and anoscopy/sigmoidoscopy procedures, where nurses or physicians are better suited by virtue of tradition if not training and experience. Obvious exceptions are phlebotomy and x-ray phases where technical staff have worked very well for many years. In some areas legal considerations will play a role in the determination of personnel requirements.

The routine testing of many subjects at a single test station becomes tedious and uninteresting for most personnel. Two immediate effects are a decrease in quality of test results (including increasing error rates in data handling) and progressive personnel dissatisfaction. Therefore, many laboratories establish a plan of training and operation whereby technical personnel may rotate among several different phases.

B. SCHEDULING AND REGISTRATION

1. Scheduling

The rate at which patients can be scheduled is a function of several variables, including age, sex, level of understanding of procedures (e.g., following instructions, dealing with questionnaires), and whether or not selective screening is practiced within the same program; i.e., whether different groups of patients to be screened receive different groups of tests, and whether these different patient groups are screened as cohorts or mixed together. For a given set of conditions, average times per procedure per patient can be measured and appropriate numbers of patients scheduled for a given number of operating hours. Consideration must be given to the possibility of testing more than one patient at a time in those stations where the procedure requires longer periods of time, e.g., audiometry, ECG, history-taking. (See Chapter Five.)

Scheduling of mixed men, women, and children has been done; adequate arrangements for privacy must be made where appropriate. It is the general experience that perfectly smooth patient "flow" is not possible to attain; accordingly, waiting areas near the test stations will be required.

Long and short appointment lead times and dealing with unscheduled arrivals are a function of program objectives. In large programs, a narrowly fluctuating rate of "no-show" patients can be measured; in many programs a certain fraction of the predicted no-shows are "double-booked" in order to maintain a high utilization rate and minimize costs per unit patient. Depending upon the environment of the screening program, and the ulterior needs of people being served, operations and therefore scheduling may have to be planned for evenings or weekends in addition to more traditional times.

When an appointment is being made for a patient, sufficient information must be obtained to provide subsequently necessary confirmation of appointment (date, time, and place) and any other documents the patient may require prior to the visit, e.g., instructions concerning diet and forms to be completed in advance of testing.

2. Registration

Correct identification of the patient is a key procedure in order to initiate correctly his entrance to the screening procedures and arrange for appropriate followup.

Primary patient identification usually includes (a) a unique number, which may vary with the screening facility or program, (b) patient's name, (c) sex (also an important variable in the interpretation of certain tests), (d) birthdate (some programs use only month and year; also an important variable for test interpretation).

Secondary identification includes: (a) home and/or business address, (b) home and/or daytime telephone numbers, (c) names, addresses, and telephone numbers of followup physician and/or clinic facility/department, and (d) as indicated by program tests and objectives, skin color, etc.

Financial information: includes Medicare or Medicaid number and identification number of any contracted prepaid health insurance program.

Consent forms, when appropriate, should be (or have been) completed by this phase for (a) parental consent for minors, and (b) release of medical information (MHTS report) to the followup physician or facility.

The registration personnel are often the first person(s) with whom the patient comes in contact. It should be evident that this first contact is one of the most important phases of the screening program. The working persons should be intelligent as well as knowledgeable about general aspects of the screening program, in addition to expected areas of patient eligibility, scheduling, followup procedures, etc. They must be understanding of patient attitudes and able to cope with usual individual questions. Multilingual capability may be a program requirement. Personnel must be aware of their responsibilities to patients and limitations with their individual problems; they must be willing to refer promptly to a supervisor as appropriate.

If mailed instructions, questionnaires, etc., have been reviewed and prepared by the patient, these might be verified at this phase. At some point in the screening program, appropriate followup arrangements must be made and/or verified. (See Chapter Ten.) Occasionally this is a two-phase process, occurring both at registration and "check-out" time (upon completion of all screening tests for that visit).

It should be evident that the registration phase is intimately involved with any formalized system of data handling; elements of these issues are discussed in Chapters Five, Eight, and Nine.

C. MEDICAL HISTORY

Most medical authorities agree that a carefully acquired medical history is a key factor in the detection of presymptomatic (occult) disease, in the identification of the cause(s) of symptomatic disease, and in the monitoring of the course and management of known disease.

Simply stated, the medical history consists of interrogating the patient. A large number of techniques have been used to elicit historical information. Virtually all of them are time-consuming. The content of the history is arbitrary and is primarily a function of program objectives and the "target" population. While the information is categorized in an arbitrary manner, most often one or both of two general types of data organization are used: the "traditional" and the "problem-oriented."

1. "Traditional" Medical History

This method of organization includes the following:

(a) Patient identification and demographic data (see above, B.2, Registration).

(b) Chief complaint—includes the main reason(s) the patient is seeking medical consultation. Sometimes this is referred to as "reason for visit."

(c) Past medical history—includes significant diseases, procedures and treatments, and known allergies.

(d) Interval history—an interrogation with the objective of updating a previously acquired medical history, wherein indicators of change in health status and related factors are sought.

(e) Family history—includes known diseases occurring in blood relatives and cohabitants.

(f) Psychosocial history—includes education, occupation, vocational activities, marital/family unit status, and habits such as smoking of tobacco or other materials, use of nonmedicinal drugs and nutritional peculiarities or "fads." More detailed psychological testing has been performed in many programs and a number of tests have been devised, such as the well-known Minnesota Multiphasic Personality Inventory (MMPI) and the California Psychological Inventory; a large literature deals with these issues and childhood and infant development[4-6] (See also Chapter Fourteen.)

(g) Review of systems—includes questions directed at eliciting recent and/or current symptoms that might indicate malfunction of specific organ systems.

2. Problem-Oriented History

Traditionally organized information may be rearranged into sets of data relating to specific patient "problems." The latter phenomena may be in the form of specific symptoms, recognized disease processes or psychosocial aberrations. The absence of problems does not in itself constitute a problem and does not interfere with this method of data organization. The relative merits of these two methods have been discussed extensively[7-9] and will not be pursued here.

Traditionally, the interrogation process has occurred on a one-to-one doctor-patient basis. Economic considerations render this method unacceptable for purposes of testing relatively large numbers of people. Accordingly, a number of technological methods have been developed to elicit selected historical data. Wakefield and Yarnall[10] have discussed different design approaches for medical history acquisition; each principal method is considered separately, with descriptions of methods, data handling characteristics, performance-cost relationships where known, and names and locations of individuals or centers having experience with each method. Methods discussed include self-administered questionnaires, punch-card devices, visual or graphic displays using programmed film strips, slide projection, television or cathode ray tube (CRT) technology and linear, multilevel, and branched question sequences.

McLean et al. have compiled a bibliography (720 entries) of manual, automated, and computer-assisted history-taking techniques.[11] None of the "automated" techniques completely substitutes for the individually conducted history, where the nuances of speech behavior and subjective chronological relationships are of a complexity beyond the scope of any current technological methods. None of the techniques is optimal for all patients.

As the content of the history is a function of the target population and MHTS program objectives, so are the methods by which it is acquired.

The social and educational characteristics of the patients will affect the validity and reproducibility of data for each level of complexity of the data collection method(s). Language content and the structuring and interrelationship of the questions will have further implications as to the methods of presentation of questions to patients. A detailed analysis of these issues, and of the technological support for obtaining clinical history information in MHTS, has been made by Johns.[12]

Self-administered patient questionnaires pose special problems of reliability. Reliability can be affected by the precision of words used, the avoidance of ambiguous terms, the degree of motivation of the patient, and the physical format and length of the questionnaire.[13]

Many questionnaires contain built-in tests of reproducibility, usually by repetition of some of the questions; alternatively, consistency can be assessed by multilevel or branching techniques. If these are reviewed by a knowledgeable person, with the patient at hand, some assessment of validity can be made. At present there are no known automated (programmed) methods of question validation that weight responses in any way that is clinically useful. Conversely, automated weighting of responses based upon such validation tests may improve accuracy of statistical research.

Presentation of historical information to the followup clinician poses a singularly difficult problem. Long detailed histories are difficult to read and evaluate in the times usually allotted for followup, while short summary historical statements imply a prior interpretation of more information or an abbreviated history, both of which the clinician finds difficult to accept at face value. The principal advantages of MHTS histories include the potential for improved standardization across large numbers of patients, multilingual capability with attendant increased validity and acceptance (economically difficult and very seldom taken advantage of), and marked reduction in the ratio of examiners to examinees.

D. CARDIOVASCULAR TESTS

Only noninvasive tests have been used in screening programs to date. In addition to the medical history, the following tests are used to estimate functional status of parts of the cardiovascular system. Taken as a whole they are, with the exception of the electrocardiogram, imprecise. They do not provide detailed measures of cardiac function such as cardiac output, peripheral arterial resistance, oximetric or other specific information. Thus, cardiovascular screening tests as currently employed are not detailed diagnostic studies per se; rather they serve as indicators of the possible presence of cardiovascular malfunction.

1. Electrocardiogram (ECG)

Several variations of electrocardiographic recording are done currently. Three, six, nine, and 12-lead scaler ECGs have been done. Standard limb and augmented unipolar leads (I, II, III, aVR, aVL, aVF) can be recorded simultaneously, as can even the precordial leads (V_{1-6}), if appropriate multichannel recording equipment is available. The higher the number of simultaneous leads, the higher the unit cost and the longer the time required for completion. Testing is most commonly done in the supine resting position. This is the ECG technique least sensitive to the presence of coronary heart disease,[14] although treatment of normal ECGs by mathematical/computer techniques may enhance their sensitivity.[15] Masters

Two-step,[16] "step" ergometry,[17] treadmill,[18] or other form of stress condition[19] are not normally considered MHTS procedures, requiring longer time for patient selection, preparation, and test execution, and in most instances requiring the presence of a physician. Sensitivity of such tests is generally low, with a relatively higher specificity in asymptomatic patients; indeed, the ECG is but one indicator of coronary artery disease.[20] Patient relaxation during the procedure is important. Some laboratories utilize such environmental adjuncts as pictures on the ceiling and soft music and lighting.

The majority of ECGs are interpreted by visual inspection. Automated (computer-programmed) interpretation methods are available[21] and have both advantages and disadvantages over the human interpreter, the principal advantages being virtually unerring recognition of the "normal" ECG, and systematic inspection of the tracing data. Disadvantages include the requirement (in most places) that a human reexamine all (or most) abnormal tracings and that interpretive programs are not yet available for (1) comparing ECGs of one individual through time, and (2) altering decision criteria to account for historical data and, to a lesser degree, drug effects and nutritional status (e.g., nonspecific morphologic changes of ST-T complexes may follow the hyperglycemia induced by the patient having ingested a glucose "challenge" dose prior to the ECG test).

2. Vectorcardiography

Technical requirements of test execution and difficulty of interpretation continue to prevent the use of vectorcardiography as a screening method.

3. Phonocardiography

Phonocardiography is another technique that is difficult to standardize and execute reproducibly. Previous experience has suggested more accuracy in children, but with relatively moderate sensitivity and low specificity.[22]

4. Echocardiography

Echocardiography is a relatively new noninvasive method of measuring or estimating a variety of heart dimensions (wall thickness of right and left ventricles and interventricular septum, chamber "diameters"), functions (motion of valve leaflets, valve stenosis or insufficiency), and hemodynamics (estimated cardiac output).[23] Principal disadvantages are difficulty in standardization and reproducibility coupled with long time of execution.

5. Arterial Blood Pressure

This is the one cardiovascular screening test that is relatively cheap, noninvasive, of minimum risk, and generally recognized as one of the few indicators of controllable and sometimes curable disease.[24] Screening efforts are increasing the rate of detection of cases, and current emphasis on treatment rather than detailed evaluation is increasing the incidence of control.[25] Patient understanding and compliance is important, however, since current public awareness of the presence and course of the disease is less than desirable,[26] and both are required for adequate management of the disorder.[25] The tendency toward elevated blood pressure may be discernible at a very early age. (See Chapter Fourteen.)

The test is usually conducted in the supine position, but may be done with the patient seated. Careful standardization of conditions, e.g., test station environment, patient position, and cuff position (same relative level of same arm), and use of recognizable end-points are essential. Cuffs should be of adequate width to minimize variability due to arm thickness. Cuffs should be inflated rapidly to above the systolic level, then deflated at 3 mm/second or less until the Korotkoff sounds disappear, then rapidly deflated. The degree of precision required is debatable—the nearest two millimeters is usual in the United States; the nearest five millimeters is commonly used in Europe. Mechanical/automated methods are available. If properly standardized and calibrated (a problem for some instruments—see Chapter Seven), they are claimed to have the advantage of overcoming human observer variability. Whatever the technique, it is advisable to consider standard procedures as recommended by the American Heart Association.

Evaluation of orthostatic dynamics by means of a tilt table or other device to change the patient's position has not proved to be a useful screening method and remains a tool for more detailed diagnostic evaluation. More detailed, second-level or selective screening tests of patients with elevated blood pressure have been proposed in an effort to define subgroups requiring different treatment modalities,[27] but such testing requires considerably more time and facilities and carries an increased morbidity.

Hypertension is a condition of considerable magnitude in that an estimated 23 million people can be classified as definite hypertensives (over 160 mm Hg systolic or 95 diastolic), about half of whom are in the age range 35–64. This is an important problem because of the well-established association of hypertension with increased risk for myocardial infarction, stroke, and other cardiovascular diseases.

The Veterans Administration Cooperative Study of Antihypertensive Agents provides firm evidence as to the effectiveness of detection and treatment in reducing mortality of patients with diastolic blood pressure averaging 115 through 129 mm Hg. A similar study of patients with blood pressure averaging 90 through 114 resulted in mixed conclusions. Firm evidence does not yet exist to demonstrate the value of intervention in persons with mild hypertension, since patient compliance with a treatment regimen is frequently unsatisfactory; and, because the cost effectiveness of mass screening may not exceed that of the traditional medical care approach to patients with high blood pressure, some investigators have concluded that extending mass screening for hypertension into the population at large is not practical or justifiable at the present time.[28] Additional work needs to be done in identifying risk factors that help to identify specific target groups for screening, persons with mild hypertension who may be at greatest risk (including whether these persons at risk benefit from lowering of blood pressure), and to identify those who will progress to "organic" disease so as to distinguish those who should be treated. It appears more reasonable to control hypertension than to care for those who become disabled as a consequence of the disease. The exact levels of hypertension needing active treatment must be further defined. Once these issues are defined, a hypertension screening program can become an integral part of preventive medicine.

6. Tests Employing Radioactive Compounds

Imaging by means of a computer interface to a scintillation counter has been used in the investigation of myocardial perfusion ([201]Thallium salts) and ventricular ejection fraction ([99m]Technicium-Albumin complex). Neither procedure is economically or technically suitable as a screening device at this time.

7. Chest X-ray

See L.

8. Tests of Peripheral Vascular Function

There has been no important change in this domain since publication of the 1970 DHEW *Guideline*.[2,3] Techniques for measurement of cerebral and peripheral blood flow or determining structural changes in arteries are not sufficiently standardized or reproducible, nor do they have sufficient sensitivity, for routine screening of large numbers of people.

(a) The self-administered questionnaire for intermittent claudication has a relatively high specificity and moderate sensitivity[29] to the existence of occlusive ilio-femoral disease.

(b) Plethysmography, oscillometry, and pulse-wave velocity are not used in MHTS programs.

(c) Infrared thermography, tested previously for use in detection of impaired blood flow in a region (e.g., supraorbital, digital), requires carefully controlled conditions, and standards for procedure and interpretation are not reliable for large-scale screening (see M).

(d) If physical examination is a part of the screening process, palpation of peripheral pulses and of skin temperature are low-sensitivity indicators of peripheral vascular function.

(e) Venography is very costly, time-consuming, and invasive, carries a real though limited morbidity, and is not suited for screening of any patients other than a selected number of those already suspected of having lower-limb deep vein occlusive disease.

(f) Ophthalmodynamometry. (See E.)

9. Coronary Heart Disease Risk Factors

Besides the questions in the medical history, measurements of serum cholesterol and, occasionally, of triglycerides are often included in screening programs. It is generally agreed that high serum levels of cholesterol and triglycerides are associated with atherosclerotic coronary artery disease (CAD), the former possibly playing a greater pathological role than the latter in angiographically demonstrated CAD.[30] Evidence suggests that there is an autosomal dominant mechanism for type III hyperlipoproteinemia[31] and that the process of atherosclerosis probably begins in childhood.[32] It has been suggested that children of early heart attack victims be screened for hyperlipidemia.[33] Both hypercholesterolemia and hypertriglyceridemia can be controlled.[34,35] Arguments have been presented, however, that the usefulness of the protein-electrophoretic distinction between types of hyperlipidemia for clinical diagnostic classification and management is questionable.[36]

E.   CENTRAL NERVOUS SYSTEM

Although two newer methods (3 and 4 below) of detecting structural and, to a limited degree, functional abnormalities of the brain have emerged in recent years, screening tests in this area (including the medical history) are difficult to execute and interpret. The most useful are prohibitively expensive.

1.   Electroencephalography (EEG)

Efforts to reduce the considerable time and cost required to produce the standard EEG, including the recording of short (time) tracings of only a small number of bipolar leads, have not been successful enough to justify this method for MHTS use. There is variability in interpretation and, especially for short runs on selected head regions, a very low yield of recognizable abnormalities coupled with a low specificity.

2.   Echoencephalography

This noninvasive method is useful for detection of lateral shift of midline structure (falx cerebri). Ease of performance and absence of risk are outweighed by very low yield, lack of specificity, and costs.[37]

3.   Brain Scan

Imaging by means of scintillation counting of an injection of a [99m]Technicium-Albumin complex is used extensively in hospital medicine as a measure of cerebrovascular integrity and is capable of detecting some arterio-venous malformations, tumors, cysts, and inflammatory lesions.[38] Yield for unselected patients is unacceptably low, while the procedure is time consuming and requires expensive equipment and highly trained technical staff. The procedure is unsuitable as an MHTS screening test.

4.   Ophthalmodynamometry

Ophthalmodynamometry has been used as an indirect measure of ophthalmic artery pressure. The foot of a spring-loaded scale is applied to the optic bulb (both scleral and corneal surfaces).[39] The method suffers from considerable observer variability and low sensitivity.

5.   Computer-Assisted Tomography

(See L.)

F.   RESPIRATORY SYSTEM

Early detection of pulmonary diseases has been studied extensively because of their high incidence, their effects on the quality of life and human productivity, and, in the case of pulmonary tuberculosis, the additional danger of contagion. It has been demonstrated that the public will cooperate in mass ventilatory screening programs.[40] In most instances, however, excluding active tuberculosis[41] and a small number of structural pathologies (see L), the abnormalities of chronic lung disease that may be discovered are not readily amenable to control; currently available therapies reportedly have limited effect on the rate of decline in lung function.[42] Conversely, most authorities have felt that more effective public health programs relating to reduction of atmospheric pollutants, occupational hazards to respiratory function, and use of tobacco should more effectively reduce the morbidity, mortality, and possibly incidence of chronic respiratory diseases.[43]

1. History

Sets of questions relating to respiratory disease, symptoms, and occupation can be useful by suggesting the presence or absence, or risk, of malfunction. Systematized questionnaires have been devised (see C).

2. Skin Tests

a. Tuberculin skin test.   This is an established method of determining previous exposure to tuberculosis, but it does not distinguish active from inactive disease. Its greatest utility is in the detection of conversion from negative to positive reactor status in children; the yields are lower in adults. The tests are easy to administer, can be done by technical personnel, and are relatively cheap. In selected groups, self-reading or parent-reading of results may be considered as an alternative to a return patient visit.[44-46]

b. Coccidioidomycosis and histoplasmosis.   Skin testing might be considered in endemic areas.

c. Blastomycosis.   This skin test continues to be unreliable, with relatively high rates of both false positive and false negative results.

3. Spirometry

Vital capacity and timed expiratory flow rates are among the simplest of the many tests that have been used to measure various aspects of pulmonary function.[47-49] The maximum volume exhaled is the vital capacity; the most commonly used of the timed volumes is the percent of the vital capacity expelled during one second of forced expiration. Spirometers of various types (see Chapter Seven) are available at relatively low cost and are easy to operate. This test will partially differentiate obstructive from restrictive disease. In general it has very low anatomic or etiologic selectivity, although it can be of moderately high sensitivity.[50,51] Test results can be normal in individuals with some pulmonary diseases and may vary with age, sex, race, and such variables as smoking habits.[52-54]

Early problems of observer variability[55] and of establishing normal patterns[56] have been largely overcome by improved technology, including online computer-supported spirometry.[57,58]

A newer measure, that of "closing volume," has a reportedly higher sensitivity than conventional spirometric tests, but further understanding of the implications of abnormal values and improved standardization is necessary.[59,60]

The single-breath nitrogen (or oxygen) test is a low-cost and relatively simple test, a sensitive indicator of early pathological change in lung function, and perhaps can be used to predict which individuals in a high-risk group (e.g., smokers) are at increased risk of developing irreversible airways obstruction.[61]

4. Other Tests of Pulmonary Structure and Function

a. Pulmonary diffusing capacity.   The carbon monoxide (CO) diffusion test is an established means of detecting the presence of abnormalities that interfere with pulmonary alveolar-capillary gas exchange. While it is safe, simple, and painless, it requires expensive equipment and a skilled operator.

b. Single-breath xenon test.   This test yields information about distribution of inhaled gas to different regions of the lungs. While rapid and painless, it requires expensive equipment and highly skilled technical support and, like CO diffusion, is unacceptable for testing large numbers of people.

c. Bronchography.   (See L.)

d. Chest x-ray.   (See L.)

e. Videodensitometry.   (See L.)

5. Sputum Cytology

Low sensitivity as well as time and cost considerations render impractical this method for mass screening for neoplasia of the respiratory system. This type of testing has been suggested, however, for selected high-risk groups, e.g., heavy smokers with productive cough, plutonium workers, uranium miners, and those with occupational exposure to asbestos, chromates, sulfur dioxide, coal gas, etc.[62]

6. Bacteriological Tests

Smears or cultures of respiratory-tract secretions for tuberculosis are impractical on a large scale.

"Culpak" or equivalent culture of pharyngeal secretions is a moderately effective way of detecting carriers of beta-hemolytic streptococcus and might be considered for patients in regions where rheumatic fever and poststreptococcal glomerulonephritis are prevalent.

G.   GASTROINTESTINAL TESTS

The medical history remains the most practical screening tool available for detection of malfunction of this extensive system, which includes the mouth, pharynx, esophagus, stomach, small and large bowel, biliary tract, liver, and pancreas.

1. Mouth and Pharynx

(a) Inspection by a nurse or technician poses problems of interpretation.
(b) Cytological study of buccal smears has been suggested as a screening test

for cancer;[62] yields are not known in random groups, although unsuspected lesions can be discovered by this method. The technique is not appropriate for precancerous leukoplakia.

(c) Inspection by dental technicians is an accepted method of detecting dental caries and periodontal disease.

2. Esophagus

The only reasonable screening test available for visualization of this organ is x-ray fluoroscopy with contrast medium (see L).

3. Stomach

a. Test for gastric acid. The only method acceptable to patients is the Diagnex-Blue test, which indicates qualitatively the presence or absence of gastric acid. It requires that the subject swallow an ion-exchange resin tablet two hours before the screening urine sample is to be drawn.

Intubation (passing a flexible naso-gastric tube to obtain directly a sample of gastric secretions) is an invasive procedure that is judged unacceptable to patients.

b. X-ray. (See L.)

c. Gastric cytology.   Impractical because of invasive methods, high cost, and low yield.

4. Pancreas

The testing of fecal samples for evidence of pancreatic enzyme deficiencies is impractical for screening laboratories. Gastroduodenal x-ray with contrast medium carries a low specificity and very low sensitivity. Indirect evidence of adequate insulin production is provided by a blood glucose determination (see H.2).

5. Gallbladder

Visualization by x-ray with contrast medium is impractical in a general purpose MHTS program, in spite of a prevalence of gallbladder disease estimated at 6 to 9 percent of adult females,[63] because of patient preparation and radiographic requirements (see L). Simple "flat" films of the abdomen may reveal radio-opaque gallstones, which are found in an occasional asymptomatic patient and are considered to be precancerous by some.

6. Liver

(a) Indirect evidence of malfunction is provided by several available blood chemistry tests, including total and direct bilirubin, alkaline phosphatase, serum glutamic oxalacetic transaminase (SGOT), glutamic pyruvic transaminase (SGPT), lactic dehydrogenase (LDH), serum proteins, etc. (see K).

(b) Liver scan (imaging after intravenous administration of [99]Technicium) is safe and noninvasive but has very low specificity and, in the absence of abnormal blood studies, very low yield can be expected.

7.   Small Intestine

Only impractical and time-consuming x-ray procedures are available for assessment (see L).

8.   Large Intestine (Colon)

Colorectal cancer is one of the most common malignancies encountered, in both males and females, accounting for approximately 13 percent of all deaths from cancer in the United States.[64] Detection or screening centers commonly utilize up to three established testing methods, excluding the history and physical examination.

a.   Fecal test for occult blood.   Several test methods are available, with widely variable sensitivity and occasionally unacceptable numbers of false positives depending upon the subject's nutritional status and diet. Screening of random groups has been shown to result in increased yield of unsuspected colorectal neoplasm.[64] With appropriate preparations the false positive rates are from 1 to 2 percent while the positive yield is approximately 5 percent.[65] The more reliable methods require a long preparation time and careful patient cooperation, or rectal examination. The test is probably done more efficiently during the course of a routine physical examination, by physician or physician assistant/nurse practitioner.

Since bleeding from colorectal cancer sometimes may be intermittent, serial tests have been suggested in suspect groups, although there is no optimum number of tests.[66]

b.   Proctoscopy/sigmoidoscopy.   This test normally requires a physician examiner, although it would seem that a screening proctoscopy could be done by a trained physician assistant. With this technique, over 50 percent of visible cancers of the colon are detectable. The procedure is probably better done in the course of a separate visit.[67] The major drawbacks for testing large numbers of persons are time, patient preparation, and acceptability. The procedure has been generally recommended for persons over 40 years of age; the optimal frequency has not been established, and the yield of new colorectal cancer in asymptomatic persons, even over 40, is low. In one series of approximately 8,000 consecutive examinations in an eight-year period the incidence of newly detected malignant lesions by this technique alone was of the order of 0.1 percent.[68] An earlier study of 3,700 males and 3,700 females yielded the finding of single or multiple polyps (of all types) of over 3 percent, with a two-to-one dominance in males.[69] Three were shown by biopsy to be adenocarcinoma.

c.   X-ray: barium enema.   (See L.)

d.   Carcinoembryonic antigen (CEA).   Understanding of the role of this antigen reportedly contained in human colon neoplasms is incomplete. Testing methods (radioimmunoassay) are complex, and specificity is not known. At present the method is not suitable for screening large numbers of persons,[70] although it may have a useful role in the management of known colon cancers.[71]

H.   ENDOCRINE METABOLIC TESTS

1.   Phenylketonuria

Sensitive and reliable blood determinations are available today for the screening of newborn infants. (See Chapter Fourteen.) The yield is low, as it is for other disorders, such as galactosemia, but the costs of later care of unrecognized cases is very high.[72] Amniocentesis, a means of detecting a number of other inherited diseases, is not considered suitable for large-scale screening.[73]

2.   Diabetes Mellitus

This is a very common disease of carbohydrate-lipid metabolism with an increasing incidence associated with advancing age. Worldwide prevalence (in "prosperous populations") ranges from 2 to 6 percent;[74] in the age group over 60 years, the prevalence approaches 10 percent.[63] Because of increasing morbidity associated with poor control of blood glucose concentrations, particularly the desirability of avoiding episodes of ketoacidosis, it is important to detect the presence of new disease as well as to monitor management. Definition of clinically important hyperglycemia, however, has undergone reevaluation and change. In 1970 the recommended procedure was a blood glucose determination after a challenge oral load of glucose.[2] More recently, a single fasting blood glucose (FBS) has been suggested as having sufficient sensitivity to detect clinically important diabetes mellitus, with appropriate weighting of results for age, sex, and time of day.[75] If the objective of the MHTS program is to identify clinically overt diabetes, then the fasting blood glucose will be acceptable; if it is desired to study the response patterns of patients with a normal FBS but with postprandial hyperglycemia, then a blood glucose will need to be tested at specified intervals after an appropriate glucose challenge.

Intravenous glucose tolerance and plasma insulin determinations are not appropriate for large-scale screening because of time considerations and, in the case of plasma insulin, complexity of the determination. Self-testing by patients, using one of the several available urine testing methods, e.g., Clinitest (copper reduction) tablet or Clinistix (glucose oxidase) strip, has been done, with a yield in one series of about 0.3 percent new cases of diabetes.[74]

3.   Thyroid

Measurement of serum levels of total thyroxine (TT4), triiodothyronine (T3), and T3 uptake, most accurately done by radioimmunoassay methods, provides a relatively specific indicator of thyroid function in the asymptomatic adult. Individually, they are variably affected by the presence of some chronic illnesses and by any of a number of drugs (see K) that the patient may have ingested, and must be evaluated accordingly. This variability of circulating TT4 and of T3 uptake may be partly overcome by calculating the Free-Thyroxine Index, which has been shown to be a more stable "physiologic" index of the patient's metabolic status.[76]

The Achilles reflex (ankle jerk) half-relaxation time, measured by recording foot displacement via a light-beam assembly onto a strip recorder (photomotogram), has been used. The method is modestly sensitive in hypothyroid states, will not differentiate other causes of abnormal reflex, is poorly sensitive to hyperthyroid effects, and is not considered sufficiently accurate for general screening use.

4. Parathyroid and Bone

Determinations of serum calcium, phosphorus, and alkaline-phosphatase are those commonly used to identify possible disease in these categories (see K).

5. Gout

Serum uric acid testing has been included in many programs for the detection of presymptomatic gout. The specificity is very low, however, since the serum level depends upon many variables, including drug effects, weight status, certain occult or overt illnesses, etc. In the Framingham study it was found that a relatively high percent of men with uric acid levels of 8 mg/dl or more develop gout in their fifties.[77] It has been found, however, that over the short term, asymptomatic hyperuricemia can be present several years with no observable adverse effects,[78] and research is now in progress to determine whether this remains true for long periods (10 or more years).[79]

6. Hyperlipidemia-Hypercholesterolemia

Determination of fasting levels of serum cholesterol and triglycerides generally have been included in MHTS programs in an effort to detect those persons at increased risk of developing coronary heart disease (see D.9 and K). It is now generally accepted that high levels of blood cholesterol and triglycerides are definite coronary artery disease risk factors.

7. Serum "Electrolytes"

The traditional quartet of sodium, potassium, chloride, and bicarbonate comprise this group, and sodium and potassium have been included in a number of programs where there has been interest in screening for secondary hypertension. These measures are of very low sensitivity and selectivity. Ease of performing these analyses, however, and their low cost and relative accuracy, coupled with the fact that many people take drugs known to alter their values, probably explain inclusion of these tests in many programs where blood analyses are performed.

8. Fructosuria, Pentosuria, and Amino-acidurias.

Efficient testing procedures for Fructosuria, Pentosuria, and Amino-acidurias are not currently available for large screening programs.

I. GENITOURINARY TESTS

1. Kidneys, Ureter, Bladder, and Urethra

Tests are available that delineate selected aspects of structure and function and can detect the presence of possible neoplasia or infection.

a. Tests of the urinary tract

(1) *Urinalysis*.   Chemical analyses of a freshly voided urine specimen (see K) using paper-strip enzyme tests are almost always done for presence of protein, hemoglobin, glucose, and chemical evidence of the presence of significant bacteriuria. Microscopic examination of urine is not often done in large-scale screening programs because of high personnel costs and difficulties with quality control. Specific gravity is a simple, highly reproducible test but, by itself, has little clinical usefulness, having low yield in a general population and low sensitivity to most genitourinary tract diseases.

(2) *Blood tests*.   Serum creatinine and urea nitrogen are routinely done in many programs. Measurement of creatinine clearance is not feasible in a single visit because of the requirement for a timed urine collection; the test is thus prohibitively complicated for routine use for large numbers of people. The single determination of serum creatinine concentration itself, while an unreliable indicator of the adequacy of glomerular filtration (GFR), has a high specificity, i.e., if abnormally elevated is highly correlated with abnormal GFR.[63] Exceptions are in persons with active muscle-wasting pathology or recent severe muscle trauma.

(3) *Cytology*.   Cytological study of urine can be expected to have very low yield in the general population. Yields would increase if testing were confined to groups at higher risk of genitourinary cancer, such as those exposed to certain industrial chemicals, including naphthalamines, benzidine, and certain commercial dyestuffs.[62]

b. Tests of the genital tract.   Included here are tests for venereal disease and for neoplasia of the cervix uteri and female breast.

(1) *Venereal diseases (VD)*.   Gonorrhea and syphilis are, respectively, the first and second most prevalent venereal diseases in the United States. Both are curable diseases capable, in the undetected condition, of producing severe incapacity in the host. In general, the finding of test results that suggest the presence of VD must be managed with sensitivity to the potential social problems that are often associated with these diseases. State and local legal requirements must be met. At the same time, care must be taken to assure confirmation of disease with test(s) of the highest possible specificity.

(a) *Gonorrhea*.   During the calendar year 1974 more than 900,000 new cases of gonorrhea were reported; a larger number of cases (estimated at 2.5 million) exists, since not all are either discovered or reported.[80] The most effective test for screening of asymptomatic males and females involves obtaining a swab of material from either the male or female urethra or anus, or the female cervix uteri, and inoculating a culture medium (e.g., Thayer-Martin). Discussions of the efficacy of this type of testing and attendant problems have been published.[81,82] This (culture) approach requires special handling of specimens, and followup contact with patients.

A shorter method is the two-minute Gonosticon Dri-Dot test, reportedly of high sensitivity and specificity,[83] in which a disposable test slide is coated with an antigen complex of *N. gonorrhaceae* for the detection of serum antibodies. Both methods require a modified pelvic examination in the female.

(b) *Trichomoniasis and candidiasis.*   Smear tests are not very sensitive in the asymptomatic patient.

(c) *Syphilis.*   Serological tests for syphilis are discussed in K.

(2) *Carcinoma of the cervix uteri.*   This is one of the most common malignancies of the adult female and, in the view of some authorities, the early detection and eradication of dysplasia and carcinoma in situ will prevent the subsequent development of invasive cervical carcinoma.[84] While it is generally accepted that carcinoma in situ and invasive cervical cancer are related phenomena, there have been varying opinions about the percent of patients with the former condition that progress to the latter, and the reasons for observed decreases in incidence and mortality for invasive disease in some studies.[62,85,86] In contrast to carcinoma of the breast, incidence is higher in women of lower socioeconomic groups and married women.

The principal method of screening for this condition is cytological examination (Papanicolaou or Pap) of a specimen of exfoliated cervical cells, which can be obtained by the patient herself (aspiration of secretions in the posterior fornix of the vagina) or by a physician-assistant or physician (using a vaginal speculum and appropriate equipment to obtain a scraping of cervical mucosa). The latter technique yields more satisfactory specimens. Standardization of procedures and quality control programs for the cytological laboratory have been published.[87]

Interpretation traditionally is done by cytotechnologists whose primary function is to screen out the normal smears, working under the supervision of a pathologist whose function is to review all questionable or frankly abnormal smears and formulate the report for communication to those responsible for followup care. In large-scale screening programs, consideration might be given to providing "consider" recommendations for further testing or other action, particularly in those circumstances where the followup physician is not a gynecologist.

Automated interpretation of cytological smears is not yet sufficiently reliable for routine use in MHTS programs. Steady progress is being made, however, in the area of computer program interpretation of cytological preparations.[88,89]

(3) *Breast cancer.*   Techniques are available for the detection of carcinoma of the female breast before the appearance of clinical manifestations. This is an important area to consider for inclusion in MHTS programs, since early detection probably improves prognosis.[90] Increased incidence is found in white females, unmarried and/or nulliparous, and in the upper socioeconomic groups. The most effective detection method would appear to be some combination of physical examination, x-ray mammography, and xeromammography, since there is a higher rate of detection by combined physical examination and mammography than by either method alone.[91] Questions have been raised, however, as to whether the benefits are outweighed by the hazard imposed by periodic radiation exposure.[92] The optimum age for screening asymptomatic women has not been established, but it appears to be approximately 50 years and older.

(a) *Physical examination.*   Examination takes at best a few minutes and can be conducted by either a physician, physician-assistant, or nurse.

All adult women should be taught the technique of self-examination. The MHTS environment provides ample opportunity to conduct the teaching sessions and to make available appropriate literature, using physician-assistant instructors.

(b) *Mammography and xeromammography.*   (See L.)

(c) *Thermography.*   This technique involves the use of a thermographic device that produces an instantaneous image, on regular or polaroid film, of the infrared emanation from the breast (entire chest wall). Normal heat patterns, and diffuse or localized patterns of increased heat, may be observed, but specificity for neoplasm is lower than with mammography. The test may be conducted by a technician; it requires about 20 minutes and the availability of a controlled constant-temperature (cooled) environment. It has been used as one of several elements in mass screening programs and is still in the process of being evaluated.[93]

As with positive cervical cytology and other findings, where there is the possibility of the presence of serious disease, care must be taken that the information is communicated promptly to the physician who is responsible for followup care.

J.   EYE, EAR, NOSE, AND THROAT

1.   Eye

Tests of visual acuity and intraocular tension are routinely done in many MHTS programs. Other tests, such as retinal photography, perimetry, and pupillary "escape" are seldom used as screening devices.

a.   Visual acuity.   Distant, near, and color vision can be tested with various charts, e.g., Snellen, Taeger, and Ishiharu plates, respectively. Testing technique is important for reliable measurement. There must be adequate background and object illumination; distances must be correct; and the patient must be instructed carefully. Misunderstandings are not infrequently misinterpreted as visual errors. If corrective lenses are worn, the report should so state.

Mechanized equipment is available (see Chapter Seven) and, while more expensive, permits a higher degree of test standardization.

A comprehensive review of various methods for testing visual acuity, ocular tension, and other eye functions is available.[94]

b.   Tonometry (intraocular tension).   It has been recommended that all persons over the age of 40 (and who are presumed free of important eye disease) should have periodic evaluation of intraocular tension. Glaucoma, a controllable cause of progressive loss of vision, is the second highest cause of adult blindness in the United States; the incidence above age 40 approaches 2 percent, and prevalence increases with increasing age.[95]

Various modifications of two basic methods of recording intraocular tension have been devised.

(1) *Impression tonometry.*   Typified by the Schiotz tonometer, alternatively the Bailliart, the technique is safe, inexpensive, and, after instillation of two drops of topical anesthetic, can be performed reliably, in less than one minute, by a trained ophthalmologic technician.[96]

(2) *Applanation tonometry.*   Several electromechanical methods are available and offer the advantage of inducing less displacement of the corneal surface. One

of the newest methods is based on the measurement of the amount of corneal displacement induced by a puff of air (no anesthesia required) by means of a narrow light-beam reflected from the corneal surface.

c.   Retinal artery pressure.   Ophthalmodynamometry is a method of estimating ophthalmic artery pressure by means of applying the footpad of a spring-loaded scale to the optic bulb, either corneal or scleral surface.[39] The method has low sensitivity and is not generally used as a screening device in MHTS programs.

d.   Retinal photography.   This test can be accomplished safely by a trained technician. However, even under very good conditions (adequately dilated pupil, patient cooperation, properly functioning equipment) there is a high rate of rejection of photographs because of marginal or unacceptable quality and, in the remainder, a high rate of observer/interpreter variability.[97] Accordingly, both sensitivity and specificity are low and cost is high.

e.   Perimetry.   Measurement of visual fields in the patient without visual symptoms is occasionally advocated by ophthalmologists but is a low-yield procedure as well as time-consuming and expensive to administer.

f.   Pupillary escape.   The Marcus Gunn sign of pupillary escape is an unsustained contraction of the pupil in bright illumination which, when more pronounced on one side, is an indicator of possible retinal or optic nerve pathology.[98] The swinging flashlight test is safe, cheap, and easy to perform, although it has low yield (less than 1 percent in patients without anisocoria) and questionable rates of observer variability.

2. Ear

a.   Auditory acuity.   The usefulness of tests of hearing ability lies first, in the detection of hearing loss in preschool and school age children; second, in the preemployment evaluation of persons likely to be exposed to high noise levels, or whose occupations require normal hearing; third, in monitoring persons already employed in jobs with associated high noise levels; and fourth, in detection of hearing loss in others who might be helped by sound amplification.

Yields are relatively high. An estimated 13.2 million persons age three years and over in the United States have been reported to have a hearing impairment in at least one ear.[99] Significant hearing loss has been found to be more frequent in men and greater in persons reporting exposure to loud noise.[100,101] Certain companies have implemented hearing "conservation" programs.[102]

Semiautomated equipment is available (see Chapter Seven) and capable of providing graphic and digital output of hearing responses to several different frequencies in both ears, separately or together. Multichannel capability permits the testing of several persons simultaneously, provides improved standardization, and can be operated by a trained technician. The testing environment must be adequately soundproofed. Patient understanding is very important; misunderstanding may easily result in erroneous recordings. Errors of this type are particularly common in young children and the aged.

b.   Rinne and Weber tuning fork tests.   These tests are part of a traditional physician-conducted neurological examination and generally are not done in MHTS programs.

3. Nose and Throat

Examination of the nose is done by means of visual inspection only, in the course of the routine physical examination, and is not normally done as a part of MHTS. Examination of the mouth and pharynx has been discussed briefly in Section G.

K. CLINICAL LABORATORY

Historically, in clinical medicine, analyses of body fluids and tissues have been conducted as a second level of investigation, to confirm or not confirm the presence of suspected disorders. With the development of MHTS, clinical laboratory data have been utilized in two new ways: first, in the confirmation of normal function and the detection of unsuspected abnormality; second, in the context of selective screening, in the search for abnormalities in persons known to be at risk of having certain disorders.

This orientation of clinical laboratory services carries different implications for patient management[103] and, because of the need to minimize false positive findings, has been stated to require rigorous quality control measures.[104]

It is a rare laboratory test result that is pathognomonic of a specific disorder. Conversely, the definitions of normality for blood and urine tests commonly will differ as a function of many variables, including the patient's age and sex, domicile, usual diet, time, quality and quantity of nutrients last ingested, time of day, physical activity status (including body position at the time of specimen collection), medications recently ingested, the presence of certain disease processes, and, not least, the method of analysis used.

Knowledge of the patient's medication (or other drug) history is especially important, since there are many known effects upon laboratory test results, due either directly to interference by the drug(s) with test reagents, or indirectly to alteration of the patient's physiological status. Table 6-1 lists but a few commonly used prescription drugs that influence a number of hematologic and chemical blood analyses. Comprehensive listings have been published.[105] While many of

Table 6-1.   Some Commonly Used Prescription Drugs, or Drug Groups, That Are Known to Influence Hematologic and Chemical Blood Analyses

Adrenocortico-steroids	Meprobamate
Allopurinol	Methyldopa
Amytriptiline	Nitrofurantoin
Anticonvulsants	Phosphates
Ascorbic acid	Probenecid
Barbiturates	Procainamide
Cephalosporins	Propranalol
Coumarin	Rifampin
Estrogens	Salicylates
Indomethacin	Sulfonamides
Isoniazid	Tetracycline
MAO Inhibitors	

these variables may have limited direct clinical significance at present, some are important in the study of states of normal for different groups and individuals. The same test procedures, therefore, may have different "normal" range values in different laboratories and, even within the same laboratory, for different groups of people.

From the point of view of patient management, test results should be correlated both with elements of the medical history and with the followup physical examination. In the MHTS environment the opportunity exists to select a set of laboratory tests for an individual on the basis of indications derived from the medical history, and similarly for groups with common historical elements, e.g., similar occupations, diets, etc.

Standardization of units for reporting test results has not yet been achieved, either within clinical laboratories or without. There is a movement in this direction, however, with the development of an international system of units (SI, see Tables 6-2, 6-3), which is being adopted by most nations and is beginning to be used in major medical journals.[106]

Principles of function and differences in equipment used in MHTS laboratories are discussed in Chapter Seven. Detailed discussion of clinical laboratory structure, staffing, analytic procedures, and quality control may be found in classic textbooks. More detailed procedures of this section can be found in such popular reference works as Todd and Sandford, *Clinical Diagnosis by Laboratory Methods*.[107]

Table 6-2.   Systeme Internationale Base Units

Quantity	Name	Symbol
Length	meter	m
Mass	kilogram	kg
Time	second	s
Electric current	ampere	A
Thermodynamic temperature*	Kelvin	K
Amount of substance	mole	mol
Luminous intensity	candela	cd
Plane angle	radian	rad
Solid angle	steradian	sr

*Also Celsius symbol C.

Table 6-3.   Common Prefixes

Prefix	Name	Symbol
10^6	mega	M
10^3	kilo	k
10^2	hecto	h
10^1	deka	da
10^{-1}	deci	d
10^{-2}	centi	c
10^{-3}	milli	m
10^{-6}	micro	μ

In general, only two types of specimens are collected and analyzed in MHTS laboratories: blood and urine.

1. Blood Tests

a. Collection and handling of blood specimens. Most blood constituents do not change significantly after a light meal, with the exception of glucose, certain lipids, and phosphorus; however, because of the possibility of lactescence (lipemia) in the postprandial state, a larger number of chemical determinations may be affected. Accordingly, blood specimens are usually collected when patients are in a postabsorptive state, i.e., six or more hours after food ingestion. Diurnal variations affect very few constituents (mainly adrenocortical steroids and iron) in any important way.

Peripheral venous blood (e.g., from the antecubital fossa) is preferred to capillary blood, where inadequate mixing may occur for a variety of reasons.

After appropriate skin preparation and tourniquet application, venipuncture with a vacutainer system reportedly offers an efficient means of specimen collection. There is a variety of specimen container volumes and anticoagulants available in sterile disposable units.[108]

Care must be taken that the tourniquet is of adequate width (about two inches or more) and that the time it is left in place (before venipuncture) is minimized.

Accurate identification of containers, work lists, and test-result documents is critical. A variety of techniques are used, including preprinted labels, automated realtime label printing, bar codes, etc. Positive error-free linkage must exist with the patients' registration and other test-phase documents. (These considerations are discussed in Chapters Eight and Nine.)

Tubes and syringes must be chemically clean. Chemically clean ware need not be sterile; conversely, sterile ware, necessary for syringes and needles, may not be assumed to be chemically clean.

Hemolysis is to be avoided. It interferes with analyses by means of release of erythrocyte contents into plasma and by affecting certain colorimetric or photometric measurements. Common causes of hemolysis are prolonged venous stasis (excessive time of tourniquet application), contamination (chemical, moisture) of equipment, too small a needle bore (20 gauge or larger is preferred), too rapid withdrawal of blood from the vein, too rough mixing, too rapid or rough transfer of blood to other containers, and prolonged contact of serum or plasma with blood cells (excessive delay in centrifugation/separation).

Centrifugation is an important procedure, and conditions for its use for different samples should specify both time and centrifugal force (not simply time and rotational speed). Formulas and nomograms to derive relative centrifugal force are available.[109] Freshly separated serum may be stored temporarily, without invalidating most tests, at $-20°C$, after rapid freezing.

b. Hematology

(1) *Hematocrit (Hct).* Hematocrit, defined as the volume of erythrocytes expressed as percent of volume of a whole blood sample, is one indirect measure of anemia. In practice, the relative or total cell volume is measured, including the "buffy" coat of mixed leukocytes and platelets. Both macro (Wintrobe) and micro

methods are available; the latter is the more frequently used. Careful attention must be directed to capillary tube bore and to time and force of centrifugation.

(2) *Hemoglobin (Hb).*   Hemoglobin is the principal protein component of erythrocytes, is the main vehicle for transportation of oxygen (O_2) and carbon dioxide (CO_2), and is also a standard indirect measure of anemia.

Several methods are available for determination of Hb concentration. They depend upon the direct measure of oxyhemoglobin, or derivatives such as acid hematin, alkaline hematin, or cyanmethemoglobin, comparing each to a known standard. Cyanmethemoglobin has been recommended as the standard method by the College of American Pathologists.

A large number of genetically determined hemoglobin variants exists, resulting in a variety of hemoglobinopathies;[110] S-S (sickle cell anemia) and S-C (thalassemia) disease are the most popularly known. Screening for many of these disorders is possible by means of electrophoresis methods; for selected abnormalities, rapid and economical tests are available.[111] Considerable controversy exists, however, over the social and economic issues of detecting and counseling persons with Hb abnormalities.[112-114]

(3) *Blood cell counting.*   Methods for quantitative determination of the concentrations (number per unit volume of whole blood) of erythrocytes (red cells), leukocytes (white cells), and thrombocytes (platelets) have been established for a long time. For erythrocytes and leukocytes, manual (microscopic) counting chambers are still used; however, for medium- to large-volume patient loads, electronic counting methods are the most widely used. (See Chapter Seven.)

Platelets are infrequently measured in MHTS programs, as are determinations of the distribution of leukocytes (differential white cell count) and erythrocyte morphology, since all three methods require special handling, longer time for completion, and a greater amount of technician time per test.

(4) *Red cell indices.*   Three computed numbers (indices) are used frequently for the determination of the morphologic type of an anemia. They are the mean corpuscular volume (MCV), mean corpuscular hemoglobin (MCH), and mean corpuscular hemoglobin concentration (MCHC); they are computed from three values: red cell count (Rbc), hemoglobin (Hb), and hematocrit (Hct) (see Table 6-4). Error in any of the three measures is reflected in the computed indices, reducing somewhat their reproducibility and reliability.

(5) *Glucose-6-phosphate dehydrogenase (G6PD).*   This enzyme, involved in erythrocyte metabolism, is deficient in a significant number of children and

Table 6-4.   Red Blood Cell Indices

MCV (mean corpuscular volume)	=	$\dfrac{\text{HCT (\%)} \times 10}{\text{Rbc (millions/}\mu\text{l)}}$
MCH (mean corpuscular hemoglobin)	=	$\dfrac{\text{Hb (gm/dl)} \times 10}{\text{Rbc (millions/}\mu\text{l)}}$
MCHC (mean corpuscular hemoglobin concentration)	=	$\dfrac{\text{Hb (gm/dl)} \times 100}{\text{Hct (\%)}}$

adults,[115] resulting in increased susceptibility to red cell hemolysis, particularly when enhanced by the presence of certain drugs in the individual's blood. Several screening tests are available, including the Heinz body test, the dye reduction test of Motulsky, and the ascorbate cyanide test.

c. Serology (immunohematology).   Serologic methods are used generally to measure a reaction between antibody (a potential constituent of any blood specimen, elaborated by the body's immune mechanisms in response to foreign protein) and specific antigen (a foreign protein added to the specimen, causing the antibody-antigen reaction). Using antigens obtained from many different microorganisms, serologic methods have been developed to detect the presence of a variety of possible antibodies, however, only two are commonly used in MHTS programs: tests for syphilis and for rheumatoid factor (indicating possible rheumatoid arthritis or allied autoimmune process).

(1) *Syphilis.*   The standard test used in the United States is the Venereal Disease Research Laboratory (VDRL) slide flocculation test (using a nontreponemal antigen). Numerous other methods are available (Hinton, Kahn, Kolmer, Mazzini, Reactive Plasma Reagin (RPR) and Wasserman) and are used variably in different parts of the world. Since false positive results are relatively frequent, even as a function of advancing age,[116] the diagnosis of syphilis must rest on confirmatory evidence obtainable either by history and physical examination or by additional laboratory study. Even then, confidence in test results has its limits, not only because of potential laboratory error, but because of possible spontaneous reversion of some test reactions.[117] Newer tests, including the direct fluorescent antibody test for *Treponema pallidum* (DFA-TP) and the microhemagglutination test for *T. pallidum* (MHA-TP) must be selected according to the clinical situation as second-level tests.[118]

Of all available tests, the RPR card test is reported to be the fastest to execute, requiring no need to separate cells from serum, no heat inactivation, and but six minutes to complete.[119]

(2) *Rheumatoid factor.* Of the methods available, the most commonly used is the latex fixation test. The frequency of false positive tests is relatively high, however, the test being positive in a variety of other pathological conditions.[120]

(3) The need for blood grouping tests, including ABO and Rh factor types, and tests for rubella antibodies are to be considered in the context of program objectives for special populations, the greatest utility appearing to be for women planning to become but not yet pregnant.

d. Chemistry.   In the past 15 years clinical biochemistry has grown rapidly in importance in the practice of medicine. The development of automated methods for the performing of multiple tests on single specimens has made chemical analyses more economical to perform and has provided the potential for improved standardization and reproducibility of analytic procedures.

There now exists a large experience in the use of groups of chemical tests, or "test panels," in screening programs for both ambulatory-outpatient and hospital populations.[121,122]

Variation in selection of panel size has been shown to have measurable effects on followup medical care and resource utilization; with increasing panel size there is a corresponding increase in diagnoses made, additional followup visits, telephone calls, and prescriptions issued.[103] (See Chapters Seventeen and Eighteen.) Because of the potential effects of even low false positive rates, care must be exercised both in the choice of analyses and the quality of equipment and methods. Automated instruments have become progressively diversified and sophisticated over the past decade. While offering the advantages cited above, they are also known to be subject to intermittent malfunction unless meticulously and frequently serviced, calibrated, and monitored during use. Skilled technologists operating under experienced supervision are important requirements for successful implementation and operation of clinical biochemical equipment.

Standard operating procedure manuals, provided by each equipment manufacturer, are the sources of detailed information concerning specific analytic methods, amounts and types of reagents required, recommended standard operation, and quality control. The more complicated the equipment, however, the less help is provided by operating manuals for predicting, detecting, and correcting malfunctions. The effective analytical capacity of an instrument system will be reduced materially (in some cases by as much as 30 to 50 percent) by the demands of the laboratory quality assurance program, including calibration runs, processing of known control samples, and process-reprocess handling of "blind" control specimens obtained from external proficiency programs. Adequate time must be provided in the total laboratory workload for all of these activities and, in large laboratories that are highly dependent upon automated equipment, for recovery from the inevitable equipment failures that will happen over a period of time, and which necessitate long periods of equipment adjustment/repair and repeating of potentially large numbers of tests.

The selection of equipment and analytical methods requires detailed investigation of the capabilities of the products and the services offered by each of a number of manufacturers. Automated analytical instruments require additional important considerations, including the following:

(1) The types of tests that the instrument is capable of performing. Most manufacturers provide a number of tests (e.g., 22) that can be performed on a specific number of channels (e.g., 12). Once the test panel is selected, the instrument will, in most instances, perform only those tests and will perform all of them on each sample of blood. In some instruments there is the option of selecting a subset of channels for some test runs, i.e., selecting different panels as desired. Such a capability increases the flexibility of the MHTS laboratory and may reduce total program costs in view of the potential effects of both real and false positive results on followup care.

Recommendations for chemical test panel composition have been included in an overall set of screening test recommendations for MHTS use by a Task Force of the National Conference of Preventive Medicine, and compared with tests recommended by the Fogarty International Center, the Association of the Schools of Public Health and the Association of Teachers of Preventive Medicine, and the American Public Health Association. (See Chapter Three.)

Table 6-5 lists recommended tests together with the announced capabilities of six representative automated multichannel clinical instruments.

(2) For each test to be performed on an instrument, data for the specificity and accuracy of the method, for its sensitivity to expected ranges of concentrations, and for its precision and reproducibility.

Table 6-5. Comparison Between Recommended Chemistry Tests and Capabilities of Selected Automated Instruments

	Equipment*						Recommended Tests† (for middle and older aged adults)			
	A	B	C	D	E	F	1	2	3	4
Acid phosphatase	+									
Alkaline phosphatase	+	+	+	+	+	+				
Amylase	+									
Bilirubin (total)	+	+	+	+	+	+				
Calcium	+	+	+	+	+	+				
Cholesterol	+	+	+	+	+	+	+	+	+	+
Cholinesterase	+									
Creatinine phosphokinase (CPK)	+	+	+	+	+	+				
Creatinine	+		+	+	+	+			+	
Electrolytes (Na⁺, K⁺)	+	+	+	+	+	+				
Globulin						+				
Glucose	+	+	+	+	+	+	+	+		+
Hydroxybutyrate dehydrogenase (HBDH)	+				+					
Iron	+		+	+						
Lactic dehydrogenase (LDH)	+	+	+	+	+	+				
Phosphorus	+	+	+	+	+	+				
Protein (total)	+	+	+	+	+	+				
SGOT	+	+	+	+	+	+	+			
SGPT	+	+	+	+	+	+				
Triglycerides	+	+	+	+	+	+	+		+	
Urea nitrogen (BUN)	+	+	+	+	+	+			+	
Uric acid	+	+	+	+	+	+	+	+		+
Total tests available	26	18	22	22	20	20				
Number of channels	1‡	17	12	20	20	20				

*A = American Monitor KDA
 B = Hycel Super 17
 C = SMA 12/60
 D = SMAC
 E = Coulter Chemical Analyzer
 F = Ortho Basic
†1. Fogarty International Center.
 2. Association of Schools of Public Health and the Association of Teachers of Preventive Medicine.
 3. American Public Health Association.
 4. Task Force of the National Conference on Preventive Medicine.[137]
‡The single channel functions as a sequential batch processor, at a high rate of speed.

(3) Relative simplicity of operation, including serial calibrations and quality control and maintenance procedures. How much of the equipment's nominal productivity is consumed by quality control functions?

(4) Service contract provisions and associated costs. Are performance records (of operational data) available for environments where the equipment is already in use?

e. *Trace elements.* For some time, certain trace elements have been recognized as essential to human health, such as cobalt, iron, manganese and zinc, serving as cofactors for various enzyme systems or other metabolic functions. Others are known to be toxic, even in trace concentrations (e.g., arsenic, lead), while still others are suspected of playing roles in either the development of or protection against several common diseases, including fluoride, selenium, lithium, aluminum, and copper.[123]

In some areas, lead poisoning is considered an important public health problem, and screening programs have been developed accordingly.[124]

In general, testing for trace elements requires flame atomic absorption technology, although several other methods have been developed in recent years, including flameless atomic absorption spectrophotometry, anodic stripping voltammetry, and gas chromatography.[125]

2. Urine Tests

a. Collection and handling of specimens.   Freshly voided urine is necessary for valid analysis. In general, a clean mid-stream specimen is preferred for all specimens; the usual procedure is to wash the genitalia (periurethral area only) with a swab of cotton wetted with an appropriate solution (sterile water and/or quaternary ammonium compound), void and discard about one ounce of urine, then collect the next two to three ounces into a sterile widemouth container, and seal. The technique is satisfactory for males for all phases of urine testing. In females there is higher risk of contamination of the specimen with epidermal debris and vaginal secretions, resulting in a higher rate of false positive tests for bacteriuria. The only alternative is to obtain a catheterized specimen in females, a procedure easily accomplished by a trained nurse or technician, but less acceptable to patients. If a pelvic examination is to be done for purposes of a Pap test, urethral catheterization could be incorporated into the procedure with little additional expenditure of time.

Urine pH and bacterial counts change over short periods of time; urine tests should therefore be done shortly after collection.

b. Specific urine tests

(1) *Glucose, protein, acetone, and pH.*   Paper strip tests are usually used for these substances. Glucose is measured by copper reduction (Clinitest tablet) or glucose oxidase (Clinistix strip) methods. Acetone strip tests are based upon a nitroprusside reaction, and protein by a tetrabromophenol blue reaction. The results are reported in semiquantitative units and are of relatively low precision. Timing of strip immersion or exposure to the specimen should be carefully controlled, and the interpretation conducted by someone with adequate color vision under good lighting conditions.

Measurement of urine specific gravity has not proved a useful screening test.

(2) *Bacteriological testing.*   Urinary tract infection in women is a common source of morbidity and is causally related to chronic pyelonephritis and chronic renal failure. Asymptomatic bacteriuria has been reported as present in as many as 3 to 5 percent of both pregnant and nonpregnant women.

Standard bacteriological procedures for the detection of bacteriuria require excessive time and personnel for routine MHTS operations. More economical methods are available. The triphenyltetrazolium chloride (TTC) test compares favorably with standard methods.[126] The dip-strip combination nitrate/culture test has reportedly good reliability for both Gram-positive and Gram-negative organisms, and may be used as a self-administered test if desired.[127]

(3) *Hemoglobin (Hb).*   Dip-stick tests for Hb are readily available (Hemastix) and are based upon the peroxidase-like activity of Hb to form blue oxidized orthotolidine. Caution in interpretation and accurate knowledge of time and method of specimen collection is required in females of menstruating age.

(4) *Microscopic examination of urine sediment.*   This test is more time-consuming, requiring centrifugation and slide preparation. Both sensitivity and specificity in the asymptomatic patient are very low and the test is not generally done in large MHTS programs.

L. X-RAY

1. Chest

In general, x-ray examinations may be conducted by a technician except where fluoroscopy is indicated. All interpretations require a trained radiologist. Automated image-processing interpretation techniques are not sufficiently advanced for routine use. As with clinical laboratory instruments, x-ray equipment must be carefully calibrated periodically and monitored for radiation "leak."

a. Chest x-rays. Chest x-rays have been used extensively in screening laboratories since the development of mass tuberculosis detection programs in the 1940s.[128] Chest x-ray, without contrast media, on both 70 and 100 mm as well as 14 × 17 in. film is a routine component of nearly all MHTS programs. Usually a single postero-anterior view is done in deep inspiration; occasionally lateral views are incorporated, especially for high-risk groups or for individuals known to have preexisting abnormal x-ray findings. There is no optimum frequency of chest x-ray screening; ideally, the frequency should be determined for each individual, and may range from a few months to two years, depending upon such variables as age, habitat, occupation, and current and past medical history.

b. Videodensitometry. This method provides quantitative measurements of physiological events, such as pulmonary blood flow, that are not available on static chest x-rays.[129] It requires two to three minutes of fluoroscopic time, but special image intensifier equipment is required, and the method is not yet used in large-scale MHTS programs.

c. Bronchography. Up to the present time, bronchography has not been acceptable as a screening test, since it requires introduction of contrast material into the patient's lungs by invasive means (transtracheal needle or endotrachial tube). A powder insufflation method has been devised that can be accomplished in a few minutes, but it requires further evaluation as to yields and possible long-term deleterious effects of the inhaled substance.[48]

2. Mammography and Xeromammography

As noted in I.3, these closely related techniques offer increased sensitivity over physical examination in the detection of asymptomatic breast cancer. Both methods are effective in the hands of experienced technologists and physicians, but it has been claimed that skill in xeromammography is more easily acquired and offers greater ease in information retrieval, for reasons including high resolution, edge enhancement, and wide latitude in the images.[130,131]

The use of these techniques in different age groups is debated, however, and concern has been expressed about possible adverse effects of too-frequent examination.[132]

3. X-Ray Tests Using Contrast Materials

In general these tests are not done except in relatively few "executive" and special occupational screening programs.

Barium contrast is used by oral ingestion in studies of the esophagus, stomach, and small intestine, and by rectal enema in studies of the colon. All studies are time-consuming, require special patient preparation, fluoroscopy, and static films, and are generally low-yield expensive procedures.

Intravenous pyelography, while not requiring fluoroscopic examination, carries with it the added risk of hypersensitivity reactions to the iodinated contrast medium, which is administered intravenously. Untoward reactions have been reported to occur in about 8 percent of patients[132] and result in death in about one case per 15,000 examinations.[133,134]

Cholecystography requires special patient preparation, as do the other contrast studies, including the need to dispense tablets to the patient for ingestion approximately 12 hours prior to the test. There is lower incidence of less serious hypersensitivity reactions, which are generally not considered a significant risk. A plain film of the abdomen (KUB), while not usually done in MHTS, is capable of detecting a variety of disorders, including cholelithiasis (see G.5), nephrolithiasis, calcific vascular disease, and a rare asymptomatic neoplasm of both bony and soft tissues. The test is easy to perform; the only risk is that it necessitates exposure of the reproductive organs to radiation. Its cost effectiveness has not been determined.

M. MISCELLANEOUS TESTS

1. Skin

The basic "test" for skin pathology is the followup physical examination, which is not usually a part of MHTS programs. The opportunity exists in the MHTS environment, however, to inform the patient of the importance of periodic self-inspection, and of the conditions, both occupational and recreational, that are known to predispose to skin cancer.

2. Anthropometry

Quantification of the physical measurements of the individual (height and weight) is an important component of the health care of growing children. (See Chapter Fourteen.) In adults, correlations between obesity and certain cardiovascular diseases have been found.[135,136]

a. Height.   Standard positioning is a requirement for reproducibility; the eye and the tragus of the ear should be on the same level, feet flat and back straight. Units have traditionally been in inches, though some centers use metric measures.

b. Weight.   A balance is preferable, calibrated to the nearest half-pound, or 250 grams.

N. MHTS REPORTS

The essential link between the MHTS laboratory and followup medical and health care is the MHTS report to the patient's physician or other appropriate medical agency, as indicated by the patient's personal request or by need for nonroutine medical intervention. (See Chapter Ten.)

In many MHTS environments several general types of reports are produced, both internally and externally.

1. Internal Reports

These reports, which can be generated by the discovery of an unexpected result at any of the test phases, are variously described as "advice" reports. They are intended to alert appropriate MHTS personnel to the presence of one or more possible abnormalities, so that action can be taken in accord with the laboratory's standard operating procedures.

2. External Reports

Following the completion of MHTS laboratory tests, the individual patient's data is collated and prepared for reporting. The time interval varies from hours to many days, depending upon which tests have been done and the data handling capabilities of the MHTS laboratory. Not infrequently the interpretations of x-ray examinations and electrocardiograms are the rate-limiting factors. Several types of reports may be issued, depending upon the time sequence of data collation and the relative urgency of possibly abnormal findings. In all cases, the report is directed to a followup physician or appropriate medical care agency.

(a) *"Alert" reports* are generated promptly in response to detection of potentially serious medical problems. Assurance that the report was received is an important consideration. Alert as well as routine reports may, in appropriate cases, be accompanied by "consider" statements, effectively requesting that the followup physician consider one or more specific actions.

(b) *Routine reports* are generated at the conclusion of all data collection and collation. In cases where some of the test data may be available significantly earlier than others, a preliminary (partial) report may be produced.

All reports should contain appropriate identification of the patient, the tests done, and the results, and be complemented by appropriate codes or other indicators that a given test was (1) not done. (2) not indicated, (3) refused by the patient, and (4) is to be interpreted in the light of additional information, such as: blood specimen lactescent, hemolyzed, etc.

REFERENCES

1. *Provisional Guidelines for Automated Multiphasic Health Testing Services,* Vol. 1. *Planning Principles.* U.S. DHEW, Health Services and Mental Health Administration, National Center for Health Services Research and Development, or N.T.I.S. PB 195 654, 1970.

2. *Ibid.,* Vol. 2. *Operational Principles* N.T.I.S. PB 196 000.

3. *Ibid.,* Vol. 3. *Proceedings of Invitational Conference on AMHTS* DHEW Publication No. (HSM) 72–3011, 1970.

4. Barnard, K., and Douglass, H. *Child Health Assessment.* Part 1. Washington, D.C.: DHEW, 1974.

5. Goldberg, D. "Screening for Disease: Psychiatric-Disorders." *The Lancet* 2(1974):1245–1247.

6. Meir, J. *Screening, an Assessment of Young Children at Developmental Risk.* Washington, D.C.: President's Committee on Mental Retardation, 1973.

7. Feinstein, A. R. "The Problems of the 'Problem-Oriented Medical Record.' " *Ann. Intern. Med.* 78(1973):751–762.

8. Goldfinger, S. E. "The Problem-Oriented Record: A Critique From a Believer." *N. Eng. J. Med.* 288(1973):606–608.

9. Weed, L. L. "Medical Records That Guide and Teach." *N. Eng. J. Med.* 278(1968):593–600.

10. Wakefield, J. S., and Yarnall, S. R. *The History Database.* 3d ed. Seattle: Medical Computer Services Association, 1975.

11. McLean, E. R., et al. "The Collection and Processing of Medical History Data—A Bibliography of Manual, Automated, and Computer-Assisted Techniques." *Method. Inform. Med.* 14(1975):150–163.

12. Reference 3, p. 125.

13. Collen, M. F., et al. "Reliability of a Self-Administered Medical Questionnaire." *Arch. Intern. Med.* 123(1969):644–671.

14. "How Helpful are Resting ECG's?"—Forum, in *Mod. Med.,* 56–60, June 1, 1975.

15. Teichholz, L. E., et al. "The Omnicardiogram. New Approach to Detection of Heart Disease in Patients With a Normal Resting Electrocardiogram." *Am. J. Cardiol.* 35(1975):531–536.

16. Robb, G. P., and Seltzer, F. "Appraisal of the Double Two-Step Exercise Test." *J.A.M.A.* 234(1975):722–727.

17. Figarola, T. R. "Evaluation of a New Step Ergometer." *J. Occup. Med.* 16(1974):615–618.

18. Froelicher, V. F., et al. "Epidemiologic Study of Asymptomatic Men Screened by Maximal Treadmill Testing for Latent Coronary Artery Disease." *Am. J. Cardiol.* 34(1974):770–776

19. Schiffer, F., et al. "The Quiz Electrocardiogram: A New Diagnostic and Research Technique for Evaluating the Relation Between Emotional Stress and Ischemic Heart Disease." *Am. J. Cardiol.* 37(1976):41–47.

20. Kannel, W. B. "Some Lessons in Cardiovascular Epidemiology from Framingham." *Am. J. Cardiol.* 37(1976):269–282.

21. Pipberger, H. V., et al. "Clinical Applications of a Second Generation Electrocardiographic Computer Program," *Am. J. Cardiol.* 35(1975):597–608.

22. Klatsky, A. L., et al. "Auscultation of the Adult Heart by Machine." *N. Eng. J. Med.* 279(1968):230–234.

23. Feigenbaum, H. "Clinical Applications of Echocardiography." *Prog. Cardiovasc. Dis.* 14(1972):531–558.

24. Hussey, H. H., "Hypertension: Value of Treatment." *J.A.M.A.* 230(1974):441.

25. Sheps, S. G., and Kirkpatrick, R. A. "Subject Review: Hypertension." *Mayo Clin. Proc.* 50(1975):709–720.

26. Oakes, T. W., et al. "Social Factors in Newly Discovered Elevated Blood Pressure." *J. Health Soc. Behav.* 14(1973):198–204.

27. Wallach, L., et al. "Stimulated Renin: A Screening Test for Hypertension." *Ann. Intern. Med.* 82(1975):27–34.

28. Sackett, D. L. "Screening for Disease: Cardiovascular Diseases." *The Lancet* 2(1974):1189–1191.

29. Rose, G. A. *Bulletin of the World Health Organization* 7(1962):645–658.

30. Cohn, P. F., et al. "Serum Lipid Levels in Angiographically Defined Coronary Artery Disease." *Ann. Intern. Med.* 84(1976):241–245.

31. Hazzard, W. R., et al. "Broad-B Disease (Type III Hyperlipoproteinemia) in a Large Kindred." *Ann. Intern. Med.* 82(1975):141–149.

32. Berenson, G. S., et al. "Serum Lipoproteins and Coronary Heart Disease." *Am. J. Cardiol.* 34(1974):588–593.

33. Chase, P. H., et al. "Screening for Hyperlipidemia in Childhood." *J.A.M.A.* 230(1974):1535–1537.

34. Murphy, B. F., "Management of Hyperlipidemias." *J.A.M.A.* 230(1974):1683–1691.

35. Smith, L. K., et al. "Management of Type IV Hyperlipoproteinemia." *Ann. Intern. Med.* 84(1976):22–28.

36. *Internal Medicine News.* 8(Mar. 15, 1975):1.

37. Klinger, M., et al. "Clinical Experience With Automatic Midline Echoencephalography: Cooperative Study of Three Neurosurgical Clinics." *J. Neurol. Neurosurg. Psychiatry* 38(1975):272–278.

38. Whelan, C. A., et al. "Nuclear Medicine and Ultrasound in the Evaluation of Neurological Diseases." *Seminars in Nucl. Med.* 6(1976):419–431.

39. Sisler, H. A. "Comparative Ophthalmodynamometry Using Scleral Pressure, Suction, and Corneal Pressure Units. A Pilot Study of 56 Normal Subjects." *Am. J. Ophthalmol.* 74(1972):964–966.

40. Barclay, W. R. "The Practicality of Case Finding in Pulmonary Emphysema." *Am. J. Pub. Health* 53(1963):16–17.

41. Edwards, P. Q. "Screening for Tuberculosis." *Chest* 68(1975):451–455, Supplement.

42. Higgins, I. T. T. "The Epidemiology of Chronic Respiratory Disease." *Prev. Med.* 2(1973):14–33.

43. Merrill, M. H. "Public Health Responsibilities and Program Possibilities in Chronic Respiratory Diseases." *Am. J. Pub. Health* 53(1963):25–33.

44. MacLean, R. A. "Tuberculin Testing Antigens and Techniques." *Chest* 68(1975):455–458, Supplement.

45. Agnes, R. S., and Maqbool, S. "Parent Reading and Reporting of Children's Tuberculin Skin Test Results." *Chest* 68(1975):459–462, Supplement.

46. Furclow, M. L. "Tuberculosis Case Finding by Tuberculin Testing a Complete Population, with Follow-up." *Chest* 68(1975):443–445, Supplement.

47. Kagemi, H. "Pulmonary Function Tests." *J.A.M.A.* 206(1968):2302–2304.

48. Comroe, J. H., and Nadel, J. A. "Screening Tests of Pulmonary Function." *N. Eng. J. Med.* 282(1970):1249–1253.

49. Green, M., et al. "Analysis of the Forced Expiratory Maneuver." *Chest* 63(1973):335–355, Supplement.

50. Webster, I. W., and Logic, A. R. "The Sensitivity of Spirometry to the Symptoms of Respiratory Disease." *Respiration* 30(1973):517–528.

51. Sobol, B. J. "Early Detection of Airways Obstruction." *Chest* 65(1974):239–241.

52. Ashley, F., et al. "Pulmonary Function: Relation to Aging, Cigarette Habit, and Mortality." *Ann. Intern. Med.* 82(1975):739–745.

53. Seltzer, C. C., et al. "Differences in Pulmonary Function Related to Smoking Habits and Race." *Am. Rev. Respir. Dis.* 110(1974):598–608.

54. Schlesinger, Z., et al. "Pulmonary Ventilatory Function Values for Healthy Men Aged 45 Years and Over." *Chest* 63(1973):520–524.

55. Rosner, S. W., et al. "Observer Variation in Spirometry." *Diseases of the Chest* 48(1965):265–268.

56. Sobol, F. J. "Some Cautions in the Use of Routine Spirometry." *Arch. Intern. Med.* 118(1966):335–339.

57. Dickman, M. L., et al. "On-Line Computerized Spirometry in 738 Normal Adults." *Am. Rev. Respir. Dis.* 100(1969):780–789.

58. Protti, D. J., et al. "Computer Assistance in the Clinical Investigation of Pulmonary Function Studies." *Method. Inform. Med.* 12(1973):102–107.

59. Sonia Buist, A. "Early Detection of Airways Obstruction by the Closing Volume Technique." *Chest* 64(1973):495–499.

60. Hyatt, R. E., and Rodarte, J. R. " 'Closing Volume,' One Man's Noise—Other Men's Experiment." *Mayo Clin. Proc.* 50(1975):17–27.

61. Sonia Buist, A. "Current Concepts: The Single-Breath Nitrogen Test." *N. Eng. J. Med.* 293(1975):438–440.

62. Randall, K. J. "Screening for Disease: Cancer Screening by Cytology." *The Lancet* 2(1974):1303–1304.

63. Beeson, P. B., and McDermott, W., eds. *Cecil-Loeb Textbook of Medicine.* 14th ed. Philadelphia: W. B. Saunders Company, 1975.

64. Hastings, J. B., "Screening for Colorectal Cancer." *Am. J. Surg.* 127(1974):228–232.

65. Medical News Section, *J.A.M.A.* 234(1975):137.

66. Neuhauser, D., and Lewicki, A. M. "What Do We Gain From the Sixth Stool Guaiac?" *N. Eng. J. Med.* 293(1975):226–228.

67. Powers, J. H. "Current Concepts in Cancer: Cancer of the GI Tract: Colon, Rectum, Anus." *J.A.M.A.* 231(1975):750–751.

68. London, F. Personal Communication: Unpublished results of the Kaiser-Permanente AMHTS Program, San Francisco, 1968–1974.

69. Molofsky, L. C., and Hayeshi, S. J. "Proctosigmoidoscopy As a Routine Part of a Multiphasic Program." *Am. J. Med. Sci.* 235(1958):628–631.

70. Turner, M. D. "Carcinoembryonic Antigen." *J.A.M.A.* 231(1975):756–757.

71. Gold, P., and Freedman, S. O. "Tests for Carcinoembryonic Antigen: Role in Diagnosis and Management of Cancer." *J.A.M.A.* 234(1975):190–192.

72. Raine, D. N. "Screening for Disease: Inherited Metabolic Disease." *The Lancet* 2(1974):996–998.

73. Lawrence, K. M. "Screening for Disease: Fetal Malformations and Abnormalities." *The Lancet* 2(1974):939–941.

74. Malins, J. M. "Screening for Disease: Diabetes." *The Lancet* 2(1974):1367–1368.

75. Siperstein, M. D. "The Glucose Tolerance Test: A Pitfall in the Diagnosis of Diabetes Mellitus." *Adv. Intern. Med.*20(1975):297–323.

76. Nusynowitz, M. L. "Free-Thyroxine Index." *J.A.M.A.* 232(1975):1050.

77. Hall, A. P., et al. "Epidemiology of Gout and Hyperuricemia; A Long Term Population Study." *Am. J. Med.* 42(1967):27–37.

78. Fessel, W. J., and Siegelaub, A. B. "Correlates and Consequences of Asymptomatic Hyperuricemia." *Arch. Intern. Med.* 132(1973):44–54.

79. Fessel, W. J. Personal communication.

80. Sacha, D. D. "Routine Screening of Asymptomatic Women for Gonorrhea." Editorial in *West. J. Med.* 123(1975):395–396.

81. Holmes, K. K. "Screening and the Detection of Gonorrhea." *West. J. Med.* 123(1975):367–371.

82. Rothenberg, R. B., et al. "Efficacy of Selected Diagnostic Tests for Sexually Transmitted Diseases." *J.A.M.A.* 235(1976):49–51.

83. Quigley, M. M., et al. "Screening for Gonorrhea in a Low Risk Population." *Am J. Obstet. Gynecol.* 120(1974):106–109.

84. Nelson, J. H., et al. "Detection, Diagnostic Evaluation and Treatment of Dysplasia and Early Carcinoma of the Cervix." *CA* (A Cancer Journal for Clinicians) 25(1975):134–151.

85. Breslow, L. "Early Case-Finding, Treatment and Mortality from Cervix and Breast Cancer." *Prev. Med.* 1(1972):141–152.

86. "Papanicolaou Testing—Are We Screening the Wrong Women? Statement of the Massachusetts Dept. of Pub. Health," *N. Eng. J. Med.* 294(1976):223.

87. Hindeman, W. M. "An Effective Quality Control Program for the Cytology Laboratory." *Acta Cytol.* 20(1976):233–238.

88. Bartels, P. H., et al. "Modeling of Histologic Images by Computer." *Acta Cytol.* 20(1976):62–67.

89. Gaub, J., et al. "Cytophotometry of Feulgen-Naphtol Yellow S Stained Liver Cells—A Computerized Method for the Calculation of Nuclear Protein." *Acta Cytol.* 20(1976):356–360.

90. Irwig, L. M. "Screening for Disease. Breast Cancer." *The Lancet* 2(1974):1307–1308.

91. Griesbach, W. A. "Screening for Breast Carcinoma." *Oncology* 23(1969):167–171.

92. Bailar, J. C. "Mammography: A Contrary View." *Ann. Int. Med.* 84(1976):77–84.

93. Strax, P. "Control of Breast Cancer Through Mass Screening." *J.A.M.A.* 235(1976):1600–1602.

94. Borish, I. M. *Clinical Refraction.* 3d ed. Chicago: Professional Press, Inc., 1970.

95. Friedman, E., and Simons, L. "Diseases of the Eye and Ocular Manifestations of Systemic Diseases." In Keefer, C. S., and Wilkins, R. W., eds., *Medicine.* Boston: Little, Brown & Company, 1970.

96. Spector, R. S. "Should Tonometry Screening Be Done By Technicians Instead of Physicians?" *Arch. Intern. Med.* 135(1975):1260–1262.

97. Unpublished data from the Kaiser-Permanente MHTS Program, 1969.

98. Levatin, P., et al. "The Swinging Flashlight Test in Multiphasic Screening for Eye Disease." *Can. J. Ophthalmol.* 8(1973):356–359.

99. "Persons With Impaired Hearing." Vital and Health Statistics Data from the National Health Survey, Series 10, No. 101, U.S. DHEW Publ. No. (HRA) 76–1528, 1975.

100. Siegelaub, A. B., et al. "Hearing Loss in Adults." *Arch. Environ. Health* 29(1974):107–109.

101. Martin, R. H., et al. "Occupational Hearing Loss Between 85 and 90 dBA." *J. Occup. Med.* 17(1975):13–18.

102. Righthand, N., et al. "A Computer-Oriented Hearing Conservation Program." *J. Occup. Med.* 16(1974):654–658.

103. Friedman, G. D., et al. "Biochemical Screening Tests." *Arch. Int. Med.* 129(1972):91–97.

104. Reference 3, p. 83.

105. "A Bibliography of Drug Interferences with Clinical Laboratory Tests," *Clinical Chemistry* 18(1972):1041–1303.

106. Barclay, W. R. "Standardizing Units of Measurements." Editorial in *J.A.M.A.* 236(1976):1981.

107. Davidson, I., and Henry, J. B., eds. Todd-Sandford *Clinical Diagnosis by Laboratory Methods.* 15th ed. Philadelphia: W. B. Saunders Company, 1974.

108. *Ibid.,* Table 9-1, p. 518.

109. *Ibid.,* Figure 9-6, p. 521.

110. *Ibid.,* Table 4-7, p. 209.

111. Asakura, T., et al. "A Rapid Test for Sickle Hemoglobin." *J.A.M.A.* 238(1975):156–157.

112. Bennis, E. L. "Optimal vs. Optional Testing for Sickle Cell Disease." Editorial in *J.A.M.A.* 234(1975):855–856.

113. Hussey, H. H. "Sicklemia: To Screen or Not To Screen." Editorial in *J.A.M.A.* 229(1974):192.

114. Schmidt, R. M. "Hemoglobinopathy Screening: Approaches to Diagnosis, Education and Counseling." Am. J. Pub. Health 64(1974):799–804.

115. Oski, F. A., and Naiman, J. L. *Hematologic Problems in the Newborn.* 2d ed. Philadelphia: W. B. Saunders Company, 1972.

116. Taskind, M. A., and Eisdorfer, C. "Screening for Syphilis in an Aged Psychiatrically Impaired Population." *West. J. Med.* 125(1976):361–363.

117. Burns, R. E. "Spontaneous Reversion of FTA-ABS Test Reactions." *J.A.M.A.* 234(1975):617–618.

118. Jaffe, H. W. "The Laboratory Diagnosis of Syphilis: New Concepts." *Ann. Intern. Med.* 83(1975):846–850.

119. Medical News Section, *J.A.M.A.* 229(1974):508.

120. Reference 107, Table 23-7, p. 1233.

121. Bailey, A. "Biochemistry of Well Populations." *The Lancet* 2(1974):1436–1439.

122. Whitehead, T. P., and Wootton, J. D. P. "Biochemical Profiles for Hospital Patients." *The Lancet* 2(1974):1439–1443.

123. Maugh, T. H. "Trace Elements: A Growing Appreciation of Their Effects on Man." *Science* 181(1973):253–254.

124. Eidsvold, G., et al. "The New York City Department of Health: Lessons in a Lead Poisoning Control Program." *Am. J. Pub. Health* 64(1974):956–962.

125. Lisk, D. J. "Recent Developments in the Analysis of Toxic Elements." *Science* 184(1974):1137–1141.

126. Resnick, B., et al. "Mass Detection of Significant Bacteriuria." *Arch. Intern. Med.* 124(1969):165–169.

127. Kunin, C. M. "Self-Screening for Significant Bacteriuria." *J.A.M.A.* 231(1975):1349–1353.

128. Breslow, L. "An Historical Review of Multiphasic Screening." *Prev. Med.* 2(1973):177–197.

129. Medical News Section, in *J.A.M.A.* 23(1975):693.

130. Cooperman, L. R., et al. "Xeromammography in the Early Detection of Breast Cancer." *West J. Med.* 123(1975):360–366.

131. Kalisher, L., and Schaffer, D. L. "Xeromammography in Early Detection of Breast Cancer." *J.A.M.A.* 234(1975):60–63.

132. Medical News Section, in *J.A.M.A.* 236(1976):541.

133. Ochsner, S. F., et al. "Untoward Reactions Observed in 10,000 Consecutive Excretory Urographies." *J. La. State Med. Soc.* 114(1963):150–155.

134. Pendergrass, H. D., et al. "Reactions Associated With Intravenous Urography: Historical and Statistical Review." *Radiology* 71(1958):1–12.

135. Kannel, W. B., et al. "The Relation of Adiposity to Blood Pressure and the Development of Hypertension; the Framingham Study." *Ann. Intern. Med.* 67(1967):48–59.

136. Thomas, H. E., et al. "Obesity: A Hazard to Health." *Med. Times* 95(1967):1099–1106.

137. Breslow, L., et al.: "Theory, Practice, and Application of Prevention in Personal Health Services." Pages 257–359 in *Preventive Medicine USA*. New York: PRODIST, 1976.

CHAPTER SEVEN

Bioengineering for Test Phases

Joseph F. Terdiman

A. INTRODUCTION

An MHTS is dependent upon a variety of instruments for the collection of patient data. These instruments are used to measure and display physiological, biochemical, or anatomical characteristics of the patient, or serve as data entry terminals for patient identification, demographic data, and medical history. They contain the sensors, transducers, and displays to which the patient or specimen is exposed, and are the visible tip of the MHTS. They must be capable of independent operation or of interfacing with a computer. The bioengineering characteristics and design features of these instruments must satisfy the rigorous requirements of the MHTS environment in terms of accuracy, reliability, safety, and ease and efficiency of operation.

The following sections discuss these bioengineering considerations.

B. INSTRUMENT CHARACTERISTICS

A test instrument can be considered to have three basic components: input, signal conditioning, and output (Figure 7-1). The input component senses an electrical, mechanical, electromagnetic, thermal, or chemical signal produced by a patient, a specimen obtained from the patient, or an external source. The signal conditioning component amplifies or otherwise processes the input signal, extracts the necessary information, and converts it to a form suitable for output. The output component usually consists of a display device (such as a recorder, meter, or digital display) and/or an electrical interface with a computer or other data pro-

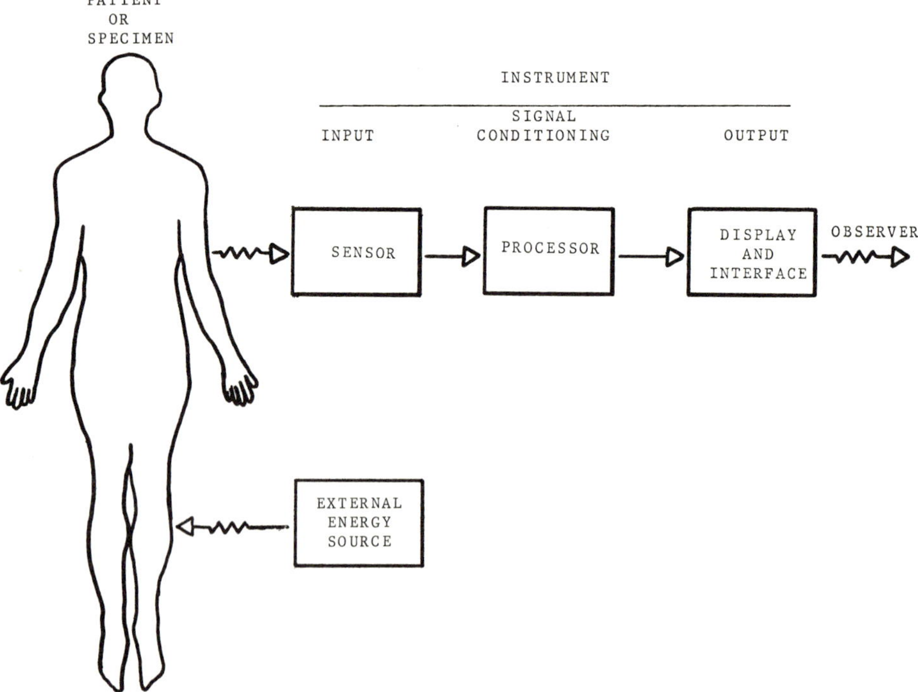

Figure 7-1. Basic components of a test instrument.

cessing equipment. Not every instrument will contain all three components, and the relative complexity of each component may vary considerably. For example, the input and output components of an x-ray machine are the x-ray tube and film, respectively. A signal conditioning component, such as an image intensifier, is rarely used in an MHTS setting. In other devices the signal conditioning component may be as simple as a lever (e.g., in skinfold calipers) or as complex as a computer (e.g., in automated chemistry analyzers, which calculate test values from light-absorption curves).

Each component operates on a signal, which may be in either analog or digital form. In the following discussion an analog signal is defined as a time-varying waveform whose amplitude is proportional to a continuous physical variable (e.g., voltages, pressures, x-ray beam intensities—see Figure 7-2). A digital signal is

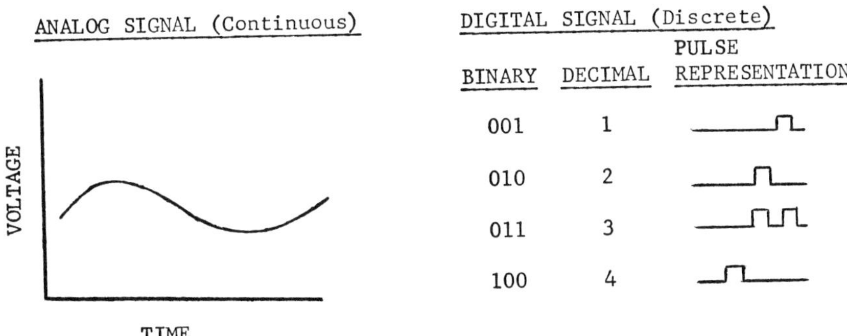

Figure 7-2.   Comparison of analog and digital signals.

defined as a series of binary digits (1's and 0's) that represent the state of a physical variable expressed as a number, at any instant of time (e.g., systolic blood pressure). An analog signal can be converted to digital form by a process called analog-to-digital conversion, in which the analog signal is sampled at uniform intervals and the instantaneous amplitude converted to its binary representation, with a suitable scale factor. Figure 7-3 illustrates the concept of analog-to-digital conversion with an electrocardiogram waveform. In Figure 7-3A the analog waveform is sampled at 25 conversions per second. The numeric values of the waveform voltage at various sampling times are shown in the table next to the figure. A waveform, reconstructed from the sampled data, is shown in Figure 7-3B. In Figure 7-3C the reconstructed waveform is shown for a sampling rate of 250 conversions per second.

1. Input Components

There are two categories of input components: passive input devices that receive signals produced by the patient (e.g., electrocardiogram, temperature, response to a history question, etc.) or by an external energy source (e.g., x-ray, ultrasound, etc.); and active devices that serve as external sources of energy (e.g., x-ray tubes, piezoelectric crystals, etc.). There are two classes of passive input devices: analog and digital.

An analog input device is a detector or transducer that receives analog signals produced by the patient or by an external energy source. The device may be in

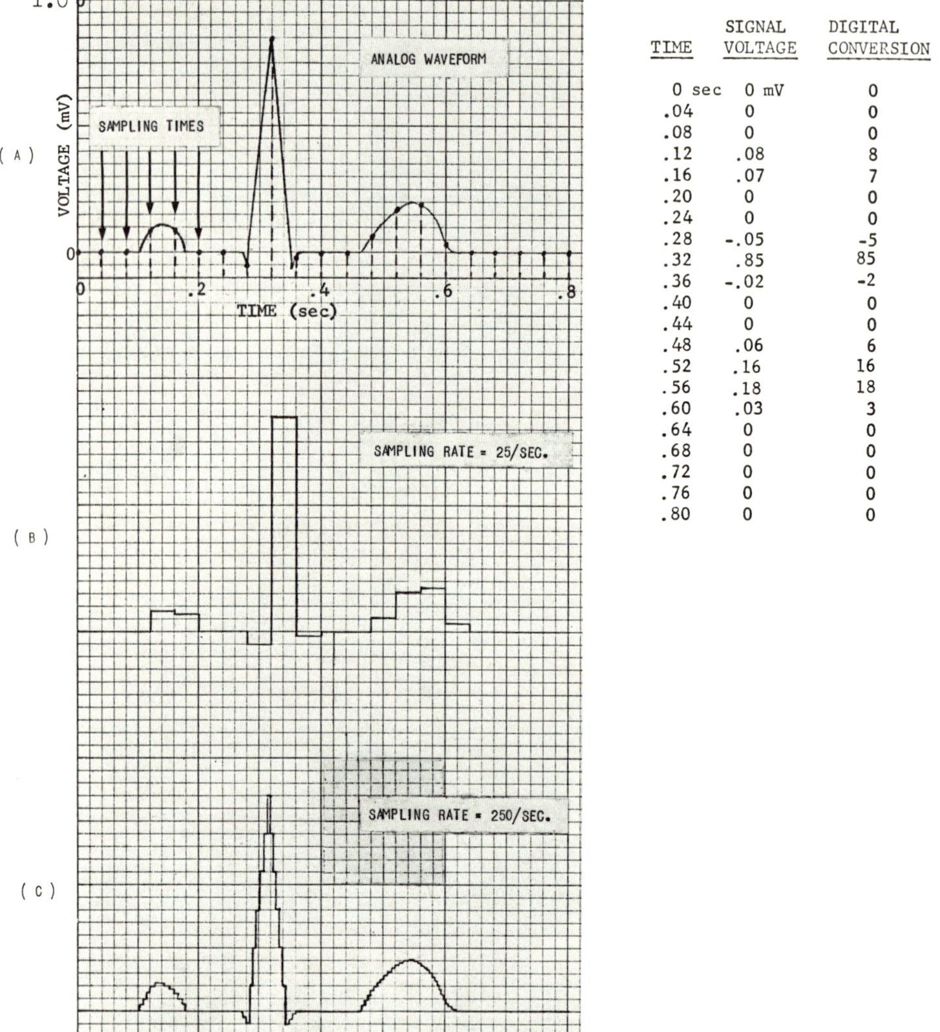

TIME	SIGNAL VOLTAGE	DIGITAL CONVERSION
0 sec	0 mV	0
.04	0	0
.08	0	0
.12	.08	8
.16	.07	7
.20	0	0
.24	0	0
.28	-.05	-5
.32	.85	85
.36	-.02	-2
.40	0	0
.44	0	0
.48	.06	6
.52	.16	16
.56	.18	18
.60	.03	3
.64	0	0
.68	0	0
.72	0	0
.76	0	0
.80	0	0

Figure 7-3.   Analog-to-digital conversion of electrocardiogram. (a) Analog waveform of an electrocardiogram sampled at 25 conversions per second. (b) Waveform reconstructed from sampled data at 25 conversions per second. (c) Waveform reconstructed from sampled data at 250 conversions per second.

physical contact with the patient or specimen being measured. A detector is a device that samples a physiological signal for transmission to the external environment. An example of a detector is an electrode used to record an electrocardiogram. The small voltage generated by the heart (of the order of millivolts) is detected by metal electrodes in contact with the skin and is transmitted through shielded cable to the signal conditioning component of the instrument. A transducer is a device that detects a physiological signal as one form of energy (heat, chemical, mechanical, etc.) and converts it to another form (usually electrical) for transmission to the external environment. Examples of transducers are microphones, air flow detectors, chemistry electrodes, photocells, thermometers, mechanical switches, etc. An example of a transducer used in an automatic blood pressure instrument is a microphone placed under a blood pressure cuff to monitor Korotkoff sounds generated by turbulence of blood coursing through the brachial artery of the arm. The mechanical vibrations in the tissue of the arm induced by turbulence are detected by the microphone, where they are transduced to an electrical signal by a sensor (usually a piezoelectric crystal) in the microphone.

Digital input devices include keyboards, switches, card readers, and badge readers. More advanced devices, not yet in widespread use in MHTS, include wand readers for reading bar code (such as the Universal Product Code found on retail store packages), light-pens (used in conjunction with visual display terminals), and optical character readers (capable of reading printed alphabetic and numeric characters from paper documents). Digital input devices are used to collect patient identification, demographic data, history or test results. Instruments that contain digital input devices are computer terminals (e.g., visual displays, typewriters, card readers), unit record equipment (e.g., keypunches), and hybrid instruments (e.g., an electrocardiograph with a keyboard for computer interfacing).

These devices may be operated by multiphasic technicians and, for certain terminals, by patients themselves. A technician at a phase may enter a patient's identification through a keyboard, switches, or a badge reader. The latter device is used in certain online MHTS in which the patient is issued, upon registration, a card with a machine-readable identification number, which he carries to all phases. At each phase the card is inserted into a badge reader connected to a data entry terminal to identify the test results entered as belonging to that patient. Demographic data and test results may be entered through a variety of digital input devices. If the MHTS provides online data entry to a computer, a visual display terminal, typewriter, or special-purpose keyboard terminal may be used. Such terminals are usually programmed to provide interactive responses to each data entry transaction. Responses may appear on display lamps or as a line of text on a typewriter or visual display screen, and may be used to validate patient identification, provide online checking of test results, indicate receipt of data transmission, or for any other programmable function. Patients may operate digital input devices in the form of automated history consoles. Typically, the patient is presented with a series of questions with multiple-choice answers on a screen, and is required to press a button on a keyboard corresponding to his answer.

An active input component is an energy source such as an x-ray tube, light source, or piezoelectric crystal (which generates sound waves at ultrasonic frequencies). These components generate signals that are modulated by intrinsic anatomical and physical properties of the patient or specimen. The modulated signals are received, conditioned, and displayed by methods appropriate to the type of signal (e.g., an x-ray image).

2. Signal Conditioning Component

Once the signal is received by the input device, it must be processed in order that the signal itself or the information it contains can be output to the external world. Signal conditioning is a general term that includes any analog or digital processing of signals. It is most easily performed on electrical signals, which is why most instruments convert a physiological signal to an electrical representation regardless of its original energy form.

Analog signal processing refers to operations on an analog input signal including amplification, filtering, modulation, demodulation, peak detection, rectification, and other transformations designed to extract information from the signal.[1] For example, signal conditioning in an electrocardiograph is performed by amplifiers that magnify and filter signals detected by the electrodes and transmit them to a strip chart recorder. If a tape recorder is used to retain a permanent electrical record of the electrocardiogram, the signal must be conditioned further to produce a signal suitable for recording on magnetic tape.

Digital signal processing refers to logical and arithmetic operations performed on a digital signal.[2] If the input signal is in analog form, it must be converted to digital form before it can be digitally processed. Input signals from keyboards and other digital input devices are already in digital form. Digital signal processing in an instrument may be performed by discrete digital logic modules or by a small computer programmed to perform a complex series of digital operations (e.g., automated chemistry analyzers).

3. Output Component

The output of an instrument is usually displayed for visual examination and may be transmitted to other instruments through an interface. Display devices are either analog or digital. An analog display device is one that displays continuous signals. Thus, electrocardiographs, blood pressure manometers, and x-ray films are analog display devices. A digital display device is one in which a measurement is displayed as a series of digits, either on a visual display screen or on a digital panel meter. Thus, spirometers usually present computed volumes and flow rates as a set of numbers on a digital display. Blood pressure (which consists of two measurements, systolic and diastolic) may be displayed either digitally as two three-digit numbers or in analog form as two heights on a mercury manometer.

A display device may produce a permanent analog or digital record or a transient record that must be visually observed and transcribed. Examples of permanent analog records are electrocardiogram tracings and x-ray films. Permanent analog tracings are usually recorded on a strip chart recorder. Modern recorders produce tracings by three different methods: photographically, with a spot of light on light-sensitive paper; with a hot stylus on heat-sensitive paper; or with pressurized ink on chemically treated paper. For high-volume MHTS in which the cost of paper may be a significant factor, the pressurized-ink system is probably the most economical. Some instruments provide permanent digital displays by means of self-contained printers, which print numeric test results (e.g., blood cell counters). The accuracy of a physiological measurement depends, to a large part, on the type of display. Manual transcription introduces an additional source of error, as discussed in Chapter Nine.

C. INSTRUMENT SELECTION CRITERIA

Selection criteria for MHTS instruments are based on requirements for input, output, signal conditioning, and overall performance, and on compatibility with the requirements of the MHTS system as a whole. The criteria to be used in evaluating MHTS instruments are shown in Table 7-1. While these divisions are somewhat arbitrary, they have proved useful for the Kaiser-Permanente MHTS.

Table 7-1.   List of Criteria for MHTS Instrument Selection

Input	Output	Instrument	MHTS System
Patient or specimen preparation	Display: digital vs. analog	Validity	Compatibility
Rapidity and ease of patient interface	Permanent record readability	Accuracy	Speed
Stress on patient	Reproduction	Precision	Future modifications
Safety	Visual display characteristics	Reliability	
Device characteristics		Cost and time to repair	
		Availability of spares	
		Modularity	
		Construction	
		Documentation	
		Operation	
		Engineering modifications	
		Specifications	
		Maintenance	
		Calibration	
		Safety	

1.   Input

a.   Patient or specimen preparation.   An efficient input device for an MHTS will require little or no preparation of the patient or specimen. The more preparation required, the longer will be the time per patient or specimen at the phase and the smaller will be the patient capacity of the MHTS. Types of patient preparation include skin preparation for electrocardiograph electrodes, sterilization of instruments and use of topical anesthetic in eyes for tonometry, blood drawing, and instructions in the use of spirometers, audiometers, automatic history terminals, and other equipment. Certain blood specimens require centrifugation to prepare them for analysis. Where there is a trade-off between ease of preparation and quality of data (such as the quality of an electrocardiogram as a function of degree of skin preparation), a compromise between system flow and data quality requirements may have to be made.

b.   Rapidity and ease of patient interface.   Following preparation of patient or specimen, the input device must be suitably positioned. The most efficient systems for positioning detectors or transducers either are automatic or else simplify the task of manual application. A suitable mechanical framework may provide rapid alignment of instruments. Such devices include electrocardiogram tables with built-in electrodes, blood pressure cuffs in fixed sleeves through which the arm is inserted, or air-applanation tonometers in which the head is rested against a positioning frame and the sensor positioned near the eye with a ''joystick'' control. For spirometers, the use of disposable mouthpieces, through which patients can blow, removes the need for cleaning the blow tube after each test.

c. Stress on patient.   An input device that increases the anxiety of the patient may cause abnormal or inconsistent readings and increase the length of time the patient must remain in the phase. An example is a direct-contact tonometer, which requires placing an anesthetic and an instrument in physical contact with the cornea, as opposed to a noncontact tonometer.

d. Safety.   Instruments that contact or pass energy through the patient are potential safety hazards. Devices that do not contact the patient are usually preferable, if there is no decrease in accuracy or ease of operation. If patient contact is necessary, electrical instruments should be checked periodically for possible electric shock hazard and current leakage (see E). Patients must be screened for allergy to topical anesthetics for tonometry. X-ray machines should be monitored for radiation leakage and unsafe levels of radiation.

e. Input device characteristics.   Detectors such as ECG electrodes should be either disposable or reusable after simple and rapid cleaning. Reusable electrodes should be mechanically strong and able to tolerate frequent changing without wear or corrosion. Transducers should be rugged and able to resist mechanical inpact (such as being dropped) without changing their characteristics. They should also be resistant to changes in temperature and humidity and to aging.

Keyboards, switches, and other digital input devices should be reliable for one hundred thousand to one million contact closures. Keys and switches should be designed for ease and accuracy of operation. Positive feedback, such as a mechanical click or visual indicator from a contact closure, is desirable.

2. Output

a. Type of display.   Where a measurement can be displayed in either analog or digital form, a digital display is usually preferable, because it is easier and more accurate to read numbers than to read and interpolate an analog display. Certain instruments, such as automated chemistry analyzers, provide optional digital outputs in addition to standard analog outputs. Important digital display selection criteria are the readability of digits and the precision (number of digits) of the display. For analog displays selection criteria include readability of scales on indicator dials, separation of scale divisions, and interpolation required to obtain desired precision. Permanent recordings of analog data, such as electrocardiograms, should provide thin, sharp tracings, nonsmearing and nonfading, that reproduce well on reproducing machines. Certain ink pigments reproduce poorly, while photographically produced tracings tend to fade. Display devices using pressurized ink or ribbon will require refills with a frequency dependent on test volumes.

Digital display devices used by patients, such as automated history terminals, require careful selection. Criteria include the size and clarity of display characters, ability to display graphical data, complexity of controls, response time, ability to recall previous questions, privacy of the interview from external observation, question capacity of the terminal, and ability to use languages other than English.

b. Interfacing.   For MHTS that use computers to print multiphasic reports, the ability to interface an instrument to data processing equipment may be an important selection criterion (see F). If an interface is required, it will be necessary to obtain an electrical output from the instrument. If the instrument does not provide an output connector for interfacing, it will be necessary to tap a signal from some internal point. The manufacturer's advice should be sought before such modifications are attempted, especially if the instrument is under warranty or maintenance agreement. Instruments that provide for external interfacing are clearly preferable in MHTS that use data processing.

3. Instrument

a. Validity. No instrument should be purchased until the validity of its results have been tested, preferably in the MHTS environment, and received medical approval. Validity testing is necessary to insure that an instrument is measuring the same variable as measured by the standard technique. Frequently, an automated instrument will measure a physiological variable by indirect means and then convert that reading to the expected value of the standard manual measurement. For certain patients the results may be quite accurate; for others there may be a considerable difference. A measure of the magnitude and frequency distribution of the differences, and an understanding of the cause of the discrepancies are required before such an instrument can be judged acceptable.

Validity testing is performed by running the new instrument against a series of known standards covering a wide dynamic range. If the instrument values are plotted against the standard values and the test results are valid, the points should lie on a straight line with a slope of 45° that passes through the origin. The deviation of these points from a straight line is a measure of the validity of the instrument method.

For example, to insure that blood pressure measured by an automatic instrument that uses an ultrasonic Doppler-shift technique is equivalent to blood pressure measured by the standard manual Korotkoff method, both methods were used on a series of patients with a wide range of blood pressures, alternating the order of measurement. Figures 7-4 and 7-5 show the results for systolic and diastolic pressures. The points lie close to the 45° line, indicating the validity of the method.

b. Accuracy. The accuracy of an instrument is tested by running it against a series of known standards. Assuming the test method is valid, accuracy is measured by the distribution of test results around the standard values. In Figures 7-4 and 7-5 the automatic and manual pressures were nearly equal for most systolic and diastolic measurements, demonstrating the accuracy of the instrument. An instrument may perform accurately on certain patients or specimens but not on others, owing to the influence of certain physiological and anatomical variables. Often, the influence of these variables is not recognized until long after the instrument is purchased and an occasional erroneous result is noted. In all cases payment for an instrument should be contingent on satisfactory installation and demonstrations of validity and accuracy.

c. Precision. The precision of a measurement is the number of significant digits in the result. The precision required for a particular measurement is governed by the clinical utility of the measurement, the accuracy of the instrument, and intrinsic physiological variability. For example, although weight can be mea-

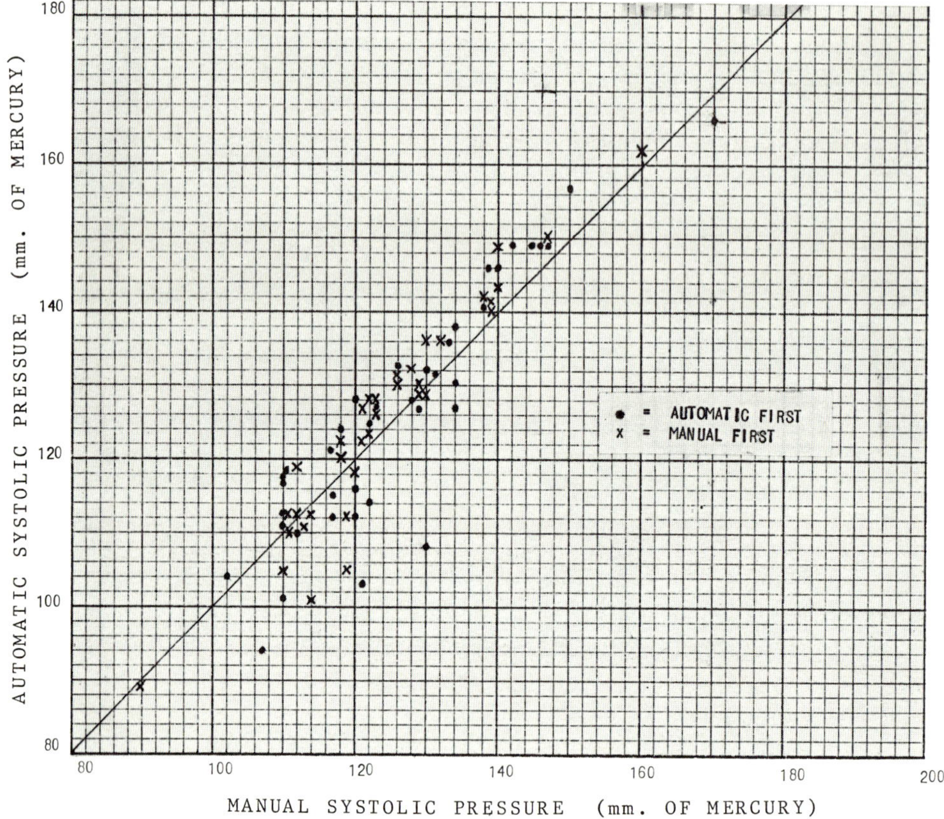

Figure 7-4.   Comparison of systolic blood pressures measured by manual and automatic methods on the same patients, and alternating the order of measurements.

sured to the nearest millionth of a gram, for an MHTS it is adequate to weigh adults to the nearest one-half pound. While pressure in a blood pressure cuff can be measured in tenths of a millimeter of mercury, this degree of precision is unnecessary because the physiological variability of blood pressure in an individual is of the order of millimeters over an interval of a few seconds. Instruments that provide unnecessary precision of measurements at increased expense are unjustified.

d.   Reliability.   An instrument operating in an MHTS environment must be extremely rugged. This is no place for fragile or unstable equipment. An important instrument specification is mean-time-before-failure (MTBF). Equipment with delicate components or many mechanical parts should be avoided, if possible, because of the increased maintenance required and decreased MTBF. Mechanical failures are usually more frequent than electrical failures.

e.   Cost and time to repair.   When a failure occurs in a multiphasic instrument, it is important to have a replacement at hand and to repair the defective instrument as soon as possible. If a duplicate backup instrument is not available, it may be possible to continue to run the phase with alternate instrumentation or with manual procedures. Without suitable backup the phase will have to close down

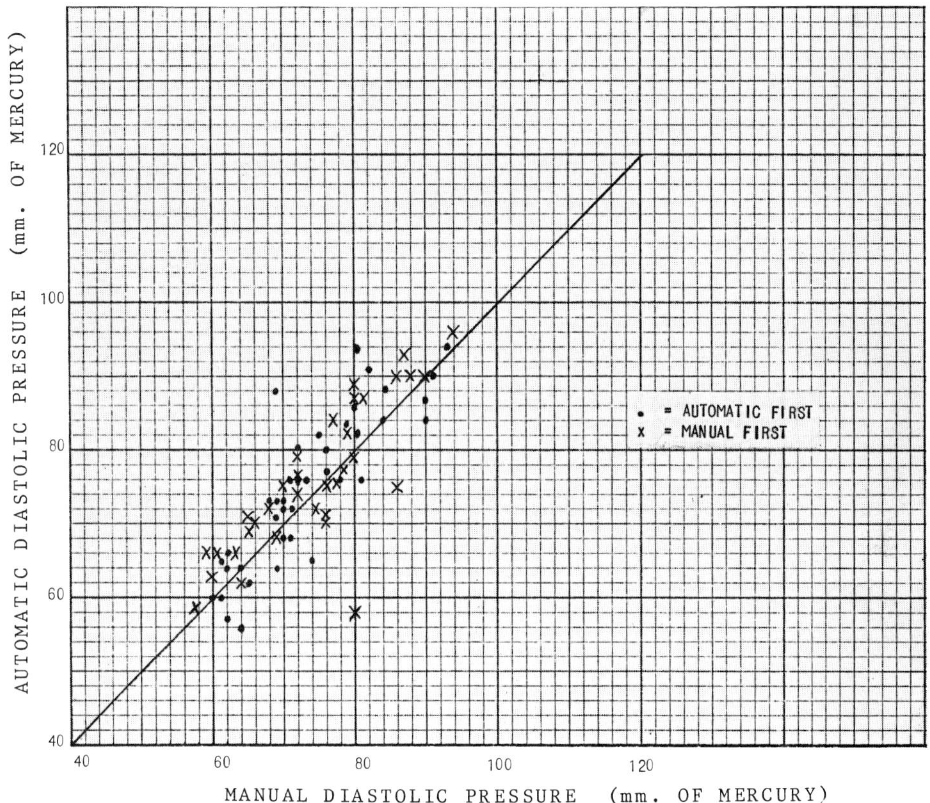

Figure 7-5.   Comparison of diastolic blood pressures measured by manual and automatic methods on the same patients, and alternating the order of measurements.

until the instrument is repaired. Types of failures vary considerably, from a burnt-out lightbulb to a defective power supply, and the difficulty of repair varies correspondingly. Ideally, fuses, lightbulbs, and other easily replaceable items should be located near the instrument for ready access. Internally, the instrument should be constructed modularly so that defective components can be easily removed and replaced with working components. If qualified maintenance personnel are available on site, it may be feasible to have a set of replacement components for the more delicate items. If maintenance personnel are not available, then a manufacturer's repair shop or maintenance service should be readily available. If the instrument cannot be repaired on site, then it may be possible to persuade the manufacturer to provide a loaner instrument while the defective one is being repaired. Such agreements may be specified in the maintenance contract, as well as a time limit for repair. If delicate mechanical parts are involved, repairs can be extremely expensive. The cost of repair replacement for these components should be ascertained prior to purchase of the instrument.

4.   Overall system considerations.   An MHTS instrument must be compatible with the general requirements of the system in terms of its patient throughput, staffing requirements, and interfacing. It must be carefully integrated into the multiphasic facility in order to maintain an even flow pattern and not create patient bottlenecks. If it takes longer to perform a measurement on an instrument than is required to maintain a given patient flow, it may be necessary to duplicate the equipment and staffing and to run two instruments in parallel. For example, it may be useful to have two electrocardiograph tables, each with a set of electrodes connected to a single instrument by means of a selector switch. While electrodes are being applied to a patient by a technician at one table, another technician may be recording an electrocardiogram from a patient on the other table.

Instrument characteristics should be compatible with plans for future system modifications, which may include increased patient volumes or conversion to online operation. If an instrument is operating at its maximum capacity or is unable to furnish an electrical output signal, a new instrument will have to be purchased if either modification is implemented.

D. MAINTENANCE

The key to trouble-free operation of multiphasic instruments is an effective program of preventive maintenance. Instruments should be cleaned and calibrated at regular intervals. Components with a known lifetime, such as batteries and lightbulbs, should be scheduled for replacement prior to their expected date of failure. Mechanical parts should be cleaned, lubricated, and checked for wear. Checking individual electronic components is not feasible, but if an instrument is showing an increasing rate of drift, or erroneous results, the instrument should be checked for impending failure or returned to the manufacturer for repair. The frequency and type of preventive maintenance must be geared to the specific instrument and will be discussed in G below. Complete documentation for the instrument should be obtained from the manufacturer. This includes instructions regarding operation, calibration, and maintenance as well as schematic diagrams of electronic and mechanical components. The latter documentation should be specified in the purchase order, since certain manufacturers are reluctant to distribute these items.

E. SAFETY

Electrical safety of medical instruments is a significant bioengineering problem. It has been shown that relatively small amounts of electrical current, of the order of tens of microamperes, are sufficient to cause cardiac arrhythmias in patients with intracardiac catheters, and rigorous current leakage standards have been adopted for instruments used in intensive care units and coronary care units.[3-6] However, patients with cardiac catheters or patients with external transvenous pacemakers are very unlikely to appear in the multiphasic environment, and therefore multiphasic instruments do not have to conform to these rigorous standards. Current leakage of 100 microamperes through a standard test load with the instrument ungrounded is acceptable. Periodic testing of instruments for increased current leakage, frayed or cracked insulation on external wires, and faulty grounding should be performed.

Multiphasic instruments should be rigidly mounted in such a way that a patient cannot pull them over or trip over them. This prevents not only injury to the patient but instrument damage and theft as well. A variety of other safety factors are related to the operation of specific instruments. Other noninstrument considerations include the ingestion or application of drugs associated with specific test phases.

F. INTERFACING

A multiphasic instrument usually must be capable of operating as a standalone device, completely independent of any other instrument. Signals or measurements are displayed by the output component of the instrument. However, in certain MHTS it may be desirable to transmit the data from the instrument to some other device. It is therefore necessary to have a suitable interface between the two devices that matches the output characteristics of one to the input characteristics of the other. Since either device may have an analog or digital input or output, interfaces may be purely analog or digital, or a hybrid with analog-to-digital or digital-to-analog conversion. An interface with digital-to-analog conversion is rarely used in an MHTS setting.

An analog interface is required between two analog instruments. Its functions may include any of the following: signal buffering, filtering, inversion, amplification, attenuation, modulation, demodulation, direct current offset, instrument isolation, impedance matching. An example is an interface between an electrocardiograph and a telephone line for remote transmission of electrocardiograms. Usually, an analog signal is not transmitted directly but is used to modulate a carrier signal at audio frequencies, which can then, be transmitted over voice-grade telephone lines.

A digital interface is required between instruments with digital outputs and inputs, such as between a blood cell counter with digital output and a computer or unit record device. The interface must transform the output signal of one into the input signal of the other with respect to voltage levels, pulse widths, data codes, data format, and transmission rate. In addition, one or more digital control signals between both instruments and the interface are usually required.

A hybrid interface is required when the output of one instrument is analog and the input to the other is digital. It combines the characteristics of pure analog and digital interfaces and contains, in addition, an analog-to-digital converter. An example is an interface between a blood pressure device, which outputs analog voltages proportional to systolic and diastolic pressures, and a keypunch machine. The interface enables numeric values of the measurements to be punched automatically into a data card. Digital or hybrid interfaces may transmit data in serial or parallel form. A serial interface transmits bit strings representing coded numeric data along a single channel. The bit string is converted back to coded numeric data by the computer or other digital device at the receiving end. While data are in serial form they can be transmitted over telephone lines through the use of modems (modulator-demodulator) at each end of the line. A parallel interface transmits coded numeric data as binary signals on multiple parallel lines, typically four lines for BCD (binary coded decimal) and eight lines for ASCII (American Standard Code for Information Interchange).

G. INSTRUMENTATION FOR TEST PHASES

In this section the characteristics of some specific MHTS instruments will be discussed. Instrument manufacturers will not be mentioned by name, but unique features of instruments of specific vendors will be described.

1. Electrocardiography

An electrocardiograph records electrical signals generated by the heart. The signals are detected by electrodes placed at various locations on the body and are combined in different ways to produce a series of standardized waveforms known as the electrocardiogram (ECG—see Figure 7-6). Each particular signal combina-

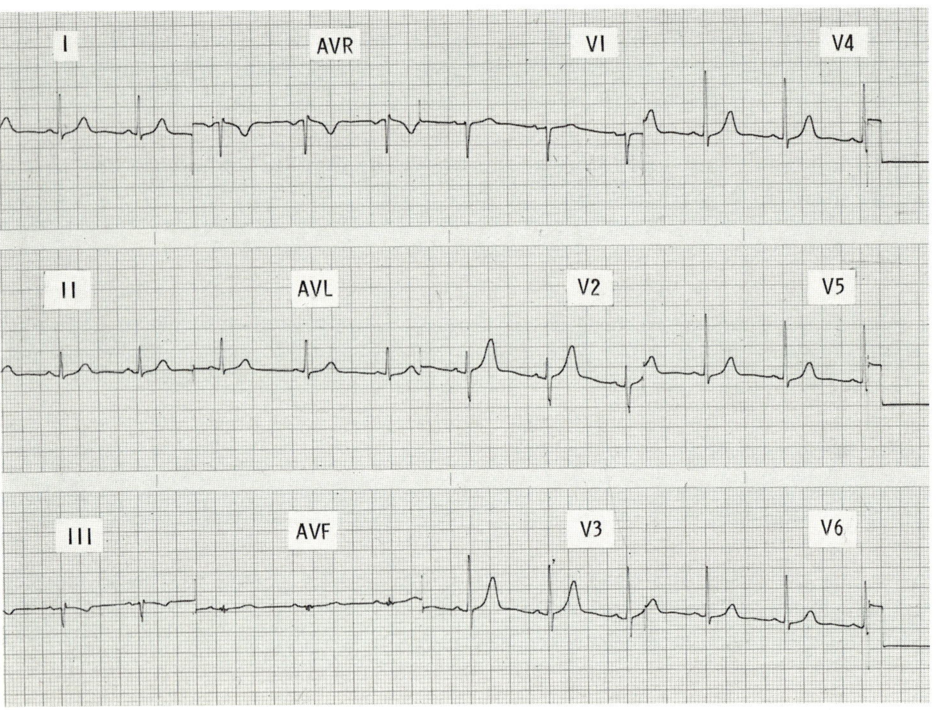

Figure 7-6. Normal electrocardiogram, consisting of 12 standard leads. The limb leads, I, II, III, AVR, AVL, AVF, are derived from four limb electrodes, and the chest leads, VI–V6, are derived from the six chest electrodes and an indifferent electrode, derived from the limb electrodes.

tion is known as a lead. The most widely used lead sets are the twelve standard leads and the three orthogonal leads. Standard leads are derived from ten electrodes, one on each limb and six on the chest. The orthogonal leads are derived from eight body electrodes, of which four correspond to standard lead electrodes. Cardiologists are generally more familiar with standard than orthogonal ECGs, and they are, therefore, the most widely used; however, several computer ECG analysis programs require orthogonal leads.

Electrodes may be applied to the patient in a variety of ways. The patient's skin must first be prepared for electrode placement. Rubbing the skin with alcohol alone is often adequate to produce a satisfactory tracing, if the electrodes have a sufficiently large surface area.[8] The use of electrode jelly may produce a better tracing but requires more time to apply and wipe off. Electrodes may be applied to the patient using straps or suction cups to hold them in place. More efficient methods for attaching limb electrodes are to mount them on spring clamps or build them into arm and leg rests on the ECG table. Use of a patient selector switch connecting to two or more sets of electrodes at separate ECG tables to the electrocardiograph permits recording of a patient's ECG from one table at the same time electrodes are being attached to patients at other tables.

Two kinds of electrocardiographs are now used in the MHTS environment: single-channel and three-channel instruments. A single-channel electrocardiograph records one lead at a time; a three-channel electrocardiograph records three leads at a time and, therefore, requires one-third the time of a single-channel instrument to record the same number of electrical complexes. Most three-channel instruments optionally provide orthogonal leads in addition to the standard leads. The advantage of a three-channel electrocardiograph is that the tracing can fit on a standard $8\frac{1}{2} \times 11$ in. document with minimal or no trimming. A single-channel recording must be cut and mounted on a standard-sized document. Almost all modern electrocardiographs have been designed to pass the most rigid electrical safety requirements, including current leakages of under 10 microamperes.[4] Maintenance and repair costs depend on the particular vendor.

There are two basic approaches to the interpretation of the ECG in an MHTS: rapid manual screening by a cardiologist and screening by automated instruments.

For manual screening ECGs are labeled with patients' identification and sent to a cardiologist for review. He may simply divide the ECGs into two categories, normal and abnormal, or give a more detailed interpretation. As a rule he will require less than one minute per ECG for interpretation. For computer-based MHTS, a physician's interpretation may be entered on a marksense card or through an online computer terminal.

For automated ECG analysis, two different approaches have been used. In the first method a digital computer is programmed to measure parameters of the ECG waveform and provide an interpretation. A second, newer method uses an electronic device that distinguishes between normal and abnormal ECGs on the basis of waveform measurements; it does not provide an interpretation.

a. Computer analysis. Several vendors provide computer interfaces for their electrocardiographs. To identify the patient to the computer system, the electrocardiograph is provided with a data entry terminal consisting of digital switches or a numeric key pad. This terminal permits the entry of a patient identification number as well as coded data regarding height, weight, diagnosis, drugs, and other data required by the computer analysis programs. ECG signals and patient data may then be transmitted directly to the computer for analysis in realtime, or they may be recorded on a storage device for subsequent offline analysis.

The usual method for transmission of ECG data is to transform the ECG into a frequency-modulated (FM) signal, which can be carried by a voice-grade telephone line, using a modulator-demodulator instrument (modem) mounted on the electrocardiograph. On the receiving end of the line, a data receiver with a similar modem demodulates the signal and provides an interface to the computer. Computer programs analyze the waveform, measure its parameters, check for arrhythmias, and provide ECG interpretations. Several ECG analysis programs are commercially available.[9-12] For online computer systems ECG interpretations may be ready for printout in a minute or less; however, physician over-reading is usually required, especially for abnormal tracings. Results may be printed on a remote terminal in the ECG facility, or on a central terminal and sent to the facility. Results may also be stored in a computer file for inclusion in the multiphasic summary report. One vendor has built a computer and printer into the electrocardiograph cart, so that tracings and interpretations are available almost immediately at the bedside.

As an alternative to realtime data transmission, ECGs may also be recorded on analog or digital tape for subsequent offline analysis. Analog FM tape units may be mounted either on the electrocardiograph cart or on the data receiver.

b. Screening instruments.   These devices electronically measure parameters of the ECG waveform and compare them with internal preset limits.[13] They inform the operator whether the ECG pattern is normal or abnormal, indicating by means of display lamps the basis for any abnormality detected. These devices are useful only for screening, since they do not provide interpretations.

2. Blood Pressure

Four techniques are in common use in MHTS to measure blood pressure: the traditional manual method and three automatic methods.

The traditional noninvasive measurement of blood pressure is usually performed by a trained health professional.[14,15] A cuff is wrapped around a patient's upper arm and inflated to a high pressure. Then it is allowed to deflate at a standard rate of 3 mm mercury/sec. A stethoscope placed over the brachial artery is used to detect the onset (systolic point) and disappearance (diastolic point) of Korotkoff sounds produced by pulsatile blood flow. Systolic and diastolic pressures are read from a manometer connected to the cuff. Values of systolic and diastolic pressure obtained by this procedure will depend not only on the patient's true blood pressure, but also on the observer's acuity of hearing, quickness of reflexes in reading and interpolating the manometer scale, ability to hold cuff deflation at the prescribed rate, extraneous noise, and cuff and stethoscope placement.[16-18] These factors and others introduce a large subjective component that often leads to inaccuracies of 10 percent or more in pressure measurements. Despite the obvious inaccuracies, this traditional method has become the standard for the measurement of clinical blood pressure against which all automated methods must be compared.

Several types of automated blood pressure instruments are commercially available, each using a different principle of detection: acoustic, pulse-wave, and ultrasonic.

a. Acoustic detection.   Acoustic blood pressure devices attempt to duplicate the operation of the traditional manual method by automated means. Inflation and deflation are controlled by an electrical pump and valves. A microphone replaces the stethoscope for detecting Korotkoff sounds. Cuff pressures are measured with a strain gauge or pressure transducer. Electrical pulses produced in the microphone by Korotkoff sounds trigger pressure readings at systolic and diastolic points. Although earlier devices were subject to false triggering by noise artifacts and auscultatory gaps (temporary disappearance of Korotkoff sounds followed by reappearance at a lower frequency), newer devices contain sophisticated electronic circuitry to minimize this effect. Pressure values may be displayed on dial indicators or as a digital display. Results are made available for transmission to data processing devices as analog or digital signals.

An advantage of this class of device is that it replicates most closely the traditional standard measurement. These instruments provide a constant level of audio detection compared to the variability of the human ear and can provide more precise control over cuff deflation rate than can a human operator. Disadvantages are that these devices are subject to many of the same error sources that affect human operators. Noise artifacts and auscultatory gaps still cause false triggering. As the microphone ages, its characteristics change, resulting in poorer reliability. Accurate positioning of cuff and microphone are critical for reliable results.

b.   Pulse-wave detection.   The operation of this type of device is based on the detection of a pulse wave generated by the pumping action of the heart and transmitted through the blood stream to the brachial artery.[19] The pulse-wave detector is a cuff placed on the upper arm that contains three inflatable balloons instead of a single one, as found in the standard cuff. One balloon serves as the systolic detector, while the other two serve as diastolic detectors. Vascular pulsations in the arm are transmitted to each balloon and from there to detector modules in the instrument. Each pulsation produces a minute puff of air in the detector that is registered by a thermistor. The function of each cuff in detection of systolic and diastolic points will not be described here in detail; however, through a combination of fluidic and electronic circuitry, systolic and diastolic points are identified and the pressure in one of the balloons is sampled and recorded. Results may be displayed and interfaced in the same manner as for acoustic instruments.

An advantage of this type of instrument is that it does not rely on the detection of Korotkoff sounds, so it is not subject to noise artifacts or changes in microphone characteristics. The major disadvantage is that systolic and diastolic pressures determined by pulse-wave detection must be compared with results of the standard auscultatory measurements, and the results do not necessarily coincide. However, some studies have shown that pulse-wave pressures more closely match systemic pressures than does the standard method. Another disadvantage is that cuff placement is even more critical with this method and requires considerable practice before consistent results are obtained. Reliable data are difficult to obtain in patients with fat or muscular arms.

A more significant problem is in the construction of the instrument. The systolic and diastolic modules contain complex and expensive mechanical apparatus; when these parts fail, they must be sent back to the manufacturer for repair and recalibration. Preventive maintenance is quite difficult because of the large number of moving parts.

c.   Ultrasonic detection.   These devices detect vascular pulsations directly by recording the change in Doppler frequency shift of an ultrasonic beam, reflected from pulsating arterial walls.[19-21] The ultrasonic transducer is mounted on a standard cuff whose pressure is monitored by a pressure transducer. As cuff pressure is decreased, the onset of pulsations marks the systolic point, and the reduction in pulsation amplitude below a threshold marks the diastolic point. This technique correlates very well with the standard manual method, as demonstrated in Figures 7-4 and 7-5. In most patients there is some deviation (e.g., in patients with fat arms), but in these cases it is probably the manual method that produces erroneously high results.[18] Inaccurate readings may result from patient movement artifacts.

3. Spirometry

There are many measures of pulmonary function.[22-26] The ones usually accepted for multiphasic screening are vital capacity, forced expiratory volume at 1 second and 2 or 3 seconds, and peak flow rate. Several types of spirometers are commercially available. They compute the parameters from two basic types of measurements: volume displacement and flow rate.

a. Volume detectors. In this class of devices, air is blown into an easily expandable enclosure such as a bellows or cylinder with water seal or piston. As the flow of air expands the volume of the enclosure, the change in volume is converted to linear motion through a mechanical linkage. Suitable transducers and timing circuits record volumetric and flow parameters. Results may be displayed on dial indicators, graphically, digitally, or interfaced with data processing equipment. The analog output of the transducers may also be connected directly to a computer interface. Computer programs can be used to calculate the four parameters, as well as other pulmonary function parameters.

b. Flow detection. The operation of spirometers with this type of detector is similar to those with volumetric detection, but they depend on direct measurement of flow rate and integrate flow over time to derive volumetric parameters. Flow rate is determined either by a pressure transducer, hot-wire anemometer, or turbine. In the first case, air is blown through a fine mesh or an array of capillary tubes known as a pneumotachograph. The pressure drop across the capillary tubes, which is proportional to flow, is measured by a pressure transducer. In the case of a hot-wire anemometer, air is blown past a platinum wire heated to a constant temperature. The slight change in temperature produced by the moving air is recorded by a thermistor and is proportional to flow rate. A new type of flow transducer consists of a finned turbine blade that spins on jeweled bearings to sense expired air flow. The rotational velocity, which is proportional to air flow, is measured photoelectrically.

The two types of spirometers have about the same accuracy. The volume spirometer is easier to calibrate. The air-flow spirometer requires for calibration a constant known air flow, which is more difficult to obtain. Maintenance is more of a problem in the enclosed-volume spirometers because of the accumulation of condensed moisture inside the air chamber. In hot-wire air-flow spirometers, saliva and moisture eventually coat the wire and change its characteristics. Air-flow spirometers provide less resistance to forced expiration than do volume spirometers, since the air tube opens into the room.

4. Anthropometry

Height and weight may be measured mechanically or electronically. Mechanical measurements are read from scales and must be manually input to computer-based MHTS. For electronic height measurement, the sensor is a measuring arm mounted on a vertical slide, which is mechanically coupled to a displacement transducer such as a variable potentiometer or shaft encoder. The transducer signal, proportional to height, is conditioned, scaled, and output as a digital display or interface signal.

For electronic weight measurement, the sensor is usually a load cell (a type of strain gauge), which is mechanically linked to the weighing platform. The load-cell signal, proportional to weight, is conditioned, scaled, and output as a digital display or interface signal.

Another possible anthropometric measurement is skinfold thickness; this measurement is made with spring-loaded calipers, which apply a standard force to a thickness of skin at a specified anatomical site. The separation of the tips of the calipers is equal to the skinfold thickness. This measurement is usually read manually, but it is possible to mount a displacement transducer on the calipers.

5. Chest x-rays

Standard 14×17 in. chest x-rays are taken in most MHTS. Some facilities use a mini-film x-ray machine, which produces a $2\frac{1}{2} \times 2\frac{1}{2}$ in. film that can be inserted into the patient's chart along with the rest of his multiphasic report. However, the resolution of this type of x-ray is not as good as that of the standard size film, and in some cases the patient receives greater x-ray exposure. X-ray machines should be checked periodically for radiation leaks and electrical hazards.

Interpretations of x-rays are made by radiologists. In computer-based MHTS, radiologists' diagnoses may be entered through marksense cards or through computer terminals.[27] Automated x-ray screening systems are under development.

6. Mammography

Mammography may be performed with conventional x-rays, xeroradiography, or thermography. There is considerable medical controversy as to which method furnishes the most clinically useful results. (See Chapter Six.) Conventional low-energy x-rays (soft x-rays) permit visualization of relatively small differences in tissue density such as are found between tumors or cysts and surrounding normal tissue. Xeroradiography uses x-rays and a xerographic process that enhances the boundary between tissues of different densities. Thermography is a process that produces a photographic mapping of skin surface temperature from infrared radiation emitted by the body. The skin temperature overlying lesions with increased blood flow, such as tumors, may be greater than the surrounding skin temperature by a fraction of a degree. Extremely sensitive infrared detectors are capable of recording these slight differences.

The same safety considerations apply to mammography as to chest x-ray. In computer-based MHTS radiologists' interpretations of mammograms may be entered as for chest x-rays. Automated mammography screening has been developed, but is not commercially available.[28]

7. Visual acuity

Except for certain experimental devices, testing of visual acuity is done manually. A standard or modified wall chart may be used, but usually a special display device is used to test other aspects of vision, such as depth and color perception, as well. Test results may be entered on marksense cards or through a computer terminal.

8. Tonometry

A tonometer is a device used to measure intraocular pressure. Tonometry is used as a screening test for glaucoma, a disease of unknown etiology, in which intraocular pressure becomes elevated and may lead to blindness, if pressure is uncontrolled.

Several types of tonometers are available. The simplest and most widely used is the Schiotz tonometer. It is a mechanical device that applies a known weight to the surface of the cornea and measures the deflection produced, which is proportional to intraocular pressure. Since the device is applied directly to the eye, it must be sterilized and topical anesthetic drops administered. Patients must be screened for possible allergic reactions to the anesthetic.

A more accurate instrument is the Goldmann applanation tonometer, which measures the force that is required to flatten (applanate) a specific optically determined area.[29] It is the currently accepted standard for measurement of intraocular pressure. However, it also contacts the eye and requires a topical anesthetic.

Recently a new applanation tonometer has been developed that measures intraocular pressure without contact between the instrument and the eye.[30,31] Applanation is produced by a controlled air-pulse of linearly increasing force impinging on the cornea. The instant of applanation is determined by a monitoring system that senses light reflected from the corneal surface. The interval of time required for the air-pulse to produce applanation is proportional to intraocular pressure. Pressure is output directly in millimeters of mercury on a digital display. No anesthetic or sterilization of instruments is required. Clinical evaluation has demonstrated good correlation between noncontact and Goldmann tonometer readings. Because of the complexity of its optical system, most maintenance and repair work on the air-pulse tonometer must be done by the vendor. Since the instrument puts out a pulse of air, an occasional patient will complain of eye irritation. This device usually produces much less anxiety in patients than tonometers that contact the eye. Patient relaxation is particularly important in tonometry, because tense, anxious patients may bear down (i.e., perform a "Valsalva maneuver") and produce transient elevation of intraocular pressure.

Test results are usually entered manually on marksense cards or into a computer terminal. It is possible to interface the digital output signal directly to data processing equipment, although existing instruments do not provide an output connector.

9. Audiometry

An audiometer tests a patient's thresholds for pure tones over the normally audible frequency range. Most MHTS facilities use automatic audiometers in which the test is self-administered.[32,33] At each test frequency the patient controls the intensity of the tone by means of a push button. Contact closure or release causes intensity to gradually decrease or increase, respectively, on a logarithmic

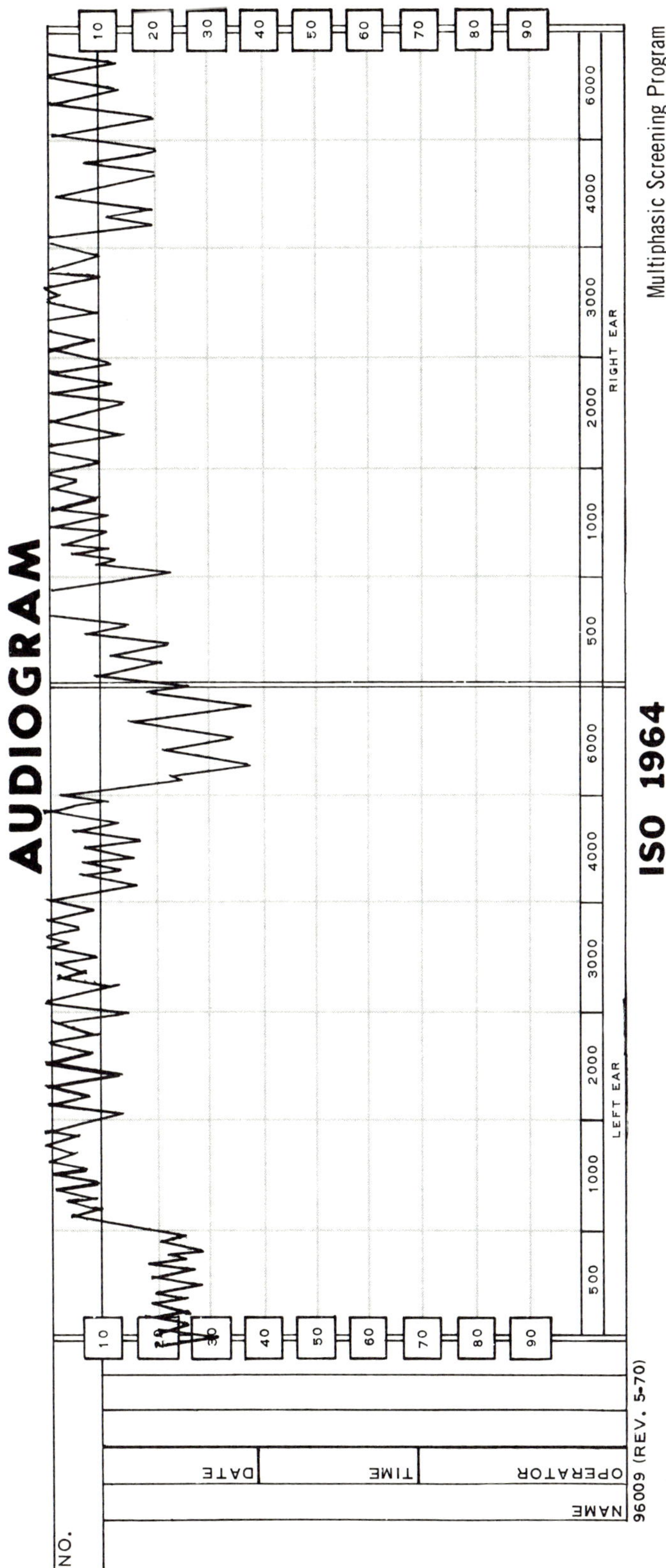

Figure 7-7. Screening audiogram, recorded on a self-administered autiometer for six different frequencies in both ears. Vertical axis is in decibels of hearing loss relative to normal thresholds (ISO 1964 standards). Horizontal axis is the frequency of tone in each ear in hertz.

scale. The audiometer automatically steps through each test frequency for each ear, providing about one minute of each tone. Typical frequencies are 500, 1,000, 2,000, 3,000, 4,000, and 6,000 hertz. A tracing is made of the relative intensity of the tones, showing the points at which the patient pressed and released the button (see Figure 7-7). This audiogram is interpreted by a technician and translated into decibels of hearing loss at each frequency. Some audiometers are capable of running tests on several patients simultaneously. While automatic audiometry is not as accurate as standard audiometric testing, the results are satisfactory for screening. Abnormal or poor-quality audiograms may be due to patients' not understanding instructions or having tinnitus (ringing or buzzing in the ears) or extraneous noise. Results are usually entered on marksense cards or into a computer terminal. Some automatic audiometers provide digital output signals for interfacing. Instrument calibration with respect to sound frequency and amplitude should be checked with an audiometric tester about once a month.

10. Hematology

Hematology testing for an MHTS usually includes the following seven tests: white blood cell count (WBC), red blood cell count (RBC), hemoglobin (HGB), hematocrit (HCT), and the three red cell indices—mean corpuscular volume (MCV), mean corpuscular hemoglobin (MCH), and mean corpuscular hemoglobin concentration (MCHC). (White cell differential counts are rarely performed.) Most clinical laboratories now use automated instruments to perform these tests.[34-36] These instruments are faster and more accurate than manual methods. Typically, test results are available less than one minute after the specimen is sampled. The results are output in digital form, which may be printed by a printer attached to the instrument, or interfaced to data processing equipment.

Hematology tests are unique in that of the six red cell measurements, RBC, HGB, HCT, MCV, MCH, and MCHC, there are only three independent variables; the remaining three variables are computed from the others. Thus, the instrument must perform only three physical measurements on the specimen (plus a fourth for WBC); the other three are computed electronically. Various instruments measure and compute different combinations of variables depending on the techniques used. For example, one instrument measures WBC, RBC, HGB, and MCV directly, and computes HCT, MCH and MCHC; another measures WBC, RBC, HGB, and HCT and computes MCV, MCH, and MCHC.

These instruments use a variety of techniques to perform the measurements. One device passes an electric current through a diluted sample as it flows through a small aperture.[35] As the cells stream through, they produce small variations in the current, because of the difference in electrical conductivity between red cells and diluted plasma. The number and amplitude of these variations are used to determine the RBC and MCV, respectively. HGB is determined by a colorimetric method. Another device counts cells photoelectrically as they pass through an aperture. A photocell detects light scattered by the cells as they move across a dark-field background.[36]

Computations may be performed by analog or digital methods. Digital computation is preferred because, barring instrument malfunction, the results are always precise. Analog computation is less accurate, has poorer precision, and requires frequent calibration; however, it has been commonly used because of its simpler design and lower cost. With recent developments in digital technology, the latter point may no longer apply.

For differential cell counts, if desired for an MHTS, several instrument manufacturers offer semiautomated and automated differential counters.[37] These instruments contain built-in computers that automatically locate white blood cells on a microscope slide and display the image on a television or microscope screen. Identification and counting of the type of white cell is done by a human operator in the first case, and by the computer in the second case. Results are output digitally for printing or interfacing.

11. Blood Chemistry Analyzers

Blood chemistries for an MHTS are usually performed as a panel, or fixed set of tests, on an automated chemical analyzer. The criteria for inclusion of specific tests in a multiphasic panel are discussed in Chapters Three and Six. The requirements of an automated chemical analyzer for multiphasic screening include:

(a) Appropriate capacity to process a number of samples per hour consistent with the rate at which the screening program processes patients. This flow may be as high as 25 patients an hour, or a total of 200 patients a day. Another operational characteristic of the multiphasic screening program is the relatively slow rate and the constant interval between the input of samples into the laboratory throughout the day, in contrast to a clinical laboratory, where batches of specimens arrive during certain periods of the day.

(b) A multichannel analyzer, in order to do a full panel of tests simultaneously.

(c) Rapid throughput time, if tests are to be completed before the patient leaves the laboratory.

(d) Consistent accuracy. This is extremely important in multiphasic screening, since the early determination of disease requires great precision at boundary limits so as to accurately separate normal from abnormal and avoid false positive and negative test results. Too many false negatives tend to defeat the main purpose of multiphasic screening, i.e., early detection of disease. Too many false positives lead to unnecessary costs for patient followup testing and physical examinations. (See Chapter Seventeen.)

All automated chemical analyzers involve most of the following steps, in a typical analysis: (1) volume measurements of sample and reagents, (2) measured volume transfers, (3) mixing, (4) incubation for a measured time at a controlled temperature, (5) precipitation by filtration or centrifugation, (6) extraction or washing of a precipitate, or extraction of an aqueous solution with an organic solvent, (7) light absorbency or other physical measurement, and (8) data recording. Moving and transfer of samples and reagents is accomplished by (1) a continuous-flow analysis system using peristaltic pumps, which force fluids in a continuous stream, separating samples by air bubbles, (2) discrete sampling, in which piston-pump syringes, pneumatically or mechanically operated, eject fluids into discrete containers, or (3) centrifugal force, which moves fluids into cuvettes located in the edge of a rotor.

Sample identification is usually by sequencing. Specimens are loaded onto the instrument sampling tray in known patient order. They are sampled sequentially, and the test results are output in the same order. In addition, some instruments provide a sample identification system in which a specimen is identified by an accession number, which may appear on a prepunched card that accompanies the sample or be printed on machine-readable labels affixed to the sample container and the corresponding patient requisition form. This number is read from the container by the instrument at the time the specimen is sampled, and it appears on the output together with the test results.

Test results may be output in analog form as a graphical display or as a digital printout on typewriter or printer. A digital output signal is available for interfacing to data processing equipment.

An automatic calibration feature permits periodic adjustment for instrument drift by interspersing standard pooled serum samples of known composition between batches of patient specimens. The calibration cycle is started either manually or automatically when the pooled serum is sampled.

Continuous-flow analyzers are the instruments most commonly used because of their high speed and relatively low cost.[38] All tests are performed on each sample; no random test selection is possible once the panel has been defined. Because of the nature of continuous-flow systems, there is a greater possibility of carryover of contamination from the preceding sample than in discrete-sampling systems. The analysis methodologies that can be used are restricted because they must conform to the special requirements of continuous-flow systems, which have longer start-up times and use greater amounts of reagents.

Discrete-sampling analyzers are more expensive than continuous-flow systems but have greater flexibility in selection of analysis methodology and in operational characteristics.[39] Some of them provide the capability of individual test selection, if a full test panel is not desired. Because every analysis channel is independent, maintenance and troubleshooting are simpler. These instruments generally have less down time and shorter start-up times.

Centrifugal analyzers run one test at a time on a batch of specimens.[40,41] To run a test panel, each specimen must be manually aliquoted into as many sample trays as there are tests; then each tray is run sequentially. These instruments require the smallest amounts of serum and have the fastest analysis times per test but require the largest amount of specimen handling. They cannot perform flame photometry tests such as sodium and potassium. Their operation appears to require more special training than any of the other instruments.

12. Achilles Reflex

The Achilles reflex measures the latency of the stretch reflex of the gastrocnemius muscle of the leg. The reflex is initiated by tapping with a hammer the Achilles tendon, which anchors the muscle to the heel. This stimulates stretch receptors in the muscle, which transmits nerve impulses to the spinal cord via sensory nerves. These nerves synapse with motor neurons that transmit nerve impulses back to the muscle to produce contraction, followed by relaxation. The Achilles reflex time is defined as the time from hammer contact to 50 percent relaxation of the muscle. It is prolonged in old age, hypothyroidism, and neurological disorders and is decreased in hyperthyroidism; however, its use as a screening tool is of doubtful clinical value.[42]

Two types of instruments are available to measure Achilles reflex: analog and digital.[43,44] In both instruments foot movement is recorded photoelectrically by having the foot interrupt a beam of light incident upon a photocell, as it rotates about the ankle. The analog device displays foot position as a tracing on a strip chart recorder; the Achilles reflex time is measured from the tracing. The digital device performs the measurement in the same manner but presents the result as a digital display in milliseconds.

13. History

Medical history can be obtained in a variety of ways as described in Chapter Six.[45,46] The simplest approach is to present the patient with a questionnaire to be filled out. The completed document may be inserted in the chart along with the multiphasic report. If it is desirable to enter the data into a computer for inclusion with the report instead of retaining a separate document, the information on the questionnaire may be keypunched or manually input through a computer terminal. In a more efficient approach to data entry, the questionnaire itself serves as a computer-readable document.[47,48] Several options are available:

a. Marksense documents. The questionnaire is constructed so that the patient responds by placing a mark in an appropriate answer field. An optical mark reader transfers the data to a computer or an intermediate storage medium. Disadvantages are that transcription of patient identification numbers to the document is error prone, entry of free text is not possible, document readers are expensive, and documents are easy to bend and readily jam the document-handling equipment.

b. Optical character readers. It is technologically possible for an optical character reader to recognize block-lettered responses written in an answer field on a questionnaire. However, the cost of such devices is prohibitive for a MHTS.

c. Marksense cards. Questions are presented on preprinted marksense cards. The patient marks the selected answers in the appropriate fields. A marksense card reader transfers the data to a computer or produces punched cards for subsequent data entry. Patient identification numbers can be pre-punched. Disadvantages are lack of flexibility of design and inability to enter free text.

d. Port-a-punch cards. These cards are similar to marksense cards except that a patient punches out his response with a stylus in a device similar to a voting machine. Disadvantages are similar to those of marksense cards. In addition, error correction is more difficult (requiring patching of punched holes) and, because the holes are perforated to allow manual punching, mechanical manipulation by card readers and personnel will result frequently in the creation of additional holes.

e. Sort-box cards. The patient is given a deck of cards, each card presenting a single question requiring a yes or no response. The patient sorts the cards into bins according to the response. Each card has a punched code to identify the question. Responses represented by the cards in a bin may be tabulated and punched by unit record equipment into a single card containing the patient's identification number. Disadvantages are similar to those of marksense cards. In addition, the presentation of multiple-choice questions is awkward.

f.   Interactive computer terminals.   An interactive computer terminal provides a flexible medium for the administration of a medical history questionnaire.[49,50] A fully branched questionnaire may be used, which most closely mimics the human interviewer. The patient is presented with a question on a display device, such as a typewriter, visual display cathode ray tube terminal (CRT), or special-purpose visual display device. He enters his response by pressing the appropriate key or button. An online computer is usually required to provide the logic that recognizes a patient's response and selects the appropriate subsequent questions. The major drawback of this approach is the cost involved in automated history terminals. Many MHTS facilities have found that the cost outweighs the benefits that accrue from the use of a branching questionnaire. Depending on the patient load and length of each interview, as many as 20 terminals have been required in a single facility.

A typewriter terminal is generally unsatisfactory as a history terminal. The printing rate of the lower-cost terminals is slow (10 to 30 characters per second). The standard full alphanumeric keyboard is not a suitable patient-response device. Special-purpose keyboards are available, but expensive.

CRTs are better than teletypewriters because of their more rapid writing rate and silent operation. However, they have the same disadvantages for patient responses.

Visual display terminals that use random-access slides and film strips are probably the most satisfactory history terminals from the patient's point of view. Displays are completely flexible and can use pictorial material. Responses to multiple-choice answers are usually entered by pressing buttons aligned to the right of the various answers. Numeric keypads can be provided for responses requiring numeric answers. Operation is virtually self-explanatory. Less computer access is required, since most of the information for the visual displays is stored in the slide or film strip at the terminal. Only control signals for frame selection and patient responses must be transmitted. Disadvantages are higher cost and difficulty in revision of questionnaire contents, since a photographic process is involved. Also, a relatively limited number of questions are possible with each terminal, and the time delay between question frames is a function of the mechanical separation of display images. As with any system involving mechanical components, maintenance and repair costs are high.

REFERENCES

1. Geddes, L. A., and Baker, L. E. *Principles and Applications of Biomedical Instrumentation.* New York: John Wiley & Sons, 1968.

2. Malmstadt, H. V., and Enke, C. G. *Digital Electronics for Scientists.* New York: W. A. Benjamin, 1969.

3. "Report of Inter-Society Commission for Heart Disease Resources. Electronic Equipment in Critical Care Areas. Part II: The Electrical Environment. Part III: Selection and Maintenance Program." *Circulation* 44(1971):A237–A261.

4. Association for the Advancement of Medical Instrumentation. Subcommittee on Electrical Safety. "Recommended AAMI Safety Standard for Electromedical Apparatus. Part I: Safe Current Limits." *J. Assn. Advan. Med. Instru.* 5(1971):314–321.

5. Whalen, R. E., and Starmer, C. F. "Electric Shock Hazards in Clinical Cardiology." *Mod. Concepts Cardiovasc. Dis.* 36(1967):7–12.

6. Dalziel, C. F. "Electric Shock Hazard." *IEEE Spectrum* 9(1972):41–50.

7. Grant, R. P. *Grant's Clinical Electrocardiography: The Spatial Vector Approach.* New York: McGraw-Hill, 1970.

8. Bergey, G. E., Squires, R. D., and Sipple, W. C. "Electrocardiogram Recording with Pasteless Electrodes." *IEEE Trans. Biomed. Eng.* BME-18(1971):206–211.

9. Pipberger, H. V., et al. "Clinical Applications of a Second Generation Electrocardiographic Computer Program." *Am. J. Cardiol.* 35(1975):597–608.

10. Elliot, R. V. *Demonstration and Evaluation of Computer-Assisted Analysis and Interpretation of the Electrocardiogram. A State of the Art Report.* Progress Report, Health Care Technology Division, National Center for Health Services Research and Development. September, 1972.

11. Bonner, R. E., and Schwetman, H. D. "Computer Diagnosis of Electrocardiograms—A Computer Program for EKG Measurements." *Comp. Biomed. Res.* 1(1968):366–386.

12. Pryor, T. A., Russel, R., Budkin, A., and Price, W. G. "Electrocardiographic Interpretation by Computer." *Comp. Biomed. Res.* 2(1969):537–548.

13. Walker, W. J. "A Small Portable Digital-Analog Device for Electrocardiographic Screening." *J.A.M.A.* 200(1967):313–316.

14. King, G. E. "Taking the Blood Pressure." *J.A.M.A.* 209(1969):1902–1904.

15. Kirkendall, W. M., Burton, A. C., Epstein, F. H., and Fries, E. D. "Recommendations for Human Blood Pressure Determination by Sphygmomanometers. Report of a Subcommittee of the Postgraduate Education Committee. American Heart Association." *Circulation* 36(1967):980–988.

16. Eilertson, E., and Humerfelt, S. "The Observer Variation in the Measurement of Arterial Blood Pressure." *Acta Med. Scand.* 184(1968):145–157.

17. Holland, W. W., and Humerfelt, S. "Measurement of Blood Pressure: Comparison of Intra-Arterial and Cuff Values." *Brit. Med. J.* 2(1964):1241–1243.

18. King, G. E. "Errors in Clinical Measurement of Blood Pressure in Obesity." *Clin. Sci.* 32(1967):223–239.

19. Gruen, W. "An Assessment of Present Automated Methods of Indirect Blood Pressure Measurement." *Ann. N.Y. Acad. Sci.* 147(1968):107–126.

20. Hochberg, H. M., and Salomon, H. "Accuracy of an Automated Ultrasonic Blood Pressure Monitor." *Curr. Therap. Res.* 13(1971):129–134.

21. Tahir, A. H., and Adriani, J. "Usefulness of the Ultrasonic Technique of Blood Pressure Determination." *Anesth, and Analg. Current Researches* 52(1973):699–702.

22. Comroe, J. H. *The Lung.* Chicago: Year Book Medical Publishers, 1962.

23. Comroe, J. H., and Nadel, J. A. "Screening Tests of Pulmonary Function." *New Eng. J. Med.* 282(1970):1249–1253.

24. Dickman, M. L., et al. "Online Computerized Spirometry in 738 Normal Adults." *Am. Rev. Respir. Dis.* 100(1969):780–789.

25. Protti, D. J., et al. "Computer Assistance in the Clinical Investigation of Pulmonary Function Studies." *Meth. Inform. Med.* 12(1973):102–107.

26. Green, M., et al. "Analysis of the Forced Expiratory Maneuver." *Chest* 63(1973):335–355, Supplement.

27. Porter, T. J., Logie, A. R., Ryan, J. F., and Webster, I. W. "A Computer Based System for Handling Radiological and Thermographic Data." *Australasian Radiol.* 17(1973):78–90.

28. Ackerman, L. V., and Gose, E. E. "Computer Interpretation of Xeromammogram Lesions." *Proc. San Diego Biomed. Symp.* 11(1972):341–342.

29. Goldmann, H. "Applanation Tonometry." In Newell, F. W. *Glaucoma: Transactions of the Second Conference.* Madison: Madison Printing Co., 1956.

30. Grolman, B. "A New Tonometer System." *Am. J. Optom.* 49(1972):646–660.

31. Forbes, M., Pico, G., Grolman, B. "A Noncontact Applanation Tonometer." *Arch. Ophth.* 91(1974):134–140.

32. Rudmose, W. "Automatic Audiometry." In Jerger, J. *Modern Developments in Audiology.* New York: Academic Press, 1963.

33. Davis, H., and Kranz, F. W. "The International Standard Reference Zero for Puretone Audiometers and Its Relation to the Evaluation of Impairment of Hearing." *J. Speech and Hearing Res.* 7(1964):7–16.

34. Wintrobe, M. M. *Clinical Hematology*. Philadelphia: Lea & Febiger, 1974.

35. Coulter, W. H. "High Speed Automatic Blood Cell Counter and Cell Size Analyzer." Presented at the National Electronics Conference. Chicago, October 1956.

36. Gochman, H. "Simultaneous Determination of White Cell Count, Red Cell Count and Hemoglobin with the Autoanalyzer Cell Counting System." In *Automation in Analytical Chemistry*. Technicon Symposia. New York: Mediad, 1965.

37. Pierre, R. V., and O'Sullivan, M. B. "Evaluation of the Hemalog-D Automated Differential Leukocyte Counter." *Mayo Clin. Proc.* 49(1974):870–874.

38. Smythe, W. J., Shanos, M. H., Morgenstern, S., and Skeggs, L. T. "SMA 12/60: A New Sequential Multiple Analyses Instrument." *Automation in Analytical Chemistry*. Technicon Symposia. New York: Mediad, Inc., 1968.

39. Horowitz, R. N., and Stewart, L. "The Hycel 17—an Evaluation." *Lab. Med.* 5(1974):46–49.

40. Schenken, J. "The Union Carbide Centrifuchem." *Lab. Med.* 5(1974):52–53.

41. Blume, P. "Experience with the Electro-Nucleonics Gemsaec Analyzer at the University of Minnesota." *Lab. Med.* 5(1974):34–40.

42. Rives, K. L., Furth, E. D., and Becker, D. V. "Limitations of the Ankle Jerk Test." *Ann. Intern. Med.* 62(1965):1139–1142.

43. Gilson, W. E. "Achilles Recording with a Simple Photomotograph." *New Eng. J. Med.* 260(1959):1027–1029.

44. Bowley, A. R., Digineed, J., Hedley, A. J., and Young, A. C. "A New Simple Detector for Achilles Reflex Measurement." *Med. and Biol. Eng.* 9(1971):351–357.

45. Wakefield, J. S., and Yarnall, S. R. *The History Database*. 3d ed. Seattle: Medical Computer Services Assoc., 1975.

46. McLean, E. R., et al. "The Collection and Processing of Medical History Data—A Bibliography of Manual, Automated and Computer-Assisted Techniques." *Meth. Inform. Med.* 14(1975):150–163.

47. Mayne, J. G., Martin, M. J., Morrow, G. W., Turner, R. M., and Hisey, B. L. "A Health Questionnaire Based on Paper-and-Pencil Medium Individualized and Produced by Computer. I. Technique." *J.A.M.A.* 208(1969):2063.

48. Martin, M. J., Mayne, J. G., Taylor, W. F., and Swenson, M. N. "A Health Questionnaire Based on Paper-and-Pencil Medium Individualized and Produced by Computer. II. Testing and Evaluation." *J.A.M.A.* 208(1969):2064–2068.

49. Slack, W. V., and Slack, C. W. "Patient Computer Dialogue." *New Eng. J. Med.* 286(1972):1304–1309.

50. Gottlieb, G. L., Beers, R. F., Bernecker, C., and Samter, M. "An Approach to Automation of Medical Interviews." *Comp. Biomed. Res.* 5(1972):99–107.

Data Processing

Lou S. Davis

A. INTRODUCTION

This chapter discusses a teamwork approach to the specification, economic justification, design, and implementation of the data processing aspects of an automated multiphasic health testing service (MHTS) laboratory. It covers some of the major problems of applying data processing to the MHTS application but will not explore the internal technical computer details for a multiphasic application; those details are covered elsewhere.[1-3] Because data processing systems need to be designed and specified from the perspective of the user as well as the data processor, the discussion will concern the requirements of these two different viewpoints rather than computers and computer equipment. (See also Chapter Three, F.)

To specify and design an efficient MHTS laboratory, expertise is necessary in each of several disciplines. The team specialists in each of these disciplines must be able to interact competently with one another. Consequently, interaction must be repetitive and frequent to allow cross-disciplinary learning. This process is a prerequisite to developing effective specifications and efficient design. It is not a linear process; it goes by spurts or leaps and bounds as studies, literature reviews, visits to other MHTS system sites, vendor presentations, and other steps occur and overlap. There are many things to do in parallel. The various topics discussed one by one in this chapter may in fact overlap, repeat, or be omitted as circumstances dictate.

B. DATA SERVICES: PROCESSING OBJECTIVES

A multiphasic health testing laboratory, within and together with the multiphasic health testing services (MHTS), will generate many various sets and subsets of data.[4] Not only do patient test data have to be processed, but also appointment data, registration data, work-list data, "tickler-file" data, administrative data, demographic data, followup data, laboratory operational data, etc. The different sets of data must be copied, sorted, collated, rearranged, and combined for different operational needs and reports. Test data themselves must be inspected (quality control), analyzed, and prepared (e.g., sorted and posted in charts) for reporting to the medical professional users. Historically, this work has been done by a clerical staff under varying degrees of control by supervisory and professional workers.

The extent to which the data themselves are processed is limited by the cost of hiring enough personnel to handle the paper work. For example, it may be thought desirable to produce legible, printed summaries of the multiphasic examinations for utilization by patients' physicians. However, typists in the quantity and quality needed to produce accurate summaries from each day's laboratory test results represent a significant service cost. Consequently, printed summaries are not usually provided in those clinics in which the paperwork is entirely manual.

Many sophisticated data management services also are possible. These would require direct handling and review of the data by the professional staff. Because it is difficult and costly to keep sufficiently competent professional personnel interested in doing complex, responsible, but highly repetitive work, these more sophisticated services are not commonly provided. For example, it is often thought desired to review each patient's test results at the end of the MHTS examination before he leaves the clinic and before his physician followup examination. This review would include checks for reasonableness of the test data, with repeat testing being initiated where necessary. More importantly, checks could be made for combinations of individual test results (normal and abnormal) to see if the patient should have additional tests, tests that are too expensive or time-consuming to do within the routine MHTS procedure. Such tasks, however, require technical expertise, guided by prescribed protocols, checking each patient's results thoroughly and consistently, patient after patient. This service, consequently, is costly and difficult to control or monitor for accuracy.

In summary, the data services that could be provided range from the simple to the most complex. Provision of such services would require additional personnel of varying skills, from the untrained clerk to the mostly highly trained professional.

What data processing objectives should be set for multiphasic services? In the manual mode, a level of data service has evolved that is compatible with direct costs vis-à-vis the user market. Current justification analysis procedures, incognizant of indirect benefits, often disallow extending services beyond the established level. This is particularly true when benefits are remote from the service area itself. For example, one could argue that if a summarized printed MHTS report would save 1.8 minutes of a physician's time in his not having to go through multiple handwritten test slips, history questionnaire, etc., and if an MHTS clinic turned out 100 such reports a day, an overall saving of three physician-hours per day could result. Assuming physician-hours at $50, each report would have a break-even value of 3 × $50/100, or $1.50. At today's clerical costs in the United States, a carefully checked, manually typed report could not be produced for only $1.50. Furthermore, it is difficult to prove that $150 would actually be saved each day by 100 typed reports, since a physician might choose to use his extra 1.8 minutes either in some nonproductive way or in giving the examinee an extra 1.8 minutes' attention. Who can estimate the dollar value of the latter and show that it warrants taking out-of-pocket dollars to pay for typed reports? Even an estimate of time savings, such as 1.8 minutes, is suspect because of the difficulties and delays involved in getting personnel to give up old habits and to learn new procedures. Any proposed extension of data service is difficult to justify because of the softness of highly subjective value judgments.

Because "it costs too much," opponents take the position:"No budget for the new data service until it is cost justified." Proponents insist: "We can't prove the benefits of the new service until it is implemented." This is not a real stalemate, however, since the old way perseveres and the new remains untried. The conservative attitude regularly prevails because it is safe and also, unfortunately, because too many new data service ideas are not well thought out; their overall impact is not investigated or they are not sufficiently planned. Still, the it-costs-too-much attitude is frequently biased by narrow thinking based on experience with manual systems. New manual improvements to manual systems are often incremental in nature, are not far-reaching, and have few additional benefits. Their cost is compared primarily to the direct quantifiable tangible benefits; hence, we have become accustomed to narrowing our cost-justification vision to immediate benefits rather than including far-reaching aggregates of qualitative intangible benefits. It is too easy to dismiss qualitative intangible benefits and stay with the immediate and the direct. Thus, new, potentially worthwhile services are often excluded by the it-costs-too-much attitude, especially when it restricts investigation. Finally, even if savings can be demonstrated, they are often in a different cost center and cannot be applied so as to pay for the additional service. Where is there an administrator who would transfer $150 per day of his physician budget to a test center just to receive printed reports?

This long preamble, hopefully, may motivate serious consideration of the following questions about the MHTS data services to be provided:

(1) What level along the continuum of data services is it feasible (practical and economical) to achieve?

(2) What are more sophisticated levels of service worth?

(3) What *are* the processing objectives for the data?

In designing the processing system, one should attempt to consider these questions in reverse order. First, ignoring temporarily the practical constraints of budget dollars, what total data services, internal and external to the MHTS, would it be desirable to furnish? Second, what cost trade-offs and cost benefits can be identified, along with studied and reasonable estimates of the probability of achieving the desired service levels? Last, how many of the trade-off dollars is management willing to spend (or reassign) to implement and operate the data service system?

In designing a new, or upgrading an existing MHTS, if the above questions are only superficially considered, and instead (as per custom) the budget is determined largely by quantifiable dollar savings obtained in reducing the MHTS clerical and technical personnel, then the level of data services will remain simple and low on the continuum. The introduction of new technological developments to aid the processing will be difficult to achieve, because the significant step increase in costs exceeds the salaries of a few clerks. Hence, the efficiencies possible in automated data processing do not normally provide enough savings in personnel alone to offset the initial costs of newer technology, especially when the volume of data (number of patients processed per time unit) is low. Where volume is high, savings in personnel will often justify implementing some new technological developments. Once given a system, justified solely on greater efficiency at a low end of the service continuum, it generally has enough surplus capability to provide additional services further up the scale, at small increments in costs, e.g., printed summaries of the multiphasic examination. The real value of the added services (such as printed examination reports), however, is still indeterminate, since the services are by-products, albeit supposedly worthwhile. Because the by-product data services usually remain unevaluated, savings may go unnoticed, or be ignored, and additional funds to move further up the service continuum remain as elusive as ever.

The data processing team is forced, by this incremental, evolutionary process, to build the strictly volume-justified system in a bottom-up patchwork mode. Because question 3 above was never answered, the system was not originally planned with an overall top-down logical approach. Ultimately, the patchwork will reach the point that the adding of one more service would require a new, more sophisticated programming system approach—which is expensive to implement. Because most of the added-on higher levels of services still remain unevaluated, there is no dollar trade-off to exchange for the reprogramming; hence, once again, "it costs too much" to do. A system developed under these conditions reaches only a slightly higher level of service than a manual system. Also, a cloud of suspicion may hover over it because "expensive" services are being furnished that have never been shown to be cost beneficial.

In summary, as many potential near- and long-term data services as possible should first be delineated. This will enable the data processing system designers to consider a hardware and software framework that would be more flexible and amenable to future additional incremental data services. Next, the proposed data services should be evaluated in terms of medical desirability and dollar trade-off, and implementation priorities should be established. Finally, a budget for the data processing services can be set that will fix the initial levels of services to be implemented.

C. USER OVERVIEW

What data services does the potential user want, ask for, or need? What additional services are possible but, because they are outside the user's frame of reference or experience, are either not considered or else dismissed without adequate consideration? Many an experienced data processing analyst has had a user ask for one thing and subsequently, upon seeing the results for the first time, realize and declare: "I know I asked for that, but that is not what I really wanted." While studying these programmed results, the user gets sudden insight into other system capabilities—often to the degree that his next request is for a complete revision of requirements. The data processing analyst, all too often, lacks sufficient insight into the user's problems to grasp the full connotation of his stated requirements. Thus, it is important that a sufficient mixture of multidisciplinary experience, training, insight, and discussion go into the preliminary consideration of potential MHTS data services, before any attempt is made to implement a system.

The MHTS has at least five general classes of users of its data: the patient, the operational personnel (nurses, technicians, clerks), the physicians (and nurse practitioners), the facility administration (for registration statistics, chart-request lists, financial reports, etc.), and the medical research staff.

It is important to consider each class and to delineate each user's near- and long-term data service requirements from his own viewpoint—all considerations initially to be unencumbered by budgetary and technical constraints. To start, a short paragraph or two describing each potential data service should be written and its meaning agreed upon by an appropriate multidisciplinary group. This will be a first step in the ultimate production of a document—an external design—that will represent a set of user functional specifications to be implemented on the target system. As discussed in E, an iterative procedure is necessary to produce the final specification document. (See also Chapter Five, F.)

Once a sufficiently large set of services is defined, the group can start consideration of medical desirability, technical implementation difficulty, retraining problems, user acceptance probability, etc., for each service. The data processing designer can begin evaluating total system complexity for specific subgroupings of the various services.

Agreement must be reached with management as to the extent and depth to which studies will be made to initially estimate, and subsequently evaluate, cost benefits of various data services. Agreement should also be reached as to which cost benefits can be translated into budget dollars to balance costs of a data processing system (B above).

The synthesis process to produce the final external design is discussed further in E and F.

The data service functions to be considered (some examples are given below) should first be specified in terms of *what* they are (rather than *how* they are to be implemented), and for which user class.

1.   Patient Identification and Administrative Information Services

Provide timely retrieval of patient identification information such as name, birthdate, sex, medical record number, insurance coverage, address, telephone number, with inquiry by either name or medical record number.

Users: MHTS appointment desk, registration desk, test phases.

2.   Health Care Entry Services

Provide a programmed branching technique to combine incoming telephone patient requests with medical record information to direct patient to the appropriate health care clinic, including MHTS.

Users: MHTS appointment desk, other referral service centers.

3.   MHTS Appointment System Services

(a) Provide timely retrieval of unfilled appointment slots by criteria such as day, time of day, approximate time-period away, reason for examination, sex, age, medical history, health care entry protocol, etc.

Users: Appointment desk, other referral service centers.

(b) Perform posting, canceling, general housekeeping of MHTS appointment files.

User: MHTS appointment desk.

(c) Provide preappointment lists and future appointment lists.

Users: Chart room (for pulling charts), MHTS registration desk, MHTS operations control.

(d) Provide mailable appointment-verifications for patients. Include personalized examination instructions, past history on followup history questionnaires (depending on what information is in system medical record), and personalized missing-data history questionnaire.

Users: Appointment desk, other referral service centers, patients.

4.   MHTS Operations Control

(a) Provide current-day appointment lists, working lists by type of appointment, special examinations, etc. Perform preparation of specimen labels, preparation of various data collection forms initialized with appropriate patient identification and other pertinent patient information.

Users: MHTS operations control, test phases.

(b) Check patient examination results for completeness, signal (potential) missing test results, analyze combinations of data for inconsistencies and signal (potential) test errors, analyze combinations of data according to physician-specified rules to signal additional tests and procedures, including referral to specialty clinics or to immediate sick care.

Users: MHTS operations control, test phases.

(c) Provide audit trail for test data sent outside multiphasic laboratory for interpretation. Prepare missing data followup lists. Prepare list of summary reports delayed due to missing data.

User: MHTS operations control.

(d) Provide daily, monthly financial reports, usage reports, statistical reports.

Users: MHTS operations control, facility administration.

(e) Provide programmed quality control procedures. Analyze standard sample data sets from various phase testing devices to signal equipment adjustment, maintenance, and repair.

Provide instream data sample procedures to adjust patient test results.

User: MHTS operations control.

(f) Provide archival and backup services for data retention, retrieval, and recovery. Provide audit control and listings for data record retention.

Users: MHTS operations control, facility administration, data processing staff.

5. Test-Phase Services

(a) Collect and record test data in a manner amenable to processing requirements. Furnish timely, appropriate feedback to the test-phase technician concerning data errors or data incompatibility with test limits or patient physiological characteristics.

Users: Test phases, MHTS operations control.

(b) Perform programmed, branching-type history questionnaires. Limit questions to information not already in system medical record. Perform in-depth branching for combinations of reported symptoms, test results, and physiological characteristics, according to physician decision rules.

User: History test phase.

(c) Perform programmed ECG analyses. Provide timely feedback to cardiologists as appropriate for validity checking. Compare current results to prior ECG results according to programmed decision rules.

Users: ECG test phase, cardiologists.

(d) Describe data service requirements for each of the remaining test phases to be implemented in this particular MHTS laboratory.

6. Medical Services

(a) Provide examination summary reports. Generate reports in medical problem orientation, time orientation, or other format. Include comparisons of test results with previous results or trend of previous results. Signal abnormal findings based on physician-generated rules. Signal diagnosis considerations ("consider" rules) based on physician-generated rules. Compare history questionnaire with previous results and signal any new symptoms reported for first time.

Users: Physicians, nurse practitioners.

(b) Provide medical data base services. Furnish timely, appropriate medical data retrieval information in appropriate format for authorized requesters. Provide for timely replacement of misplaced hard-copy reports.

Users: Referral services, health care services, nonappointment clinics, physicians, nurse practitioners, facility administration (insurance claims, back-to-work examinations, etc.).

7. Research Data Services

(a) Provide sequential files of specified, selected subsets of data (across patients) in hard-copy or machine-readable form.

Users: Physicians, research staff, facility administration.

(b) Provide direct retrieval and manipulation of data subsets to produce summary information, statistical comparisons and reports.

Users: Physicians, research staff, facility administration.

D. THE DATA PROCESSING PROBLEMS

As the major effort in exploring the potential services (B and C) culminates and the iterative process (E) of defining a statement of functional requirements (F) begins, general data processing capabilities, constraints, and costs will progressively impact the deliberations. Although the goal of the study process is to define the requirements of the MHTS data services from the user's viewpoint, and not to define the manner of implementation, certain data system problems must be recognized. What major variables will affect the data services specifications? We will discuss these as (1) problem definition, (2) problem magnitude, and (3) basic implementation direction.

1. Problem Definition

a. System responsiveness. Several of the preliminary requirements stated in C specify "timely." Hence, one of the major considerations of medical data services is the problem of response time. Response time is generally considered to be the time between the submission of a work unit to a processing system and the return of a result.

Three terms, *realtime, online,* and *offline,* are often used in data processing.[5] Although these terms are used somewhat differently by various writers and definitions overlap, they are convenient for this discussion of response time. *Realtime,* as used here, will refer to those cases where system response to input is fast enough to affect subsequent input. For example, a system is operating in realtime if, during the time it is connected directly to a test instrument for input of patient test samples, it will respond to interspersed input standard test samples for instrument calibration. Realtime will also include here conversational terminals where direct system responses vary significantly with user input. For example, visual display devices for displaying medical history questions, featuring in-depth branching penetration of detailed history levels dependent on patient input, would be considered as operating in realtime.

Online, as used here, includes direct entry of data to the system from the point of origin, with the output transmitted directly back to where it is used. This is similar to realtime, but for online the variety of system responses and entry of subsequent input is limited. For example, if the user enters a test result into the terminal, the system may respond only with a signal or message indicating the result is satisfactory or is outside established limits. In the latter case, the technician checks the test result and repeats the procedure to reenter the correct data. The tendency is to use the term "online" in those cases where the patient is still at the test station and the test can be immediately monitored and repeated, if necessary, before the patient leaves. *Offline* is used where test results are entered into the system at some point other than where originally generated, and after the patient leaves the clinic. Often it refers to batched data entered into the system's computer in a time period subsequent to patients' visits.

There are many advantages to timely data services. However, *timely* often connotes achieving capabilities high in the service continuum with the additional requirement of online or realtime processing or both. Online and realtime processing, as discussed in the examples above, result in better error checking and data correction. Signaling errors to the medical technician and getting data problems corrected while the patient is still in the clinic is superior to processing the data offline and having data processing personnel involved in subsequent error procedures. Other advantages of online processing, such as reduction of paperwork, improved quality control, generation of additional tests to perform (according to physician rules), etc., are discussed by Ariet.[1]

Unfortunately, data processing systems, including hardware and software components, become increasingly (often exponentially) expensive as the requirements for timely data services progress from offline to online to realtime performance. High patient and data volumes greatly increase the costs by requiring expanded processor capability to achieve appropriate response time. Thus, requirements for "timely" performance require careful analysis as to how the degree of system responsiveness relates to cost benefits.

Other requirements also imply a high degree of responsiveness for satisfactory implementation. The specification for a programmed, branching type history (C.5.b) would require interactive visual display terminals displaying programmed selection material, for patient entry of history data. The full high-cost import of this, including the needs for multiple terminals to avoid queuing, a communication system, a more powerful computer, direct-access files, sophisticated programming, and the development of extensive, well-tested medical branching decisions, must be carefully weighed against benefits.

In summary, one of the major problems affecting data processing is selection of the degree of system responsiveness needed for each service. Each data service requirement must be carefully defined and evaluated with regard to response time needed.

b.   Patient data files.   Two significant problems relate to the patient data files: (1) how to organize the files, (2) whether to keep a short-term or long-term data base.

(1) *Patient data file organization.* Medical information processing is difficult because the underlying medical data are variable and complex. The set and number of data elements stored from visit to visit are variable. Also, many data

elements (variables) change in definition over time. Because data must be stored in a manner (by storage location, by label, etc.) such that they can be meaningfully retrieved, it must be decided how the data base program is to track variable content of data items and items whose definitions may change from one visit to the next. At what point does a test change enough to become a different test? For example, is the reported test result for a glucose test by potassium ferricyanide reduction the same as a glucose test result by glucose oxadase? Over time the clinical laboratory may have used both methods. Is it important, on MHTS summary reports to physicians, to distinguish the two test results? Is it important to distinguish the two for research purposes? The answers to the last two questions for this example are likely to be ''no'' and ''yes,'' respectively. For other examples the answers will vary. Thus, considerations of total data services and of *all* users' needs are vital to data element definition and storage strategy.

Processing rules for medical data services contain many exceptions and too few generalities. Adjustments and changes in the rules occur with high frequency and sometimes seem arbitrary. The data storage organization and technique chosen will absolutely limit the degree of flexibility the system will have, not only for current changes, but also for subsequent changes needed for evolution to higher levels along the service continuum. Consequently, the record design should allow as much data item storage flexibility as possible within the confines of cost, response time, and implementation time. Generally, the more flexibility and capability required of the data base, the more difficult it is to program, and (for a given computer) the longer it will take the system to retrieve data. A data base strategy that has capability beyond immediate requirements makes the system more amenable to subsequent data service changes. This would avoid a complete reprogramming effort, as well as an entire data base translation, when requirements change. At best, it is a difficult trade-off to judge. Medium- to long-range goals for the data service system are necessary prerequisites for a judicious decision.

Because the set of data items encompassed by an MHTS examination represents many areas of medicine—history, clinical laboratory tests, ECG, x-ray, visual tests, auditory tests, etc.—a comprehensive data storage strategy is required. Even if the initial data service requirements are minimal, the complexity and extent of the examination data require a storage strategy entry point significantly beyond elementary solutions.

(2) *Short-term or long-term data base.* A short-term data base is a system in which data for single current active visits are kept on direct-access files for processing. After all data for a patient's current visit are collected and processed, the visit record is purged to magnetic tape. No effort is made either to collate the patient's previous visits or to retrieve previous data for use during the current active visit. Such a system is relatively easy to implement at moderate cost but precludes from further consideration many of the services listed in C.1–7.

An elementary long-term data base is a system in which data for single current active visits are kept on direct-access files along with selected prior data retrieved from the tape files. After all data for a patient's current visit are received and processed, the visit record is purged to magnetic tape. An active effort is made to collate the patient's previous visits. Selected prior data are retrieved from the tape files and moved to the direct-access files before the patient revisits the clinic. While this system has clear advantages over the short-term data base, such as making available comparisons to previous data for summary reports (C.6.a), it also precludes many of the services proposed in C.1–7. Ease and cost of implementation may be moderately greater than with a short-term data base system. However, unless patient volume is low, it will be difficult and expensive to operate. With high volume, the set of history tapes becomes larger and larger over time; and the collating, updating, retrieval, backup, and general housekeeping problems create a very large and error-prone overhead. Also, in this case, if the MHTS processes patients appearing on a drop-in (i.e., nonappointment) basis, retrieval of their old data for current data service requirements may not be possible within the response-time requirements.

A long-term data base that keeps predefined "essential" medical data from all visits, on a direct-access basis over long periods of time, represents a significant step-function increase in costs and difficulty of implementation. However, this step is essential if the data services listed in C.1–7 are to be implemented. Ideally, if the organization has a distributed data base facility already in existence, the MHTS function could implement the higher-level service functions as a distributed processor and relegate long-term data storage and retrieval to the organization data base service. This would allow individual medical applications such as the MHTS to be implemented at a very high level of data service and at a more easily justified cost (if the organization data base service has been already justified). However, in 1976 such facilities did not exist; therefore, some very difficult and complex trade-off decisions must be made between desired data services and data base management system implementation costs.

(3) *Volume.* A third problem is that of patient volume—the number of patient records to be input, processed, and stored. The impact of high volume on response time and data base has already been discussed. Volume also impacts data entry design, data processing staffing, and considerations involving techniques to improve flow and keep track of patient status and data result status. Since many estimates of needed data processing capability are based on estimated processing volume, accurate patient volume estimates for the near and long term are necessary.

2. Problem Magnitude

At some point in the system analysis, a tentative budget range for data processing must be recognized. This budget must encompass the expected life cycle of the system so that capital and development costs (if any) are prorated over the years. This tentative budget, established by cost-benefit expectations, will set an approximate limit to hardware and software capability, thereby establishing the preliminary scope of data services that can be provided.

3. Basic Implementation Direction

As the system analysis progresses, various assumptions can be made as to how the data service system could be implemented, given a specified budget as in D.2 above. For example, will the facility develop the system with its own data processing and engineering staff, or is an outside vendor to develop it and turn it over for operation? Within these two basic divisions there are many alternatives for implementation. Is the system to be developed from the specifications, or will a vendor-supplied turnkey system fit the specifications satisfactorily? Is the computer system to be freestanding or connected to a larger system? Will the clinic have terminals that are operated by a remote computer on a time-sharing basis?

Although it would be premature at this point to settle on any one alternative, because there are so many permutations of ways of implementation, it is necessary to consider the more desirable alternatives and computer cost range expectations.

With a budget range set, the feasibility of the preferred alternatives (as well as response time and data base consequences) can be better evaluated.

E.   ITERATION PROCEDURE

Having progressed through this much work, the multidisciplinary team will have a better understanding of the relationships between data service objectives, costs, benefits, functions to be performed, problem size, and basic implementation directions. Although many of the individual problems will have been studied and restudied, the process needs to be iterated many times. It will be necessary to discuss the interrelationships between proposed data services and implementation consequences. If the tentative decisions made in choosing the basic direction (D.3) turn out to require a budget range greater than cost benefits, a reexamination of requirements (and cost benefits) is in order. Compromise, adjustment, and repeated review are necessary. This process must be conducted resolutely to lead up to a final, documented definition of requirements.

It will help, in this iterative procedure, to use as many development tools as possible to keep track of proposed design and progress. Good documentation of meeting minutes, the use of written reports for all proposals, of HIPO[6] for specification of functions, and of critical path diagrams for development sequences are all helpful. Mock-ups of all proposed input formats, data service displays, and hard-copy reports are invaluable in reducing communication misunderstanding about what is wanted.[7]

In order to help keep all the desired services in mind, the committee should especially aim for as complete and well-documented a list of desired data service functions as possible (C). During the iterative procedure the team could even keep two such lists, one a theoretical no-cost-constraints and no-implementation-constraints list, and the other a practical target list for implementation. The latter, in effect, becomes a requirements list.

F.   USER REQUIREMENTS

Eventually there will come a time when the iteration must stop and a set of user requirements be specified. (A deadline date should have been set when the study was first initiated.) This user requirements specification should be a document that spells out a set of functions of *what* is to be provided (as opposed to *how* the functions are to be implemented).

From these requirements a preliminary *external design* set of specifications is prepared, in diagrammatic form. These are divided into the functions, indicating all input data to each function, the logical process within each function, the output of each function, and the relationship of the functions. (See also Chapters Five and Twenty.) Expected response times must be specified, and mock-ups of all displays and reports prepared. It is to be emphasized that the external design reflects the *users'* views and does not address implementation.

Finally, this total set of specifications should be presented (walked through) for completeness and accuracy by the multidisciplinary team to as many concerned, appropriate, and responsible users as feasible.

Armed now with a well-defined set of user requirements, the preliminary external design, and a tentative budget range, the team can begin serious consideration of implementation.

The fundamental choice of either purchase an outside vendor's system or develop the system within-house can be a labyrinthic one.[8] Unavailability of in-house technical talent, limited time to implement, and amortization of development costs over many systems are considerations that could lead to choosing a vendor with a turnkey system. The vendor may also have developed easy-to-use terminals for specific online data use at the various MHTS test stations. On the other hand, the vendor's system may present a wide variance from the user requirements, may not have a data base compatible with other organizational needs such as administrative or research use, or may not be amenable to large (or small) patient volume. If the organization has (or plans to have) other medical data processing applications, the vendor's system is likely to have an incompatible interface to the other system. These questions must all be evaluated.

G. VENDOR-SUPPLIED SYSTEMS

The choice here is either to consider an already developed system that can be brought in, installed, and tuned (or tailored, insofar as possible) to the user requirements, or to have an outside vendor develop a system in substantial accordance with the requirements. The former case (the so-called turnkey system) will be discussed here. The latter case will not be discussed specifically but is covered by a combination of this section and the next (H).

1. Completion of the External Design

The first step is to use the preliminary external design to compare, point-by-point, each difference (positive as well as negative) between the data service requirements and the capabilities of each vendor's system.

A final external design, representing what each particular vendor system *will* furnish for the user, must be prepared. It must contain the actual specifics tied to services, including displays, reports, hardware, etc. It should also include system response times, implementation time, system maintenance, and backup procedures.

The final external design specification process will also be iterative and lengthy, as each vendor will offer to add to or tailor his system to meet as many requirements as possible. Consequently, it may be necessary to abbreviate the process by broadly reviewing several vendors' products to narrow down to two or three vendors for in-depth studies. One way to do this is to give the preliminary external design documentation to the vendors and let each prepare a final external design (i.e., in the form of a proposal).

Just as the user requirements (in the form of the preliminary external design) were reviewed by appropriate personnel, so should each vendor's external design that will be considered for implementation be reviewed.

2. Contract Negotiations

The most important point is to get all vendor verbal promises made during the final external design phase specified in the final external design document. The external design document then becomes that part of the contract which specifies the services and performance level to be met by the vendor. Making this documented, expected performance a part of the contract generally forces a high-level review and approval in the vendor's company.[9-11]

More detailed advice about computer hardware and software contracts is available in other references.[12,13] There are even consulting firms that advise in negotiating computer contracts.[14]

Important considerations that should be included in the contract are:

(1) The vendor should provide (and keep up to date) source listings of all programs used in the supplied system.

(2) Specific procedures should be established regarding requests for program changes and implementation of such changes, including format of request, response-time allowance to vendor to provide estimate for changes, and establishment of priorities for revisions.

3. Installation, Checkout, Acceptance

Every effort should be made to satisfy (after a critical review) the environmental conditions recommended by the vendor for his system, including power, space, air conditioning, and construction, and have these ready when the system is delivered.

A large number of complete sample patient-test-data protocols should be pre-specified and ready for entry when the system is released by the vendor for use. These protocols should include checks for abnormal findings, tests for results outside of reasonable limits, combinations of history questions to include all questions answered, combinations of results to force all medical decision rules in the system, etc. Any data result or combination of data results in which a program error could lead to subsequent erroneous medical action and/or medical liability should be expressed in a patient test protocol. At a very minimum, the system should not be accepted until it processes all sample patient protocols correctly.

Because of the large number of test permutations, it will be impossible to have complete assurance that the system is error-free. Consequently, errors will be discovered during the life cycle of the system. Whenever an error is found and corrected, the test conditions that generated the error should become part of another sample patient protocol. The set of protocols should be saved and used each time the computer system (hardware and software) is revised to insure that any revisions have not caused new problems.

4. Operation, Program Malfunction, and Maintenance

As the system is operated, discrepancies between the user requirements as documented, the vendor's implementation interpretation, and the user's expectations will surface. There will probably be many users, who for one reason or another did not participate in the original requirements specification or review, for whom the system will be a surprise, and some of whom consequently will not be ready to change to any new procedures or new work habits forced by the system. The latter group will have many suggestions (hopefully constructive) to change or modify the system. In addition, the need for new data services will arise, and requests will continually be made to change the system.

Because of the costs and long lead times often entailed in adding new services and making changes, it is imperative that the revised requirements be correctly specified, clearly documented, and agreed upon by all concerned prior to implementation. It is imperative that all documentation, user requirements, external design, program listings, etc. be updated at appropriate times in the revision process.

Because the addition and changes must be tested, additional sample patient protocols are necessary. If the data processing system is a realtime operation system, it may be necessary to do some of the testing while the system is in actual operation processing patients. Thus, one of the criteria in system specifications is the ability to do such testing in a "safe" manner—i.e., to protect the integrity of patient processing and not damage the system or data base.

In spite of the best of efforts, however, system failures due to either hardware or software problems will arise. Consequently, backup procedures allowing continuing operation of the clinic must be ready (and demonstrated before system acceptance). While breakdown of an offline system may not impact the clinic processing significantly, the more online or realtime components a system has, the more essential and complex satisfactory backup procedures become. An abrupt and rare interruption of the regular operation of a realtime data entry terminal, in which many data collection decisions are directed and confirmed under programmed rules to a backup paper-and-pencil recording of data, may lead to severe degradation in quality of data collection. Since the operations personnel are not as familiar with the backup system, however regularly practiced, slowdown of patient processing and general disruption of patient flow and progression through the MHTS will ensue. To reduce the time spent in back up mode operation, spare "plug-in" parts, such as terminals, printers, etc., should be readily available. Vendor field engineering support should be locally available for quick response to repair hardware failures.

H. SELF-DEVELOPED SYSTEMS

1. First Internal Design and Data Processing Requirements

Just as the external design, reflecting the user's view of the MHTS system, was developed iteratively, so also will be the sets of documents that specify the programming view of the data processing system requirements and design.

The preliminary internal design, the functional specification expressing *what* is to be accomplished in the MHTS from the programmer's viewpoint, will be completed after the user requirements and external design are set. The overall logic, input, processing, output, and interconnection of each data service function must be specified, documented, and iteratively reviewed. The internal design efforts are likely to lead to a more detailed version of the external design.

As the major parts of the internal design are completed, the detailed questions of *how* the system is to be implemented will be addressed. Thus must begin the consideration of overall strategies for file design, decision and logic table handlers, input/output drivers, interrupts processing, operating systems, data base management, telecommunication processing, etc. Hardware capabilities, selection of programming languages, availability of software packages, etc., must also be considered. Then in relation to the tentative budget a first set of the data processing requirements can be documented.

2.   Final External Design

The preliminary external design (the user's view of the system) should now be reviewed against the capabilities and constraints uncovered in the internal design and data processing requirements step (H.1 above) and a final external design prepared. This final design should express functionally the system as the physicians, operations personnel, and other users will see and use it. It should again be reviewed, service by service, and a complete walk-through of the specifications performed. At this point, the system requirements for the first implementation should be frozen; at least no changes should be considered unless their full impact on the implementation schedule (H.3) is understood and approved.

3.   Computer Selection and Order; Implementation Schedule

If the organization already has a computer system, it may be desirable to consider its use, providing it has sufficient processing time and software operating system capability to handle the MHTS data processing requirements as defined. Another option would be to use a time-sharing or a remote job entry service or both. Many systems use freestanding minicomputers to run MHTS systems. Newer ideas involve using a minicomputer in the MHTS to perform much of the application logic, but connected by communication lines to a large computer system for supplemental computing and long-term data base storage and retrieval. The choice between the alternatives must encompass the specified MHTS requirements, the budget, and the long-term organization goals for medical data processing. Alternatives that encompass the leading edge of technology must be recognized as such, and proper allowances for costs and implementation time made.

When one alternative is chosen, then proposals for the implied hardware (computer, terminals, communication equipment, etc.) from many vendors should be invited for consideration.

A detailed schedule, including factors such as equipment delivery time, construction for installation (wiring, air conditioning, etc.), staff hiring and training, software design, programming, coding and testing, etc., should be documented. A project control technique, such as the critical path method, is most helpful in establishing the project schedule and the subsequent monitoring for project progression.

4. Detailing Internal Specifications

Following completion of the final external design and selection of the specified hardware, the programmer's internal design specifications can be put in final form and frozen. Other documentation such as flow charts, input/output formats, error messages, preliminary program writeups, etc., should be prepared. All functional and flow documentation should be reviewed by the data processing staff and approved by the computer processing management.

Backup procedures should also be similarly covered, including walk-throughs by all concerned. If the design is for an online system, the impact of hardware and software failures must be carefully examined and appropriate procedures for operational personnel delineated.

5. Coding and Testing

Following preparation of all the above documentation and adequate program training of the staff, then (and only then) should the coding of the programs start.

It is difficult to restrain the individual programmers from starting coding the moment each receives some information about what is wanted. Typically, when programs are started before the problems are well specified, the programmer ends up making many small assumptions (and decisions) about how "things" should be, and these get expressed in the code while he is writing it. Later, when these decisions are found to be inadequate or in error, they are difficult to change and may even require rewriting large segments of code.

Complete specification of the problems often reveals common requirements and generalities that can be coded as service or library routines for the overall program system, thereby saving enormous amounts of coding.

Organized and rational procedures of testing have been developed and written about over the last few years. The data processing management should decide on the testing procedures and require the staff to follow them. In addition, sets of test decks (sample patient protocols, as discussed in G.3) should be prepared and extensively used.

6. Installation

During the period between the order for hardware and the delivery of the system, the physical site should have been prepared according to the requirements of the vendor's specifications. Depending upon the sophistication of the equipment, an adequate set of equipment test procedures and programs (agreed upon earlier in the contract with the hardware vendor) should be applied to the equipment before it is accepted.

If the software has already been partially tested on another system (at the vendor's local office or elsewhere), final program testing and checkout can be completed.

Careful coordinated planning will be required if the system is to be inserted into an already operating MHTS. An intensive program of training for all those who enter data into the system, receive output, etc., preceding the cutover will be necessary. If the MHTS has a heavy volume, it may be wise to reduce the number of appointments for the first few days of running in order to allow the MHTS personnel to get used to the new work procedures.

It is likely that the MHTS personnel will also have to cope with learning and using the backup procedures during this period, as the data processing system will undoubtedly suffer early hardware and software failures.

7.   Operation, Program Modification, and Maintenance

As the system is operated, discrepancies between the user's requirements as documented, the data processing staff's interpretation, and the user's expectation will surface. These problems and subsequent program modifications are discussed in G.4. However, now the facility's own programming staff will make the modifications. Because of this, there is a great temptation to correct problems informally on a person-to-person demand basis. Except for serious errors, which must be changed immediately (e.g., reporting a given test result erroneously), all requested changes should go through a formal review and approval cycle before they are implemented. (System modification requests are also discussed in Chapter Five, B.2.) This will allow review, by many, of the impact on various types of users, as well as any necessary training and coordination of the changes. Sometimes this review procedure inserts some delay that in turn provides a desirable cooling-off period, allowing a more rational look at a new (enthusiastically supported) idea.

To maintain satisfactory hardware performance, the vendor should provide quick-response service from a local office to repair hardware failures (see G.4).

I.   OTHER CONSIDERATIONS

1.   Privacy, Confidentiality, and Security

The increasing interest in and legislation for control of personal data banks[15] requires proper supporting security procedures. The fact that the records are magnetically recorded (and hence not easily readable to the roving human eye) does not decrease the need to protect them from unauthorized disclosure, erroneous modification, or loss and destruction.[16,17] Analogous techniques used in securing conventional medical records, as have been developed in the long tradition of confidentiality between patient and physician,[18] must, as a minimum, be implemented.

Indeed, an important part of the external design specification is to spell out the *security* measures that will be necessary to maintain *confidentiality* to protect patients' *privacy*.[19] Both physical and logical security measures must be specified. Physical measures include locked access to the computer and computer data storage areas, fire protection, remote terminal protection, etc. Logical measures, such as program password checking at terminals, limiting the type of terminal information displayed to class of user, etc., are recommended. Automated data processing can create new security problems.[17] For example, because various patient reports are so easy and quick to produce, many copies are often produced for work use. These copies eventually are thrown away or filed away in places other than the conventional medical chart. Hence, security measures for these data as well as waste paper disposal must be planned.

2. Mobile MHTS Systems

The requirement that the MHTS be mobile[20] does not change the need for planning the data processing system as already described. Because of the limited space of the mobile lab, the number of different test procedures and the volume of patients is probably reduced. Consequently, the data processing requirements are likely to be less, and systems simpler. Long-term storage and recall of the data for future examinations may not be needed, as the mobile center is less likely to be a part of a given population's regular ongoing health care. If these lessened needs do indeed obtain, the data processing costs should be greatly lessened.

3. Use of the Computer for Other Applications

If it is decided that the MHTS is to have its own computer system, then it may be desirable to have the ability to process other applications, such as accounting, payroll, etc., on the same computer system that handles the MHTS data. For a small increment in hardware costs (for memory, additional input/output units, etc.), many computers offer this capability. However, an operating system program to control the overlapping processing of multiple applications is needed. The degree of sophistication needed for the operating system by a particular set of applications must be determined. This added criterion will reduce the hardware choices.

Some vendors with turnkey MHTS systems do not provide capabilities for processing other applications (background jobs) while the MHTS programs are operating.

4. Technology Changes

The revolution that is occurring in electronics is going to have far-reaching influences in computer applications. The costs of processors, main memories, and direct-access storage devices are dropping dramatically. The availability of greatly increased computing capacity for far less money will make many desirable computer application services feasible. Although these advanced services require sophisticated software (more expensive than ever), operating systems, data base systems, etc., will also become available just as they have on today's large, complex, and expensive computers. The availability of these programming tools (which represent many years of manpower effort), together with very low-cost but powerful computer systems, will accelerate development of general management information systems.[21] These systems, hopefully, will be able to be used for medical records, since, from an information science viewpoint, medical data are just data. In the next few years, emphasis will change from freestanding medical applications, such as MHTS, clinical laboratory, etc., to integrated information systems, where there is a distributed processing and distributed data base capability. As hardware costs continue to fall and as programming sophistication increases, these systems will be built. It isn't too early to consider now the kinds of

MHTS services that are possible only in such systems. As systems are developed under current constraints, keeping in mind those data services that cannot yet be implemented may allow building the current system in such a way that it can be more easily transformed into a future system.

ACKNOWLEDGMENTS

The author wishes to acknowledge and thank N. Bell, M. Collen, J. Duncan, D. Hueter, and E. Van Brunt for their contributions.

Thanks are also extended to the following persons or companies for responding to information requests regarding implemented MHTS systems: M. Ariet, University of Florida; G. Collings, New York Telephone; F. Failing, Pelam, Inc.; S. Gort, International Business Machines, Inc.; L. Schneider, International Health Systems, Inc.; R. Shoen, AML International; P. Wharton, Charlotte Medical Clinic; K. Yamaguchi, Toshiba; W. Yamamoto, George Washington University.

REFERENCES

1. Ariet, M., and Clark, E. M. "Multiphasic Screening: Computer Principles." Chapter 11 in Haga, E., ed. *Computer Techniques in Biomedicine and Medicine*. Philadelphia: Auerbach Pub., Inc., 1973.

2. Gillis, A. "Data Processing Requirements for Multiphasic Health Screening Centers." In *Automated Multiphasic Health Testing and Services*. U. S. DHEW, N.T.I.S., Springfield, Va., Vol. 3(1970):99–124.

3. Scott, M. R., and Frederik, W. S. "Electronic Data Processing (EDP) and Multiphasic Health Screening." *J. Occup. Med.* 14(1972):457–461.

4. "Data Processing, Provisional Guidelines." In *Automated Multiphasic Health Testing and Services*. U.S. DHEW, N.T.I.S., Springfield, Va., Vols. 1 and 2 (1970):17–20, Reports Nos. PB 195654 and 196000.

5. IBM Corp. *Data Processing Glossary*. White Plains, N.Y., 1972.

6. Stay, J. F. "HIPO and Integrated Program Design." *IBM Sys. J.* 15(1976):143–154.

7. Donelson, W. S. "Project Planning and Control." *Datamation* 22(1976):73–80.

8. Polli, G. "Medical Computing in the Small Clinic: Data Processing Alternatives and Their Economic Impact." *Computers & Medicine,* March 1976.

9. Bucci, R. A. "Beware the Standard Lease." *Datamation,* March 1973.

10. Bucci, R. A. "Avoiding Hassles with Vendors." *Datamation,* July 1974.

11. Nelson, N. "Laboratory Data Standards." In *Proc. ECHO Spring Mtg.,* San Francisco, April 1973.

12. Brandon, D. H., and Segelstein, S. *Data Processing Contracts.* New York: Van Nostrand Reinhold Co., 1976.

13. Bigelow, R. P. *Guide to Negotiating a Computer Contract.* Newton, Mass.: Computerworld, 1969.

14. "Company Specializes in Negotiating Contracts for Users." *Computerworld,* Oct. 22, 1975, p. 40.

15. Westin, A. F., and Baker, M. A. *Databanks in a Free Society.* New York: Quadrangle Books, 1972.

16. Davis, L. S. "Data Security Considerations in a Medical System." In *IBM Data Security Symp.* IBM Corp., White Plains, N.Y. Form No. G520–2838, April 1973.

17. Davis, L. S., and Terdiman, J. F. "The Medical Data Base." Chap. 4 in Collen, M. F., *Hospital Computer Systems.* New York: John Wiley & Sons, 1974.

18. Gabrieli, E. R. "Data Center Ethics." *Computers & Medicine,* Nov. 1975.

19. Renninger, C. R., and Branstad, D. K. "Government Looks at Privacy and Security in Computer Systems." *NBS Technical Note No. 809,* Nat'l Bureau of Standards, U.S. Dept. of Commerce. Washington, D.C.: U.S. Govt. Print. Off., Feb. 1974.

20. Fitzpatrick, M., and Zaves, N. A. "Mobile Multiphasic Health Screening—Mediclinic." *J. Occup. Med.* 14(1972):450–456.

21. Floam, G. "Putting a Data Base on a Mini." *Datamation* 22(1976):97–100.

CHAPTER NINE

Quality Control

Joseph F. Terdiman

A. INTRODUCTION

An MHTS requires a program of quality control to insure the accuracy of patient identification and of test results.[1-5] Quality control provides assurance that the data on a multiphasic report belong to the patient whose name appears in the heading, that quantitative measurements (such as blood pressure and serum glucose) are accurate within a few percent, that qualitative results (such as x-ray and EKG interpretations) were made from the correct source documents and are clinically accurate and reliable, and that answers to personal and medical history questions were accurately recorded.

Adequate quality control is especially important for multiphasic testing, in which a battery of tests is performed on a large number of patients in a short period. If an instrument begins to produce erroneous results, many patients may receive inaccurate measurements before the malfunction is detected. The cost of these errors in terms of a patient's health and additional medical services required may be considerable, depending upon the type of test and the nature of the error. For example, a 10 percent error in height or weight is usually of little clinical significance. If necessary, these tests can be quickly and inexpensively repeated. On the other hand, an error in a tonometry measurement (a test for glaucoma in which intraocular pressure is measured) may prove expensive and be of grave significance. If the test result was falsely high (a false positive), the patient may be referred to an ophthalmologist for one or more followup visits to recheck the measurement. If the measurement was falsely low or normal (a false negative) when intraocular pressure was actually high, permanent visual impairment or blindness (and a possible lawsuit) may occur because the patient did not receive the early treatment that would have been started had the condition been detected during multiphasic testing. (See Chapter Seventeen.) Therefore, a heavy burden is placed on health professionals responsible for the multiphasic facility: the system must always provide accurate, reliable data for each patient.

The clinical utility of multiphasic health testing depends to a large extent on physicians' confidence in the accuracy of the data. A physician will develop this confidence only after a period of time during which he has received consistently accurate and reliable multiphasic reports. Frequent errors in test data or patient identification will decrease his confidence in the results, thereby decreasing the effectiveness of multiphasic health testing as a component of a health care delivery system.

The value of multiphasic data for epidemiological research depends on their quality. Because of the large numbers of patients that receive multiphasic examinations and the broad spectrum of medical testing performed, a multiphasic data base provides a vast potential resource for a variety of epidemiological studies. If the data are inaccurate or unreliable, however, statistical analyses will provide meaningless or erroneous conclusions.

A complete multiphasic quality control system checks both testing procedures and data processing procedures. Quality control of testing procedures assures the proper calibration, functioning, and operation of test instruments. Quality control of data processing procedures assures that patient identification and test data will be accurately entered into and reported out from the computer system.

A quality control system can be divided into six basic components:

(1) *Patient identification checking* is necessary to insure that test results are linked to the correct patient.

(2) *Data monitoring* is necessary to check the accuracy and reliability of the measurements.

(3) *Personnel monitoring* is necessary to insure that multiphasic technicians and clerks are consistently following proper testing procedures and not inadvertently affecting the measurements.

(4) *Instrument standardization and calibration* are necessary to maintain the accuracy of test instruments.

(5) *A reporting system* is necessary to communicate equipment malfunctions or personnel problems to appropriate individuals.

(6) *Error correction procedures* are necessary when inaccurate test results have been inadvertently reported to a user.

B. PATIENT IDENTIFICATION CHECKING

Each piece of multiphasic data must be linked to a specific patient. This linkage is usually provided by assigning the patient an identification number, which is associated with each test result. The number may be a permanent one, such as a health plan medical record number or a social security number, or it may be a sequential accession number assigned to the patient at the time of the multiphasic visit. This number is the primary patient identifier for the MHTS. Secondary identifiers, including patient's name, sex, and date of birth, are used for verification of the primary identifier. They also are required to appear in the heading of the multiphasic report, and age and sex are necessary for some normal value calculations.

Because of the importance of accurate patient identification, an additional check digit is sometimes entered into the system at the same time as the identification number. The value of the check digit is computed from the other digits of the identification number by an algorithm such that, if an error is made during transcription or computer input, such as an incorrect digit or a transposition of two adjacent digits (the most common numerical transcription errors), the check digit computed from the erroneous number will differ from the original check digit. Comparison of the computed check digit with the value entered will reveal the error. In this manner, a computer can be programmed to check the accuracy of the primary identifier.

The method by which a patient's identification number is associated with his test data depends upon the mode of data entry for the MHTS. In some online computer systems the registering patient is assigned an accession number, which is entered into the system through a computer terminal together with his name and other identifying information. The patient is handed a machine-readable identification badge, which contains the accession number (with or without check digit) in the form of punched holes, magnetic strip, or bar code. At each phase the accession number is read by a suitable badge reader connected to the computer, which identifies the patient to the system and signals that the data that follow (from instrument or terminal) belong to that patient. These systems usually provide feedback from the computer to the phase for verification of the accession number. Although this linkage method seems highly reliable, patients, on occasion, will misplace their badges or inadvertently switch badges with another patient.

In online computer systems without badges an identification number must be keyed in through a terminal at each phase. Entry of a check digit and suitable feedback for verification are especially important in these systems to prevent erroneous data linkages.

In some offline multiphasic computer systems data cards are the principal data entry documents. Both identification number and test results are usually keypunched and/or marksensed into the cards, which are then read into a computer terminal. A patient's identification number (possibly including a check digit) and secondary identifiers may be keypunched into a header card from information provided by the patient at the time the appointment was made, and verified, if possible, against the patient's administrative record. Minor discrepancies in the verified data, such as a minor misspelling of a name or a small difference in birth year, may be ignored, but major discrepancies, such as a difference in sex or in first or last name, may indicate an error in the patient identification number and should be checked with the patient. From the header card the identification number can be gang-punched into a pack of test cards by unit record equipment. The patient carries the prepunched pack with him throughout the testing. At each phase the appropriate test card (which now contains the patient's identification number) is withdrawn from the pack and the test data entered via keypunch or marksense entry. Thus, all data cards will contain the correct patient identification number.

C. DATA MONITORING

The purpose of data monitoring is to check the functioning and calibration of test instruments[6,7] and the multiphasic technicians' operation of these instruments by means of statistical analyses of the test data the instruments produce. Deviations of test results from established baseline patterns indicate either equipment malfunction, incorrect operation, or poor calibration.

Data monitoring is usually performed on a daily basis. Individual test results are stored by computer in a separate quality control file, from which age- and sex-specific means and standard deviations are computed. In addition, daily numbers of abnormal test results, unsatisfactory tests, and tests omitted are recorded (see Figure 9-1). The results are compared with previous days' runs to detect variations in the normal patterns. Variations may appear as shifts in means, increases in standard deviations, or increases in the number of abnormal values, unsatisfactory tests, or tests omitted. Changes in patterns of data are most easily recognized from graphical displays. For example, a plot of the daily average value of a measurement as a function of time can be used to monitor test performance (see Figure 9-2). Random variations in the mean are normally expected, owing to day-to-day variability in patient age and sex distribution and in the characteristics of individuals within these population subgroups. A sudden shift in the mean may indicate instrument malfunction or change in measurement technique. A gradual monotonic shift in average measurement usually indicates poor instrument stability or improper calibration procedures.

Data monitoring, as described above, cannot detect errors in measurements on individual patients; it only provides statistical information about test performance for a large number of measurements. Therefore, individual random errors may still occur, and additional checking is necessary for their detection. Manual or automatic checking of abnormal test results and appropriate retesting will reduce considerably the number of false positive tests. The incidence of false negative tests can be determined only by retesting a random sample of patients with normal test values.

Occasionally, an erroneous result will escape detection and will be printed on a report for distribution to a nurse or physician. When such errors are discovered, appropriate means of reporting and correcting them must be established (see F and G below).

Data monitoring in a computer-based MHTS can be performed in either online or offline modes. In an online system test data are entered into the computer, either automatically by the instrument, or manually by a technician through a computer terminal. A computer program can scan the data for abnormal values and signal the technician if an abnormality has been detected. More complex logical checking by the program can detect invalid entries (e.g., an alphabetic character in a numeric field), impossible test results (e.g., a hemoglobin of 99), and illegal combinations of entries (e.g., a valid test result together with "test omitted"). If the patient is still at the test phase, the test can be repeated. In offline data monitoring systems the data are usually analyzed at the end of the day after all multiphasic test data have been collected. Repeat testing is usually not possible, and errors discovered in the data must be corrected by other means.

The results of data monitoring can also be used to compare similar measurements performed at different medical facilities. Differences in instruments, calibration or operating procedures, or reference standards may appear as differences in daily averages or standard deviations of test results (provided the patient populations are similar).

For qualitative tests such as the electrocardiogram (EKG) and chest x-ray, variations in the daily pattern of diagnoses may indicate that different physicians are reading the EKG or x-ray and may be using different criteria for interpretation.

D. PERSONNEL MONITORING

In performing various multiphasic measurements, technicians must consistently follow a set of standard procedures. Variations in technique may be revealed by data monitoring as shifts in the mean or standard deviation of a test result. When such changes are observed, the responsible technician should be notified and the procedure corrected. A change in multiphasic technicians at a phase is often accompanied by a shift in the mean or standard deviation of the measurement performed, unless the standard procedures for the phase were precisely followed by both old and new personnel.

A standard procedures manual is a necessity for a MHTS. It must describe in great detail the procedures necessary to calibrate and operate each instrument at each phase. Technicians should be monitored by their supervisor on a regular basis to assure that they are following the standard procedures correctly.

```
TEST: POTASSIUM
```

			FEMALE			
AGE	<35	35-44	45-54	55-65	>65	<35
LO LIM	3.50	3.50	3.50	3.50	3.50	3.50
HI LIM	5.50	5.50	5.50	5.50	5.50	5.50
NUMBER	38	16	20	11	10	19
%_TOTAL	24.5	10.3	12.9	7.1	6.4	12.3
AVERAGE	4.38	4.36	4.39	4.29	4.67	4.49
ST DEV	0.36	0.35	0.46	0.47	0.35	0.45
MINIMUM	3.86	3.74	3.46	3.50	3.99	3.79
MAXIMUM	5.62	4.92	5.68	5.03	5.23	5.36
#ABN_HI	1	0	1	0	0	0
#ABN_LO	0	0	1	0	0	0
#TND	0	0	0	0	0	0
#PRT	0	0	0	0	0	0
#TNI	0	0	0	0	0	0
#TUS	0	0	0	0	0	0

```
TEST: CALCIUM
```

			FEMALE			
AGE	<35	35-44	45-54	55-65	>65	<35
LO LIM	8.50	8.50	8.50	8.50	8.50	8.50
HI LIM	10.50	10.50	10.50	10.50	10.50	10.50
NUMBER	38	16	20	11	10	19
%_TOTAL	24.5	10.3	12.9	7.1	6.4	12.3
AVERAGE	9.55	9.52	9.69	9.77	9.82	9.91
ST DEV	0.44	0.31	0.40	0.16	0.28	0.32
MINIMUM	8.75	9.03	8.96	9.40	9.41	9.23
MAXIMUM	10.65	10.16	10.59	9.99	10.25	10.57
#ABN_HI	2	0	1	0	0	1
#ABN_LO	0	0	0	0	0	0
#TND	0	0	0	0	0	0
#PRT	0	0	0	0	0	0
#TNI	0	0	0	0	0	0
#TUS	0	0	0	0	0	0

```
TEST: CHOL
```

			FEMALE			
AGE	<35	35-44	45-54	55-65	>65	<35
LO LIM	140	140	150	150	150	140
HI LIM	240	240	260	260	300	240
NUMBER	38	16	20	11	10	19
%_TOTAL	24.5	10.3	12.9	7.1	6.4	12.3
AVERAGE	171.79	193.31	219.55	227.00	259.30	181.16
ST DEV	34.49	32.15	34.74	26.46	42.68	27.68
MINIMUM	99	141	147	197	162	128
MAXIMUM	252	283	299	276	315	228
#ABN_HI	1	1	2	2	2	0
#ABN_LO	6	0	1	0	0	1
#TND	0	0	0	0	0	0
#PRT	0	0	0	0	0	0
#TNI	0	0	0	0	0	0
#TUS	0	0	0	0	0	0

Figure 9-1. Daily quality control report for potassium, calcium, and cholesterol. Table shows low and high limits, number of patients, percent of total patients, average test values, standard deviations, minimum and maximum values, number of high abnormals

	MALE					
35-44	45-54	55-65	>65	T MAL	T FEM	TOTAL
3.50	3.50	3.50	3.50			
5.50	5.50	5.50	5.50	60	95	155
11	11	13	6	60	95	155
7.1	7.1	8.4	3.9	38.7	61.3	100.0
4.36	4.42	4.34	4.64	4.43	4.40	4.41
0.34	0.37	0.41	0.24	0.40	0.40	0.40
3.55	3.94	3.49	4.30	3.49	3.46	3.46
4.79	5.44	4.84	5.05	5.44	5.68	5.68
0	0	0	0	0	2	2
0	0	1	0	1	1	2
0	0	0	0	0	0	0
0	0	0	0	0	0	0
0	0	0	0	0	0	0
0	0	0	0	0	0	0

	MALE					
35-44	45-54	55-65	>65	T MAL	T FEM	TOTAL
8.50	8.50	8.50	8.50			
10.50	10.50	10.50	10.50	60	95	155
11	11	13	6	60	95	155
7.1	7.1	8.4	3.9	38.7	61.3	100.0
9.64	9.60	9.55	9.52	9.69	9.63	9.65
0.26	0.48	0.42	0.63	0.44	0.38	0.41
9.19	8.83	8.87	8.83	8.83	8.75	8.75
10.18	10.80	10.61	10.70	10.80	10.65	10.80
0	1	1	1	4	3	7
0	0	0	0	0	0	0
0	0	0	0	0	0	0
0	0	0	0	0	0	0
0	0	0	0	0	0	0
0	0	0	0	0	0	0

	MALE					
35-44	45-54	55-65	>65	T MAL	T FEM	TOTAL
140	150	150	150			
240	260	260	300			
11	11	13	6	60	95	155
7.1	7.1	8.4	3.9	38.7	61.3	100.0
203.27	224.91	213.69	194.83	201.65	201.07	201.29
32.84	38.23	29.71	16.52	34.58	45.13	41.36
149	164	173	170	128	99	99
258	290	277	219	290	315	315
1	2	1	0	4	8	12
0	0	0	0	1	7	8
0	0	0	0	0	0	0
0	0	0	0	0	0	0
0	0	0	0	0	0	0
0	0	0	0	0	0	0

(ABN_HI), number of low abnormals (ABN_LO), number of tests not done (TND), number of patients refusing tests (PRT), number of tests not indicated (TNI), and number of tests unsatisfactory (TUS), for each age and sex category, and totals.

TEST:OC TENS-NCT-R

MAR	TOTAL NO	TOTAL AVER	MALE NO	MALE AVER	FEMALE NO	FEMALE AVER
1	159	17.52	74	17.65	85	17.41
2	126	17.30	66	17.75	60	16.80
3	161	17.13	84	16.94	77	17.34
4	87	16.71	40	16.30	47	17.06
5	164	16.88	77	17.10	87	16.68
8	160	17.56	71	17.66	89	17.48
9	172	17.34	81	17.37	91	17.30
10	169	17.88	75	17.80	94	17.95
11	92	17.25	46	17.61	46	16.89
12	169	16.56	87	16.68	82	16.44
15	171	17.39	75	17.43	96	17.38
16	163	16.81	77	17.30	86	16.38
17	163	16.54	67	16.97	96	16.25
18	91	17.23	45	17.60	46	16.87
19	178	15.88	73	15.77	105	15.96
22	169	16.80	79	16.80	90	16.81
23	167	16.85	73	16.59	94	17.05
24	172	16.70	60	17.35	112	16.36
25	92	17.68	43	18.11	49	17.30
26	185	16.54	90	16.98	95	16.14
29	177	17.11	72	17.75	105	16.68
30	177	17.12	74	17.38	103	16.94
31	165	16.98	66	17.56	99	16.61

```
MAR                      10.0                            20.0
     ----------------------------------|----------------------------
 1                                      |                    F
 2                                      |                 F     M
 3                                      |                 MF
 4                                      |               M  F
 5                                      |                  F  M
 8                                      |                     F
 9                                      |                    F
10                                      |                      F
11                                      |                  F  M
12                                      |               FM
15                                      |                  FM
16                                      |                F  M
17                                      |                F  M
18                                      |                  F  M
19                                      |              MF
22                                      |                   F
23                                      |                 MF
24                                      |                F  M
25                                      |                 F     M
26                                      |              F  M
29                                      |                 F     M
30                                      |               FM
31                                      |                F  M
```

Figure 9-2. Monthly quality control report for ocular tension by noncontact tonometer. Table shows daily totals for males, females, and all patients, for number of patients

TOTAL TND	MALE TND	FEMALE TND	TOTAL ABN	MALE ABN	FEMALE ABN
0	0	0	1	1	0
30	13	17	1	1	0
0	0	0	0	0	0
0	0	0	0	0	0
0	0	0	0	0	0
0	0	0	1	0	1
0	0	0	0	0	0
0	0	0	1	1	0
0	0	0	0	0	0
0	0	0	0	0	0
0	0	0	0	0	0
0	0	0	0	0	0
0	0	0	0	0	0
0	0	0	2	1	1
0	0	0	0	0	0
0	0	0	0	0	0
0	0	0	0	0	0
0	0	0	0	0	0
0	0	0	0	0	0
0	0	0	1	1	0
0	0	0	3	2	1
0	0	0	0	0	0
0	0	0	1	1	0

30.0

(NO), average test values (AVER), number of tests not done (TND), and number of abnormal test values (ABN). Daily average values for males and females are plotted below.

E. INSTRUMENT CALIBRATION AND STANDARDIZATION

Calibration is a procedure by which an instrument or its components are adjusted to give a standard output for a known calibration input.[8] Standardization is a procedure by which an instrument is adjusted to give the correct output when performing a measurement on a known standard input.

These two procedures are identical for some instruments, such as blood chemistry analyzers, in which the input used for calibration is a known standard. In some instruments (such as electrocardiographs) calibration is usually performed by means of an internal calibration signal of known amplitude; the instrument is then adjusted to produce the appropriate output signal. Calibration is often synonymous with adjusting the gain and offset of the amplifiers in these instruments. In other instruments a physiological signal is simulated, either mechanically or electrically, to produce a known response. An example is a spirometer, in which a known volume of air is introduced over a fixed time interval. The instrument is calibrated to give the correct volume and flow rate. In the case of a blood chemistry analyzer the instrument is calibrated for a baseline reading (offset) with a blank sample, and for a standard reading (gain) with a reference standard whose composition has been accurately determined. Quality control standards of known composition are usually run with each batch of samples to check the instrument calibration. In other types of instruments, such as blood pressure monitors, there is no standard simulator that can be used to calibrate the instrument. Instead, the monitor is standardized by performing a blood pressure measurement on a patient with a known blood pressure determined by the traditional standard method. Individual components of a blood pressure instrument, such as the pressure gauges, may be calibrated independently with suitable instruments. This type of standardization is not completely satisfactory, since the standard input is a biological signal whose intrinsic variability is significant, and whose measurement is partially subjective; but until a suitable mechanical device is available that can simulate an arm with a pulsating artery, this method will have to suffice.

Instruments should be checked against a standard at least once a day. The frequency of recalibration will depend on the stability of the instrument and the difficulty of the procedure. Some instruments (such as chemistry analyzers) may be recalibrated with each batch of samples. Other instruments (such as audiometers) may be calibrated once per month. Calibration procedures for specific instruments will be discussed in H below.

F. REPORTING SYSTEM

An effective quality control system must provide a means by which reports of data errors, instrument malfunctions, or procedural errors can be transmitted to appropriate multiphasic personnel. Data monitoring by itself is valueless unless individuals responsible for the accuracy of the instruments and their proper operation are notified when errors are detected, so they can take appropriate action to correct the errors and prevent their recurrence. Similarly, if the recipient of a multiphasic report discovers an error, he should be able to initiate a procedure that will result in correction of the error. Therefore, appropriate formal or informal reporting procedures should be provided. Such procedures should include data monitoring, user reports, and technician reports. Daily quality control printouts should be provided by the data monitoring system. User reports should be filed whenever erroneous patient identification or test results are noted on a multiphasic report. Multiphasic technicians should report suspected instrument malfunctions or difficulties in operation.

A detailed quality control system developed at Kaiser-Permanente is shown in Figure 9-3. The primary pathway for information flow is represented by heavy

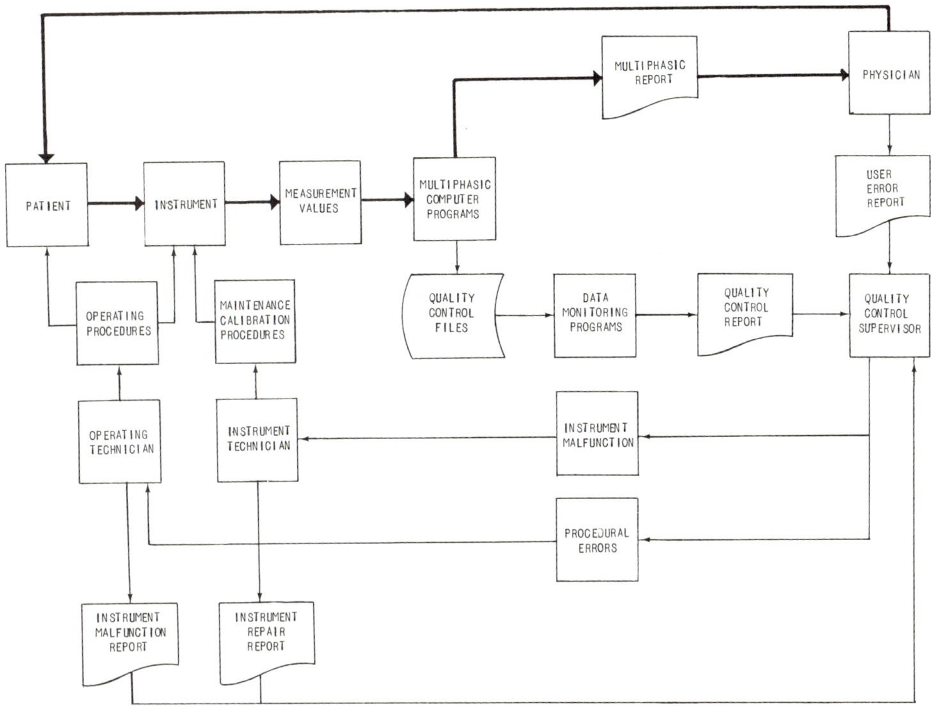

Figure 9-3. Quality control system developed by Kaiser-Permanente. Heavy arrows show the primary flow of multiphasic information. Thin arrows show the flow of information for quality control.

arrows and includes patient, test instrument, data collection system, multiphasic report, and physician. Thin arrows show the flow of information for quality control. The multiphasic computer programs provide data to the quality control file for monitoring. Statistical analyses are performed on the data, and a report is sent to the quality control supervisor. If an instrument malfunction is suspected, the instrument technician is notified. If an error in operating procedure is suspected, the responsible multiphasic technician is notified. On the other hand, problems detected by operating technicians, instrument technicians, or users can be reported to the quality control supervisor by means of instrument malfunction reports, instrument repair reports, and user error reports, respectively.

G. ERROR CORRECTION

A suitable error correction procedure is necessary for MHTS data, consistent with state regulations governing the correction of data in a medical record. The correction procedure used depends on whether the data have been printed on a report and distributed, and whether the patient is available for repeat testing.

In the first and simplest case, an error is discovered while the patient is still within the multiphasic facility; the test can be repeated and the erroneous result deleted from his file. In the second case, the patient is no longer available, but a report of the test results has not yet been printed; the erroneous result can be deleted from the patient file and replaced with a suitable comment, such as "test unsatisfactory." In the third case, which is the most difficult and the most expensive to correct, the report has been printed and distributed. If the error is discovered by multiphasic personnel, an amended report should be printed showing the erroneous result suitably flagged and the corrected result (or "test unsatisfactory" if the patient is not available). This report should be sent immediately to the original recipient, or, depending on the nature of the error and its possible clinical significance, the individual should be telephoned. The multiphasic data file should be modified to reflect the corrected information, but the original wrong data should not be erased. As on the report, the erroneous data should be flagged and the corrected data appended. If additional reports are requested at some later time for any reason, these new reports will contain both the erroneous and corrected data. This procedure is necessary for medico-legal reasons.

If the user detects an error, it may not be necessary to print an amended report, provided the existing report is suitably annotated; however, the multiphasic data files should still be changed for the reasons stated above. Any subsequent reports printed from these files should contain both the error and the correction.

H. QUALITY CONTROL FOR TEST PHASES

This section will discuss quality control for specific MHTS instruments, including calibration and standardization, data monitoring, and error correction. The physical characteristics of these instruments are described in Chapter Seven.

Data monitoring for quantitative measurements refers to computation of daily means and standard deviations by sex and age group (usually 10-year intervals). In addition, the numbers of high and low abnormals, unsatisfactory tests, and tests omitted are tabulated.

1. Electrocardiography

Calibration of an electrocardiograph is usually performed by adjusting the gain of the amplifiers until an internal electrical calibration pulse produces a deflection five millimeters high on the EKG tracing. In some instruments the width of the pulse is also five millimeters or 200 milliseconds at a standard paper speed of 25 millimeters per second. Since there is usually no adjustment for paper speed of the recorder, any deviation of the pulse from five millimeters implies poor regulation of recorder speed and may require factory adjustment. Calibration pulses are normally recorded at the beginning or end of each patient's EKG.

An electronic EKG simulator may be used to check instrument performance.

This is a device to which the limb electrodes and one chest electrode may be connected. It produces a consistent standard electrocardiogram tracing, against which instrument calibration may be checked.

Data monitoring consists of tabulating the EKG interpretations. Variations in the pattern of diagnoses may reflect differing criteria used by different cardiologists. Observer variability in the interpretation of EKGs can be measured by having an individual read a set, then reread them after an interval of several weeks. If the EKG interpretation is performed by a computer program, all abnormal results should be verified by a cardiologist.[9] EKG tracings may be identified by attaching preprinted labels or by writing or imprinting identifying information on the tracing. Occasionally, an EKG will be mislabeled, resulting in erroneous data on the multiphasic report. Appropriate error correction procedures should be performed on the report and the tracing.

Large numbers of unsatisfactory tests may indicate problems with electrodes, skin preparation, loose connections, or instrument malfunction. In particular, baseline wandering indicates problems with electrode placement. An EKG containing high-frequency noise components may indicate electrical interference, a loose connection, or, occasionally, muscle tremor or shivering in the patient. Sixty-cycle noise indicates poor grounding, a broken cable shield, or a nearby source of sixty-cycle interference (power lines, fluorescent lights, or other electromechanical equipment). Voltage fluctuations on the power lines may also cause baseline variations.

2. Blood Pressure

Blood pressure instruments cannot be calibrated directly, because there is as yet no suitable mechanical simulation device. Certain components of a blood pressure instrument, however, can be calibrated. For example, the pressure gauge can be calibrated by inserting a T-tube in the air tubing between the instrument and the cuff balloon. One side of the tee can be connected to a mercury or aneroid manometer. By this means, the systolic and diastolic pressure points may be read directly from the manometer and compared with the instrument readings, which can be adjusted to agree with the external manometer. There may also be internal electrical calibration controls.

Instrument standardization should be performed daily by measuring systolic and diastolic blood pressure on a standard patient, usually a technician whose blood pressure is known, using manual and automatic methods either simultaneously or sequentially.[10,11] The instrument should be adjusted so that the two pairs of readings agree within 5 percent. Because of observer variability, a five-millimeter error in manual measurements can be expected.[12]

Data monitoring consists of recording systolic and diastolic blood pressures for the different age and sex subgroups. In addition, if it is possible to record both manual and automatic blood pressure measurements on a few patients each day, comparison of the two sets of values will provide a good indication of instrument accuracy.

Generally, if an abnormal blood pressure is recorded by an automatic instrument, the measurement should be repeated by manual testing. It should be noted that a second measurement of blood pressure will generally tend to be lower than the first, because the patient has a longer time to relax and adjust to the procedure.

3. Spirometry

The method of calibration depends upon the type of spirometer used. In spirometers that operate on the principle of volume displacement, calibration is performed by injecting a standard volume of air over a known period of time. If volume increases linearly with time, the usual parameters of vital capacity, forced expiratory volume at one, two, or three seconds, and peak flow rate may be calculated and the spirometer adjusted to agree with the calculated values. In spirometers that operate on the principle of direct measurement of air flow, an air pump with a standard flow rate is required for calibration, and from the flow rate the various volume parameters can be calculated. Some spirometers have an internal calibration device that substitutes a standard calibration voltage for the signal from the volume or flow transducer. The instrument is electrically calibrated when it is adjusted to give a standard reading when the calibration signal is applied. However, this type of calibration does not permit compensation for the changing characteristics of the transducers and is, therefore, less accurate than calibration by mechanical simulation of a spirometry measurement.

If a mechanical device is not available for calibration, a standard patient, usually a technician whose pulmonary function parameters are known, should test the device at the beginning of each day's operation.

Data monitoring consists of recording each spirometry parameter for the different age and sex subgroups.[13] A nomogram, which is a function of age, height, and sex, may be used to calculate the expected values of some of the parameters. Consistent deviation from the expected values may indicate the need for recalibration.

4. Anthropometry

Calibration of an automatic height instrument requires two rods of different lengths. The gain and offset of the instrument should be adjusted to give the correct readings for each rod. If the device is linear, it should give accurate measurements for any height within its range of motion. Calibration of weight measurements for mechanical or electronic scales is performed in the same way, with several standard weights placed on the weighing platform. Data monitoring of these measurements is as described above for quantitative measurements.

5. Chest X-Rays

X-ray tube voltage, current, and possible radiation leakage should be checked periodically by qualified x-ray technicians. X-ray diagnoses are monitored by tabulating the results daily. Unusual patterns of diagnoses may indicate use of differing criteria by different radiologists.[14] As with EKG's, observer variability in reading chest x-rays may be measured by having an individual read a set, then reread them after an interval of several weeks. Unsatisfactory x-rays may indicate equipment malfunction, poor-quality x-ray film, or problems with the developing procedure.

6. Mammography

The same considerations apply to mammography as to chest x-ray.

7. Visual Acuity

Most visual acuity devices do not require calibration. If a wall chart is used, a standard observation distance must be marked. If an optical testing device is used, a technician with normal vision should test the device periodically.

8. Tonometry

Tonometry instruments cannot be calibrated directly, because as yet no artificial eyeball is commercially available to simulate the mechanical properties of the eye. Calibration of the device is normally done by the manufacturer. Mechanical devices, such as the Schiotz tonometer, need no further recalibration, although the zero setting may require adjustment. Electronic devices may have internal electronic calibration checks. Standardization may be performed on a technician with a known normal intraocular pressure. Since the Goldmann applanation tonometer, which measures the force required to flatten a specific optically determined area, is the currently accepted standard for measurement of intraocular pressure, the technician's pressure should be determined on this device.[15]

9. Audiometry

An audiometer requires periodic calibration of the frequencies and intensities of the tones it generates.[16,17] Frequency is easily calibrated with an oscilloscope, or, for greater accuracy, with a frequency counter. Intensity is more difficult to calibrate and requires a special audiometric calibration instrument, an electronic ear, which is accurately calibrated to standard audiometric intensities.

Measurement of sound intensity on an absolute scale is difficult, because sound is a subjective sensation, which corresponds physically to the amplitude of the pressure wave generated in air by the vibrations of a diaphragm in headphones or a loudspeaker. On a relative scale the intensity of sound can be readily measured relative to the intensity at the normal threshold of hearing. These threshold intensities vary with frequency and correspond to specific amplitude values of the pressure waves, which have been determined empirically for a large number of patients with normal hearing. Threshold intensities measured by the International Standards Organization in 1964 are known as the ISO 1964 standards. The intensity of sound at hearing threshold is arbitrarily defined as zero decibels (db), and all values of sound intensity are expressed in decibels, relative to this standard intensity. Electronic ears are themselves calibrated to audiometric standards to give a zero reading when a sound of threshold intensity is present. To calibrate an audiometer with an electronic ear, the audiometer headphones are placed on the device, and the audiometer controls are adjusted to give a reading of zero decibels at each test frequency.

Audiometer calibration should be checked once per month. Standardization should be performed daily by measuring the hearing of a standard patient with normal hearing.

Data monitoring consists of recording the average decibel loss for each ear and frequency for the different age and sex subgroups. A gradually increasing decibel loss at all frequencies may indicate decreasing output power of the audiometer. Older age groups should show higher decibel losses. Large numbers of unsatisfactory tests for self-administered audiometry testing may indicate poor instructions given by the technician to the patient. The first ear tested may show a greater average decibel loss than the second ear, because of the additional testing experience the patient has received by the time the second ear is tested. Another possible reason for consistent differences between the two ears is that external noise may be louder in the direction of one ear than the other.

10. Hematology

Automatic hematology instruments require initial daily calibration, and then frequent calibration checks with each batch of samples.[18-20] Initial calibration consists of various checks and adjustments to mechanical and electronic systems, as required by the particular instrument. After adjusting pressures, voltages, and timing functions, the instrument is checked for background count with a blank sample (containing no blood cells) and then is calibrated with a reference control standard, provided by the manufacturer, whose hematologic parameters have been accurately assayed. The instrument is adjusted to give the expected values for all parameters. Reproducibility is checked by repeated measurements on the same specimen. Linearity is checked by measurements on specimens with high and low parameter values.

Calibration checks are performed during patient runs by including with each batch of patient specimens a quality control sample (a pooled blood specimen) whose hematologic parameters are known. The measured quality control sample parameters are compared with the expected values and, if the differences are sufficiently large, recalibration is performed.

Data monitoring consists of recording the values of each parameter for the different age and sex subgroups. Of the seven hematology parameters usually determined by these instruments, only four are actually measured. The remaining three values are computed by the instrument from three of the measured variables. This computation, which is usually performed by analog methods, can be checked by the data monitoring program. Errors of a few percent are not uncommon. Variation in the average values of the parameters implies problems with the instrument, the reference control standard, or the reagents.

Data produced by the instrument are usually scanned by a technologist before they are released from the laboratory. If the instrument is connected online to a computer, provision must be made to permit editing of test results, rejection of erroneous ones, and retesting, if necessary. Only after the technician has verified the results should the data be released to the multiphasic system.

11. Blood Chemistry Analyzers

The same considerations apply to blood chemistry analyzers as to hematology instruments.[18, 20-27] Initial mechanical and electronic checks and adjustments are performed, followed by baseline calibration with a blank sample and measurement calibration with a reference control standard provided by the manufacturer, whose composition has been accurately assayed.[28] The instrument is adjusted to give the expected values for all parameters. Depending upon the instrument, several dilutions of the reference control standard may be used to obtain a calibration curve.

Calibration checks are performed during patient runs by including with each batch of specimens a quality control sample (usually a pooled serum specimen) whose chemistry values are known. Some instruments have an automatic calibration cycle, in which they recognize the standard and blank specimens from their accession numbers or positions on the specimen tray and automatically recalibrate themselves to give the expected values. For manual instruments recalibration is performed whenever the instrument reading on a standard specimen differs from its true value by a significant amount.

Data monitoring consists of recording the values of each chemistry for the different age and sex subgroups. Variation in the average values of a parameter implies problems with the instrument, reference control standard, or reagents. Average values can be strongly affected by outliers—values that lie far outside the normal range. A data monitoring program can choose to ignore outliers in computing averages.

Another source of error is in patient identification.[29] Most instruments process samples in a sequence that corresponds to their order on a work list, which contains the specimen identification. If a specimen is loaded onto the tray out of sequence, the test results of an entire batch may be associated with incorrect patients. To eliminate this problem, machine-readable accession numbers can be entered on cards or labels on the specimen containers, which are read by the instrument as the sample is withdrawn and are printed along with the test results.

12. Achilles Reflex

Achilles reflex instruments record foot movement in response to tapping the Achilles tendon, by having the foot interrupt a beam of light incident upon a photocell, as it rotates about the ankle.[30]

Analog instruments display foot position as a tracing on a strip chart recorder. If the speed of the recorder is accurate, as measured by a calibration pulse of known duration, no further instrument calibration is necessary, since the Achilles reflex time is measured from the tracing.

Digital instruments are more difficult to calibrate. If an analog signal can be obtained from the output of the photocell, it can be displayed on a strip chart recorder, and the reflex time measured from the tracing can be compared with the digital value. Otherwise, standardization can be checked by daily measurements of the reflex time of a standard patient.

Data monitoring is as described above for quantitative measurements.

13. History

Although a program of preventive maintenance for mechanical and electronic equipment used in automated history takers is a necessity, history-taking equipment does not require the kind of calibration or data monitoring needed by other multiphasic test instruments. However, some degree of quality control is required for processing of these data, which depends on the method of data acquisition.[31-35]

For marksense and optically readable documents, a random comparison of data entry on source documents with the corresponding printout on the multiphasic report should be made. Discrepancies are usually due to stray marks on the documents, marksense or optical reader malfunction, or error in patient identification. An estimate of the error rate can be obtained only by sampling.

For automated history takers that use slides or film strips to display history questions, the order of the photographic material must be checked against the branching logic of the computer program. An error in placement of a slide of a projector tray may lead to illogical sequences of questions or erroneous history data on the report.

REFERENCES

1. Discher, D. P., Massey, F. J., and Hallett, W. Y. "Quality Evaluation and Control Methods in Computer-Assisted Screening." *Arch. Environ. Health* 19(1969):323–333.

2. Spooner, R. B. "Automated Instruments for Multiphasic Testing and Their Maintenance." In *Automated Multiphasic Health Testing and Services,* Vol. 3. U. S. DHEW, Health Services and Mental Health Administration, National Center for Health Services Research and Development, 1970.

3. Friedman, G. D. "Reliability and Validity of Automated Multiphasic Health Testing Data." Unpublished report, 1975.

4. Frederik, W. S. "Medical Quality Control in a Computerized Multiphasic Health Screening System." Presented at Technicon International Congress, New York, June 1972.

5. Collen, M. F., and Terdiman, J. F. "Technology of Multiphasic Patient Screening." In *Annual Review of Biophysics and Bioengineering,* Vol. 2(1973):103–113.

6. Hoffmann, R. G. "Statistics in the Practice of Medicine." *J.A.M.A.* 185(1963):864–873.

7. Hoffmann, R. G., and Waid, M. E. "The 'Average of Normals' Method of Quality Control." *Am. J. Clin. Path.* 43(1965):134–141.

8. Geddes, L. A., and Baker, L. E. *Principles and Applications of Biomedical Instrumentation.* New York: John Wiley & Sons, 1968.

9. Elliot, R. V. *Demonstration and Evaluation of Computer-Assisted Analysis and Interpretation of the Electrocardiogram. A State of the Art Report.* Progress Report, Health Care Technology Division, National Center for Health Services Research and Development, September 1972.

10. King, G. E. "Taking the Blood Pressure." *J.A.M.A.* 209(1969):1902–1904.

11. Kirkendall, W. M., Burton, A. C., Epstein, F. H., and Fries, E. D. "Recommendations for Human Blood Pressure Determination by Sphygmomanometers. Report of a Subcommittee of the Postgraduate Education Committee. American Heart Association." *Circulation* 36(1967):980–988.

12. Eilertson, E., and Humerfelt, S. "The Observer Variation in the Measurement of Arterial Blood Pressure." *Acta Med. Scand.* 184(1968):145–157.

13. Dickman, M. L., et al. "Online Computerized Spirometry in 738 Normal Adults." *Am. Rev. Respir. Dis.* 100(1969):780–789.

14. Yerushalmy, J. "The Statistical Assessment of the Variability in Observer Perception and Description of Roentgenographic Pulmonary Shadows." *Radiological Clinics of North Amer.* 7(1969):381–392.

15. Goldmann, H. "Applanation Tonometry." In Newell, F. W., *Glaucoma:* Transactions of the Second Conference. Madison, Wis.:Madison Printing Co., 1956.

16. Rudmose, W. "Automatic Audiometry." In Jerger, J., *Modern Developments in Audiology.* New York: Academic Press, 1963.

17. Davis, H., and Kranz, F. W. "The International Standard Reference Zero for Puretone Audiometers and Its Relation to the Evaluation of Impairment of Hearing." *J. Speech and Hearing Res.* 7(1964):7–16.

18. Wintrobe, M. M. *Clinical Hematology.* Philadelphia: Lea & Febiger, 1974.

19. Coulter, W. H. "High Speed Automatic Blood Cell Counter and Cell Size Analyzer." Presented at the National Electronics Conference, Chicago, October 1956.

20. *Quality Control Manual.* Council on Clinical Chemistry of the American Society of Clinical Pathologists, 1960.

21. Smythe, W. J., Shanos, M. H., Morgenstern, S., and Skeggs, L. T. "SMA 12/60: A New

Sequential Multiple Analyses Instrument." *Automation in Analytical Chemistry.* Technicon Symposia, Mediad, Inc., White Plains, N. Y., 1968.

22. Taylor, P. C., and Carter, A. B. "Experience of Processing Results for Quality Control Offline." *J. Clin. Path.* 26(1973):391–392.

23. Flokstra, J. H., Varley, A. B., and Hagans, J. A. "Reproducibility and Accuracy of Clinical Laboratory Determinations." *Am. J. Med. Sci.* 251(1966):646–655.

24. Freier, E. F., and Rausch, V. L. "Quality Control in Clinical Chemistry." *Am. J. Med. Technology* 24(1958):195–200.

25. "A Discussion of Quality Control in the Clinical Laboratory." *Bull. Lab. Med.* 16(1967):1–2.

26. Foote, E. K., Baker, E. R., and MacDonald, A. H. "The Establishment of a Clinical Chemistry Quality Control Program." *Mass. J. Med. Technology* 1(1959):13–19.

27. Newell, J. E. "Achievement and Control of Quality in Clinical Chemistry." *Bull. Coll. Amer. Pathologists* 14(1960).

28. Benenson, A. S., Thompson, H. L., and Klugerman, M. R. "Applications of Laboratory Controls in Clinical Chemistry." *Am. J. Clin. Path.* 25(1955):87–94.

29. Rubin, M. "A laboratory sample identification system." *Rev. Informatique Med.* 2(1971):91–96.

30. Rives, K. L., Furth, E. D., and Becker, D. V. "Limitations of the Ankle Jerk Test." *Ann. Intern. Med.* 62(1965):1139–1142.

31. Collen, M. F., Cutler, J. L., Siegelaub, A. B., and Cella, R. L. "Reliability of a Self-Administered Medical Questionnaire." *Arch. Int. Med.* 123(1969):664–681.

32. McLean, E. R., et al. "The Collection and Processing of Medical History Data—A Bibliography of Manual, Automated, and Computer-Assisted Techniques." *Meth. Inform. Med.* 14(1975):150–163.

33. Mayne, J. G., Martin, M. J., Morrow, G. W., Turner, R. M., and Hisey, B. L. "A Health Questionnaire Based on Paper-and-Pencil Medium Individualized and Produced by Computer. I. Technique." *J.A.M.A.* 208(1969):2063.

34. Martin, M. J., Mayne, J. G., Taylor, W. F., and Swenson, M. N. "A Health Questionnaire Based on Paper-and-Pencil Medium Individualized and Produced by Computer. II. Testing and Evaluation." *J.A.M.A.* 208(1969):2064–2068.

35. Slack, W. V., and Slack, C. W. "Patient Computer Dialogue." *New Eng. J. Med.* 286(1972):1304–1309.

Physical Examinations and Referrals

Stephen L. Taller

A. REFERRAL FOR PHYSICIAN EXAMINATION AND FOLLOWUP CARE

1. Introduction

If automated multiphasic health testing services (MHTS) are to be of significant clinical value to patients, then the historical and laboratory data must be evaluated, a physical examination performed, and all of the information integrated and related to each specific patient.[1,2] The results of the evaluation must be promptly and accurately communicated to the patient, who must be informed of any action decisions made. When necessary, provision must be made for the patient to receive further testing and referral for followup care as indicated.

2. Specific Requirements for Followup after MHTS

a. Patient processing requirements.   If results are online (i.e., available before the examinee leaves the MHTS unit), initial contact concerning followup may occur at the end of the examination. At that time the patient may be told a test should be repeated immediately or may be given an appointment to come back at a later date. A repeat test may be one of several types. It may simply be a repetition of an original procedure, i.e., a second screening; or it may be a test of another sort, i.e., a supplemental test. Explanation and reassurance that retesting is regular practice should be given to help allay natural concern.

If results are not online, the examinee may be requested by letter or phonc to return to MHTS for a repeat test. Again, efforts should be made to allay concern.

If repeat testing is to be done and it involves one of the regular MHTS procedures, then it is advisable that arrangements be made to send the examinee directly to the appropriate station. If the repeat testing requires equipment available at a regular MHTS station but constitutes a special procedure, then an appropriate card designating the procedure is necessary to alert the station personnel to the change from routine.

It is important that when an examinee makes a return visit for repeat testing, registration procedures allow for identification and coding so that the results can be incorporated with the examinee's earlier findings.

Most followup procedures will be done offline and at some time after results have been sent to a designated physician or clinic. The first step in followup, of course, will be verification that such a source of medical care has been designated. It is advisable that such verification be established, if at all possible, before the examinee leaves the MHTS unit. After an appropriate lapse of time (the exact length depending upon the type of examination and the results), the examinee should be contacted to see whether he has been in touch with the source of medical care. Some examinees will not wish to avail themselves of followup medical care, but reasonable effort should be made to persuade them to do so.

b. Personnel requirements.   Many of the followup procedures can be carried out without direct personal contact between MHTS personnel, the examinee, and the physician. Followup may, however, include contact between MHTS personnel and both examinee and physician. Consideration should be given to the requisite attributes of those MHTS personnel who will be dealing with each of these two groups. Those dealing with the examinees must be very personable and understanding, and they may have to be bilingual. They must be well aware of the anxiety the examinee may have. Those dealing with the physicians must have a practical grasp of the confirmatory and diagnostic tests doctors may employ after seeing the MHTS results, as well as some of the therapy they may institute; these personnel should be thoroughly conversant with the normal ranges and variations of MHTS test results, in order to be prepared to answer questions posed by the physicians.

If the examinee does not name a source of medical care or does not set up a followup appointment, the number of followup contacts to insure compliance with requests for repeat testing may be limited. Some flexibility is necessary, depending on the results of the MHTS in individual cases. Obviously, if a life-threatening condition has been found, the utmost persuasion to seek medical care should be used. Arguments based solely on professional knowledge may not be sufficient to persuade a person to put himself under medical care. Family or community resources should be utilized in this effort at persuasion. If suggestions for physician followup care are undertaken by MHTS personnel, the same attempt to insure compliance is recommended.

The supervisor of the followup personnel should be aware of all followup "failures" and should be available to assume direct responsibility in these cases before they are lost to view. For example, if a physician is disturbed about receiving a followup form, he should be referred to the supervisor.

c. Quality control. It is advisable to monitor the followup experience with respect to both test results and referral practices, so that use of resources may be planned for greatest efficiency. Followup attempts that are finally designated as failure to comply with referrals should be grouped and analyzed regularly. Efforts should be made to uncover the underlying reasons for these failures to get repeat tests or make and keep followup appointments.

Adequate provision for these essential steps is sometimes neglected, despite emphasis on their importance in the literature.[3,4,5] Sometimes the MHTS report never reaches the patient's physician, or the patient has no physician to whom the report can be sent, or he requests that it be sent to a physician who does not know him.[2,5,6] The physician unfamiliar with MHTS computer printout format for the data presented may ignore or misinterpret them.[7,8] It has been shown that physicians, buried in an avalanche of data, may make little clinical use of them,[7,9,10,11] and do not respond to requests by the MHTS unit for followup information.[12,13]

Patient failure to comply with instructions is a ubiquitous problem.[14,15,16] All too frequently, once the testing is over, patients tend to postpone the action phase.[4] The patient may not obtain followup tests;[17] or, thinking that MHTS is "all he needs," he may never see a physician.[2,6,7,11,12] Some MHTS units have attempted to solve these problems by restricting their services to patients who are directly referred by physicians.[5,18,19] Other efforts have included extensive public relations campaigns among physicians,[20] and the preparation of extensive patient explanatory material as well as physicians' manuals to accompany printouts.[19,20,21,22]

3. Usual System of Referral to Physicians for Followup Care

a. Report referral. All MHTS units produce a summary data report, either handwritten or computer printed. This report is sent to the physician identified by the patient as his physician, or to the referral source other than a physician (an insurance company for example). In most cases some source documents are forwarded together with the MHTS report (particularly electrocardiograms, but also audiograms, spirograms, x-ray minifilms, etc.). Freestanding MHTS units commonly send data by mail, but in-house units may use hand delivery, interoffice mail, etc. Some units will also telephone the physician or referral source if significantly abnormal laboratory results are found.[12,18,20,21,23]

b. Patient referral for physician examination. In MHTS units that provide an online physical examination, no referral for this phase is necessary. Immediately upon completion of testing, the patient undergoes physical examination. The examining physician may then make further referrals for additional testing and followup.[21,24]

The majority of MHTS units operate with an offline physical examination and vary considerably in their modes and methods of patient referral for this phase of the multiphasic study. Some make no referral, assuming that since the patient was referred by a physician, the patient or his physician will provide for followup, if necessary.

Some automatically refer every patient back to his physician or referral source at the time of the MHTS. Many others take no action at the time the patient is seen, but notify the patient later when all data are available; they may then refer all patients,[11,19] or only those in whom abnormalities were found.[20,23] Other units telephone or write the patient about the results of MHTS only if abnormalities are found during testing.[12] If a patient does not have an identified physician and needs referral, several units assist him in obtaining a physician.[20,23]

Most units do not persist beyond the initial referral, but some send followup letters or make followup telephone calls urging patients to complete the evaluation,[19] paying particular attention to patients with significant abnormalities in test results.[20] Several units assign health workers specifically to this followup activity[19,20] and use computer record-keeping to make sure the patients do not "get lost."[23]

c. Data and patient followup. Many MHTS units, particularly freestanding commercial organizations, make no attempt to ascertain whether the patient actually returned to the physician or referral source, or to obtain data concerning the final outcome of the evaluation.[18,21]

Some units enclose blanks with the data summary sent to the physician, requesting that he return them with a record of further actions taken, diagnoses made, etc.[12,19,25] Others do this only if abnormalities are found on MHTS.[20] Some make these contacts also by telephone[23] or by personal interview.[11] Several units make repeated efforts to obtain followup data,[19,20,23] and at least one pays physicians to return evaluation forms.[20] Those units that are involved in research projects usually are much more persistent than others in this endeavor.[19]

4. Physician Referral and Followup Care in KPMC Oakland

a. Early method. Before the introduction of the new Nurse Practitioner Section with its provision for patient followup, the Kaiser-Permanente Medical Center (KPMC) Oakland MHTS unit's followup and referral methods were somewhat similar to community offline "in-house" MHTS programs. At the completion of the testing phases, patients were asked to wait briefly for a preliminary review of available data to be sure that no urgent action was necessary. All laboratory reports available before the patient actually left the MHTS area were reviewed by the MHTS supervisor. If potentially serious abnormalities were found (as identified in Table 10-1), the patient was sent directly to the emergency clinic, or his regular physician was telephoned immediately and asked for instructions.

Table 10-1. Current MHTS STAT Advice Rules
Patient's regular physician to be contacted or patient sent to emergency clinic the day of multiphasic health checkup, when test result as follows:

Chemistries	Results	Hematology	Results
Calcium	> 12.0	Hemoglobin	< 8.0
	< 7.5		> 18.0
Creatinine	> 10.0	WBC/with low	
Glucose	> 350	HgB	< 2,000
(if urine sugar			> 25,000
3+ or 4+ and			
acetone positive)		B/P diastolic	> 125
Potassium	> 6.4		
	< 2.9	Intra-ocular	≥ 30 mm
Sodium	< 120	pressure by non-	
		contact tonometer	
		(refer to eye	
		clinic that day)	

EKG—action per directive of cardiologist reading electrocardiograms

Patients without serious abnormalities were then instructed by a receptionist to call the central appointment desk and make an appointment for a "multiphasic return visit" with an internist in the Department of Medicine (Figure 10-1).

If the patient had an identified regular physician, that visit was to be with him; if he had none, the appointment was to be made with any available physician. The patient was told that this additional appointment was necessary in order for him to have a physical examination and for a physician to review the test results. Patients who qualified were also asked to make an additional appointment for a sigmoidoscopic examination (with an internist) (Figure 10-2), and for a pelvic examination and Papanicolaou smear (with a gynecologist) (Figure 10-3).

The day following the MHTS examination, a preliminary computer printout was produced for each patient and reviewed immediately by the MHTS staff. If any abnormalities were found that were felt might call for quick action, an emergency notification form was prepared and, with the patient's chart and the preliminary printout, was hand delivered to the patient's physician within 24 hours (Figure 10-4). Eight to 10 days after the MHTS the physician also received a carbon copy of the completed computer printout for his review. This also served as a backup copy if, for some reason, the patient's chart was not available at the time of the return visit.

The appointment for the multiphasic return visit was made four to six weeks from the date the patient was seen in the MHTS, partly to allow time for all MHTS

MULTIPHASIC FOLLOW-UP APPOINTMENT

PLEASE MAKE THE FOLLOWING MULTIPHASIC FOLLOW-UP APPOINTMENTS.

1. ☐ MHC RETURN APPOINTMENT WITH DR.______________________

2. ☐ MHC SIGMO APPOINTMENT (ALL PATIENTS OVER 40) WHO HAVE NOT
HAD A SIGMO IN THE PAST 2 YEARS.

3. ☐ MHC CANCER DETECTION ("PAP") TEST
-FAMILY PLANNING - For women who are using birth control pills.
-GYN CLINIC - For women who are not using birth control or are having a
problem.

FOR OAKLAND PATIENTS		
FOR	GREEN APPOINTMENT PHONES IN HOSPITAL	FROM YOUR PHONE
MHC Follow-up Appointment with Doctor (1)	6984	658-8220
MHC Sigmo (2)	6984	658-8220
MHC GYN (3)	5080	645-5080
Family Planning Closed; 12 - 1:00	6797	645-6797

PATIENTS RECEIVING FOLLOW-UP CARE FROM OTHER
KAISER-PERMANENTE MEDICAL CENTERS SHOULD CALL:

DIAL:

Antioch	757-7680
Hayward	782-3456
Napa	255-3942
Richmond	234-3131
San Rafael	479-3400
Vallejo	644-5631
Walnut Creek	933-3000

Refer to this date______________________ when making the above appointment.

07259 (REV. 8-75)   M35-8-73

Figure 10-1. Instruction form given to patient for routine followup visit.

data to reach the internist and partly because of congestion in the internist's
schedule.

In his regular daily schedule, each full-time internist at Kaiser-Permanente
Medical Center, Oakland, had five 15-minute multiphasic followup appointments.
When the patient was seen, the physician had available the completed MHTS
computer printout as well as the audiogram, the electrocardiogram, and the
patient's history questionnaire.

The physician interviewed the patient and reviewed the computer-collected
history, the history questionnaire, and any other pertinent information in the
patient's clinic chart. He then performed a complete general physical examination
(omitting the pelvic). Following this, he reviewed and interpreted to the patient
the MHTS laboratory results, ordered any indicated followup testing or referrals,

PERMANENTE MEDICAL GROUP
3772 Howe Street
Oakland, California 94611

PLEASE REGISTER WITH THE RECEPTIONIST AT SECOND FLOOR WEST ABOUT TEN (10) MINUTES BEFORE YOUR APPOINTMENT TIME.

Examination of the rectum is an important part of your regular health check-up and helps the physician to detect significant disease of the rectum.

Special preparation is necessary for this examination:

    1. On the day preceding the examination avoid fruits and vegetables.

    2. On the day of your appointment **omit** the meal preceding your examination.

    3. **Do Not Take Any Laxatives Before The Examination.**

    4. Enema, see instructions below.

Just before you leave home for your appointment use a disposable Fleet Enema Kit. Follow instructions on the package. A Fleet Enema Kit may be purchased at the Pharmacy.

INSTRUCTIONS FOR TAKING AN ENEMA

When giving yourself an enema, lie on your back with legs raised (Figure 1) **or** on your left side with left knee slightly bent and right leg drawn up toward chest (Figure 2). After taking the enema in either position, the knee-chest position (Figure 3) should be assumed, and the solution should be retained until the urge to evacuate is **strong.**

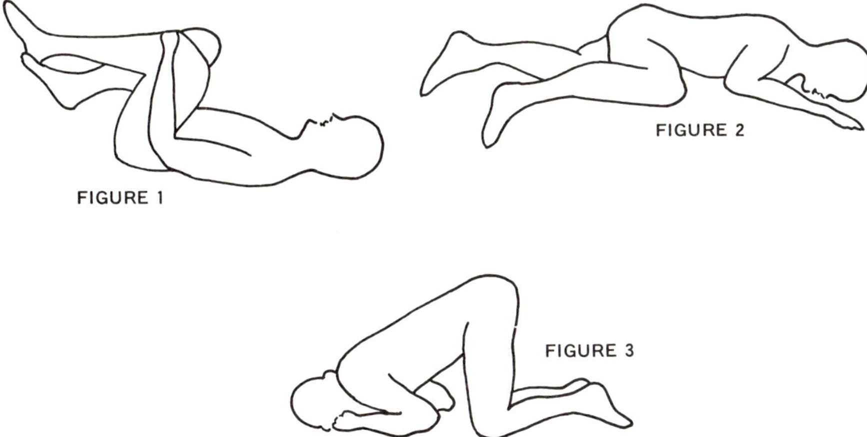

If you have any questions, or wish to cancel your appointment, please call 658-8220, ask for FUTURE MEDICAL APPOINTMENTS, Monday through Friday, 9:00 A.M. to 5:00 P.M., or Saturday, 9:00 A.M. to 12:00 Noon.

Charges for this examination are based on your coverage.

97162 (REV. 11-71)

Figure 10-2. Instruction sheet given to patient at the time appointment was made for sigmoidoscopic examination.

MULTIPHASIC GYN EXAMINATION INSTRUCTIONS

This clinic is not for treatment. The purpose of this examination is to search for diseases without symptoms.

If you have symptoms of possible pelvic difficulty, we advise you to seek help by means of a regular Gyn. appointment.

Please Read and Follow Carefully:

1. Omit all douching for 24 hours before the examination.

2. The day of the examination, it would be helpful if you will bring with you a slip of paper containing the following information:

   a. Date of last menstrual period, or date of menopause.

   b. Date and type of Gyn (female) surgery done, if any.

   c. Medicines you are taking -- hormones -- or birth control pills.

If you have any questions, or wish to cancel your appointment, please call 645-5080, Monday through Friday, 9:00 A.M. to 5:00 P.M.

07374 (REV. 5 73)

Figure 10-3.   Instruction sheet given to patient when appointment was made for pelvic examination and Papanicolaou smear.

answered the patient's questions, began or continued treatment as necessary, and instructed the patient when to return. All data obtained by the physician were entered on both sides of the Multiphasic Diagnosis Form (Figures 10-5 and 10-6).

b.   Drawbacks to this system

(1) The system included an unavoidable delay of four to six weeks between the performance of MHTS and the physician return visit (although it also included an acceptable method for taking rapid action on markedly abnormal laboratory findings).

(2) On average, 25 percent of patients going through MHTS never appeared for the physical examination.[26] Some never made a followup appointment; some failed to appear; and some canceled the return visit appointment and did not reschedule. Even when reached by letter or telephone, some patients declined to come in for the physical examination. The physician had no practical way of following up on these incomplete evaluations.

B.   NURSE PRACTITIONER PHYSICAL EXAMINATION

1.   Rationale for Using Nurse Practitioners

With the development of the "new entry mode" (see Chapter Fifteen) a nurse practitioner section was designed to immediately complete the health evaluations, providing physical examinations by nurse practitioners under physician supervision.[27]

MHC SUMMARY REPORT
PRELIMINARY

DATE

| MHC NOTICE |

THE ATTACHED PRELIMINARY MHC SUMMARY REPORT LISTS THE FOLLOWING ABNORMALITY FOR YOUR EARLY CONSIDERATION

TO	LOCATION
FROM	LOCATION
RE (PATIENT'S NAME)	MEDICAL RECORD NUMBER	DATE OF MHC
ADDRESS - NO. STREET CITY	ZIP CODE	HOME PHONE	BUSINESS PHONE

☐ **BLOOD CHEMISTRIES**
  ☐ Alk Phos Greater Than .125 Units, Age Over 21
  ☐ BUN Greater Than 50 MG%
  ☐ Calcium Greater Than 12.0 MG%
  ☐ Calcium Less Than 7.5 MG%
  ☐ Creatinine Greater Than 2.5 MG%
  ☐ Glucose 2 Hr Greater Than 200 MG%
  ☐ Potassium Greater Than 6.4 MEQ/L, Not Hemolyzed
  ☐ Potassium Less Than 2.9 MEQ/L
  ☐ SGOT Greater Than 100 Units
  ☐ Sodium Less Than 120 MEQ/L
  ☐ Total Bilirubin Greater Than 4.0 MG%

☐ **CHEST X-RAY**
  ☐ Follow-up 14 x 17 X-Ray Ordered by X-Ray Department

☐ **OTHER FINDINGS (Listed Below)**

☐ **HEMOGLOBIN**
  ☐ Less Than 10.0 GM and Female
  ☐ Less Than 12.0 GM and Male
  ☐ Greater than 18.0

☐ **WHITE CELL COUNT**
  ☐ Greater Than 15,000
  ☐ Less Than 3,000

☐ **EKG**
  ☐ Consider Early Alert To Physician

☐ **MAMMOGRAPHY**
  ☐ '. . . Suspicious For Cancer'

☐ **BLOOD PRESSURE**
  ☐ Greater Than 125 MM Diastolic

☐ **BLOOD IN URINE FOR MALES**

NURSE'S SIGNATURE

R.N.

A MHC FOLLOW-UP APPOINTMENT HAS BEEN MADE WITH YOU BY THE PATIENT.

PLEASE REQUEST **YOUR NURSE** TO CONTACT THIS PATIENT FOR ANY FURTHER ACTION YOU MAY DEEM NECESSARY.

RECOMMENDED ACTION:

DOCTOR'S SIGNATURE

M.D.

06649 (5-75)   PLEASE FILE IN CHART WHEN COMPLETE

Figure 10-4. Emergency notification form, hand-delivered (with patient's chart and preliminary printout) to the patient's physician within 24 hours after MHTS staff review of this material.

PERMANENTE MULTIPHASIC DIAGNOSIS RECORD

PLEASE INDICATE THE STATUS OF ALL CONDITIONS OR FINDINGS BY INSCRIBING ONE OF THE FOLLOWING LETTERS IN THE APPROPRIATE BOX.

N - NEW DIAGNOSIS OR FINDING
R - RECURRENCE
C - CONTINUING-ESSENTIALLY UNCHANGED
I - IMPROVED
W - WORSENING OR EXACERBATION
O - OLD - NO LONGER ACTIVE OR PRESENT
D - DELETE - CONDITION NO LONGER VALID
P - PROVISIONAL

NFS = NOT FURTHER SPECIFIED

PHYSICIAN NAME CODE

MR. NO.

LOCATION
HAY OAK RICH S.F. S.S.F VJO S.RAF

NAME:

DATE OF VISIT
MONTH   DAY   YEAR

BIRTHDATE:

TIME OF VISIT   A.M. P.M.

SEX

MEDICAL CHART COPY

DISABILITY

PATIENT'S GENERAL CONDITION TODAY IS ASSOCIATED WITH THE FOLLOWING LIMITATION IN HIS USUAL ACTIVITIES:

- NONE
- MILD
- MODERATE
- SEVERE
- COMPLETE

GENERAL

- NO SIG. ABNORM.
- NO DIAGNOSIS MADE
- PENICILLIN DRUG REACT
- POSS ADV DRUG REACT
- FATIGUE CHRONIC
- FEVER NFS
- LUPUS ERYTH SYSTEMIC
- OBESITY
- SARCOIDOSIS
- SYPHILIS LATENT
- SYPHILIS PRIMARY
- SYPHILIS SECONDARY
- WEIGHT LOSS NFS

ENDOCRINE METABOLIC

- DIABETES MELLITUS
- GLYCOSURIA RENAL
- HYPERCALCEMIA
- HYPERCHOLESTEROLEMIA
- HYPERTRIGLYCERIDEMIA
- HYPERURICEMIA
- HYPOGLYCEMIA

THYROID

- ENLARGED DIFFUSE
- HYPERTHYROIDISM
- HYPOTHYROIDISM
- NODULE(S)
- THYROIDITIS

HEMATOLOGY

ANEMIA

- IRON DEFICIENCY
- PERNICIOUS
- THALASSEMIA
- HEMOGLOBIN C
- HEMOGLOBIN S
- HEMOGLOBINOPATHY NFS
- ANEMIA NFS
- HODGKIN'S DISEASE
- INFECTIOUS MONO
- LEUK CHRON LYMPH
- LEUKEMIA NFS
- LYMPHADENOPATHY NFS
- LYMPHOSARCOMA
- MULTIPLE MYELOMA
- POLYCYTHEMIA VERA
- POLYCYTHEMIA RELATIVE
- THROMBOCYTOPENIA

SKIN

- ACNE VULGARIS
- CARCINOMA BASAL
- CARCINOMA NFS
- CELLULITIS

DERMATITIS
- CONTACT
- MEDICAMENTOSA
- NEURODERMATITIS
- RHUS
- SEBORRHEA
- STASIS
- DERMATITIS NFS

- ECZEMA
- FUNGUS INFECTION
- FURUNCLE(S)
- HERPES ZOSTER
- HERPES SIMPLEX
- KERATOSIS
- LIPOMA
- NEVUS
- PEDICULOSIS
- PITYRIASIS ROSEA
- PRURITUS NFS
- PSORIASIS
- SEBACEOUS CYST
- SUNBURN
- URTICARIA
- VERRUCA VULGARIS
- XANTHELASMA
- XANTHOMA

EYE

- ARCUS SENILIS
- CATARACT
- CONJUNCTIVITIS
- GLAUCOMA
- EOM ABNORMALITY
- IRITIS
- PTERYGIUM
- STYE

RETINOPATHY
- DIABETIC
- HYPERTENSIVE - A/S
- RETINOPATHY NFS

ENT

- CERUMEN
- HEARING LOSS
- MENIERE'S SYND
- OTITIS EXTERNA
- OTITIS MEDIA
- TINNITUS
- EPISTAXIS
- RHINITIS: ALLERGIC
- RHINITIS NFS
- SINUSITIS ACUTE
- DENTAL DISORDER
- GLOSSITIS
- LARYNGITIS
- LEUKOPLAKIA
- PHARYNGTIS: BACT
- STOMATITIS APHTHOUS
- TONSILLITIS
- TUMOR ORAL NFS

CHEST

- ASTHMA BRONCHIAL
- BRONCHIECTASIS
- BRONCHITIS ACUTE
- BRONCHITIS CHRONIC
- CA LUNG PRIMARY
- CA METAST TO LUNG
- EMPHYSEMA
- PNEUMONIA: ATYPICAL
- PNEUMONIA: BACTERIAL
- PNEUMONIA NFS

TUBERCULOSIS
- ACTIVE PULMONARY
- INACTIVE PULMONARY
- ACTIVITY UNCERTAIN
- NON-PULMONARY
- CONVERTER

ETIOLOGY UNKNOWN
- UPPER RESP INFECTION
- CHEST PAIN
- COUGH
- DYSPNEA
- HEMOPTYSIS
- INTERSTITIAL DISEASE
- PULM LESION(S)

CARDIOVASCULAR

- ANGINA PECTORIS
- ARTERIOSCL HEART DISEASE
- AORTIC INSUFFICIENCY
- AORTIC STENOSIS

ARRHYTHMIA
- ATRIAL FIBRILLATION
- ATRIAL FLUTTER
- PAROXYSMAL TACHY NFS
- PREM BEATS-ATRIAL
- PREM BEATS-VENTR
- SINUS BRADYCARDIA
- ARRYTHMIA NFS
- COR PULMONALE
- HT FAILURE CONGESTIVE
- HT MURMUR SYST NFS
- HT MURMUR FUNCT
- HYPERTENSIVE HEART DIS

HYPERTENSION
- ESSENTIAL
- RENAL
- HYPERTENSION NFS
- LABILE BLOOD PRESSURE
- HYPOTENSION ORTHOSTATIC
- MITRAL INSUFFICIENCY
- MITRAL STENOSIS
- MYOCARDIAL INFARCT
- MYOCARDOPATHY-ITIS
- PERICARDITIS
- RHEUMATIC HEART DISEASE
- SEPTAL DEFECT: ATRIAL
- SEPTAL DEFECT: VENTR
- VALVE PROSTHESIS
- WOLF-PARK'N WHITE

PERIPHERAL VASCULAR

- ARTIOSCLER OCCL DIS
- INTERMITTENT CLAUD'N
- LEG CRAMPS NFS
- PERIPHERAL EDEMA
- RAYNAUD'S
- THROMBOPHLEBITIS
- VARICOSE VEINS

GASTROINTESTINAL

ETIOLOGY UNKNOWN
- ABDOMINAL PAIN
- MASS
- BLEEDING
- DYSPHAGIA
- NAUSEA
- PYROSIS
- CONSTIPATION
- DIARRHEA

UPPER GASTROINTESTINAL
- DUODENAL ULCER
- ESOPH HIATUS HERNIA
- FUNCTIONAL DISTRESS
- GASTRIC CARCINOMA
- GASTRIC ULCER
- GASTRITIS
- GASTROENTERITIS
- CHOLELITHIASIS
- GALL BLADDER DIS
- HEPATITIS
- HEPATOMEGALY NFS
- LIVER CARCINOMA
- LIVER CIRRHOSIS
- LIVER TEST ABN
- PANCREAS CARCINOMA
- PANCREATITIS CHRONIC

LOWER GASTROINTESTINAL
- REGIONAL ENTERITIS
- COLITIS ULCERATIVE
- COLON NEOPLASM
- DIVERTICULOSIS
- DIVERTICULITIS
- IRRITABLE COLON
- HEMORRHOIDS
- MELENA
- POLYP(S)
- PRURITUS ANI
- RECTUM: BLEEDING
- RECTUM: CARCINOMA
- RECTUM: FISSURE
- HERNIA-VENTRAL
- HERNIA-UMBILICAL
- HERNIA-INGUINAL
- HERNIA-FEMORAL

GYNECOLOGY

- CERVIX CARCINOMA
- MENO-METRORRHAGIA
- MENOPAUSAL SYND
- PREGNANCY
- PREMENS EDEMA
- PREMENS TENSION
- VAGINITIS MONILIA
- VAGINITIS TRICH
- VAGINAL DISCH'G NFS
- OVARY CARCINOMA
- UTERUS: CARCINOMA
- UTERUS: LEIOMYOMA(S)

BREAST

- ABSENT
- CARCINOMA
- FIBROCYSTIC
- NODULE(S)

GENITO - URINARY

GENERAL
- AZOTEMIA
- CALCULUS
- DYSURIA
- HEMATURIA
- IMPOTENCE
- BACTERIURIA ASYMPT
- URINARY TRACT INF
- ART NEPHROSCLEROSIS
- GLOM NEPHR CHRONIC
- NEPHROPATHY DIABETIC
- NEPHROTIC SYNDROME
- PYELONEPHR ACUTE
- PYELONEPHR CHRONIC
- CYSTITIS
- GONORRHEA
- HYDROCELE
- SPERMATOCELE
- PROSTATE BPH
- PROSTATE CARCINOMA
- PROSTATITIS
- TESTIS ABS/ATROPHIC
- URETHRITIS NFS

MUSCULOSKELETAL

ARTHRITIS
- ARTHRALGIA
- ANKYLOSPONDYLITIS
- GOUT
- OSTEOARTHRITIS
- RHEUMATOID
- ARTHRITIS NFS
- BACK PAIN LUMBO SACRAL
- BACK PAIN POSTURAL

BURSITIS TENDINITIS
- ELBOW
- HIP
- SHOULDER
- OTHER
- CARPAL TUNNEL SYND
- CHEST WALL PAIN
- CLUBBING
- CONTUSION
- DISC DIS: CERVICAL
- DISC DIS: LUMBAR
- DUPUYTREN'S CONTR
- EPICONDYLITIS ELBOW
- GANGLION
- JOINT EFFUSION
- KYPHOSIS
- MUSCULO SKEL PAIN
- MYALGIA
- MYOSITIS
- OSTEOPOROSIS
- SCOLIOSIS
- SPONDYLOSIS CERV

NERVOUS SYSTEM

- BELL'S PALSY
- CEREB VASC INSUFF
- CHRON BRAIN SYND
- CVA RESIDUA
- DIZZINESS

HEADACHE
- MIGRAINE
- TENSION
- HEADACHE NFS

NEUROPATHY
- DIABETIC
- NUTRITIONAL
- HERPES ZOSTER
- NEUROPATHY NFS

- PARKINSONISM
- SEIZURE DISORDER
- SYNCOPE
- VERTIGO

PSYCHOLOGICAL

- ALCOHOLISM: ACUTE
- ALCOHOLISM: CHRONIC
- ANXIETY REACTION
- DEPRESSION
- DRUG DEPENDENCE
- HYPERVENT SYND
- HYSTERIA
- INSOMNIA
- PERSONALITY DISORD
- PSYCHOTIC BEHAVIOR

REFERRED TO:

- ALLERGY
- DERMATOLOGY
- DIETICIAN
- NON APP'T
- EMERG. RM
- ENT
- OB-GYN
- HOSPITAL ADMISSION
- MEDICAL
- NEUROLOGY
- OPHTHALMOLOGY
- OPTOMETRIST
- ORTHOPEDIC
- PHYS. MED.
- PSYCHIATRY
- SIGMO
- SOC. SERVICE
- SURGERY
- UROLOGY
- OTHER _______

PREVENTIVE MAINT. CLINICS

- ARTHRITIS
- BACK CARE
- LIPID
- DIABETES
- FAMILY PLANNING
- GASTROINTESTINAL
- HYPERTENSION
- IMMUNIZATION
- SMOKING CESS PROG
- SPECIAL KIDNEY
- TEENAGE CLINIC
- WT REDUCTION
- WORRIED WELL
- OTHER _______
- HEALTH EDUCATION

STATUS   PRINT CONDITIONS PRESENT NOT LISTED ABOVE

RETURN
- _____ DAYS
- _____ WEEK(S)
- _____ MONTH(S)
- PRN

PL 1/72 (REV) 06-6-11/74
COPYRIGHT 1972

C MARFAN SYNDROME

Figure 10-5. MHTS diagnosis form: Part 1.

PHYSICAL EXAMINATION

BLOOD PRESSURE ____/____ MM HEIGHT ____ WEIGHT ____

(√) INDICATES NO ABNORMALITIES FOUND

SKIN		
NODES		
EENT		
NECK AND THYROID		
THORAX AND BREASTS		
LUNGS		
HEART		
ABDOMEN		
BACK AND EXTREMITIES		
NEUROLOGICAL		
RECTUM		
GENITALIA		

MULTIPHASIC FOLLOW UP

ADDITIONAL STUDIES ____

TREATMENT ____

REMARKS ____

____ M.D.

Figure 10-6. MHTS diagnosis form: Part 2.

The overall objectives of the health evaluation in the new entry mode were to convert patients' wants into medically defined needs, to allow more efficient allocation of medical and paramedical resources, and to minimize unnecessary physician involvement, thus freeing physician time for the care of the sick. It was also designed to satisfy the health care needs of essentially well persons, thereby conserving physician visits.

The specific objectives of the nurse practitioner section were to:

(1) Increase the entrance capacity and accessibility of the medical care delivery system by entering patients through comprehensive testing and online nurse practitioner examinations with physician consultation, rather than through a physician appointment.

(2) Achieve prompt and appropriate referrals of the patients to specific services of the medical care delivery system, through triage protocols that would identify medical need as determined by the comprehensive health evaluation.

(3) Provide for secondary testing where initial findings were positive to accurately determine the patient's health status.

(4) Perform some preliminary workup of patients directed to the sick care services, thus conserving physician time for medical decision making and treatment.

(5) Establish a basic patient health profile for future reference.

(6) Provide education for health care and disease prevention and for the most effective use of the medical care delivery system, through educational displays, printed materials, and nurse practitioner teaching.

(7) Direct patients' return for their next comprehensive health evaluation, at intervals determined by age and health status, thus establishing a concept of continuous health care that emphasizes optimizing health, and disease prevention, rather than episodic, crisis-oriented sick care intervention.

(8) Offer the above services in a manner that would prove satisfactory both to the patients and to the referring physicians.

Registered nurses were assumed to be the best type of personnel to work with physicians for the attainment of these objectives. They are basically prepared in many of the requisite skills and have the background knowledge for quickly learning the others.[28,29,30] They tend as a group to be warm, compassionate people, trained and interested in counseling and teaching. In the United States there is a large pool of registered nurses, many of whom are interested in moving into new fields of endeavor that will utilize their skills in an outpatient setting to a higher degree than has been possible heretofore.[31,32,33,34] Existing licensure is now broad enough in most states to allow nurses to perform these new functions.[28,35,36,37,38] The salary scales for physicians and nurse practitioners provide for three or more nurse practitioners for one physician's salary.

In the nurse practitioner section of the MHTS, the following functions were developed as necessary and appropriate:

(1) Obtain a screening health history, including chief complaint, present illness, review of systems, past medical history, social history and family history (securing this directly from the patient, or by reviewing with the patient written or computer-collected materials). Summarize the history and record or present it in a clear, organized manner.

(2) Perform a complete general physical examination (including a standard

pelvic examination, with the taking of Papanicolaou smears). In these examinations, be able to differentiate between normal, normal variant, and abnormal. Record these findings in a systematic, organized manner.

(3) Using defined criteria, screen the results of laboratory examinations and order further testing as needed.

(4) Using defined criteria, act on the results of history taking, physical examination, and laboratory tests by making appropriate referrals for further evaluation or care.

(5) Instruct, teach, and counsel patients in the routine care of specified health problems as outlined in protocols.

(6) Work collaboratively with physicians and other members of the health team in planning to meet adult patients' health needs.

An important question was whether registered nurses, trained as nurse practitioners, could provide the same quality of care as physicians for the duties outlined above.[39] Some data were available from evaluations by others of the quality of care provided by nurse practitioners. Duncan et al.[40] had found that pediatric nurse practitioners did not miss diagnoses "any more often than could be expected in the usual routine pediatric practice." Charney et al.,[41] Fine et al.,[42] and Hinman[43] confirmed this with particular reference to history and physical examination, as did Stehbens et al.[44] with cardiac murmurs. Lewis et al.,[45] Runyan et al.,[46,47] Stein,[48] Gordon,[49] and Spector et al.[50] observed that nurse practitioners could replace physicians in outpatient health maintenance clinics for the surveillance of chronic diseases without loss of quality. Kaku et al.[51] observed that well-trained nurse practitioners nearly equaled physicians in accuracy of adult physical examinations. Ostergard[52] reported a similar degree of accuracy achieved by a group of nurse practitioners performing pelvic examinations, and Schlesinger et al.[53] noted the same for prenatal care. Papers from the Burlington randomized trial reported equal outcomes in practices that did, and those that did not, utilize nurse practitioners.[29,31,54,55,56]

2. The Training Program for Nurse Practitioners

Only the recent literature contains documentation of training programs for pediatric nurse practitioners.[57,58,59,60,61,62] Reports have appeared lately of training programs for general practice family nurse practitioners. Some courses have been informal.[63,64,65] Some formal courses are short-term,[66,67,68,69,70,71] and others lead to a master's degree after completion of one or two years' training.[70,72] However, until very recently (and well after our training program was developed), little attention has been paid to documentation of the training of nurse practitioners for adult health care. Some reports of programs utilizing nurse practitioners in this field have given no details about their training;[73,74,75] some preparation has been informal and on-the-job.[57,76,77] Some training programs have utilized existing courses in physical diagnosis intended for medical students.[51,78] Some reported programs are brief (3 to 4 months),[79,80] others mid-length (six to 12 months);[81,82,83] and, as noted above, there are graduate programs leading to a master's degree.[57,70] Some attention has also been paid of late to the possibility of including training for such work in the basic registered nurse's training course,[84,85,86] and to the general methods needed to train nurse practitioners to work in an expanded role.[87,88,89]

Considerable differences among the types and lengths of training and orientation given to nurse practitioners have resulted from lack of agreement with regard to the level at which they should perform, and to how much basic knowledge is needed for the tasks and responsibilities given them.[35,90] Our need was specifically to train nurses to perform a defined complex of functions that were conceived as an adjunct to an MHTS unit.

A formal six-month full-time training program designed to fulfill this requirement was developed in 1970.[91] The training was conducted in the Kaiser-Permanente Medical Center, Oakland, which has a 300-bed general hospital and is staffed by 125 full-time physicians of the Permanente Medical Group, representing all major medical and surgical specialties. The director of the course was a board-certified internist; the instructors were qualified specialists, subspecialists, or trained nurse practitioners.

The course consisted of four basic sections:

(a) Techniques of performing and evaluating the physical examination.
(b) History taking and evaluation.
(c) Evaluation of laboratory data; methods and procedures of referral for further care.
(d) Evaluation of patients' needs for health education and counseling.

a. Techniques of performing and evaluating the physical examination. The distribution in time of the following six methods of instruction over the 24-week training period is indicated in Table 10-2.

(1) *Basic studies.** Twenty-five hours of formal lectures on the basic techniques of physical examination of the major anatomic systems were given by specialists in the specific areas (see Table 10-3). Thirty-three hours of supervised practice laboratories were integrated with the lectures; these were supplemented by 27 hours of unsupervised practice sessions (see Table 10-4). Students performed physical examinations on each other and on healthy volunteers. Assignments were given in standard textbooks of physical diagnosis. Pamphlets, charts, and audiovisual aids were employed. Emphasis was on the parts of the physical examination that would be useful in initiating referrals for further evaluation. After the first group of nurses had completed the course, these trained nurse practitioners provided considerable assistance in the practice laboratories and allowed a significant decrease in utilization of physician time in the training.

(2) *Internal medicine preceptor training.* Students spent two days weekly for five weeks in the office of a board-certified member of the Department of Medicine. They first observed techniques of physical examination, then demonstration of abnormal findings. They subsequently performed complete physical examinations on selected patients. The doctor then repeated the examination, demonstrated and discussed abnormalities the student had missed, and corrected improper examination techniques.

(3) *Hospital ward experience.* Students spent one and a half days weekly for 10 weeks on the medical wards of the hospital, observing the wide range of abnormal physical findings available in a hospital setting. Abnormalities were demonstrated to the students, each of whom then examined the patient. Students were taught to improve their examination techniques on patients with abnormal physical findings

---

* A detailed outline of the lecture and laboratory series, assignments in textbooks and other sources, and a schedule of the total course are available from the author on request.

Table 10-2. Outline of Six-Month Training Course for Nurse Practitioners in Adult Health Appraisals

Week:	1	2	3	4	5	6	7	8	9	10	11	12	13	14	15	16	17	18	19	20	21	22	23	24
Basic lectures	x	x	x																					
Preceptorship				x	x	x	x	x	x															
Ward rounds							x	x	x	x	x	x	x	x	x	x								
Specialty rotations									x	x	x	x	x	x	x	x								
Supervised clinical practice																	x	x	x	x	x	x	x	x
Staff meetings	x	x	x	x	x	x	x	x	x	x	x	x	x	x	x	x	x	x	x	x	x	x	x	x

Written ↑ Examination (after week 15/16)   Practical ↑ Examination (after week 22)

Reprinted from *Medical Care* [91] by permission of publisher.

Table 10.3.   Lectures in the Basic Techniques of Physical Examination (25 Hours)

Lectures (60 to 90 minutes per lecture)	Number of Lectures
Introduction	1
Ear, nose, and throat	1
Eye	2
Back and extremities	1
Neck and thyroid gland	1
Heart and lungs	3
Breasts	1
Abdomen	1
Nervous system	1
Skin	1
Rectum and male genitalia	1
Female genitalia	2
The integrated physical examination	1
Total lectures	17

Table 10-4.   Laboratories in the Techniques of Physical Examination (60 Hours)

Laboratories (three-hour sessions)	Supervised Practice	Unsupervised Practice
Ear, nose, throat, neck, thyroid	2	1
Eye	2	1
Back and extremities	1	1
Heart and lungs	3	2
Abdomen	1	1
Nervous system	1	1
The Integrated physical examination	1	2
Total sessions	11	9

and to describe their findings accurately and completely, using proper medical terms. Senior medical residents were instructors in this portion of the course.

(4) *Specialty clinic training.* The students spent 215 hours in outpatient specialty clinics such as dermatology and ophthalmology (Table 10-5), where they received further experience in the use of examining instruments such as the ophthalmoscope and in the methods of physical examination. They observed a wide range of common abnormalities. Differentiation was emphasized between benign and malignant lesions and between normal, normal variant, and abnormal findings.

(5) *Supervised clinic experience.* The nurses performed physical examinations on patients being seen in the nurse practitioner section of the Department of Medicine. Early in this portion of the training period the supervising physician completely repeated each nurse's examination. As each student gained experience, the doctors began to omit checking parts of the examination. Eventually, they checked only "critical areas" such as heart and lungs, and abnormal findings.

Table 10-5. Specialty Clinic Assignments for Training in the Techniques of Physical Examination (215 Hours)

Specialty Clinic	Days of Training
Dermatology	7
Ophthalmology	5
Ear, nose, and throat	4
Gynecology	4
Surgery	3
Urology	2
Nuclear medicine	2
Total days	27

(6) *Staff conferences.* At weekly meetings with the course director, teaching films were shown, and students' problems or uncertainties were discussed.

b.   History taking and evaluation.   The essentials of history taking were taught in an introductory series of four lectures supplemented by selected reading assignments. Further practice and training were given during the preceptorship in internal medicine, during the students' rotation through the specialty clinics, at the staff conferences, and in the supervised clinical experience (see *a* above). Emphasis was placed on categorizing items in the history as significant or nonsignificant by a standard pattern of questioning, and on identifying items that necessitated referral for further evaluation. Students were taught to ascertain the severity, duration, frequency, and progression of symptoms, and to record previous treatment.

c.   Evaluation of laboratory data; methods and procedures of referral for further care.   Two introductory lectures outlined the normal values, basic significance, and followup procedures for the multiphasic laboratory examinations used in the health evaluations. The information was reinforced during the instruction listed in *a* above.

d.   Evaluation of educational needs and health counseling.   Lectures by physicians, nurse practitioners, and health educators were given weekly on:

(1) Recognition and evaluation of patients' health needs.

(2) The teaching process (including educational methods and audiovisual techniques).

(3) Instruction in specific aspects of patient education, such as breast self-examination and teaching patients what to do about specific medical problems and common conditions such as varicose veins, hemorrhoids, and chronic constipation.

(4) The functions of a nurse practitioner and the process of role change.

e.   Certification.   No legally constituted body or published method of examination and certification for nurse practitioners exists at present, with the exception of the examination given by the National Board of Medical Examiners (which is primarily established for non-nurse physician assistants)[90] and the proposed certification by the American Nurses' Association.[35] We therefore developed an examination and certification procedure specifically for our program. The procedure was improved and refined with experience in subsequent examinations of 35 additional nurse practitioners trained in a similar manner at other Kaiser-Permanente facilities. The methods employed were based on established systems for testing health professionals who were performing similar tasks.

The expected tasks outlined above were analyzed and judgments made as to the specific skills and knowledge required for the performance of each. The nurse practitioners were expected to replace internists or generalists in limited tasks, but under supervision. Therefore, on examination, levels of performance of these tasks were expected to equal those of senior medical students or junior house staff, but it was not expected that the nurse practitioners would possess their integrative skills. After the first group of nurses had been certified, their performance at work provided us with an additional standard for gauging the test performance of future groups. Kay[83] and Gilbert[80] have developed testing systems that resemble ours.

The examination was divided into written and practical sections. The written examination, given at the end of four months of formal training, was 90 minutes in length. The nurses were examined for their understanding of anatomy, physiology, techniques of physical examination and history taking, interpretation of laboratory findings, and patient teaching and counseling. The types of questions included requests for term definition, true/false choice, multiple choice, fill-in, and short essay.* The questions given to the first group of trainees were selected from a large pool of suggestions submitted by the course faculty. In selecting questions for subsequent examinees, questions submitted by the first group of nurse practitioners were added to the pool. The level of difficulty was set so that a grade of 75 percent was passing, but a well-trained nurse practitioner should score 90 percent or higher. Achieved scores have ranged from 84 to 98 percent, with an average of 94 percent.

The practical examination, given at the end of the additional two months of supervised clinical experience, was modeled after the practical bedside examination formally given to physicians by the National Board of Medical Examiners. Most of the patients examined had numerous physical abnormalities, some evident and some subtle. Each student examined two patients under the direct observation of physicians not associated with the nurse practitioner training course. Students were observed for their general approach to the patient and for proper techniques of history taking and physical examination. Each was expected to find and accurately describe all abnormalities.

3. Operational Procedures of the Nurse Practitioner Section

a. Scheduling appointments.   Physical examinations by the nurse practitioners were scheduled through a central appointment desk, for those patients who (1) required or requested a comprehensive health checkup, (2) were not clearly acutely ill, (3) had not been seen by a physician within the preceding year, and (4) accepted an appointment for a physical examination by a nurse practitioner. A detailed protocol was developed to assist the appointment clerk in this appointment procedure (Figure 10-7).

---

*A copy of a typical examination is available from the author.

To facilitate the entry into the health care system of patients who needed to be seen promptly, some appointments were held open until 48 hours before the examination date, and a programmed mix of "easy" (code 3), "intermediate" (code 2), and "difficult" (code 1) patients was booked each day for examinations in the nurse practitioner section (see Figure 5-4).

b.   Physical facilities and staffing.   The nurse practitioner facilities at Kaiser-Permanente Medical Center, Oakland, were adjacent to the MHTS area. They consisted of 17 examining rooms, two doctors' and nurse practitioners' consultation offices, a clerk's office, and two waiting areas for patients. At any one time the staff comprised eight to 10 nurse practitioners, one supervising physician, one licensed vocational nurse, one clinic aide, and two health testing clerks. The licensed vocational nurse and clinic aide introduced the patient to the unit, initiated forms, directed patients to examining rooms, and performed other such duties. The health testing clerks maintained records, collated the data for the final health evaluation report, telephoned patients when necessary, sent letters informing them of the results of their health evaluation, aided in arranging referrals, and forwarded the completed health evaluation report to the patient's personal physician.

Physician supervisors for the medical nurse practitioners were internists and generalists from this medical center who worked an average of a half-day weekly in this section.

c.   Outline of nurse practitioner physical examination and referral triage. The nurse practitioner when seeing the patient had available:

(1) The patient's clinic chart containing all previous hospital and outpatient medical records.

(2) A computer printout of the patient's history obtained via an interactive terminal (see Figure 10-8).

(3) A preliminary online report of MHTS laboratory data (Figure 10-9).

The nurse practitioner saw the patients individually, reviewed the present and past history in enough detail to bring the patient's problems into proper focus, then performed a complete physical examination including pelvic examination and Papanicolaou smear. The physical examination was similar to that performed by a primary care physician; however, emphasis was primarily on identifying physical findings that were important in triage for patient referral, and secondarily on documenting the presence of other significant physical findings. The basic items to be covered in the physical examination were printed on a checklist; provision was also made for additional written entries (Figure 10-10).

After completing the physical examination the nurse practitioner reviewed the available laboratory reports, interpreted them to the patient, and, following a detailed protocol, ordered retests and further laboratory evaluations where appropriate. Special patient instruction forms were used to facilitate retesting (Figure 10-11). When appropriate, the nurse practitioner gave general advice about common minor medical problems.

Racks of health pamphlets were available in the examining rooms. Patients with specific problems received specific referrals to the patient audiovisual library in the health care center for information on family planning, hypertension, diabetes, obesity, and a wide variety of other health-related subjects. (See Chapter

NURSE PRACTITIONER SECTION
Standard Orders for Use of Patient Triage Code System

I. Patients of the following types, or with the following complaints or
problems can be given appointments in the Nurse Practitioner Section.

Code 1 ("Difficult" Patients)
1. Colostomy or ileostomy patients (without problems)
2. Patients under the care of a psychiatrist
3. Slow thinkers
4. Slow talkers
5. Patients with a moderate language barrier
6. Moderately anxious teenagers or adults
7. Patients who are nervous or depressed
       or who have an emotional problem.
8. Patients who complain of dizziness or blacking out
9. Patients with liver trouble
10. Patients claiming significant weight loss
       over a short period of time.
11. Patients with many questions who seem to want to talk a lot.

Code 2 ("Intermediate" Patients)
1. Patients being followed regularly but with no present complaints
2. Elderly (>60 years) patients with no complaints
3. "Tired or rundown" patients
Patients who have:
4. Headache - not longstanding
5. Eye or ear problems
6. Coughing
7. Abdominal pain, gas or indigestion
8. Bright blood in stool
9. Changes in bowel habits (diarrhea, constipation)
10. Urinary problems with no infection
11. Swelling of ankles
12. Back problems
13. Obesity
14. Joint pains, swelling or arthritic problems
15. Thyroid trouble
16. Anemia
17. Diabetes under followup and with no complaints
18. Old stable cerebrovascular accidents without major disability
19. Gout
20. Cancer with no problems
21. Mild language barrier
22. Mild anxiety
23. Patients >45 years who have not had a physical for 5 years
24. Patients >45 years who have never been seen at Kaiser
25. Patients referred by private M.D. or dentist

Code 3 ("Easy" Patients)
1. Teenagers
2. Patients requesting a regular physical
3. Persons who want a physical examination
       or need prescriptions
4. Patients with hayfever, allergies or asthma with no acute symptoms
5. Patients needing routine physical examinations
       and having no health problems.
6. Persons requesting "annual physical"
7. Persons requesting "routine checkup"

Figure 10-7a. Protocol for guidance of nurse practitioner section appointment clerk in
making appointments for examination of patients by nurse practitioner.

Twelve.) As an additional health education measure, a teaching and counseling
outline was developed by the staff of the nurse practitioner section, giving the
nurse practitioners guidance in proper and acceptable counseling of patients with
respect to selected frequent, benign conditions (Figure 10-12).

In accordance with established guidelines the patients were referred when
necessary to appropriate divisions of the medical center for further evaluation or

II. Patients who are <u>not</u> <u>eligible</u> for appointment with Nurse Practitioners

    <u>Code 5</u>
      Patients who are (or have):
      1. Blind
      2. Deaf
      3. Language barrier - severe
      4. Physical handicap - moderate to severe
          (or with complicated appliances or pacemakers).
      5. Multiple problems, being followed by a doctor
      6. Mentally retarded - moderate to severe
      7. Severe mental illness
      8. Patients with acute and urgent problems of possible serious import.
          Examples: Angina pectoris
                  Longstanding cardiac disease with recent problems
                  Longstanding emphysema with recent problems
                  Severe gastrointestinal complaints (or black stools)
                  Cirrhosis with recent problems
                  Seizures
      9. Patients who insist on seeing their regular doctor
     10. Patients younger than 14 years
     11. Patients who have had a physical examination within the last 12 months
     12. Patients with a private physician they intend to continue to see.
     13. Patients with a colostomy or ileostomy who have problems.

The exclusion criteria are set up with these factors in mind:

    1. Exclude patients whom the nurse practitioners could not help;
       whose new medical problems are such that a nurse practitioner
       could not handle them even for triage, or who have a chronic
       medical problem or history so complex that a nurse practitioner
       could not add to patient's care.

    2. Exclude patients who insist on receiving the same service again
       from their regular physician or another source, and in whom any-
       thing the nurse practitioners would do would be mostly duplicative.

    3. Exclude patients to whom the nurse practitioners might be able to
       offer service to but who, because of technical problems (such as
       blindness), would take so much time to evaluate that the nurse
       practitioners' efficiency would be significantly decreased.

Figure 10-7b.

followup. They could be referred when appropriate to the Department of Internal Medicine, to any of 11 specialty clinics (ENT, urology, etc.), or to any of the preventive maintenance or health care services. (See Chapter Eleven.) Each patient received a special wallet card (Figure 10-13), which provided direction for future use of resources within the medical center.

The amount and type of physician-nurse practitioner-patient interaction depended on protocol and the patient's health status. Many patients were dismissed from the unit without seeing the physician unless they asked to see him. For some others there was no direct interaction; after completing the evaluation, the nurse practitioner went on to the next patient while the physician separately reviewed the findings and saw the patient briefly. For other patients there was a brief discussion between physician and nurse practitioner, or a more detailed consultation during which the physician and nurse practitioner spent time together with the patient. The doctor confirmed all significant physical findings and major diagnoses, provided medical direction and counsel for the nurse practitioner,

```
                    PERMANENTE MEDICAL GROUP - OAKLAND
                         Multiphasic Health Checkup
                          Final Report of History


Patient:                                  MR#
Phone No:                                 Female Born:   12/42
Bus. Ph.:                                 Visit date:    4/21/1975
                                          Visit time:    Ø9:38
                                          Print date:    Apr 28  75
Doctor:  Unknown
         Oakland                          Rec. ser. no.   Ø-ØØ57


Medical History:  Initial visit, full.

Reason for visit: Annual physical.

PRIMARY PROBLEMS (patient's estimate):
     She reports premenstrual tension.

SYMPTOMATIC REVIEW, POSITIVE RESPONSES:

   GENERAL HEALTH:
      She feels her health is generally good.  TB skin test negative over a year
ago.  Has had tetanus booster or series in the past 10 years.  She is overweight.
      Coffee:  Drinks 1-2 cups/day.
      Smoking habits:  Has smoked 2 or more packs of cigarettes (inhaled) a day
for 1Ø-2Ø years.
      Drinking habits:  Seldom or never drinks.
      Weight change:  Has lost and is overweight by about 1Ø pounds without dieting.

   C.N.S.
      Has been having ordinary headaches.

   SKIN:
      Has had an unspecified dermatologic problem.  This is located on the scalp.

   E.E.N.T.:
      Wears dentures and they cause no difficulties.

   UPPER G.I.:
      Appetite is described as 'too good'.

   LOWER G.I.:
      Believes she has hemorrhoids.

   GYN:
      Menstruation began at 1Ø-14 years old.  Her periods occur regularly (every
26-3Ø days) and last 4-5 days.  She menstruated within the past month.  She is
currently using birth control pills and is experiencing headaches associated with
this.  She wants or needs contraceptive advice.  She has had a Pap test within
the past year.  She has breast pain associated with her periods.

   PSYCHOLOGIC:
      She worries a great deal.  Has never seen a psychiatrist or psychologist.
```

Figure 10-8a. Computer printout of patient's history, available to nurse practitioner at time of patient examination.

wrote prescriptions, and reviewed patient triage and referral decisions that were not covered in "standing order" protocols. The nurse practitioners recorded all actions taken and diagnoses made on special forms (Figures 10-5 and 10-14).

A most important part of the overall operation, and one that underwent continuous improvement, was the mechanism of triage for referral, which was designed to insure that all necessary actions and notifications were accomplished. A

MR#   4/21/1975   Page 2

SYMPTOMATIC REVIEW, NEGATIVE RESPONSES:

No known current symptoms relative to vision or eyes, E.N.T., pulmonary, chest pain, cardiac or hypertensive disease, dyspepsia, abdominal distress, urinary or hematologic problems.

PAST PROBLEMS:
Has had caesarian section. Reports anemia.

GENERAL INFORMATION:
Marital status:	Married.
Birthplace:	North America.
Children:	One; 1–3 years old.
Home situation:	Single family house with spouse or children.
Education:	Completed high school.
Occupation:	Involves sitting or walking; Finds it satisfactory.
Exercise:	Under one hr./week bicycling, jogging or walking No time/week in sports or exercise program Less than one hr./week in active hobbies.

Family history: Father is living and in good health. Mother is living and ill with cancer. Other blood relatives have had cancer, diabetes and high blood pressure.

Number of previous multiphasic exams: none.
Referral: self.

Patient's statement of accuracy: honest as possible.

I: 3.
P: 5.

Figure 10-8b.

multiple-copy triage slip was used to monitor and control this process and to serve as a transmittal document by which other divisions were notified of actions taken. It was also useful for statistical analysis (Figure 10-15).

The rules for patient referral triage and secondary testing by the nurse practitioners were developed empirically after consultations with physicians of the medical center's Department of Medicine, specialty clinics, and preventive maintenance clinics. Initially, patient triage was performed without computer assistance. Results of laboratory tests were reported offline; and in that early period patient triage was performed in three stages:

(1) First-level triage was accomplished on the day of health evaluation on the basis of history and physical examination.

(2) Second-level triage was accomplished a few weeks later, when the final computerized summary report was received together with the patient's complete medical record. The nurse practitioner reviewed this information and, using a detailed protocol, arranged the final disposition of the patient. One of a series of appropriate letters was then sent to the patient, giving him the results of his health evaluation and suggesting further tests or referrals where indicated (Figure 10-16).

(3) Third-level triage was completed on the basis of the results of subsequent or repeated tests such as glucose tolerance, lipid studies, or thyroid function tests, which confirmed or negated the presence of various disease states. The repeated

ON-LINE REPORT
PHYSIOLOGICAL DATA

ANTHROPOMETRIC MEASUREMENTS:
     height   65.3 in
     weight   178.0 lbs

CARDIOVASCULAR:
     B.P.   Godart   132/69   (usual range: 90-159/50-89)
               manual   data not entered
     pulse   Godart   **50   (usual range: 60-95)
               manual   data not entered

ACHILLES REFLEX:
     data not entered

HEARING:
     test not done
     NOTE(S): patient does not wear hearing aid
               patient is not under the care of the ear dept.

VISION ACUITY:
     right eye   20/40 or better
     left eye   20/40 or better
     NOTE(S): patient is not under the care of eye dept.

OCULAR TENSION: (non-contact)
                         value   usual range
     right eye   13   4 - 25
     left eye   15   4 - 25

RESPIRATORY:
     Peak flow   7.3 l/sec
     Fevb-is   3.9 liters
     Fevb-2s   4.1 liters
     Vital cap   4.1 liters

CHEST X-RAY INTERPRETATION:
     no significant abnormality

ECG INTERPRETATION:
     no significant abnormality
     ** sinus bradycardia

URINALYSIS:
     ph   6
     glucose   negative
     protein   negative

Figure 10-9a. Preliminary online report of MHTS laboratory data, available to nurse practitioner at time of patient examination.

```
                          MR #                        4/23/1975


        HGB                   negative
        clinitest             data not entered
        acetone               data not entered
-----------------------------------------------------------------------

SEROLOGY:
        VDRL:                 data not entered
-----------------------------------------------------------------------

HEMATOLOGY:
        wbc      t/cmm        9.6           3.5 - 12.Ø
        rbc      m/cmm        5.1           4.5 - 6.Ø
        hct      gm%          47.3          4Ø.Ø - 54.Ø
        hgb      g            15.3          13.Ø - 17.Ø
        mcv      cu mic       92            8Ø - 1ØØ
        mch      mcmcg        3Ø.1          26.Ø - 34.Ø
        mchc     gm%          32.6          32.Ø - 36.Ø
-----------------------------------------------------------------------

BLOOD CHEMISTRY:
                             value         usual range
        NOTE:  Blood drawn Ø hours since last food - 75 gm. diet not taken
        sodium    meq/l       143           135 - 146
        pot       meq/l       5.Ø           3.5 - 5.5
        calcium   mg%         9.8           8.5 - 1Ø.5
        chol      mg%         181           14Ø - 24Ø
        gluc      mg%         1Ø6           5Ø - 155
        bun       mg%         14.6          5.Ø - 25.Ø
        uric      mg%         5.2           2.Ø - 7.5
        creat     mg%         1.Ø           Ø.3 - 1.4
        bili      mg%         Ø.9           Ø.1 - 1.4
        alk ph    mu/ml       41            1Ø - 95
        ldh       mu/ml       154           8Ø - 24Ø
        sgot      mu/ml       16            1Ø - 5Ø
-----------------------------------------------------------------------

**8Ø1 ADVICE RULES ISSUED:
        none
-----------------------------------------------------------------------
** = outside usual range
-----------------------------------------------------------------------
```

Figure 10-9b.

laboratory studies were usually carried out within a few weeks of second-level triage. When the results were received in the nurse practitioner section, the health testing clerk arranged appropriate referrals to the preventive maintenance or internal medical clinics in accordance with defined rules.

Offline reporting of results obviously delayed patient triage. Especially where third-level triage was required, the process might extend from three to six weeks. Later, the availability of most of the test results online made it possible to combine first- and second-level triage and to perform them on the day of examination. Referrals to sick care services or preventive maintenance clinics were scheduled in accordance with the urgency of need. The reasons for the referral were documented and were included in the permanent medical record, so that when the patient arrived at the referral clinic the reason for the visit was clear.

HEALTH EVALUATION SECTION
PHYSICAL EXAMINATION

M.R. NO.

NAME:

DATE OF BIRTH:

SEX:

SYSTEMS NEGATIVE

- BACK AND SPINE
- SKIN
- EARS
- EYES
- NOSE
- MOUTH AND THROAT
- NECK
- BREASTS
- LUNGS
- HEART
- ABDOMEN
- RECTAL
- GENITALIA
- EXTREMITIES
- NEUROLOGICAL

BACK AND SPINE

- NOT EXAMINED
- LORDOSIS
- PILONIDAL CYST (INFLAMED)
- PELVIC TILT
- BACK OR SPINE ABNORMALITY, NFS

SKIN

- NOT EXAMINED
- DERMATOPHYTOSIS
- ECZEMA/NEURODERMATITIS: MILD
- ECZEMA/NEURODERM: MOD. OR SEV.
- KERATOSIS, ACTINIC
- KERATOSIS, SEBORRHEIC
- ACNE VULGARIS: MILD
- ACNE VULGARIS: MOD. OR SEVERE
- ACNE ROSACEA
- FURUNCULOSIS
- HEMORRHAGIC PHENOMENA
- PSORIASIS: MILD
- PSORIASIS: MOD. OR SEVERE
- XANTHOMA
- XANTHELASMA
- JAUNDICE
- INFECTION, NFS
- DERMATITIS SEBORRHEIC
- ABNORMALITY, NFS
- ABNORMALITY SUSP. FOR MALIG.

EARS

- R L NOT EXAMINED
- R L DISCHARGE
- R L CERUMEN OBSTRUCTING
- R L OTITIS EXTERNA
- R L TYMPANIC MEMBRANE PERF.
- R L ABNORMALITY, NFS

EYES

- R L NOT EXAMINED
- R L ABSENT OR BLIND
- R L SCAR IRIDECTOMY
- PUPILS UNEQUAL: LT. > RT.
- PUPILS UNEQUAL: RT. > LT.
- R L PUPIL UNREACTIVE TO LIGHT
- EXTRAOCULAR MUSCLE ABN., NFS
- LID LAG
- R L PTERYGIUM OVER CORNEA
- R L CATARACT
- R L FUNDUS NOT SEEN
- R L OPTIC DISC MARGINS INDISTINCT
- R L RETINA MICROANEURYSM
- R L RETINA EXUDATE
- R L RETINA HEMORRHAGE
- R L RETINAL ABNORMALITY, NFS
- R L ABNORMALITY, NFS

NOSE

- NOT EXAMINED
- R L OBSTRUCTION
- R L CONGESTED
- R L POLYPS
- R L NOSTRIL ABNORMALITY, NFS

MOUTH AND THROAT

- NOT EXAMINED
- DENTAL CARIES/GUM DISEASE, NFS
- HOARSENESS
- LEUKOPLAKIA
- LIP-TUMOR/LESION SUSP FOR MALIG.
- GUM/MUCOUS MEMB-TUM/LES SUSP MALIG
- TONGUE-TUMOR/LESION SUSP MALIG.
- TONSILS-TUMOR/LESION SUSP MALIG.
- PHARYNX-TUMOR/LESION SUSP MALIG.
- ABNORMALITY, NFS

NECK

- NOT EXAMINED
- R L SALIVARY GLAND ENLARGED
- R L LYMPHADENOPATHY - ANT. CERV.
- R L LYMPHADENOPATHY - POST. CERV.
- R L LYMPHADENOPATHY - OCCIPITAL
- R L LYMPHADENOPATHY - SUPRACLAV.
- R L LYMPHADENOPATHY - SUBMANDIB.
- R L THYROID, ENLARGED DIFFUSE
- R L THYROID, NODULES MULTIPLE
- R L THYROID, NODULE SINGLE
- R L ABNORMALITY, NFS

BREASTS

- NOT EXAMINED
- R L ABSENT
- LYMPHADENOPATHY AXILLARY
- R L NIPPLE ABN./DISCH. SUSP MALIG.
- R L SKIN ABNORM. SUSP FOR MALIG.
- R L MASS, UPPER OUTER QUADRANT
- R L MASS, LOWER OUTER QUADRANT
- R L MASS, UPPER INNER QUADRANT
- R L MASS, LOWER INNER QUADRANT
- R L MASS, SUB AREOLAR
- R L ABNORMALITY, NFS

LUNGS

- NOT EXAMINED
- CHEST DEFORMITY, NFS
- R L BREATH SOUNDS DIM./ABS. ANT.
- R L BREATH SOUNDS DIM./ABS. POST.
- R L RHONCHI FEW
- R L RHONCHI MANY
- R L RALES - ANTERIOR UPPER
- R L RALES - ANTERIOR LOWER
- R L RALES - POSTERIOR UPPER
- R L RALES - POSTERIOR LOWER
- R L WHEEZES - FEW
- R L WHEEZES - MANY
- RESPIRATORY DISTRESS, NFS
- R L ABNORMALITY, NFS

HEART

- NOT EXAMINED
- P2 INCREASED
- A2 INCREASED
- A2 DECREASED
- ARRHYTHMIA, NFS
- ABNORMALITY, NFS

HEART (CONT'D)

MURMUR 1

- SYSTOLIC
- DIASTOLIC
- GRADE 1
- GRADE 2/3
- GRADE 4
- GRADE 5/6
- APEX
- AORTIC AREA
- LEFT STERNAL BORDER
- NECK
- LEFT AXILLA

MURMUR 2

- SYSTOLIC
- DIASTOLIC
- GRADE 1
- GRADE 2/3
- GRADE 4
- GRADE 5/6
- APEX
- AORTIC AREA
- LEFT STERNAL BORDER
- NECK
- LEFT AXILLA

ABDOMEN

- NOT EXAMINED
- EXAM INADEQUATE
- HERNIA INCISIONAL
- R L LYMPHADENOPATHY INGUINAL
- R L HERNIA INGUINAL/FEMORAL
- R L KIDNEY ENLARGED
- LIVER PALPABLE NOT ENLARGED
- LIVER CONSISTENCY FIRM
- LIVER CONSISTENCY SOFT
- LIVER ENLARGED: 2 CM
- LIVER ENLARGED: 4 CM
- LIVER ENLARGED: 6 CM
- LIVER ENLARGED: 8 CM OR MORE
- MASS: EPIGASTRIC
- R L MASS: UPPER QUADRANT
- R L MASS: LOWER QUADRANT
- SPLEEN ENLARGED
- HERNIA UMBILICAL REDUCIBLE AND LESS THAN 2 CM
- HERNIA UMBILICAL IRREDUCIBLE OR MORE THAN 2 CM
- AORTA WIDENED
- ABDOMINAL ABNORMALITY, NFS

RECTAL

- NOT EXAMINED
- EXAM INADEQUATE
- HEMORRHOIDS
- MASS, NFS
- SKIN LESION PERIANAL
- PROSTATE ENLARGED: 1+ OR 2+
- PROSTATE ENLARGED: 3+ OR 4+
- R L PROSTATE NODULE
- PROSTATE CONSISTENCY - HARD
- ABNORMALITY, NFS

MALE GENITALIA

- NOT EXAMINED
- EXAM INADEQUATE
- R L HYDROCELE
- R L TESTICULAR MASS
- R L EPIDIDYMIS LESION, NFS
- R L TESTIS, ABSENT/ATROPHIC
- PENILE LESION, NFS
- ABNORMALITY, NFS

FEMALE GENITALIA

- NOT EXAMINED
- EXAM INADEQUATE
- BARTHOLIN CYST
- VULVITIS
- VULVA ABNORMALITY, NFS
- CYSTOCELE
- RECTOCELE
- URETHRA DIVERTICULUM/CYST
- VAGINAL DISCHARGE
- VAGINAL MUCOSA ATROPHIC
- VAGINAL ABNORMALITY, NFS
- CERVIX ABSENT
- CERVICITIS
- CERVIX POLYP
- IUD STRING IN OS
- CERVIX ABNORMALITY, NFS
- R L ADNEXAL MASS, NFS
- UTERUS: ABSENT
- UTERUS: ENLARGED LESS THAN 8 WK
- UTERUS: ENLARGED MORE THAN 8 WK
- UTERUS: PREGNANT PROBABLE
- UTERUS: PROLAPSE

EXTREMITIES

- NOT EXAMINED
- CLUBBING
- HEBERDEN NODES
- R L KNEE, OSTEOARTHRITIS-MOD./SEV.
- R L HIP, OSTEOARTHRITIS-MOD./SEV.
- R L ANKLE EDEMA: 1+ OR 2+
- R L ANKLE EDEMA: 3+ OR 4+
- R L PRETIBIAL EDEMA: 1+ OR 2+
- R L PRETIBIAL EDEMA: 3+ OR 4+
- R L DORS. PEDS/POST. TIB. PULSE ABS
- JOINT INFLAMMATORY CHANGES:•
- R L •FINGERS/HAND
- R L •WRIST/ELBOW
- R L •LOWER EXTREMITY
- R L DUPUYTREN CONTRACTURE-MILD
- R L DUPUYTREN CONTRACTURE-MOD./SEV.
- R L VARICOSE VEINS: MILD
- R L VARICOSE VEINS: MOD. OR SEV.
- R L SHOULDER ROTATOR CUFF SYNDROME
- R L DEFORMITY/AMPUTATION: UPPER
- R L DEFORMITY/AMPUTATION: LOWER
- R L ABNORMALITY, NFS

NEUROLOGICAL

- NOT EXAMINED
- MENTAL STATUS ABN., POSS., NFS
- NEUROLOGICAL ABNORMALITY, NFS

ADDITIONAL PHYSICAL FINDINGS:

PULSE:

BP:

HES 1075-50 (REVISED)

Figure 10-10. Forms used to record items to be covered by nurse practitioner in physical examination.

KAISER
PERMANENTE
MEDICAL CENTER

Department of Medicine
Health Evaluation Section

INSTRUCTIONS FOR YOUR FASTING BLOOD FAT TEST

(Lipid Panel)

It is important, but not urgent, to retest your
blood for possibly abnormal amounts of fat. This
test may be done Monday through Friday.

For accurate test results you should not change
your eating pattern or any other habits, except
when you plan to have the blood sample taken.
At that time you should be in a fasting state.
Therfore, please follow these directions:

1.   Do not have food or liquids (except water)
     from 7:30 p.m. the night before the test
     until after you have had the test.

2.   Please bring this requisition with you to
     the Clinic Laboratory located on the ground
     floor of 280 West MacArthur Blvd., Oakland,
     Calif., between the hours of 7:30 a.m. and
     7:30 p.m.

If you have any questions about this test, please
call the Hyperlipidemia Clinic at 645-6789.

If the test result is abnormal, we will contact
you again; otherwise, you may assume the retest
result is normal.

Thank You

Figure 10-11.   A typical instruction form given to patient when retesting was required.

The health testing clerk screened all returned followup or recheck laboratory tests and sent to the referring physician only those that were abnormal, thus relieving the physician of the burden of reviewing false-positive MHTS results.[24] The nurse practitioner section accepted the responsibility for attempting to follow through on patients who did not appear for retesting (Figure 10-17) and for notifying the physician if the patient declined to repeat tests (Figure 10-18). The patient's personal physician, upon receipt of the completed health evaluation report, was thus apprised that his patient had been examined and, after reviewing the results, could take any further action he deemed necessary (Figure 10-19).

4.   Experience with Nurse Practitioner Examination in Other Centers

There is little published information concerning the utilization of medical nurse practitioners in routine health assessment, and even less about their utilization as an adjunct to multiphasic health testing services in the manner described here.

14. Self Breast Examination

    1. To check for any breast changes - lumps, masses. Not difficult
        to carry out.
    2.
    3. Examination. After period stops each month (do not examine just
        before period since breasts are swollen and engorged). Observe
        in mirror for size, etc. When lying down, palpate entire breast
        for lumps, nodules, etc. Squeeze nipples for discharge (especially
        blood). Most lumps are not tumor.
    4. Health Center - film and pamphlet.
    5. Any change.
    6. Surgery Clinic.

15. Pilonidal Cyst (Not inflammed)

    1. A cyst at the base of coccyx area (tail bone).
    2. Not serious; not malignant.
    3. If becomes mildly inflamed or tender; warm compresses (moist)
        wet turkish towel covered with a plastic bag; heating pad for
        heat; Sitz bath.
    4.
    5. If becomes inflammed (red, swollen, painful, draining).
    6. Surgery Clinic.

16. Inverted Breast Nipples. (That patient can remember having all her
    life).

    1. Inverted nipples of the breasts; many women have; most can nurse.
    2. Not serious.
    3. Nothing.
    4.
    5. If condition is something new, occuring symmetrically or asymmetrically.
    6. Surgery Clinic.

17. Corns

    1. Kernels of hard tissue that form on the toes caused by pressure or
        by rubbing of shoe (bony nodule of toe joints pressing against shoe).
    2. Not serious; not tumor.
    3. Wear comfortable shoes; soak feet in warm water to soften corn and
        make it easy to extract kernel or core. (Caution: do not attempt
        shaving corn with free razor blade, except non-diabetics, after
        proper instruction. Avoid the use of over-the-counter solutions
        to remove corns.) Dr. Scholls pads without medication may be used.
    4.
    5. If corn becomes infected and painful.
    6. Surgery Clinic or local Podiatrist.

*Key to Sections:
1. What it is.   4. Where to learn more about it.
2. What it isn't.   5. When to see a doctor.
3. What to do for it 6. Which doctor to see.

Figure 10-12. Sample page from nurse practitioner's patient teaching outline.

PERMANENTE MEDICAL GROUP
OAKLAND

You have had a General Checkup and
Physical Examination on:

________________ / ____ 19 ________

Your regular medical doctor is:

Dr. ____________________ Phone: 645-6 ______

01530 (9-73)
HES-673-41

PERMANENTE MEDICAL GROUP
OAKLAND

You have had a general checkup
and physical examination on:

________________ / ________ 197 ____

IF YOU BECOME ILL, NEED PRESCRIPTION REFILLS
OR HAVE ANY OTHER QUESTIONS, CALL THE MEDI-
CAL ADVICE NURSE AT 645-6918.

07336 (9-73)
HES-673-42

Figure 10-13.   Wallet cards given to patients who completed MHTS, with instructions for use of health center facilities.

Cipolla et al.[92] outlined the use of nurse practitioners for routine preemployment physical examinations without automated testing. Duff et al.[93] briefly mentioned the use of a "health technician" to perform the physical examination, but apparently the patient so examined still saw a physician. Wright[13,94] mentioned the use of nurse practitioners for pelvic and breast examinations. Coulehan et al.[82] described the utilization of a nurse practitioner in routine health assessments, and Hinman[43] discussed the use of physician assistants for the same duties.

Gilbert and his associates pioneered in this field, using nurse practitioners for routine health assessments as early as 1969.[51,80] Experience with nurse practitioners trained and utilized in a manner somewhat similar to ours is reported by Henriques et al.[95] This concept has been applied by the Southern California Permanente Medical Group; they have also been utilizing nurse practitioners in offline non-MHTS assessments.[96]

HEALTH EVALUATION SECTION - DEPARTMENT OF MEDICINE - OAKLAND

ADDITIONAL HISTORY ☐ NEW MEMBER ☐ LANGUAGE BARRIER

LAST HEALTH EVALUATION________ OCCUPATION________

REMARKS — Discussed or Instructed

- Alcohol ☐
- Low back ache (minor) ☐
- Cerumen ☐
- Constipation ☐
- Fatigue ☐
- GI upset (minor) ☐
- Headaches (minor) ☐
- Hemorrhoids ☐
- Hygiene ☐
- Joint/muscle ache ☐
- Kegel exercises ☐
- Menopause ☐
- Obesity ☐
- Personal concerns ☐
- Rhinorrhea/Hay fever ☐
- Self breast exam ☐
- SKIN: Acne ☐
  - Dermatophytosis ☐
  - Misc. skin prob. ☐
- Sexual concerns ☐
- Smoking ☐
- Tension/Stress ☐
- Varicose veins ☐

ADDITIONAL STUDIES ☐ PAP SMEAR DONE

REMARKS AND TREATMENT ☐ OUTSIDE MEDICAL RECORDS SENT FOR ☐ IRON PROTOCOL

REFERRALS CONTINUE FOLLOW-UP WITH: ☐ REGULAR MD ☐ MAINT. CLINIC ☐ CALL: ☐ REGULAR MD PRN ☐ MED. ADVICE RN PRN

RETURN TO HES IN_____YEARS ________ R.N. MEDICAL NURSE PRACTITIONER

LETTER_____SENT ________ ________ TRIAGE DONE

HES 1275-49
06984 (1-76)

Figure 10-14. Form on which nurse practitioner recorded actions and diagnoses.

HEALTH EVAULATION SECTION KPMC-TRIAGE & REFERRAL

☐ REGULAR
☐ BY REQUEST   DR. _______________   NP _______________
☐ ASSIGNED
                PATIENT'S ADDRESS   MD SUPV. _______________

                                          MCDS ☐   MHC ☐

HOME PHONE _______________   WORK PHONE _______________

| FIRST LEVEL TRIAGE | SECOND LEVEL TRIAGE   DATE | THIRD LEVEL TRIAGE |

FIRST LEVEL TRIAGE

MEDICAL _______________
SPECIALTY _______________
____

1) HYPERTENSION _______________
2) G.I. ☐
3) ARTHRITIS ☐
BACK CARE ☐
CONCERNED WELL ☐
HEALTH COUNSELOR _______________
LIBRARY _______________
STOP SMOKING ☐
TEENAGE ☐
WT. CONTROL ☐
OTHER _______________
PAP DONE _______________
COMMENTS:

09093 (1-72)
G61-1-72

SECOND LEVEL TRIAGE   DATE

REFER: NO REFER
MEDICINE ______ WKS   MEDICINE
SPECIALTY _______________
TESTS ORDERED:

SENT LETTER # ______ _______________
LETTER SENT _______   INITIAL
REF. BP ☐   PAP, ABN-A _______________
PAP WNL ☐   PAP, ABN-B _______________
ADV RULE LAB _______________
1ST LEVEL LAB _______________
801 LAB _______________
RECORDS TO REFERRING MD _______________

THIRD LEVEL TRIAGE

PHMC RETESTS	WNL	ABN	PHMC-REF
GTT			
URIC ACID			
LIPID PANEL			
RENAL			

REF. HYPERTENSION ☐
OTHER RETESTS   WNL ☐   ABN ☐
LETTER # _______   SENT _______________
LAB TO RMD _______   PHMC _______________
LAB FOLLOW-UP _______________
RMD NOTIF. _______   PHMC NOTIF. _______
FILED _______

PHMC = PREVENTATIVE HEALTH MAINTENANCE CL.
RMD = REFERRING PHYSICIAN
                                    HES 1271-19

Figure 10-15.   Triage and referral slip originating in nurse practitioner section. Multiple copies used for monitoring, control, and as a transmittal document for notifying others of actions taken.

5.   Evaluation of the Nurse Practitioner Section

a.   Utilization of services.   The nurse practitioner section operation was analyzed in detail for the period April 1971–June 1973; most of the data outlined below are from that period. Specific areas of data have been updated as circumstances necessitated.

The results of a survey of the reasons for seeking medical care, as recorded by randomly selected patients on self-administered questionnaires, are shown in Table 10-6. While 47 percent were seeking a general checkup and mentioned no significant problem, 53 percent were seeking advice about one or more medical concerns, in the categories noted in rank order in Table 10-6. Most patients, even though they stated that they were well, recorded some symptoms in the inventory-by-systems questionnaire. These complaints do not appear in Table 10-6, but were reviewed and acted upon by the nurse practitioner section. It is thus evident that the nurse practitioner section functioned as an entry and periodic evaluation point not only for healthy persons but also for those with a broad spectrum and multiplicity of medical problems.

The nurse practitioner section in 1976 was providing health evaluations on 1,500 to 2,000 patients per month or 18,000 to 24,000 patients per year. Pelvic examinations with cervical smears were performed on approximately 6,000 women in that year. Except for 3.3 percent referrals to the gynecology clinic, each pelvic examination represented a saving of one visit to a gynecologist. The nurse practitioner section was in operation 4½ days (36 hours) a week, paralleling the hours of operation of the MHTS unit. The extra half-day was used for review of medical

ANTIOCH • HAYWARD • NAPA • OAKLAND • REDWOOD CITY • RICHMOND • SACRAMENTO • SAN FRANCISCO
SAN RAFAEL • SANTA CLARA • SOUTH SAN FRANCISCO • SUNNYVALE • VALLEJO • WALNUT CREEK

THE PERMANENTE MEDICAL GROUP

A.J. Sender, M.D., Physician-in-Chief, Oakland Division
Robert L. Cella, M.D., Assistant Physician-in-Chief, Oakland Division
280 West MacArthur Boulevard - Oakland, California 94611 - Telephone: 645-5000

Department of Medicine
Health Evaluation Section

Date:

Dear

The results of your recent examination in the Health Evaluation
Section have been reviewed by our medical staff and we are pleased to
inform you that no significant abnormalities were found.

The results have been sent to your doctor for his review. If
you have any further questions call him directly. Unless you have
been instructed otherwise, we suggest that you return for another
examination in_______________________. In the meantime, if you
develop any medical problems, call or see your doctor.

We suggest that you take advantage of the health education programs in our Audiovisual Library and Exhibits Theaters, located on
the first floor of the Health Education Center, 3779 Piedmont Avenue,
Oakland. These additional services are available without cost to you
to help keep you healthy and well.

Very truly yours,

Health Evaluation Section

HES-874-1

Figure 10-16. Letter originating in nurse practitioner section, used in second-level triage.

charts, referral triage, staff meetings, and continued nurse practitioner in-service training. This schedule also allowed time for discussion of problems as they appeared and permitted adjustments as experience was gained. In addition, it provided opportunity for the nurse practitioners to broaden their skills in health counseling and gynecology, and to work in the preventive maintenance and general medical clinics.

For the period March to October 1974, a stable operational interval, the average daily number of patients seen by the nine nurse practitioners was 106; each nurse practitioner provided comprehensive health evaluations and counsel-

THE PERMANENTE MEDICAL GROUP

A. J. Sender, M.D. • Physician-in-Chief, Oakland Division
Robert L. Cella, M.D. • Assistant Physician-in-Chief, Oakland Division
280 West MacArthur Boulevard, Oakland, California 94611 • Telephone: 645-5000

Department of Medicine
Health Evaluation Section

Date________________________

Dear ______________________,

    After your Health Evaluation Section checkup on__________________________,
you were advised to have some additional tests. Since we have not yet received the results of these additional tests, we cannot complete your evaluation.

    If you have already had the tests done, or if there are any problems
about having them done, please call us at the number given below. Otherwise,
we would suggest that you come in for the tests as soon as possible.

                          Very truly yours,

                          Health Evaluation Section

                          Telephone: 645-6850

HES-474-21

Figure 10-17. Letter originating in nurse practitioner section, sent to patients who did
not respond to notification that they should be retested.

ing for 12 patients daily, or an average of one patient every 38 minutes. This meant
that each physician supervisor reviewed the examination of 106 patients each day.
If one converts all nurse practitioner time used (in seeing patients, triage, administration, staff meetings, and in-service education) to physician equivalents in a 3:1
derived salary ratio and adds all physician time involved in supervision and
administration, then 23 to 24 patients each day are "examined" for the cost of one
physician's salary.

HEALTH EVALUATION SECTION
DEPARTMENT OF MEDICINE
KPMC - OAKLAND

Patient________________________________

MR #________________________________

Date of HES Evaluation________________________________

Date________________________________

To Dr.________________________________

This patient has had the tests listed below ordered as a follow-up of an H.E.S. Evaluation.

As of this date we have not received the results. We will not contact the patient further.

Please take any action you feel appropriate.

Tests Ordered:

PLEASE FILE THIS IN PATIENT'S CHART

HES 1075-22

Figure 10-18. Notification, from nurse practitioner section to patient's physician, that the patient had not responded to advice for repeat testing.

```
HEALTH TESTING REPORT


HEALTH EVALUATION SECTION, DEPARTMENT OF MEDICINE
PERMANENTE MEDICAL GROUP - OAKLAND, CALIFORNIA



                              Date




TO DOCTOR

Attached are the completed results of a Health Evaluation Section examination of
your patient.  This included a physical examination by a medical nurse practitioner
under a physician's supervision.

Any advice or referrals that were made on the basis of the history, physical findings,
and review of the multiphasic tests are noted on the attached diagnosis form.  Any
additional tests ordered are also noted.  We will refer all possibly abnormal retests
to you for further evaluation.  You may wish to enter additional diagnosis on the
diagnosis form.

The patient (was) (was not) instructed to make a follow-up appointment with you
in ______________ weeks.  If, after your review of the HES report, you have further
advice for your patient, please contact him directly.

Any questions concerning this report should be referred to the supervising medical
nurse practitioner, Ext. 6850 or 6964.

Please have the attached HES report and this letter filed in the patient's chart.
THIS IS THE ORIGINAL COPY.




                    Reviewed: ____________________________ M.D.

                        Date: ____________________________


HES 1275-13
09068 (REV. 12-75)
```

Figure 10-19. Transmittal letter from nurse practitioner section to physician, accompanying completed results of MHTS.

Table 10-6. Reasons for Initial Visit of Patients Requesting Physician Services and Seen in Nurse Practitioner Section

Reason for Visit	Percent
Health checkup without specific complaint	47
Specific complaint	53

Chief Specific Complaint	Percent of Patients with Complaints
Gastrointestinal	19
Headache or dizziness	17
Tired or rundown	9
Cardiovascular	9
Respiratory	7
Obesity	6
Eyes, ears, nose, throat	6
Musculoskeletal	5
Emotional problems	4
Other	18

Since January 1975 California law has permitted registered nurses to identify and record "normal" findings. Since this date, the nurse practitioners have completed the evaluation by protocol of 63 percent of the patients seen in the nurse practitioner section; no direct physician-practitioner interaction was required for those patients. A short nurse practitioner-physician discussion was required for 17 percent of the patients; for the remaining 20 percent, more detailed consultation was needed, during which the physician and nurse practitioner saw the patient together. Seventy-seven percent of patients went through the nurse practitioner section without seeing a physician, either because they had no problems or findings not covered in the protocols (69 percent) or because they were referred by protocol for further evaluation (8 percent).

The rates of referral to sick care, preventive maintenance, and health care services during the stable period, January–June 1973, are summarized in Table 10-7; the rates in this period were very similar to those for the entire period, April 1971–June 1973. Fewer than 9 percent of the patients required referral to their own internists for further evaluation and management; 91 percent did not need the services of their personal physician at the time of health evaluation. Seventeen percent were referred directly to specialty sick care clinics. Thus a large majority (75 percent) of the patients examined in the nurse practitioner section required no further direct physician care at that time. As shown, 18.5 percent of the patients were referred to the preventive maintenance services. Repeat analysis in October 1974 revealed little change in these figures. The number of patients requiring referral to more than one care service was small (Table 10-8).

The frequency of referral to the preventive maintenance clinics is shown in Table 10-9; similar details about referrals to specific specialty sick care services appear in Table 10-10.

Table 10-7. Patients Referred from Nurse Practitioner Section, Monthly Averages, January–June 1973

	Number	Percent
Average total number of patients		
examined per month	903	100.0
Patients referred to:		
Sick care services	235	26.1
Patient's internist	80	8.9
Specialty clinics	155	17.2
Preventive maintenance services	167	18.5
Health care services	501	55.4
Counseling and clinics	104	11.5
Exhibits and library	397	43.9

Table 10-8. Patients Referred from Nurse Practitioner Section to More Than One Care Service, Monthly Averages, January–June 1973

	Number	Percent
Average total number of patients		
examined per month	903	100.0
Patients referred to:		
Sick care and preventive maintenance	41	4.5
Preventive maintenance and health care	15	1.7
Sick care and specialty clinic	14	1.6
Sick care and health care	13	1.4
Sick care, preventive maintenance,		
and health care*	3	0.3

*Health care counseling and clinics only (see Table 10-11); excludes referrals to patient library and exhibits.

Referral to health care services fluctuated as the number of such services varied from time to time, and as the nurse practitioners assumed increasing responsibility for health counseling and advice about minor medical problems. On the average, 11.5 percent of the patients examined per month were specifically referred to the health care services (Table 10-11). Thirty-nine percent of the referrals were for general health counseling; these patients were primarily worried-well persons who had more than one functional problem, and who represented 5 percent of the persons examined monthly in the nurse practitioner section. Eighteen percent of these referrals were for nutritional advice and 16 percent each for aid in stopping smoking or in weight control. In addition to specific referrals, all patients seen in the nurse practitioner section were informed of the availability of the health center's patient library and health exhibits, where they could obtain information about health maintenance or about specific medical problems.

Data concerning the frequency with which secondary or diagnostic laboratory tests were required are presented in Table 10-12. For October 1974, 22 percent of the patients required subsequent testing, primarily serum chemistry, urinalysis, or hematology. For these 430 patients, 657 tests were ordered; results were abnormal

Table 10-9. Referrals to Preventive Maintenance Clinics from Nurse Practitioner Section, Monthly Averages, January–June 1973

	Number	Percent
Average total number of patients examined per month	903	100.0
Number of referrals per patient:		
1	146	16.2
2	20	2.2
3	1	0.1
Total	167	18.5

	Number	Percent of 189 referrals per month	Percent of 903 patients per month
Average total referrals per month	189*	100.0	.
Patients referred to:			
Hypertension	90	47.6	10.0
Gastrointestinal	38	20.1	4.2
Arthritis	27	14.3	3.0
Back care	10	5.3	1.1
Diabetes	9	4.8	1.0
Kidney	8	4.2	0.9
Hyperlipidemia	7	3.7	0.8

*Some patients were referred to more than one preventive maintenance clinic.

in 30 percent, normal in 39 percent, unknown, not done, or not reported at the time of review in the remaining 32 percent.

b.   Cost analysis.   The nurse practitioner section unit costs for entry into the health care system through this new mode during the period January 1–June 30, 1973, are shown in Table 10-13. The unit costs shown include direct and indirect (overhead and plant operation) expense, and are based on the 5,353 patients seen by the nurse practitioners during the relevant period. As indicated, the unit cost of $10.86 in the first six months of 1973 included nurse practitioners' services, physician supervision, wages of support personnel, computer costs, overhead, and plant operation expense. The average physician time expenditure per patient was three minutes. If one adds the cost per patient of multiphasic health testing during that period ($17.46), the total cost of entry of a patient into ambulatory care in the new medical care delivery system by multiphasic health testing and nurse practitioner appraisal is seen to have been $28.32. These figures do not include the expense of followup laboratory testing or of visits to physicians, to the preventive maintenance clinics, or to the health center. The figures were calculated assuming a ratio of four nurse practitioners to one supervising physician. The unit is presently operating with a ratio of eight or ten nurses to one physician, so that physician costs per examination have diminished considerably.

c.   Patient acceptance

(1) *Patient compliance with appointments*. Patient compliance with nurse practitioner appointments was high. Of those who fulfilled the criteria for this type of

Table 10-10. Referrals to Specialty Sick Care Services from Nurse Practitioner Section, Monthly Averages, January–June 1973

	Number	Percent
Average total number of patients examined per month	903	100.0
Number of referrals per patient:		
1	135	15.0
2	18	2.0
3	2	0.2
Total	155	17.2

	Number	Percent of 177 referrals per month	Percent of 903 patients per month
Average total referrals per month	177*	100.0	
Patients referred to:			
Optometry	31	17.5	3.4
Gynecology	30	16.9	3.3
Otolaryngology	28	15.8	3.1
Dermatology	27	15.3	3.0
Surgery	20	11.3	2.2
Ophthalmology	11	6.2	1.2
Urology	9	5.1	1.0
Allergy	8	4.5	0.9
Orthopedics	6	3.4	0.7
Neurology	4	2.3	0.4
Psychiatry	3	1.7	0.3

*Some patients were referred to more than one specialty service.

health evaluation and were offered the program by the central appointment staff, approximately 90 percent accepted. More than 98 percent of those who accepted by telephone and subsequently came in for health evaluation completed both the multiphasic tests and nurse practitioner evaluation. Fewer than 1 percent refused to undergo the nurse practitioner physical examination; their reasons for refusal included an occasional long wait due to initial errors in scheduling, not having understood that the health evaluation was to be done by a nurse practitioner, and preference for seeing their personal physician for followup. In only 0.2 percent of the cases were nurse practitioner health evaluations not indicated because the patients had been improperly assigned when they telephoned for an appointment, or because the patient had already undergone a complete examination in the medical clinic in the recent past.

(2) *Patient satisfaction with nurse practitioner examinations.* A survey was made of the degree of satisfaction expressed by patients examined in the nurse practitioner section. Their responses were compared with (a) those of patients tested in MHTS and referred to a physician for physical examination and (b) those seeing a physician for a traditional periodic health examination. Details of this survey have been described.[97] In general, there was a high degree of satisfaction with both physician and nurse practitioner physical examination across the wide

Table 10-11. Referrals to Specific Health Care Services from Nurse Practitioner Section, Monthly Averages, January–June 1973*

	Number	Percent
Average total number of patients examined per month	903	100.0
Number of referrals per patient:		
1	100	11.1
2	3	0.3
3	1	0.1
Total	104	11.5

	Number	Percent of 109 referrals per month	Percent of 903 patients per month
Average total referrals per month	109†	100.0	
Patients referred to:			
Health counseling, including concerned well	42	38.5	4.7
Nutrition	20	18.4	2.2
Weight control	17	15.6	1.9
Stop smoking	17	15.6	1.9
Family planning	11	10.1	1.2
Teenage	2	1.8	0.2

*All well patients seen in the nurse practitioner section were routinely referred to the patient health library and exhibits for information on general health maintenance.
†Some patients were referred to more than one health care service.

Table 10-12. Results of Secondary or Diagnostic Tests, Nurse Practitioner Section, October 1974

	Number	Percent	
Total number of patients examined	1,925	100	
Patients for whom secondary or diagnostic tests were ordered	430	22	
Number of secondary or diagnostic tests ordered	657	100	
Results normal	253	39	(56% of tests with results known)
Results abnormal	199	30	(44% of tests with results known)
Results unknown and/or test not done	265	32	

socioeconomic spectrum represented by the Kaiser-Permanente Health Plan membership. The patients responded enthusiastically to the high degree of compassion and obvious deep interest and understanding shown by the nurse practitioners. In addition to the summary of results displayed in Table 10-14, re-

Table 10-13. Unit Cost Per Patient Examined, Nurse Practitioner Section, January 1–June 30, 1973

		Cost per Patient $N = 5,353$
Physician supervision*		$ 2.64
Nurse practitioner*		4.30
Support personnel*		1.45
Direct nonpayroll		0.26
Computer costs		0.92
Direct equipment cost	$0.19	
Computer center recharge	0.73	
Total direct cost		9.57
Total indirect cost†		1.29
Total		$10.86

*Includes salaries and fringe benefits.
†Overhead and plant operation.

Table 10-14. Summary of Results of a Survey of Patient Satisfaction Expressed After Examination by Nurse Practitioner (NP) or by Physician (MD)

	After Examination by	
Strong Satisfaction Expressed with	NP (%)	MD (%)
Physical examination	81	68
Length of wait for appointment	72	27
Competence of examiner	86	77
Attention received from examiner	84	70
Examiner's explanation of findings	77	68
Examiner's advice	71	65

sponses to the survey indicated that 54 percent of the patients who were examined by a nurse practitioner preferred that type of checkup; 25 percent would rather have been examined by a physician, 15 percent favored a traditional (nonmultiphasic) doctor's visit, and 6 percent expressed no preference. Forty-eight percent of patients examined by a nurse practitioner stated that they would be "very satisfied" if their routine health care were given by a nurse practitioner rather than by a physician; 28 percent stated that they would be "fairly satisfied"; 12 percent expressed no preference.

Kay,[83] working in a unit similar to ours, noted a similarly high level of patient satisfaction with nurse practitioner examinations. Others have confirmed general patient satisfaction and acceptance of nurse practitioner care.[45,52,55,69,73,80,98,99]

d. Staff satisfaction with the nurse practitioner section

(1) *Physicians.* It took time and practical experience for the physicians to reorient themselves from the old system, in which they took complete responsibility for all decisions about the patient, and the nurse was a technical assistant, to the new system. Weiler[100] discussed the problems physicians have in relinquishing any portion of their "professional turf." In this new mode of practice, the nurse

practitioner is a collaborator and associate who combines skills with those of the physician to provide a unique type of care and an enhanced capacity to care for patients. Bates[101] has outlined the steps requisite to this change of professional self-image. A few of our physicians found themselves uncomfortable in this new practice mode, but the majority in our Department of Medicine have given evidence of their approval by accepting regular rotating consultative responsibility in the nurse practitioner section.

The physicians of the Departments of Medicine and Obstetrics-Gynecology were surveyed with respect to their opinions of nurse practitioner examinations. Their responses indicated that the nurse practitioners provided almost twice as many benefits as problems to them in their work, and more than twice as many benefits as problems for their patients. When given a list of positive and negative statements about the nurse practitioner section, 44 percent of physicians agreed with the positive statements and 30 percent agreed with the negative statements. When asked which medical care system gave them greater general satisfaction, 43 percent chose the nurse practitioner section; 43 percent selected the traditional periodic health checkup system; 14 percent did not answer or were not sure. Others have confirmed physician acceptance of nurse practitioners.[102]

(2) *Nurse practitioners.* The nurse practitioners showed a high degree of acceptance of this system and assumed their new role with enthusiasm and increased job satisfaction. Others have confirmed this observation.[34] The nurse practitioners proved highly capable of and interested in carrying out their responsibilities, as others also have noted.[47,73] This dedication both to the patients and to the new system contributed significantly to the success of the program. The nurse practitioners saw themselves as active partners with the physician in providing care, rather than as mere passive vehicles for providing service. They were able to integrate their traditional skills of counseling and teaching with their newly acquired skills of history review, physical examination, and health evaluation.

The nurse practitioners encouraged patients to verbalize their concerns and questions. They gave patients a fuller and more positive health counseling experience than could usually be afforded by busy physicians, who carried heavy primary responsibility for sick care.[103] In this way they added another special dimension to the checkup.[104]

When queried in a survey of opinion, the nurse practitioners replied that the nurse practitioner section system yielded 50 percent more benefits than problems for them in their work and more than three times as many benefits as problems for their patients. When the nurse practitioners were given the same list of positive and negative statements concerning the nurse practitioner section that had been presented to the physicians, 50 percent agreed with the positive statements and 14 percent agreed with the negative statements. When asked which medical care system in general gave them greater satisfaction, 83 percent replied that they preferred the nurse practitioner section system; 6 percent preferred the traditional system; 11 percent did not answer or were not sure.

While the nurse practitioners were highly satisfied with their work in the nurse practitioner section, it became clear from our experience and that of others[105] that, because of physical and mental fatigue, nurse practitioners could not indefinitely perform efficient health evaluations 40 hours a week. To maintain a successful system it proved necessary to let the nurse practitioners spend at least 40 percent of the working week in other activities, such as health maintenance of patients with chronic disease, health counseling, care for minor acute illness, etc.

6. Wider Applications of the Nurse Practitioner Concept

The concept of entry into ambulatory care and routine health evaluations through the MHTS and the nurse practitioner section described in this chapter can be translated into other formats and adapted for use in other systems, particularly those of the Health Maintenance Organization (HMO) category. Each HMO could design its own components for such a system, setting up and implementing its own standards for types of patients eligible, tests to be done, type of history review and physical examination to be performed by the nurse practitioners, amount of responsibility to be delegated to them for referral, retesting, counseling, etc., and the level, degree, and organization of physician supervision. Although this system clearly operates most efficiently in an online mode, it can be adapted easily to an offline mode.

Nurse practitioners can work with any doctor or group of doctors having a patient load sufficient to provide the nurse practitioner with 10 to 15 patients daily. They can perform preliminary evaluations of new patients, or followup on old patients. For patients with complaints, they can provide the physician with a data base and a clear idea of the urgency of the problem. For well patients, they can perform routine health evaluations. The concept of the nurse practitioner section can also be applied profitably to health evaluations required by schools, to preemployment or insurance examinations, and to physical examinations before hospital admission for elective medical and surgical procedures. Figure 10-20 illustrates a preoperative evaluation form used in the nurse practitioner section.

Our experience and data in MHTS indicate that this new mode of entry into medical care, and of routine interim health evaluation, can improve service and decrease unnecessary utilization of scarce medical resources. The reasonable cost per patient adds to the system's merit; it is an important way of containing costs of health care delivery. The actual dollar costs are lower than those of the equivalent examination performed either by multiphasic health testing followed by physician examination or by the traditional evaluation completed by our physicians in their offices. In addition, over a studied two-year period, utilization of overall medical resources by patients who had been seen in the nurse practitioner section was lower than that by patients seen in the traditional modes, further saving dollars and physician time.[97,106] (See Chapter Seventeen.)

C. SUMMARY

The physical examination and referral process is the essential final link that connects MHTS to patients' clinical care.

In previous systems this was often the weakest link and consumed considerable physician time.

A new system has been developed and implemented to perform this function more efficiently and to conserve valuable physician time. The essential ingredients of this new mode of entry and programmed health evaluation were proper appointment scheduling, multiphasic health testing services, preferably

KAISER
PERMANENTE
MEDICAL CENTER

MEDICAL RECORD NUMBER _______________

PREOPERATIVE EXAMINATION - HEALTH EVALUATION SECTION

NAME (LAST, FIRST, MIDDLE)

ADDRESS (NUMBER, STREET, CITY)

BIRTHDATE	PHONE NUMBER	CODE	GROUP

DATE TO BE ADMITTED	TYPE OF SURGERY

HISTORY:

    BLEEDING TENDENCY?

    NO . . . . IF YES, WHAT?

    REACTION TO DRUGS?

    NO . . . . IF YES, WHAT?

    PERTINENT REVIEW OF SYSTEMS:

    PERTINENT PAST HISTORY:

PHYSICAL:	NORMAL		BP	PULSE	RESP.
ENT					
EYES					
NECK					
SKIN & NODES					
BREASTS					
HEART					
LUNGS & CHEST					
ABDOMEN					
EXTREMITIES					
RECTAL					
GENITALIA					
NEUROLOGICAL					

IMPRESSIONS:

RECOMMENDATIONS: PATIENT IN OPTIMUM OBTAINABLE CONDITION FOR PLANNED SURGERY?

☐ Yes

☐ No

	R.N., MNP		S.M.D.

HES 1/75-48

Figure 10-20. Preoperative evaluation form used in nurse practitioner section.

with online reporting of results, and health evaluation by specially trained nurse practitioners supervised by a physician. The total process permitted rapid triage of sick from well patients for appropriate referral within a medical care delivery system. Appointments for such health checkups were available within a few days. The health evaluation was usually completed in a single visit, requiring about three hours of the patient's time.

Seventy-four percent of patients did not require referral to a physician for further medical care; thus physician time was freed for the care of the sick. It was striking that only 9 percent of the patients needed referral to their personal physicians for further diagnosis and management. The 17 percent who were referred to other specialty clinics did not require the usual visit to their own physician to make this referral.

The paramedically staffed preventive maintenance and health care clinics within the new medical care delivery system receive 19 and 12 percent respectively of the patients seen in the nurse practitioner section.

Approximately one-half of all patients completed evaluation and counseling in the single visit to the nurse practitioner section. This large group of patients did not enter the sick care system. When a patient of this group subsequently did require sick care, his medical record presented to his physician an organized health history and general health evaluation that served as a baseline health profile, thus conserving patient and physician time.

Our experience indicated that registered nurses could be rapidly trained to assume this expanded role. They could be integrated into a large health care program, where, in performing adult health evaluations, they carried important responsibilities on the health care team. This extensive program of physician supervision and consultation combined with carefully designed protocols and advice rules enabled us to delegate considerable responsibility to nurse practitioners after a six-month period of training.

REFERENCES

1. Shapiro, S. "The Health Care Structure and Automated Multiphasic Health Testing and Services." In *Provisional Guidelines for Automated Multiphasic Health Testing and Services*, Vol. 3, *Proceedings of the Invitational Conference on AMHTS*. DHEW Publication No. (HSM) 72–3011, 1970.

2. Hall, W. "AMHTLC." In *Health Evaluation: An Entry to the Health Care System*, D. F. Davies, ed., J. B. Tchobanoff, asst. ed. New York: Intercontinental Medical Book Corp., 1973.

3. *Provisional Guidelines for Automated Multiphasic Health Testing and Services*, Vol. 1, *Planning Principles*. DHEW Report No. PB 195 654, pp. 7, 24–27, 1970.

4. *Provisional Guidelines for Automated Multiphasic Health Testing and Services*, Vol. 2, *Operational Principles*. DHEW Report No. PB 196 000, pp. 5, 18, 76, 78, 1970.

5. "Multiphasic Testing, 1971, Socio-economic Report." California Medical Association, Bureau of Research and Planning, pp. 1–27. Mimeo report.

6. *Statement of Multiphasic Health Testing*. American Medical Association, PD 210–1804–139: 5M; 202–I: 5/72. Pamphlet.

7. Bates, B., and Yellin, J. A. "The Yield of Multiphasic Screening." *J.A.M.A.* 222(1972):74–78.

8. Driggs, M. F. "Technological Surveillance in Preventive Medicine." *Engineering Foundation Research Conferences, Automated Multiphasic Health Testing*. C. Berkley, ed. New York: The Engineering Foundation, 1971.

9. Schneiderman, L. J., DeSalvo, L., Baylor, S., and Wolf, P. L. "The 'Abnormal' Screening Laboratory Results. Its Effect on Physician and Patient." *Arch. Intern. Med.* 129(1972):88–90.

10. Williamson, J. W., Alexander, M., and Miller, G. E. "Continuing Education and Patient Care Research: Physician Response to Screening Test Results." *J.A.M.A.* 201(1967):118–122.

11. Olsen, D. M., Kane, R. L., and Proctor, P. H. "A Controlled Trial of Multiphasic Screening." *N. Engl. J. Med.* 294(1976):925–930.

12. Khoury, S. A. "Multiphasic Screening in Washington, D.C., 1968 and 1969 Results." *Health Services Reports* 87(1972):664–668.

13. Wright, H. G. "Multiphasic Screening in Britain." In *Proceedings of the Conference On A Critical Analysis of the Cost Effectiveness of Multiphasic Screening.* Seattle, Wash. Med. Computer Services Assn., pp. 39–46, 1972.

14. Gillum, R. F., and Barsky, A. J. "Diagnosis and Management of Patient Noncompliance." *J.A.M.A.* 228(1974):1563–1567.

15. Rosenstock, I. M. "Patients' Compliance with Health Regimens." *J.A.M.A.* 234(1975):402–403.

16. Vaisrub, S. "You Can Lead a Horse to Water . . ." Editorial, *J.A.M.A.* 234(1975):80–81.

17. Aller, J. C., Ayers, W. R., Caceres, C. A., and Cooper, J. K. "Systems Analysis of Operational Data from a Multiphasic Screening Center." *Proc. IEEE* 57(1969):1953–1960.

18. East Bay Screening Center, Berkeley, California. Descriptive Literature, 1970.

19. "Report covering period October 1, 1968, through December 31, 1968." Milwaukee Health Department Health Appraisal Program. Contract PH 108–66–281. Mimeo report.

20. Yedidia, A., Bunow, M. A., and Muldavin, M. "Mobile Multiphasic Screening in an Industrial Setting. The California Cannery Workers Program." *J. Occup. Med.* 11(1969):601–602.

21. The Health Maintenance Center, The American Health Corporation, New York, N.Y. Descriptive literature, 1972.

22. *Physicians' Manual.* Health Evaluation Center, French and Polyclinic Medical School and Health Center, New York, 1973. Mimeo.

23. Collings, C. H., Jr., Dupong, W. A., et al. "Multiphasic Health Screening in Industry." *J. Occup. Med.* 14(1972):433–465.

24. Holland B., Holland, P., and Hsieh, R. K. C. "Automated Multiphasic Health Testing." *Public Health Reports* 90(1975):133–139.

25. Alameda County Health Care Services Agency, Oakland, California. Descriptive literature, 1974.

26. Siegelaub, A. Unpublished data.

27. Feldman, R., Taller, S. L., Garfield, S. R., Collen, M. F., Richart, R. H., Cella, R., and Sender, A. J. "Forum: Allied Health Professionals." "Nurse Practitioner Multiphasic Health Checkups" *J. Preventive Med.* 6(1977).

28. "Extending the Scope of Nursing Practice. A Report of the Secretary's Committee to Study Extended Roles for Nurses." *J.A.M.A.* 220(1972):31–36.

29. Pickark, C. G., Jr. "Family Nurse Practitioners: Preliminary Answers and New Issues." Editorial. *Ann. Int. Med.* 80(1974):267–268.

30. Westlake, R. E. "The People-System." In *Health Evaluation: An Entry to the Health Care System,* D. F. Davies, ed., J. B. Tchobanoff, asst. ed. New York: Intercontinental Medical Book Corp., 1973.

31. Baker, A. S. "Primary Care by the Nurse." Editorial. *N. Engl. J. Med.* 290(1974):282–283.

32. Egeberg, R. O., and Pesch, L. A. "The Roles for Nurses." Editorial. *J.A.M.A.* 220(1972):1237–1238.

33. McCormack, R. C., and Crawford, R. L. "Attitudes of Professional Nurses Toward Primary Care." *Nursing Research* 18(1969):542–544.

34. Bullough, B. "Is the Nurse Practitioner Role a Source of Increased Work Satisfaction?" *Nursing Research* 23(1974):14–19.

35. "The Nurse Practitioner Feasibility Study." C. Mundy, ed. HSEC Report 73–3, Health Services Education Council, San Jose, Calif., 1973.

36. Hershey, N. "New Directions in Licensure of Health Personnel." *Economic and Business Bulletin* 24(1971):22–35.

37. Dean, W. J. "State Legislation for Physician's Assistants. A Review and Analysis." *Health Services Reports* 88(1973):3–12.

38. Barkin, R. M. "Need for Statutory Legitimation of the Roles of Physician's Assistants." *Health Services Reports* 89(1974):31–36.

39. Bailit, H., Lewis, J., Hochheiser, L., and Bush, N. "Assessing the Quality of Care." *Nursing Outlook* 23(1975):153–159.

40. Duncan, B., Smith, A. N., and Silver, H. K. "Comparison of the Physical Assessment of Children by Pediatric Nurse Practitioners and Pediatricians." *Am. J. Pub. Health* 61(1971):1170–1176.

41. Charney, E., and Kitzman, H. "The Child-Health Nurse (Pediatric Nurse Practitioner) in Private Practice. A Controlled Trial." *N. Engl. J. Med.* 285(1971):1353–1358.

42. Fine, L. L., and Silver, H. K. "Comparative Diagnostic Abilities of Child Health Associate Interns and Practicing Pediatricians." *J. Pediatr.* 83(1973):332–335.

43. Hinman, E. J. "The Importance of the Physical Examination as a Routine Part of Multiphasic Health Testing." In *Proceedings of the Conference On A Critical Analysis of Cost Effectiveness of Multiphasic Screening*. Seattle, Wash. Med. Computer Services Assn. 1972.

44. Stehbens, J. A., and Lauer, R. M. "Pediatric Cardiology: A New Role for the Pediatric Assistant." *J. Pediatr.* 81(1972):394–398.

45. Lewis, C. E., Resnik, B. A., Schmidt, G., and Waxman, D. "Activities, Events and Outcomes in Ambulatory Patient Care." *N. Engl. J. Med.* 280(1969):645–649.

46. Runyan, J. W., Phillips, W. E., Herring, O., and Campbell, L. "A Program for the Care of Patients with Chronic Diseases." *J.A.M.A.* 211(1970):476–479.

47. Runyan, J. W. "The Memphis Chronic Disease Program. Comparisons in Outcome and the Nurse's Extended Role." *J.A.M.A.* 231(1975):264–267.

48. Stein, G. H. "The Use of a Nurse Practitioner in the Management of Patients with Diabetes Mellitus." *Med. Care* 12(1974):885–890.

49. Gordon, D. W. "Health Maintenance Service: Ambulatory Patient Care in the General Medical Clinic." *Med. Care* 12(1974):648–658.

50. Spector, R., McGrath, P., Alpert, J., Cohen, P., and Aikins, H. "Medical Care by Nurses in an Internal Medicine Clinic. Analysis of Quality and its Cost." *J.A.M.A.* 232(1975):1234–1237.

51. Kaku, K., Gilbert, F. I., and Sachs, R. R. "Comparison of Health Appraisals by Nurses and Physicians." *Pub. Health Reports* 85(1970):1043–1046.

52. Ostergard, D. R. "The Potential for Paramedical Personnel in Family Planning." *A.J.P.H.* 64(1974):27–31.

53. Schlesinger, E. R., Lowery, W. D., Glaser, D. B., Milliones, M. D., and Mazumdar, S. "A Controlled Test of the Use of Registered Nurses for Prenatal Care." *Health Services Reports* 88(1973):400–404.

54. Burrows, B., and Traver, G. A. "Nurse Practitioner Programs." Editorial. *Ann. Int. Med.* 80(1974):268–270.

55. Spitzer, W. O., Sackett, D. L., Sibley, J. C., Roberts, R. S., Gent, M., Kergin, D. J., Hackett, B. C., and Olynich, A. "The Burlington Randomized Trial of the Nurse Practitioner." *New Engl. J. Med.* 290(1974):251–256.

56. Sackett, D. I., Spitzer, W. O., Gent, M., Roberts, R. S. "The Burlington Randomized Trial of the Nurse Practitioner: Health Outcomes of Patients." *Ann. Int. Med.* 80(1974):137–142.

57. Anderson, E. M., Leonard, B. J., and Yates, J. A. "Epigenesis of the Nurse Practitioner Role." *Am. J. Nursing* 74(1974):1812–1816.

58. Andrews, P., Yankauer, A., and Connelly, J. P. "Changing the Patterns of Ambulatory Pediatric Caretaking: An Action-Oriented Training Program for Nurses." *A.J.P.H.* 60(1970):870–879.

59. Silver, H. K., Ford, L. C., and Day, L. R. "The Pediatric Nurse Practitioner Program." *J.A.M.A.* 204(1968):88–92.

60. "Guidelines on Short-Term Continuing Education Programs for Pediatric Nurse Associates." *Am. J. Nursing* 71(1971):509–512.

61. Bullough, B., St. Geme, J. W., and Neumann, C. G. "Pediatric Nurse Practitioners: Issues in Training." *Health Services Reports* 88(1973):767–771.

62. Standard, R. L., and Easley, H. "D.C.'s New Pediatric Nurse Practitioners." *Health Services Reports* 87(1972):387–391.

63. Schutt, B. G. "Frontier's Family Nurses." *Am. J. Nursing* 72(1972):903–909.

64. Biggs, B. "Nurse-Clinician-Practitioner-Assistant-Associate." *Am. J. Nursing* 71(1971):1936–1937.

65. Oseasohn, R., Mortimer, E. A., Geil, C. C., Eberle, B. J., Pressman, A. E., and Quenk, N. L. "Rural Medical Care: Physician's Assistant Linked to an Urban Medical Center." *J.A.M.A.* 218(1971):1417–1419.

66. Brunetto, E., and Birk, P. "The Primary Care Nurse. The Generalist in a Structured Health Care Team." *A.J.P.H.* 62(1972):785–794.

67. Spitzer, W. O., and Kergin, D. J. "Nurse Practitioners in Primary Care. I. The McMaster University Educational Program." *C.M.A. Journal* 108(1973):991–995.

68. Munier, S. K., and Richardson, A. "Development of New Nursing Roles in a Comprehensive Health Center." *J. Nursing Admin.*, July-August 1974:44–49.

69. Merenstein, J. H., Wolfe, H., and Barker, K. M. "The Use of Nurse Practitioners in a General Practice." *Med. Care* 12(1974):445–452.

70. "Preparing Nurses for Family Health Care." *Nurs. Outlook* 20(1972):53–59.

71. Walker, A. E. "Primex—The Family Nurse Practitioner Program." *Nurs. Outlook* 20(1972):28–31.

72. Januska, C., Davis, C. D., Knollmueller, R. N., and Wilson, P. "Development of a Family Nurse Practitioner Curriculum." *Nurs. Outlook* 22(1974):103–108.

73. Schulman, J., Jr., and Wood, C. "Experience of a Nurse Practitioner in a General Medical Clinic." *J.A.M.A.* 219(1972):1453–1461.

74. Flynn, B. C. "The Effectiveness of Nurse Clinicians Service Delivery." *A.J.P.H.* 64(1974):604–611.

75. Kane, R. L., Jorgensen, L. A., Teteberg, B., and Kuwahara, J. "Is Good Nursing-Home Care Feasible?" *J.A.M.A.* 235(1976):516–519.

76. Hendrickson, R. M. "She Packs 90 Minutes into an Hour." *PRISM,* April 1974:pp. 30–38.

77. Sheedy, S. G. "Medical Nurse Practitioner in a Neighborhood Center." *Am. J. Nursing* 72(1972):1416–1419.

78. Moore, A. C. "Nurse Practitioner: Reflections on the Role." *Nurs. Outlook* 22(1974):124–127.

79. Baker, A. S., Soper, M., Keairnes, H., Farrisey, R., and Goldfinger, S. E. "Expeditious Training of Nurse Practitioners." *Mass. Physician,* September 1973:pp. 52–56.

80. Gilbert, F. I., Jr., and Nordyke, R. A. "Automated Multiphasic Health Testing in Multispecialty Group Practice." *Prev. Med.* 1(1973):261–265.

81. Bates, B., and Lynaugh, J. E. "Laying the Foundations for Medical Nursing Practice." *Am. J. Nursing* 73(1973):1375–1379.

82. Coulehan, J. L., and Sheedy, S. "The Role, Training, and One-Year's Experience of a Medical Nurse Practitioner." *Health Services Reports* 88(1973):827–833.

83. Kay, R. F. "Nurse Specialist Training and Utilization Program." Kaiser-Permanente Medical Care Entities, Southern California Region, Los Angeles, 1975. Mimeo.

84. Fagin, C. M., and Goodwin, B. "Baccalaureate Preparation for Primary Care." *Nurs. Outlook* 20(1972):240–244.

85. McGivern, D. "Baccalaureate Preparation of the Nurse Practitioner." *Nurs. Outlook* 22(1974):94–98.

86. Cawston, H. E. "Physical Appraisal: A Nursing Function?" *Canadian J. Pub. Health* 63(1972):67–68.

87. Awtrey, J. S. "Teaching the Expanded Role." *Nurs. Outlook* 22(1974):98–102.

88. Malkemes, L. C. "Resocialization: A Model for Nurse Practitioner Preparation." *Nurs. Outlook* 22(1974):90–94.

89. Lewis, E. P. "A Role by Any Name." Editorial. *Nurs. Outlook* 22(1974):2.

90. Todd, M. C. "National Certification of Physicians' Assistants by Uniform Examinations." *J.A.M.A.* 22(1972):563–566.

91. Taller, S. L., and Feldman, R. "The Training and Utilization of Nurse Practitioners in Adult Health Appraisal." *Med. Care* 12(1974):40–48.
92. Cipolla, J. A., and Collings, G. H., Jr. "Nurse Clinicians in Industry." *Am. J. Nursing* 71(1971):1530–1534.
93. Duff, W. R., and Lipscomb, H. S. "A Health Testing Concept: Simple—by Design." In *Health Evaluation. An Entry to the Health Care System*, D. Davis, ed., J. B. Tchobanoff, asst. ed. New York: Intercontinental Medical Book Corp., 1973.
94. Taylor, W. "Screening for Breast Cancer—Identifying the High Risk Patient." In *Proceedings of the Conference On A Critical Analysis of the Cost Effectivensss of Multiphasic Screening*. Seattle, Wash. Med. Computer Services Assn. 1972.
95. Henriques, C. C., Virgadama, V. G., and Kahane, M. D. "Performance of Adult Health Appraisal Examinations Utilizing Nurse Practitioners-Physician Teams and Paramedical Personnel." *A.J.P.H.* 64(1974):47–53.
96. Crisafulli, C. Personal Communication.
97. Garfield, S. R., Collen, M. F., Feldman, R., Soghikian, K., Richart, R. H., and Duncan, J. H. "Evaluation of an Ambulatory Medical Care Delivery System." *New Engl. J. Med.* 294(1976):426–431.
98. Gardner, H. H., and Ouimette, R. "A Nurse-Physician Team Approach in a Private Internal Medicine Practice." *Arch. Intern. Med.* 134(1974):956–959.
99. Martin, L. L. "I Like Being an FMP." *Am. J. Nursing* 75(1975):826–828.
100. Weiler, P. G "Health Manpower Dialectic—Physician, Nurse, Physician Assistant." *A.J.P.H.* 65(1975):858–863.
101. Bates, B. "Physician and Nurse Practitioner: Conflict and Reward." *Ann. Int. Med.* 82(1975):702–706.
102. Yankauer, A., Tripp, S., Andres, P., and Connelly, J. P. "The Outcomes and Service Impact of a Pediatric Nurse Practitioner Training Program—Nurse Practitioner Training Outcomes." *A.J.P.H.* 62(1972):347–353.
103. Thompson, H. C. "Quality Assurance of Child Health Care." In *Proceedings of the Conference On A Critical Analysis of Cost Effectiveness of Multiphasic Screening*. Seattle, Wash. Med. Computer Services Assn. 1972.
104. O'Donnell, W. E. "Who Says Annual Checkups are a Waste of Time?" *Med. Econ.*, July 8, 1974:97–108.
105. Gilbert, F. I., Jr. Personal communication.
106. Collen, M. F., Garfield, S. R., Richart, R. H., Duncan, J. H., and Feldman, R. "Cost Analysis of Alternative Health Evaluation Modes." *Arch. Int. Med.* 137(1977):73–79.

CHAPTER ELEVEN

Preventive Health Maintenance Adjuncts to MHTS

Krikor Soghikian

A. Introduction
B. Objectives
C. Preventive Health Maintenance Programs
D. Preventive Health Maintenance at Oakland Kaiser-Permanente
E. Conclusion

A. INTRODUCTION

The full potential of an MHTS cannot be achieved without effective adjunctive and followup measures to maintain the health of the well and of those with early asymptomatic disease.[1]

The World Health Organization has defined health as a state of complete physical, emotional, and social well-being, not just the absence of disease.[2] Recently, Terris has suggested a modification of this definition that includes functional ability in addition to subjective feeling of well-being.[3] He has also suggested substituting "illness," which is always symptomatic, for disease, which may be symptom-free. He postulates that "health and illness are mutually exclusive, but health and disease are not." He cites atherosclerosis, tuberculosis, histoplasmosis, and sarcoidosis as examples of diseases in healthy individuals. His proposed definition may be useful for epidemiological studies but not for health care planning. It is true that not all incipient diseases are detectable by current health evaluation techniques, but this technological gap should not detract from a holistic definition of health. One has only to look at hypertension, a very prevalent silent disease, to realize the enormous implications of its detection and treatment for continued health.

Richart's health-status model, which takes into consideration both consumer and provider perceptions, provides much more useful definitions of health and nonhealth.[4] The model, demonstrated in Figure 11-1, classifies individuals in four health groups: the "well," who are symptom-free; the "well-sick," who have symptoms but no detectable pathology, suggesting a "psychomatic" etiology for their symptoms; the "sick-well," who are asymptomatic but have a silent disease, such as hypertension; and the "sick," who have symptoms of a specific disease or

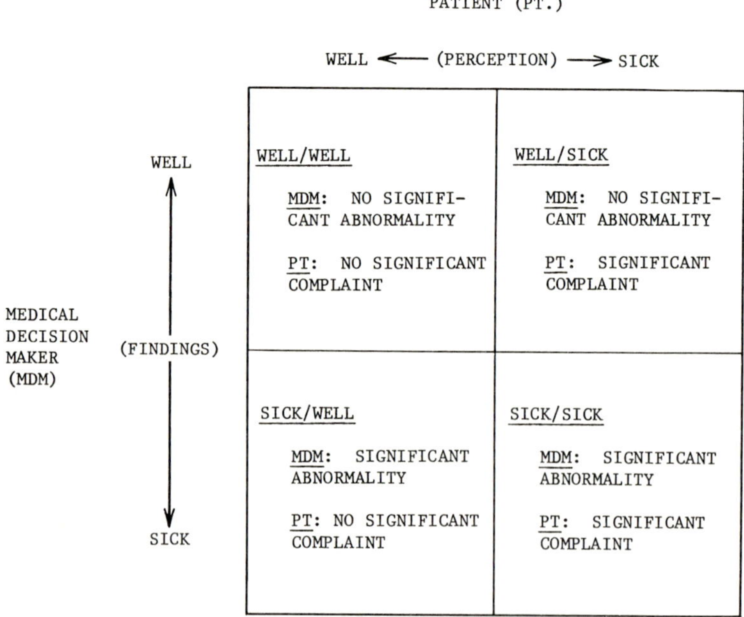

Figure 11-1.   Health status classification through medical decision maker and patient concurrence matrix.

illness. Such a classification can serve as a basis for the development of a comprehensive health care delivery system in place of the traditional "complaint-response" mode.[5] (See Chapter Two, C.)

It has been said that "good medicine includes both good preventive care and good therapeutic care, with no sharp distinction between the two."[6] This was fully recognized in the Health Maintenance Organization (HMO) Act passed by Congress in 1973, which called for preventive health services in addition to basic physician and hospital services.[7]

Many factors affect health—genetic, environmental, and cultural, to name a few. A total program for health maintenance would involve efforts directed to these factors by governmental bodies, voluntary agencies, community groups, and individuals. The discussion of preventive health maintenance in this chapter will be limited to potential interventions in personal health services within a medical care delivery system, or "that aspect of a physician's practice in which he applies to individual patients the knowledge and techniques from medical, social and behavioral science to prevent disease or its progression."[8]

B. OBJECTIVES

Historically, preventive health efforts have been directed to the control of infectious diseases by means of improved sanitation and mass immunization. These efforts have achieved notable success in reducing mortality and morbidity at all ages and in increasing longevity for the young. But they have produced relatively little gain in longevity for individuals over the age of 45, because the major causes of death in this group, atherosclerosis and cancer, have not been significantly affected. A relevant health maintenance program must therefore address itself to the prevention and control of the degenerative diseases of later life.

According to Fuchs, "the greatest current potential for improving the health of the American people is to be found in what they do and don't do to and for themselves."[9] White believes that "life style has become the prime health hazard of this country," and we should look outside the health care system to discover ways to deal with it; he does go on to say, however, that physicians have the opportunity of raising the public's consciousness about life-style-induced health problems.[10] This has been emphasized by the National Conference On Preventive Medicine: "Seeking health behavior that would prevent disease is as much the physician's job as is seeking immunity status to prevent disease."[11]

The objectives of a preventive health maintenance program could be stated as follows:

(1) The promotion of health-oriented changes in individual life style.

(2) The recognition of risk factors conducive to disease and their modification where possible.

(3) The detection of early disease, the course of which can be arrested or retarded by medical intervention.

(4) The development of preventive services that are acceptable to health care recipients and providers and are integrated within an organized delivery system.

It is believed that fulfilling these objectives will reduce disability, morbidity, and mortality and decrease societal costs resulting from preventable illness and loss of work. Indeed, such outcomes have been documented by several recent studies.[12–16]

C. PREVENTIVE HEALTH MAINTENANCE PROGRAMS

1. Scope

In adopting a health maintenance viewpoint at the level of personal health services, three basic goals have to be considered:

(a) *The promotion of health.* There is no question that health is an important, if not the most important, factor contributing to the quality of life. To communicate this notion involves the education and motivation of individuals not only to believe in health as a valuable possession but also to accept personal responsibility for its maintenance. Conceptual issues and methods to achieve these results are detailed in Chapter Twelve.

(b) *The early detection of disease.* It is generally accepted that "intervention into the natural history of disease is more likely to be effective if it is initiated early even before symptoms occur."[11] If so, provisions have to be made to offer periodic examinations to population groups to detect incipient disease.

(c) *The prevention of illness.* In addition to patient education, this goal encompasses a variety of measures such as appropriate immunizations, behavioral change interventions, and psychosocial counseling.

These goals are reflected in the traditional classification of preventive medicine into primary and secondary modes. Primary prevention consists of intervention before a disease process becomes manifest, e.g., immunization against measles, or the development of good eating habits to avoid obesity. Secondary prevention involves the early diagnosis of disease and the institution of measures to stop or modify its progression, e.g., the treatment of asymptomatic pulmonary tuberculosis to arrest it, or the control of hypertension to prevent cardiovascular target organ involvement. Sometimes the term tertiary prevention is used to describe the treatment of symptomatic disease to avoid further progression and complications, as well as rehabilitation to minimize resultant disability. In the broadest sense, of course, treatment of disease at any stage can be considered as preventive health maintenance.

2. Choice of Programs

It has been said that a health maintenance focus can be achieved by continued surveillance of several parameters of health and by intervention at the earliest sign of their deviation from the norm.[5,6,11] These parameters are listed below, with examples of surveillance measures:

(a) *Immunologic.* Obtaining a history of immunizations or of hypersensitivity reactions.

(b) *Bacterial.* Testing for early tuberculosis, latent syphilis, asymptomatic urinary tract infection.

(c) *Anatomical.* Checking for breast lumps, obtaining cervical scrapings, performing dental examinations.

(d) *Physiological.* Monitoring of hearing, intraocular pressure, pulmonary function, blood pressure.

(e) *Chemical.* Testing for certain constituents in body fluids, e.g., cholesterol, glucose, and hemoglobin in the blood, protein in the urine.

(f) *Behavioral.* Observing for precursors of emotional disorders, such as life crises, or habits hazardous to health, such as smoking, drinking, and drug abuse.

(g) *Genetic.* Screening for sickle cell trait, testing for phenylketonuria.

In considering the selection of preventive maintenance procedures to detect and modify deviations in the above parameters, we need to ask several critical questions:[11]

(1) Is the procedure effective in achieving the intended objective?

(2) Is the deviation (or condition) frequent or serious enough to justify intervention?

(3) Are there means of dealing with the condition besides the contemplated procedure?

(4) How easy is it to integrate the procedure within the existing health care delivery structure?

(5) What additional costs will the procedure engender—i.e., is the procedure cost-beneficial?

These questions have to be asked frequently, since the answers are by no means static. They depend on a great many factors, which are in a constant state of flux. Some of these factors are:

(1) Scientific and technical advances.

(2) Attitudes, knowledge, and practices of health care providers and recipients.

(3) Organizational modes of personal health services, including financial arrangements.

Based on the above considerations, the National Conference on Preventive Medicine has developed minimum batteries of preventive procedures for selected age groups, an example of which appears in Table 11-1. (See also Chapter Three, E.)

3. Current Health Maintenance Programs

Health maintenance has assumed a large role in the practice of pediatricians and obstetricians in recent years. Prenatal and child care have become standards of medical practice. A similar trend is already visible in the practice of adult medicine as well. Still calls adult preventive medicine "the fourth phase in the evolution of medicine," and he asserts its "goal is to provide adults with the same kind of high-quality, scientifically sound preventive services that pediatricians provide for infants and young children."[17]

Table 11-2 shows the percentage of persons using selected preventive care services as revealed by the 1973 United States Health Interview Survey.

It is apparent that a sizable proportion of the United States population participates in preventive health maintenance activities. In reviewing the health care literature, however, it is difficult to find references to organized preventive health

Table 11-1. Minimum Battery of Preventive Procedures,* Ages 36–64†

Procedure	Condition	Type of Prevention	Intervention
History of completed immunization or booster in past 10 years	Tetanus, diphtheria	1	Tetanus-diphtheria vaccine
VDRL	Syphilis	2	Diagnosis and treatment
Height and weight	Malnutrition and obesity	1–2	Counselling and diet; diagnosis and treatment
Blood pressure	Hypertension and associated conditions and complications	1–2	Diagnosis and treatment
Cholesterol	Coronary artery disease	1	Behavior change and diet
Hematocrit	Anemia	2	Diagnosis and treatment
Stool for blood	Occult malignancy	2	Diagnosis and treatment
Glucose tolerance test	Diabetes	2	Behavior counselling and diet
Breast exam	Breast cancer	2	Diagnosis and treatment
Mammography or xerography in all over age 50 and high-risk less than age 50	Breast cancer (more frequent than every five years)	2	Diagnosis and treatment
History/life style	Heart and lung disease	1–2	Behavior counselling
Hearing and vision testing	Hearing and vision disorders	2	Diagnosis and treatment
History and counselling	Alcoholism and drugs	1–2	Behavior counselling
History and counselling	Smoking	1–2	Counselling
Counselling	Accidents	1	Counselling
Cervical smear	Cancer cervix (high-risk groups)	2	Diagnosis and treatment
PPD	Tuberculosis (high-risk groups)	2	Diagnosis and treatment

*National Conference on Preventive Medicine, Bethesda, Md., 1975, Vol. 1, pp. 34–35.
†One visit every five years from age 40 to 60.

Table 11-2. Percent of Persons Using Selected Preventive Care Services, United States, 1973*

Type of Care	Percent Ever Had Care	Percent Had Care in Past Year
Electrocardiogram (40 years and over)	60.4	24.5
Glaucoma test (40 years and over)	53.7	23.4
Chest x-ray (17 years and over)	80.1	31.2
Eye examination (three years and over)	87.7	41.3
Breast examination (females, 17 years and over)	76.3	48.0
Pap smear (females, 17 years and over)	75.2	45.9
Routine physical (under 17 years)	86.2	50.1

*Vital and Health Statistics, Series 10, No. 95, "Current Estimates from the Health Interview Survey, United States, 1-73."

maintenance programs. Probably many exist but are not reported. Certainly the half-dozen federally approved HMOs are mandated to provide preventive medical services.[7] Most of the available information pertains to programs that deal with specific chronic diseases, such as hypertension and diabetes.[18,19] Several programs are described that provide primary care to patients with chronic disease using physician-nurse teams in university hospital settings.[20,21] Neighborhood clinics attempt to incorporate preventive health maintenance in their services.[22-24] Others use patient counseling as a program of prevention in association with periodic health examinations.[25,26] Voluntary agencies offer programs in cancer detection, respiratory care, and smoking cessation. Additionally, commercial firms have entered the obesity, smoking, and other health hazard fields with dubious benefits. Considering the degree and complexity of behavior modification required to alter today's "life-style crisis" and positively influence health, the programs referred to do not appear to measure up to the task.[27-30]

4. Design of Preventive Health Maintenance Programs

In the light of the preceding discussion it is evident that the design of a comprehensive preventive health maintenance program is a major undertaking. Nordyke has graphically illustrated the great need of individuals for preventive health action and the low level of physician involvement in such action;[31] Figure 11-2 is a modified presentation of this discrepancy. Even though part of it can be ascribed to the training and interests of physicians, a large determinant is the availability of resources. The introduction of multiphasic screening, new roles for paramedical personnel, and health care protocols have immeasurably expanded these resources.

A preventive health maintenance program can now be designed to include the following:

(a) An MHTS for the detection of subclinical conditions and risk factors amenable to modification or treatment.

(b) A triage and advice rule system for referral of patients to appropriate followup settings.

(c) Preventive maintenance clinics to provide patients with necessary instruction, care, and surveillance.

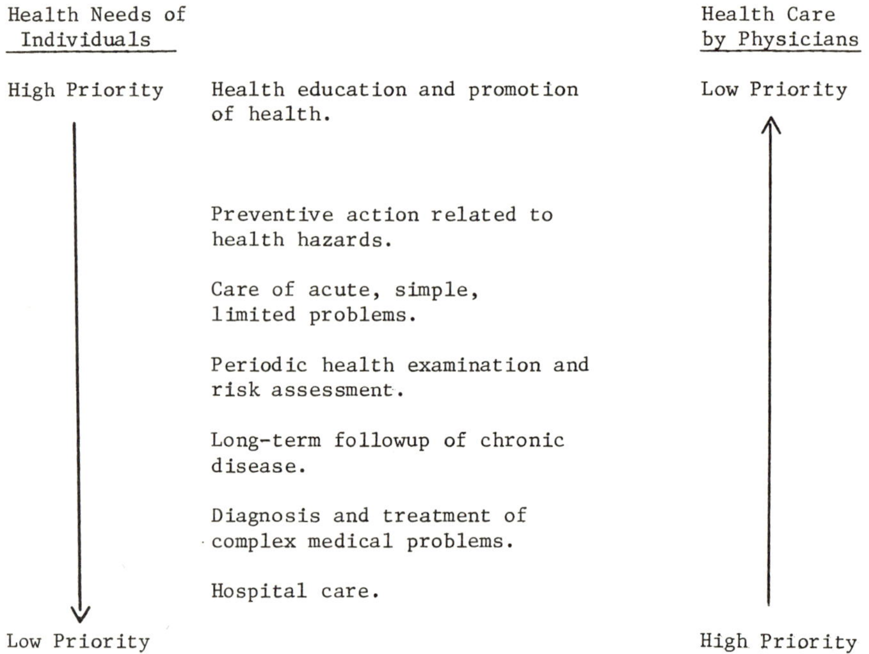

Figure 11-2. Discrepancy between health needs of individuals and health care by physicians.

(d) Physician-paramedical teams to supervise and operate these clinics.

(e) Protocols to guide paramedical personnel in carrying out their functions.

(f) A mechanism for ongoing review of the quality of care provided.

(g) Periodic evaluation and updating of the program components based on operational results, quality reviews, and new knowledge.

The first two program components have been discussed in Chapters Six and Eight. An implementation model incorporating the other components will be described in D of this chapter. Several recent articles have reviewed the utilization of paramedical personnel and of protocols in health maintenance, team practice, patient management, and quality control.[20,21,32–39]

D. PREVENTIVE HEALTH MAINTENANCE AT OAKLAND KAISER-PERMANENTE

1. Introduction

Health maintenance has been one of the fundamental premises of the Kaiser-Permanente Medical Care program since its inception. The underlying belief has been that provision of preventive health services would reduce morbidity and mortality, enhance the quality of life, and decrease utilization of health services and costs. The Multiphasic Health Testing Services (MHTS) has emerged as an outcome of this philosophic stance. (See Chapters One and Two.)

In order to facilitate understanding of the preventive health maintenance system described in this chapter, it is useful to briefly review the mode of medical practice within the Kaiser-Permanente Medical Care Program. A more detailed description of the program has appeared elsewhere.[40] The Permanente Medical Group is a partnership of physicians who take care of the health needs of the Kaiser Foundation Health Plan membership on a contractual basis. Members pay monthly dues to the health plan, which in turn pays the medical group a monthly capitation fee per member for use in providing all necessary health services. This prepayment feature removes the usual financial barrier of traditional medical care and allows for the planning and implementation of an integrated health care delivery system.

The physicians associated with the Medical Care Program practice in groups centered around several outpatient-inpatient facilities geographically located in areas of the health plan's population concentration.

The Oakland Kaiser-Permanente Medical Center (KPMC) serves approximately 130,000 members, of whom nearly 100,000 are 18 years or older. It has a 320-bed general hospital, offices for physicians, and facilities for radiology, laboratory, pharmacy, physical therapy, and other ancillary services. The physician staff is organized into departments representing the usual medical specialties. Physicians in each department render care according to their individual training, experience, and style.

It is safe to say that, by opting for prepaid group practice, physicians who joined the medical care program exhibited a more holistic perception of health care, and indeed, individually and departmentally, included prevention in their day-to-day practice of medicine. However, they did not have a formalized health maintenance program until the establishment of the New Medical Care Delivery System (MCDS). The implementation of MCDS, based on a conceptual article by Garfield, was made possible through a contract with the National Center for Health Services Research and Development in 1970.[41,42] MCDS was designed to provide a complete health evaluation to all health plan members who called in for an appointment in the Department of Medicine in Oakland, as a mechanism for triage and referral for subsequent care (see Figure 11-3). The evaluation triage was performed by a nurse practitioner-physician team based on MHTS and

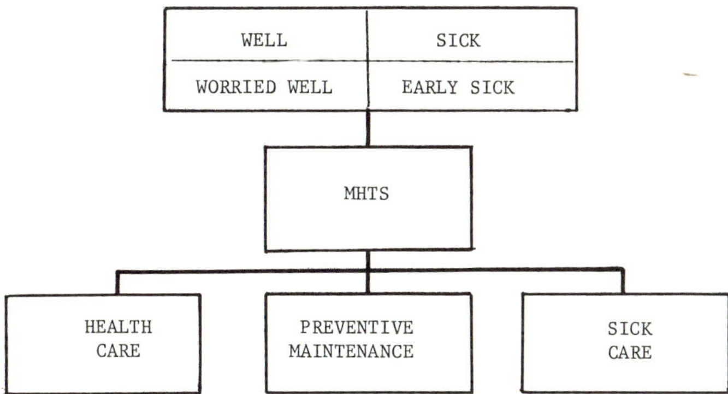

Figure 11-3.   Schematic representation of MHTS triage and referrals.

physical examination results. Decisions were then made for referral to traditional sick care or two innovative health care and preventive maintenance services. The focus of MCDS was to use health care personnel and resources more effectively to meet the medical care demand created by the removal of the fee-for-service barrier. A more detailed description of MCDS appears in Chapter Fifteen.

2.   Preventive Health Maintenance System

In this system, health care and preventive maintenance have been administratively combined in a single unit called the health center. The center is under the overall supervision of a physician and a supervisor of paramedical personnel. It is part of the Department of Medicine, an arrangement that integrates preventive and therapeutic care and facilitates communication between paramedical staff and physicians. Figure 11-4 outlines the organizational framework of the health center. The following discussion will be limited to its preventive maintenance component. The health care component, which is the educational adjunct of MHTS, will be described in Chapter Twelve.

In the choice of target conditions for preventive maintenance, the criteria mentioned earlier in this chapter were considered, including the seriousness of the condition, the effectiveness of intervention in altering it, the feasibility of including the intervention in the planned system, and the projected costs. Other factors considered were the prevalence of the condition in the Kaiser-Permanente MHTS population (see Chapter Seventeen, Table 17-6), its suitability for management by physician-paramedical personnel teams using protocols, and the acceptability of the intervention to the patients and to the providers of care. The following ten conditions were selected: arthritis, backache, diabetes, gastrointestinal diseases, hyperlipidemia, hypertension, overweight, psychosomatic problems, smoking, and urinary tract disorders.

Ten preventive maintenance clinics were established to manage these selected conditions. Consideration was also given to a geriatric clinic, but it appeared that most older patients had at least one chronic condition that would be monitored in one of the ten clinics. A respiratory clinic was added at a later date to provide preventive maintenance services to patients with bronchial asthma and chronic obstructive pulmonary disease. The gastrointestinal clinic, because of the nature of the medical problems it had to deal with, assumed more of a diagnostic than a maintenance function; its activities were therefore transferred to the Department of Medicine. The clinic was thus terminated and will not be described further. The concerned-well clinic for psychosomatic problems required more resources than were available to provide the necessary preventive mental health services. The clinic was consequently discontinued, but its concepts were implemented at the Kaiser-Permanente Medical Center in Santa Clara, which will be discussed in Chapter Thirteen.

3.   Facilities

The preventive health maintenance clinics were housed in a building separate from the Department of Medicine because of space limitations. The facility consisted of two adjacent service units and a shared waiting room. Each unit included six examining rooms and an office surrounding a work area. Patients

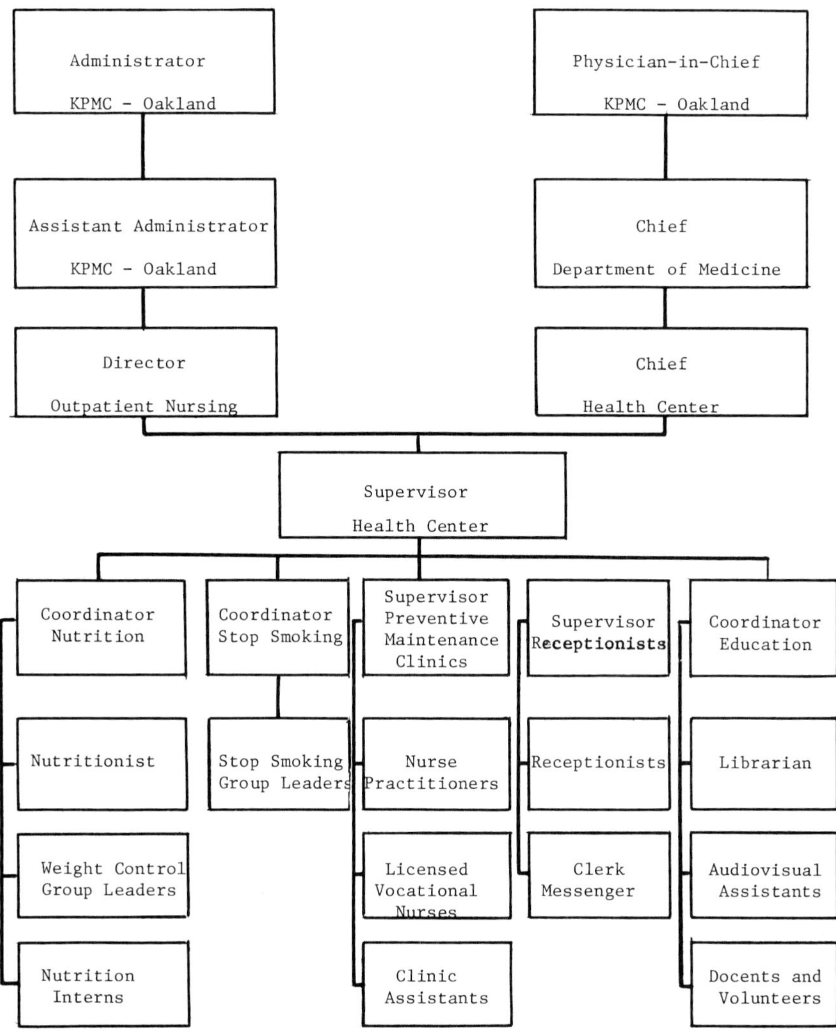

Figure 11-4. Organizational table of health care and preventive maintenance.

entered the examining rooms through a peripheral corridor, and nurse and paramedical personnel functioned within the central work area. Conceptually and operationally, it would have been beneficial to include the preventive health maintenance clinics within the geographic boundaries of the Department of Medicine, thus increasing its visibility and influence, providing easier access to physician supervision, and avoiding duplication of certain ancillary functions.

4. Personnel

At the inception of the preventive health maintenance system, it was decided to utilize registered nurses as the primary providers of care in most of the clinics. The reasons were that nurses had the appropriate background and motivation; that they were used to working with physicians; that their position within the institutional hierarchy was established; and that they were already licensed by the state to perform a variety of tasks under physician supervision. Since then, the admendment of the Nursing Practice Act in California has made it easier for registered nurses to function in an expanded role.

The criteria for the selection of nurses consisted of prior experience in an outpatient setting and an expressed interest in assuming an augmented role. No academic training was required beyond the R.N. level. Nurses were initially entered into a specially designed course, which consisted of didactic lectures, demonstrations, group practice sessions, and a supervised work period lasting nine months. They were examined at the end of the course by means of oral case presentations and discussions with the faculty, consisting of nurse educators, health educators, and physicians drawn from the Kaiser-Permanente Medical Center and the Kaiser Foundation School of Nursing in Oakland. The training program was broad in scope in order to orient the nurses to the gamut of health maintenance problems. Initially, the practical experience of each nurse was limited to two clinics to provide in-depth preparation for the assumption of responsibility of patient care in those clinics, e.g., hypertension and diabetes. In time, however, the nurses were oriented to take care of patients with other chronic conditions. Currently, most of the nurses are able to handle all health maintenance problems in the preventive maintenance clinics.

After the course was completed, requirements were established for the training and certification of nurses as nurse practitioners capable of performing complete health evaluations. (See Chapter Ten.) All nurses currently working in the preventive maintenance clinics have obtained such certification. Because of the large expenditure involved in the educational program outlined above, new nurse practitioners are now being recruited from educational institutions that offer nurse practitioner courses leading to certification. These nurses are then subjected to a relatively short period of on-the-job training before assuming their assigned roles as patient care providers.

In addition to nurse practitioners, the preventive maintenance staff comprised health educators, nutritionists, licensed vocational nurses, clinic assistants, receptionists, and clerks. Later, graduates of the stop smoking and weight control clinics were trained to assume group leadership responsibilities.

5. Preventive Maintenance Clinic Design and Operation

The design of the preventive maintenance clinics is typified by the hyperlipidemia clinic flow chart in Figure 11-5. The usual operational pattern consists of three sequential components: patient entry, management, and surveillance. Patient flow through these components is governed by decision rules. Features common to all the clinics will be reviewed now; specific details about each clinic will be given in D.10.

The clinics operate on a scheduled appointment basis, and not all are in operation every day. Figure 11-6 shows the 1975 schedule for the clinics. Nurses or group leaders are assigned to each clinic a specified number of hours per week, as seen in the schedule. Most of this time is spent in direct patient contact; some time is spent in indirect patient care, such as telephone calls, physician consultations, and documentation.

In the arthritis, diabetes, hyperlipidemia, hypertension, and special kidney clinics, the patient-provider encounters are usually on a one-to-one basis. New

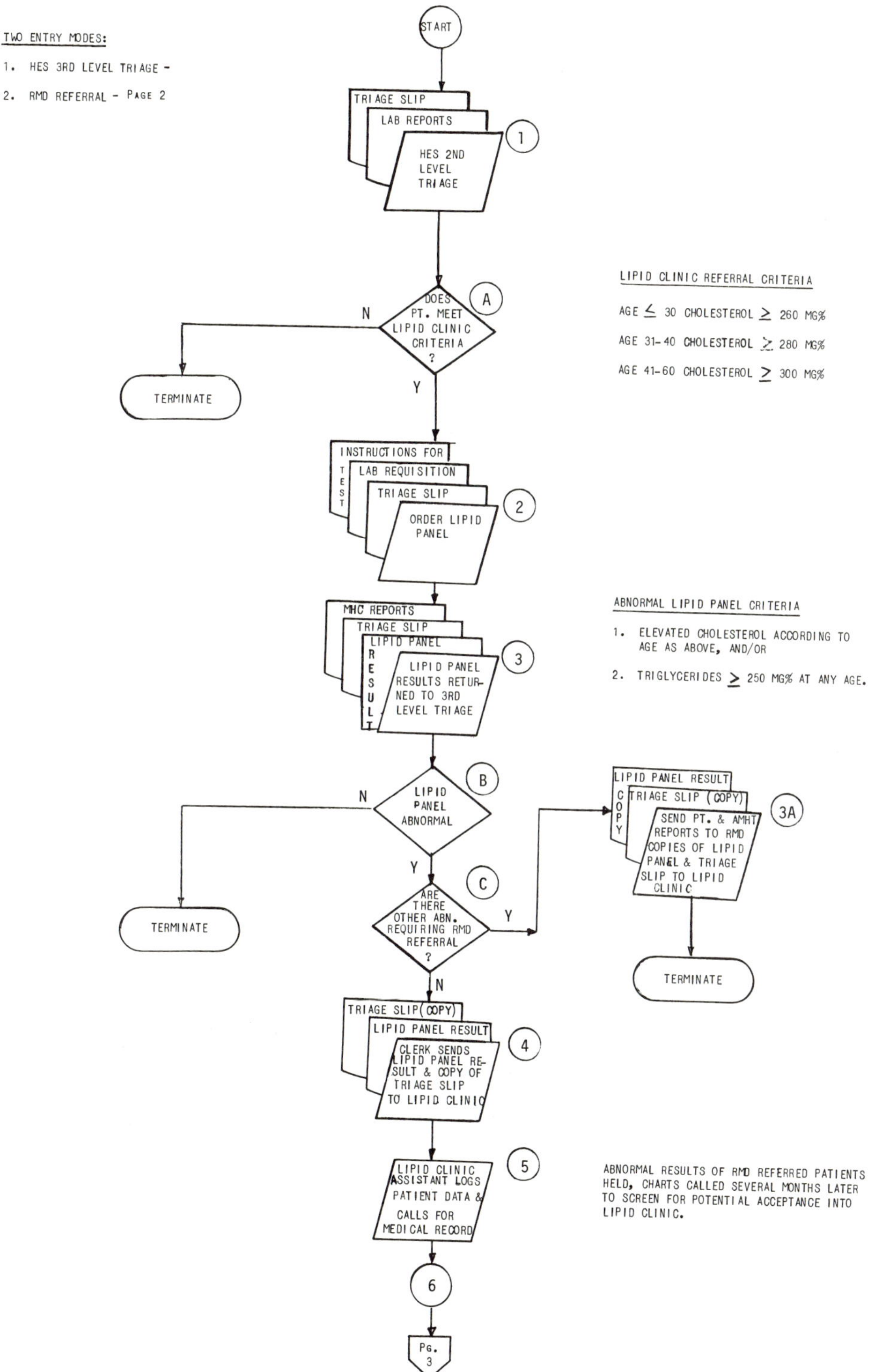

Figure 11-5a.   Hyperlipidemia clinic flow chart.

LIPID CLINIC CRITERIA
HEALTH PLAN MEMBER
M.R. LAST DIGIT 0, 1, 2, 3, 5, 6, 8
ABNORMAL LIPID PANEL RESULTS
NO ACUTE OR CHRONIC DISEASES INTERFERRING WITH TREATMENT, FOLLOW-UP, OR PROGNOSIS.
PHYSICAL EXAM IN PAST 12 MONTHS
PG. 1
2
TRIAGE SLIP
REVIEW FORM
LIPID PANEL RESULT
MEDICAL RECORD
LIPID CLINIC NURSE REVIEWS MEDICAL RECORD
6
DOES PT. MEET ALL LIPID CL. CRITERIA ?
D
N
Y
NON-ACCEPTANCE LETTER
LIPID PANEL RES.
MEDICAL RECORD
INFORM RMD, STATE REASON; FILE IN MEDICAL RECORD
6A
DOES PATIENT HAVE RMD ?
F
N
Y
ELIGIBLE FOR OTHER PMS CLINIC
E
N
Y
REQUEST FORM
LIPID PANEL RESULT
MEDICAL RECORD
REQUEST RMD APPROVAL FOR LIPID CLINIC ATTENDANCE
7
INFORM APPROPRIATE PMS CLINIC
6B
NON-ACCEPTANCE LETTER
LIPID PANEL RES.
MEDICAL RECORD
INFORM RMD THAT PT. IS NOT ELIGIBLE FOR LIPID CL., BUT IS FOR OTHER CLINIC
6C
ATTENDANCE APPROVED ?
G
N
Y
LIPID CLINIC ASSISTANT LOGS REFUSAL
7A
LETTER
CALL PATIENT TO MAKE INTAKE APPOINTMENT
8
TERMINATE
TERMINATE
INTAKE APPOINTMENT MADE ?
H
N
Y
SEND LETTER REQUESTING PATIENT TO MAKE INTAKE APPOINTMENT
8A
LIPID CL. SUM.
CHART REVIEW
MEDICAL RECORD
DIET QUEST.
DIET DIARY
FOLLOW UP AND EXAM FORMS
LIPID CLINIC
PATIENT AND SPOUSE COME FOR INTAKE VISIT
9
INTAKE APPOINTMENT MADE ?
I
Y
N
PATIENT CALLS RECEPTIONIST TO MAKE APPOINTMENT: RECEPTIONIST INFORMS CLINIC ASSISTANT WHEN APPOINTMENT MADE.
J
8N
PG. 3
PG. 3

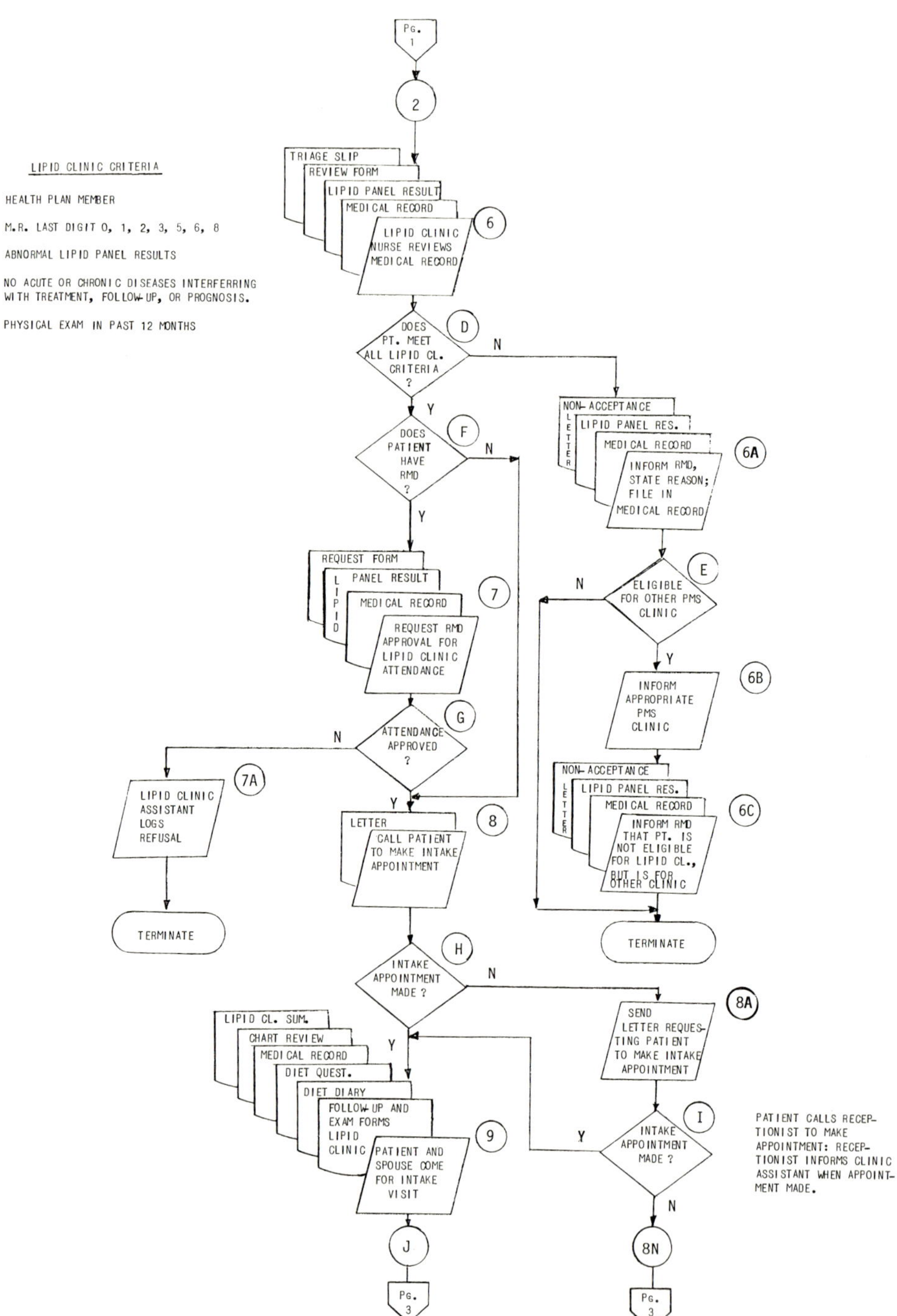

Figure 11-5b.

PG.
3

IF LIPID ABNORMALITY DUE TO
ANOTHER DISEASE, IT IS BEST
TREATED BY TREATING THE
UNDERLYING DISEASE

9

IS
THERE A
QUESTION OF
SECONDARY
ETIOLOGY
?

J

Y

N

PATIENT SCHEDULED TO
SEE LIPID CLINIC NURSE FOR RISK
FACTOR SUMMARIZATION AND RECOMMENDA-
TIONS; NURTRITIONIST FOR DIET
INSTRUCTIONS

LAB INSTRUCTIONS

REQUEST LAB
TEST TO R/O
SECONDARY
ETIOLOGY

9A

MEDICAL RECORD

FOLLOW-UP & EXAM
F
O
R
M
S

1ST FOLLOW-UP
VISIT SCHED-
ULED BY
RECEPTIONIST

10

N

SECONDARY
ETIOLOGY CON-
FIRMED ?

K

Y

NOTE TO RMD

MEDICAL RECORD

REFER PATIENT
TO RMD
FOR
FOLLOW-UP

9B

MEDICAL RECORD

DIET QUEST.

DIET DIARY

PATIENT AND
SPOUSE VISIT
WITH NUTRITION-
IST FOR DIET
INSTRUCTION

11

TERMINATION

MEDICAL RECORD

FOLLOW-UP FORM

FOLLOW-UP
VISITS AT
SCHEDULED
INTERVALS

12

PG.
3

I

MEDICAL RECORD

NOTE TO RMD

INFORM RMD
AND
LOG NO
FOLLOW-UP

8B

TERMINATE

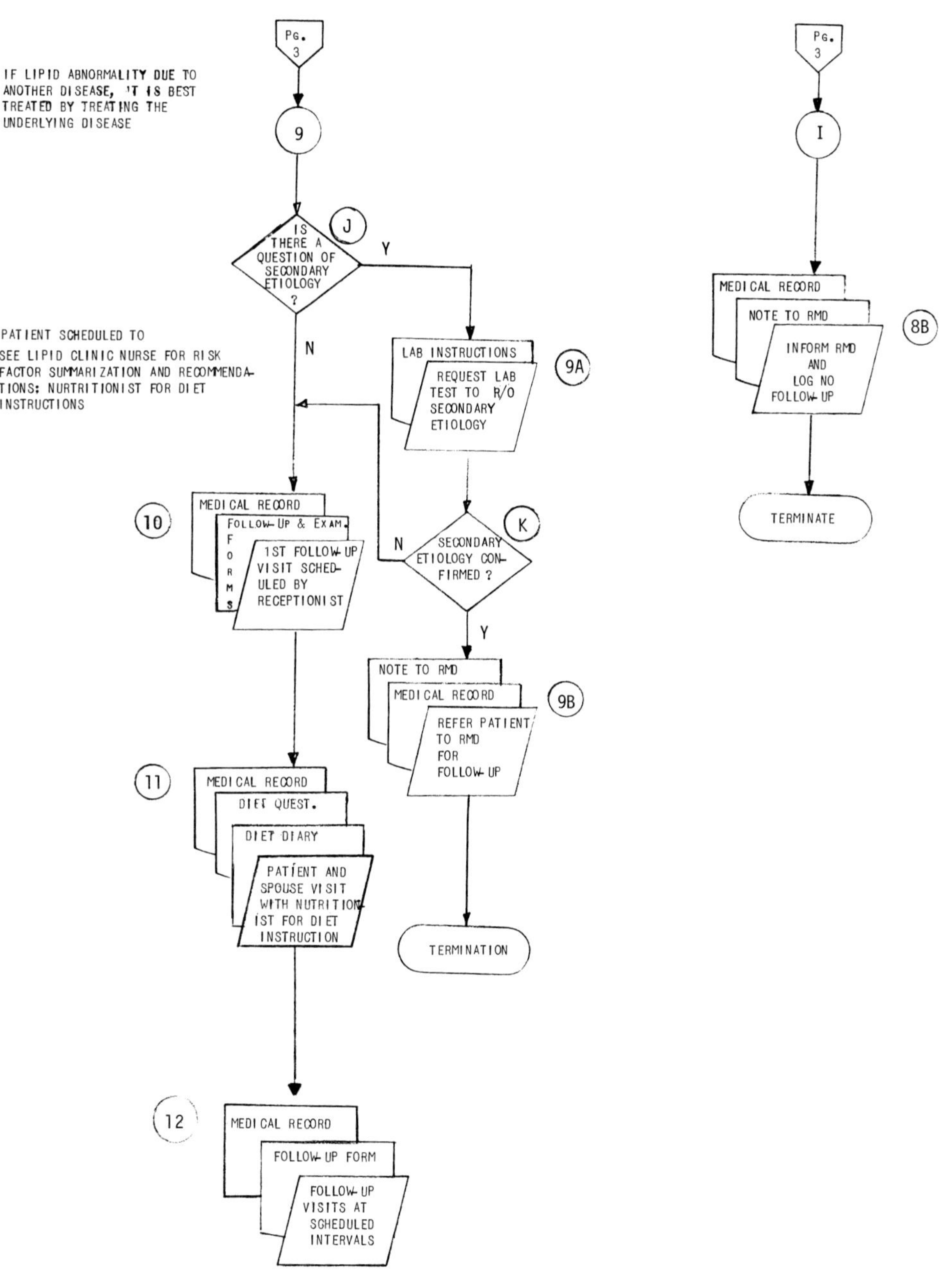

Figure 11-5c.

	MONDAY	TUESDAY	WEDNESDAY	THURSDAY	FRIDAY
A.M.	Diabetes Hyperlipidemia Hypertension Stop Smoking	Hypertension Respiratory Special Kidney	Diabetes Hypertension Stop Smoking	Arthritis Diabetes Hypertension	Arthritis Hypertension Special Kidney
P.M.	Arthritis Diabetes Respiratory Special Kidney	Diabetes Hypertension Weight Control	Back Care Hyperlipidemia Hypertension Respiratory Special Kidney	Diabetes Hypertension Respiratory Special Kidney	Diabetes Hypertension Special Kidney
EVE.	Stop Smoking Weight Control	Weight Control	Stop Smoking Weight Control	Weight Control	

Figure 11-6. Preventive maintenance clinics schedule.

patients have 30-minute appointments, and return patients have 15-minute appointments. Three of these clinics offer educational classes as part of their patient care program. The respiratory, back care, weight control, and stop smoking clinics provide an initial patient interview, followed by a series of group sessions, each lasting approximately one and one-half hour.

Each clinic is under the supervision of a physician, who has ultimate responsibility for the quality of care it renders. A physician is in attendance at each session of the clinic where individual patient care is provided. He sees all new patients, and he sees return patients at the request of the nurse practitioners. The nurses provide care according to a standard protocol, which indicates when a physician consultation is necessary. In the four group-encounter clinics, the physician is primarily a resource person and attends only one of the group sessions.

6.   Entry into the Clinics

a.   Referral sources and procedures.   Patients are usually referred to the preventive maintenance clinics from MHTS, but they may be referred from any physician or paramedical person at the Oakland Medical Center. In general, referrals are not accepted from other Kaiser-Permanente medical facilities because of the difficulty of integrating preventive services into their general health care. However, patients may refer themselves to the stop smoking and weight control clinics with no restriction as to their source of primary care, though geographic location usually acts as a natural barrier to such referrals.

Each clinic has eligibility criteria, which have been circulated to all potential referral sources within the Oakland Medical Center. These criteria take into consideration several factors such as age, attitudes, and health status. In general, patients are not eligible for referral if they have a concomitant acute or chronic disease that impairs longevity, requires frequent physician followup, or interferes with their ability to participate in a clinic program. In MHTS, the eligibility criteria have been included in the nurse practitioner triage rules, described in Chapter Ten. The flow chart in Figure 11-7 demonstrates the triage rules and priorities for referral to the preventive maintenance clinics. The priorities have been set up somewhat arbitrarily, taking into consideration the nature and seriousness of the patient's problem. Specific eligibility criteria are outlined in the description of each clinic in D.10.

Before a patient's actual entry into any of the preventive maintenance clinics, the referral criteria may require certain tests and retests. Some of these are ordered by the nurse practitioners in MHTS; for example, if a patient has an elevated serum cholesterol, a lipid panel is ordered prior to referral to the hyperlipidemia clinic. Some retests are performed in the preventive maintenance clinic itself; for example, if a patient's blood pressure (BP) is found to be elevated in MHTS, the patient is referred to the hypertension clinic for additional BP measurements; the results of these rechecks will decide whether the patient should be treated in the clinic, placed under surveillance, or discharged from the clinic. Two of the decision rule modules that govern acceptance of patients in the hypertension clinic are presented in Figures 11-8 and 11-9.

b.   Entry triage.   As shown in Figure 11-7, patients are referred from MHTS to the preventive maintenance clinics at three triage levels. At the first level, a

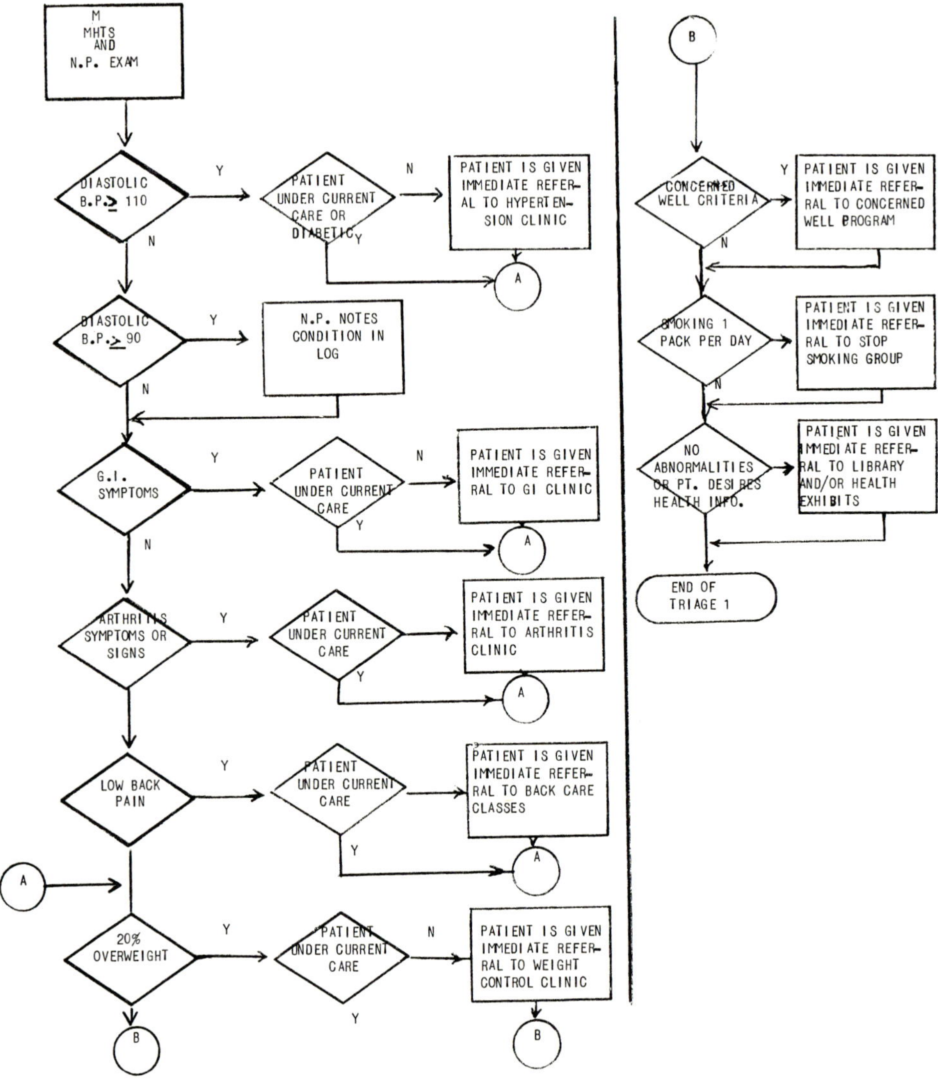

Figure 11-7a.   Triage levels and referral priorities to preventive maintenance clinics.

patient who has a distinct qualifying abnormality is referred directly to the appropriate clinic. As an example, if he is found to have elevated BP, he is asked to make an appointment in the hypertension clinic; he can do this in person at the clinic or by telephoning from home. Referrals at the second triage level are based on MHTS results that are not available online at the time of the nurse practitioner examination. An example would be the presence of significance bacteriuria, which is not reported for at least 24 hours following MHTS. No second-level decisions are made until all MHTS results are reported, usually within two weeks. Third-level triage referrals are based on repeat tests or new tests ordered on the basis of MHTS or nurse examination findings. The presence of an elevated MHTS serum cholesterol, for example, triggers a lipid panel order by the nurse practitioner

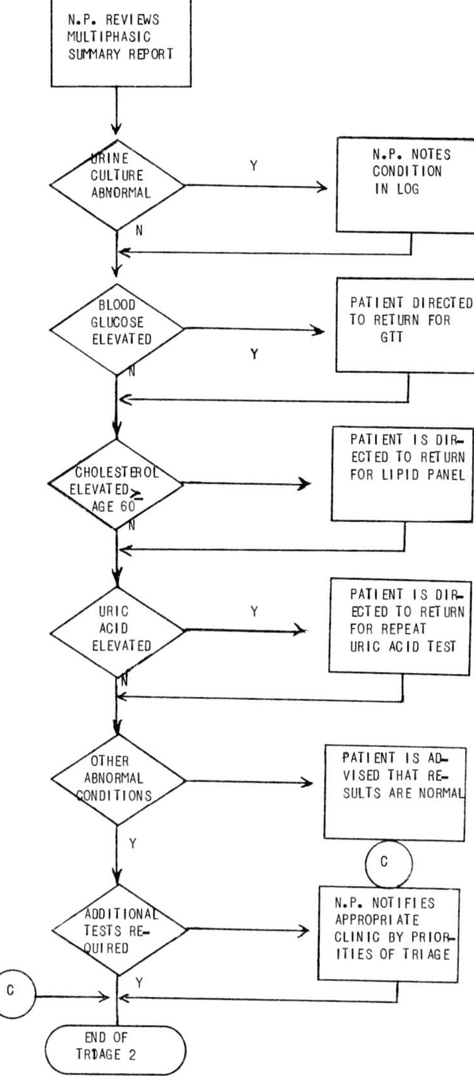

Figure 11-7b.

when she first sees the patient; at the third triage level, the lipid panel result is reviewed; if it is abnormal, the patient is sent a letter asking him to make an appointment in the hyperlipidemia clinic.

In order to keep track of all referrals and to insure that patients make their appointments and keep them, a special triage system has been set up in the preventive maintenance clinics. A designated clerk receives a copy of each triage slip, which is made out by the MHTS nurse practitioners and which specifies the level of referral (see Figure 11-10). This triage slip is logged in and, within a month following the patient's MHTS examination, the triage clerk examines the preventive maintenance clinics' appointment books to see if the patient has made his appointment. If he has not, a form letter is sent to him stressing the necessity of

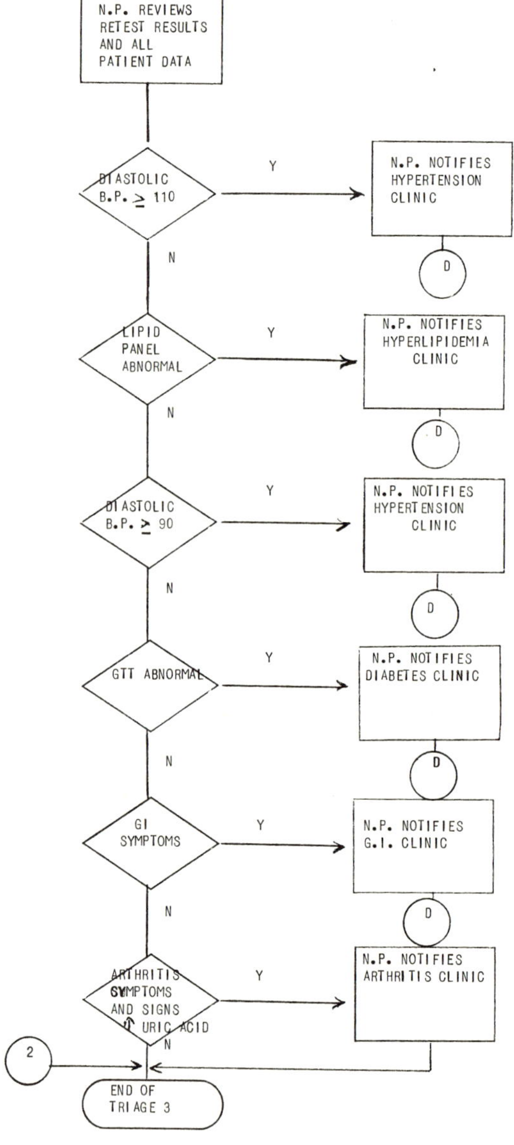

Figure 11-7c.

a followup visit. If the patient does not respond to the letter, the clerk attempts to reach him by telephone. If she is unable to reach him, or to convince him to make an appointment, she contacts the patient's physician for further disposition.

7.   Patient Care Management

a.   Intake.   This usually consists of an individual encounter with a nurse practitioner, who obtains a complete history pertaining to the patient's presenting problem, including social and psychological factors that might influence his care. She then performs a physical examination to assess the patient's health status.

BLOOD PRESSURE GROUP DETERMINATION*

	1	2	3	4	5	6	7	8	9	10	11	12	13	14	15
Sex	—	—	—	F	F	F	F	F	F	M	M	M	M	M	
Age	<20	<20	<20	20–39	20–39	20–39	≥40	≥40	≥40	20–59	20–59	20–59	≥60	≥60	≥60
Blood pressure (BP)†	<85	85–119	≥120	<90	90–124	≥125	<95	95–129	≥130	<90	90–124	≥125	<95	95–129	≥130
BP group 0	X			X			X			X			X		
BP group I		X			X			X			X			X	
BP group II			X			X			X			X			X

*For ease of tabulation, patients have been classified in three severity groups based on sex, age, and blood pressure level:

Group 0 = normal diastolic BP.
Group I = mild to moderate diastolic BP elevation.
Group II = severe diastolic BP elevation.

†BP = Casual sitting diastolic blood pressure.

Figure 11-8. Blood pressure group determination.

	1	2	3	4	5
Known hypertensive?	N	N	N	Y	—
BP Group (MHC* or RMD† referral)	0	0	1–2	—	—
BP Group (first BP)	0	1	0–1	0–1	2
Terminated from clinic	X				
Return for second BP in one week		X	X		
Do orientation		X	X	X	
Return for intake in 2–4 weeks				X	
Order intake lab tests				X	
Continue same medication if under Rx				X	
Consult with RMD or SMD§					X

*MHC = Multiphasic health testing.
†RMD = Regular physician.
§Hypertension clinic supervising physician.

Figure 11-9.   First blood pressure decision module.

The type and extent of examination vary from clinic to clinic. The nurse orders appropriate tests to complete the health assessment. During the intake she gives the patient preliminary information about his health problem and the clinic's role in its management; she answers his questions and refers him to audiovisual materials that pertain to his care.

In the stop smoking and weight control clinics, the intake is conducted by trained lay personnel and does not involve health assessment. In the hyperlipidemia clinic the intake visit is a group instruction session; health assessment is performed at the second visit.

b.   Process of care.   This is a team approach involving the patient, the nurse practitioner, and the consulting physician. Once the health assessment is completed, the nurse discusses her findings with the physician consultant, and a mutually acceptable management plan is initiated that is based on a special protocol for each clinic. The physician does not necessarily see the patient at the time of the health status evaluation unless the nurse practitioner has some questions about unusual findings or symptoms. After the physician consultant-nurse practitioner interaction the nurse reviews the management plan with the patient, outlines the reasons for the therapeutic choice, describes the side effects of medications if any are prescribed, and discusses with the patient their mutual expectations from the clinic.

Many of the patients under care in the preventive maintenance clinics have a regular physician in the Department of Medicine whom they consult for any medical problem they may have. Before a patient is accepted in a preventive maintenance clinic, his regular physician's permission is obtained. During the process of care in the clinic the nurse practitioner may contact the patient's

HEALTH EVAULATION SECTION KPMC-TRIAGE & REFERRAL

☐ REGULAR
☐ BY REQUEST   DR. ______________________   NP______________________
☐ ASSIGNED
PATIENT'S ADDRESS   MD SUPV. ______________

MCDS ☐   MHC ☐

HOME PHONE ______________________   WORK PHONE ______________________

| FIRST LEVEL TRIAGE | SECOND LEVEL TRIAGE   DATE | THIRD LEVEL TRIAGE |

FIRST LEVEL TRIAGE

MEDICAL ______________________
SPECIALTY ______________________
____

1) HYPERTENSION ______________________
2) G.I. ☐
3) ARTHRITIS ☐
BACK CARE ☐
CONCERNED WELL ☐
HEALTH COUNSELOR ______________________
LIBRARY ______________________
STOP SMOKING ☐
TEENAGE ☐
WT. CONTROL ☐
OTHER ______________________
PAP DONE ______________________
COMMENTS:

09093 (1-72)
G61-1-72

SECOND LEVEL TRIAGE   DATE

REFER: NO REFER
MEDICINE______ WKS   MEDICINE
SPECIALTY ______________________
TESTS ORDERED:

SENT LETTER #______   ______________
LETTER SENT ______   INITIAL
REF. BP ☐   PAP, ABN-A ______________
PAP WNL ☐   PAP, ABN-B ______________
ADV RULE LAB ______________________
1ST LEVEL LAB ______________________
801 LAB ______________________
RECORDS TO REFERRING MD______________

THIRD LEVEL TRIAGE

PHMC RETESTS	WNL	ABN	PHMC-REF
GTT			
URIC ACID			
LIPID PANEL			
RENAL			

REF. HYPERTENSION ☐
OTHER RETESTS   WNL ☐   ABN ☐
LETTER # ______   SENT ______________
LAB TO RMD ______   PHMC ______________
LAB FOLLOW-UP ______________
RMD NOTIF. ______   PHMC NOTIF. ______
FILED ______

PHMC = PREVENTATIVE HEALTH MAINTENANCE CL.
RMD = REFERRING PHYSICIAN

HES 1271-19

Figure 11-10.   Health evaluation section triage and referral form.

physician for a variety of reasons: the patient may have symptoms unrelated to the health problem under management in the clinic; the patient may not be following her instructions; or physician contact may be required by the protocol or felt to be important by the nurse practitioner. It is also the policy of the preventive maintenance clinics to refer patients back to their physicians periodically for a general checkup. The frequency of such referrals depends on the patient's age and predetermined clinic criteria; it may vary from once a year to every four years.

Patients who are under care in the preventive maintenance clinics may at times require consultation in departments other than the Department of Medicine; the nurse has the prerogative to refer such patients to the appropriate department, either on her own or in consultation with the preventive maintenance clinic physician consultant.

 c. Patient management protocols.   The nurse practitioners use a specific protocol to manage patients in each preventive maintenance clinic. The protocols developed by the physician consultant for each clinic with advice from members of the Department of Medicine, represent generally accepted patient care strategies. The protocols are in the form of sequential guidelines, with provisions for physician input at certain decision levels. The following is an excerpt from the arthritis clinic protocol:

 BACK PAIN: Low Back Pain Syndrome

  I. *Differentiation*
   A. If pain is located in lower back and buttocks, and
   B. There is paraspinal muscle spasm or tenderness to palpation over the
    affected level, and
   C. Straight leg raising test is positive, then
   Probable diagnosis is low back pain.

II. *Workup*

Test to order:	*Expected results:*
X-ray of lumbo-sacral spine if none done within last year, unless patient is in acute distress.	Any of the following findings: (1) normal (2) scoliosis (3) spondylolisthesis (4) spina bifida (5) decrease in intervertebral disc spaces (6) osteophyte formation

III. *Treatment*

    A. Sequence of drugs

        1. ASA gr V tabs II q 4 h prn pain; if history of GI distress or intolerance to ASA, use acetaminophen (Tylenol) gr V tabs II q 4 h prn pain.

        2. for severe pain use ASA or acetaminophen with codeine $\frac{1}{2}$ gr, tab I prn pain, no oftener than q 4 h (prescription must be in MD's handwriting).

        3. If above not adequate, use Valium 5 mg tabs, tab I tid prn in addition to the above medications.

        4. If any further medication required, consult MD.

        5. If symptoms persist beyond 10 days on analgesic therapy, consult MD regarding traction, orthopedic consult, etc.

        6. Return to clinic in 3-4 weeks as necessary.

    B. Physical therapy

        1. If pain severe, advise absolute bed rest until pain subsides.

        2. Instruct patient to apply moist or dry heat (e.g., 30 minutes with heating pad on low) 3 to 4 times per day.

        3. Instruct patient to avoid any heavy lifting until symptoms subside, to follow handout on "38 Activities to Avoid," and after pain has decreased to follow handout on exercises for low back pain.

        4. Refer patient to Back Care Clinic classes and, if appropriate, to the Health Education Center library to see back care films for reinforcement of instructions on rest and exercise.

A format as shown above appears to be more suitable for use by well-trained nurse practitioners than the more constraining decision rules referred to earlier (Figures 11-8 and 11-9). The protocols are helpful not only in insuring optimal patient management, but also in auditing nurse performance and monitoring utilization of services and costs.

d. Patient education. As mentioned above, patient education is an integral part of patient management in the preventive maintenance clinics. In the stop smoking, weight control, and respiratory clinics, patient education is the key management process. The educational program in each clinic will be detailed in D.10. A more general discussion of patient education is provided in Chapter Twelve.

e. Patient surveillance

(1) *Followup procedures.* Patients are monitored continuously in the preventive maintenance clinics until such time as they leave the health plan, are discharged from care in the clinics, choose to see a physician instead, or are referred to a physician. Each clinic has its own followup system, which is part of the patient management protocol and defines the frequency of visits and the condi-

tions under which visits are to be made. The protocol also indicates the tests and procedures the patient has to undergo at specified intervals. Whenever a patient does not show up for an appointment, or cancels it, he is reminded by mail to return for another visit; he may be contacted by telephone if the situation warrants.

(2) *Surveillance protocols.* Certain patients who are referred to the preventive maintenance clinics do not immediately qualify for intake but have a borderline abnormality that has to be kept under surveillance, such as a labile BP. These patients are not discharged from the clinics but are advised to return at periodic intervals for reevaluation. The decision table in Figure 11-11 outlines the surveillance system for labile hypertensive patients.

8. Quality Control

Quality control is closely monitored in the preventive maintenance clinics through several mechanisms.

a. Management protocols. The protocol for each clinic is written by the physician consultant to that clinic, with advice from members of the Department of Medicine. It reflects the state of the art—the highest quality—in the management of a particular disease or condition. It is updated frequently to incorporate the most current therapeutic modalities.

b. Physician-nurse practitioner interaction. Such interaction takes place constantly, either because of the requirements of the protocols or because of doubts in the nurse practitioners' minds about certain symptoms, signs, or other aspects of patient care that they observe. The nurses tend to err on the side of cautiousness, thus enhancing the quality of care they provide.

c. Peer review. This ongoing process is performed by the preventive maintenance clinics' staff on a monthly rotation basis. The peer review group consists of one nurse coordinator, one physician, and two nurse practitioners, who meet once a week to review five medical records. The records are examined for completeness and for adherence to protocols and to standards of care. The review findings are discussed with the nurse practitioners at their bimonthly meetings and are also brought to the attention of the Chief of the Department of Medicine and the Quality of Care Committee at the Oakland Medical Center.

d. In-service education. A formal in-service education program for nurse practitioners is provided through bimonthly meetings conducted by the nurses or by invited consultants. The discussion topics are based on expressed nurse practitioner needs and on the recommendations of the peer review committee, the objective being positive reinforcement of nursing skills to improve performance quality.

e. No-show and cancellation followup. This has been alluded to earlier and aims at maintaining continuity of care, an important ingredient of quality.

9. Data Collection and Processing

Forms have been designed to simplify the organization, communication, and storage of clinic information. Physical measurements, symptoms, nurse examina-

	1	2	3	4	5	6	7	8	9	10	11	12	13	14	15
BP group (first reading*)	0	0	0	0	0	0	0	0	1	1	1	1	1	2	—
BP group (second reading*)	0	0	0	0	1	1	1	1	0	0	0	0	1	—	2
Type of visit (code†)	10	11	12	13	10	11	12	13	10	11	12	13	—	—	—
Return for observation in	12 mo.	12 mo.	12 mo.	12 mo.		6 mo.				6 mo.					
Go to Module 4 (portometer availability)					X		X	X	X		X	X			
Return for intake in 2–4 weeks													X		
Order intake lab tests													X		
Consult with SMD														X	X

*During each observation visit two BP readings are obtained 30 minutes apart.
†For ease of tabulation, codes are used for type of visit:

10 = first six-month observation visit.
11 = six months off birth control (BC) pills observation visit.
12 = second six-month observation visit.
13 = 12-month observation visit.

Figure 11-11. Blood pressure observation visits.

tion findings, laboratory results, diagnoses, prescribed treatments, and telephone messages are recorded with respect to time, so that progress and response to therapy can be more clearly ascertained. Four or more visits can be recorded on a single form. Coded notations describe the progression of symptoms and diagnoses; for example, N = new occurrence, I = improved from last visit.

Initially, separate forms were used for each clinic. As time went on and the nurses were able to take care of patients with multiple disease problems, it became necessary to create a single form, which appears in Figure 11-12. The back of this form is used for patient identification and comments. However, intake data are still documented on a form that is specific for each clinic. Figure 11-13 shows the two sides of the intake form of the diabetes clinic.

All forms are entered into the patient's permanent medical record, which is identified by the patient's unique medical number and is available from a centralized chart room whenever the patient makes a visit to the outpatient clinic or is hospitalized at the Oakland Medical Center.

10.   Description of Component Clinics

a.   Preventive maintenance arthritis clinic

(1) *Objectives.* To provide diagnostic, therapeutic, and monitoring services to patients with arthritis or musculoskeletal disorders.

(2) *Referral criteria.* MHTS rererrals are based on the following criteria, as judged by nurse practitioners or physicians: (a) presence of joint, neck, or back symptoms (stiffness, pain, swelling); (b) significant musculoskeletal abnormalities on physical examination: tenderness about a joint, inflammation about a joint (heat, redness, swelling), significant noninflammatory joint changes, pelvic tilt of one-half inch or more, physical abnormality at base of the spine (hair tuft, color spot, or dimple) associated with a history of back pain; (c) the following diagnoses: arthritis, any type; musculoskeletal syndromes; osteoporosis.

(3) *Clinic operation.* (a) *Intake visit.* The nurse interviews the patient regarding his symptoms, performs an appropriate musculoskeletal examination, and explains the purpose and function of the arthritis clinic. She discusses her findings with the physician consultant, who sees the patient and establishes a working diagnosis. The nurse proceeds to order protocol-indicated laboratory or x-ray studies, initiates treatment, including articular injections, and institutes followup. She explains to the patient the nature of his problem and the rationale for treatment, answering questions and allaying anxiety in the process. Figure 11-14 shows a nurse practitioner injecting a knee joint.

(b) *Followup visit.* At this visit, the nurse reviews the patient's symptoms and physical status and the results of diagnostic studies. If the patient is responding to the therapeutic regimen, the nurse arranges further treatment and followup per protocol. If new diagnostic or patient care problems are evident, she discusses them with the physician consultant and takes action accordingly.

b.   Preventive maintenance back care clinic

(1) *Objectives.* To instruct patients suffering from chronic or recurrent back symptoms regarding good posture, proper back care, and supportive exercises.

(2) *Referral criteria.* Referrals from MHTS are accepted for patients with (a) diagnosis of low backache of any etiology, except when associated with systemic

	N - NEW I - IMPROVED W - WORSE	ADD CONT. D/C	WNL ABN △- CHANGE	✓ - LAB ORDERED X - PT. EDUCATION A - ASSESSMENT
	DATE			
	TIME			
	CLINIC			
S X				
C L I N I C A L	WEIGHT			
	PULSE			
	B.P. SITTING - L.C. - S.C.			
	STANDING			
	STANDING p̄ EXERCISE			
	FOOT EXAM			
L A B	CHOLESTEROL - PHENOTYPE			
	TRIGLYCERIDES			
	K+			
	URIC ACID			
	GLUCOSE - FASTING			
	2 HR. P.C.			
	RANDOM			
U R I N E	CLINIC - GLUCOSE			
	ACETONE			
	PROTEIN			
	HOME-METHOD			
	RELIABILITY			
	AVG. FASTING VALUE			
	AVG. P.C. VALUE			
P T. E D.	DIET			
	DISEASE PROCESS			
	FOOT CARE			
	MEDS			
	TENSION/STRESS			
	URINE TESTING			
A				
D I M E D S				
D I S P.	REFER			
	RETURN			
	M.N.P.			
	M.D.			

06161 (4-76)

Figure 11-12. Preventive maintenance flow record.

338

KAISER-PERMANENTE MEDICAL CENTER, OAKLAND
PREVENTIVE MAINTENANCE DIABETES CLINIC

Intake Data

1. Referred by: a) HES ☐ b) GMC ☐
    c) HES Regular ☐ d) RMD ☐ _______________________   BP ___/____________________

2. Age: __________ Education _______________________   Height _________ inches
                                                           Weight _________ lbs.
3. Occupation: _____________________________________   Visual Acuity Right ______/______
                                                           Visual Acuity Left ______/______
4. Highest weight ______ lbs. at age: ______________   Urine Clinitest ______________
                                                           Urine Protein ________________
5. Least adult weight ______ lbs. at age: __________   Urine Acetest ________________

6. Family history diabetes: ____

7. Personal history: ____
    ____

8. Year of onset: _________________________ Age at onset: _____________________________

9. Type of onset: ____

10. Hospitalizations for diabetes: ____
    ____

11. Episodes of acidosis: ____
    ____

12. Episodes of hypoglycemia: ____
    ____

13. Presence of:

                        No   Yes   Details

    A. Retinopathy   ☐   ☐   ____

    B. Nephropathy   ☐   ☐   ____

    C. Neuropathy   ☐   ☐   ____

    D. Perif. Vasc. Dis. ☐   ☐   ____

    E. ASHD   ☐   ☐   ____

    F. Cereb. As   ☐   ☐   ____

14. History of treatment: ____
    ____
    ____
    ____

Figure 11-13a. Diabetes clinic intake form.

Diabetes Clinic Intake Data

Page 2 of 2

Name: _________________________________

MR#: _________________________________

15. Recent blood sugars:GTT

	Blood	Urine
Fasting		
1 hr.		
2 hr.		
3 hr.		

16. Other major diseases: ☐Hypertension   ☐Obesity   ☐Hyperlipidemia, Type_______

____

____

____

17. Other significant medicines: ____

____

18. Notes: ____

____

____

INITIAL TREATMENT PLAN

19. Medication: ____

____

20. A.   Diet: _________________   Cal.: _________________   Feedings: _________ Reduction ☐

    B.   Refer nutritionist ☐   C.   Refer A/V Library: ☐

21. Urine Testing: Type: _________________   Sig: _________________

22. Routine followup with regular physician: _________________________________

23. Routine checkups: When: _________________NR with RMD   MHC/MD   HES/MNP

24. Return to DMC _______weeks. Tests ordered: _________________________________

25. Notes: ____

____

____

____

____

Signed: _________________R. N.   _________________, M.D.   _________________
        Medical Nurse Practitioner   Physician Consultant   Date

Figure 11-13b.

disease such as malignancy or the results of an industrial injury, or (b) a significant postural abnormality.

(3) *Clinic operation.* Patients are scheduled in groups of six to eight to attend one or more one-hour instruction sessions. At the first session the clinic assistant shows parts of a videotape series on back care. She proceeds with instructions on the use of heat, good body mechanics, good posture, and the use of medications if prescribed by the patient's physician. She then demonstrates a primary set of exercises and assists the patients with them. (See Figure 11-15.)

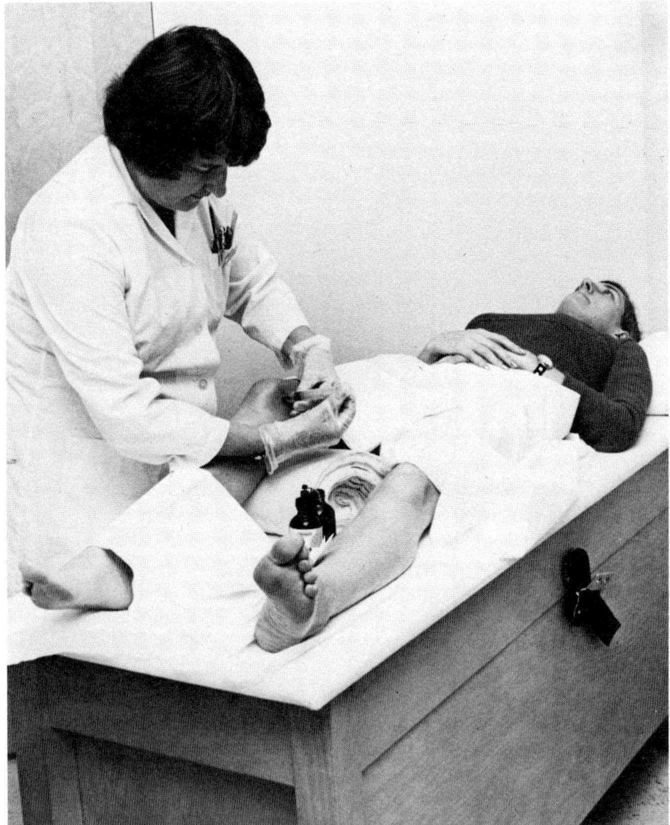

Figure 11-14.   Nurse practitioner injecting a knee joint.

At the end of the first session the patients are given an instruction sheet and encouraged to practice the exercises at home. They are asked to return in one week, at which time the number of primary exercises is increased according to tolerance. Exercise tolerance is determined by the clinic assistant, by the patient, or by direct instructions from the physician.

If the primary exercises are well tolerated, the assistant demonstrates and assists the patients with the secondary set of exercises. The patients are then asked to return every three or four weeks until they have mastered the primary and secondary sets of exercises.

Once a week the physician consultant conducts a discussion group on back care, reinforcing the information on the videotapes and the instructions of the clinic assistant. He also answers any specific questions the patients may have.

c.   Preventive maintenance diabetes clinic

(1) *Objectives.* The clinic's objectives are (a) to control the physiological aspects of diabetes and to prevent ketosis and other complications, (b) to provide knowledge and emotional support to the patient in accepting his disease and cooperating in its management.

(2) *Referral criteria.* MHTS referrals are accepted if they satisfy the following criteria:

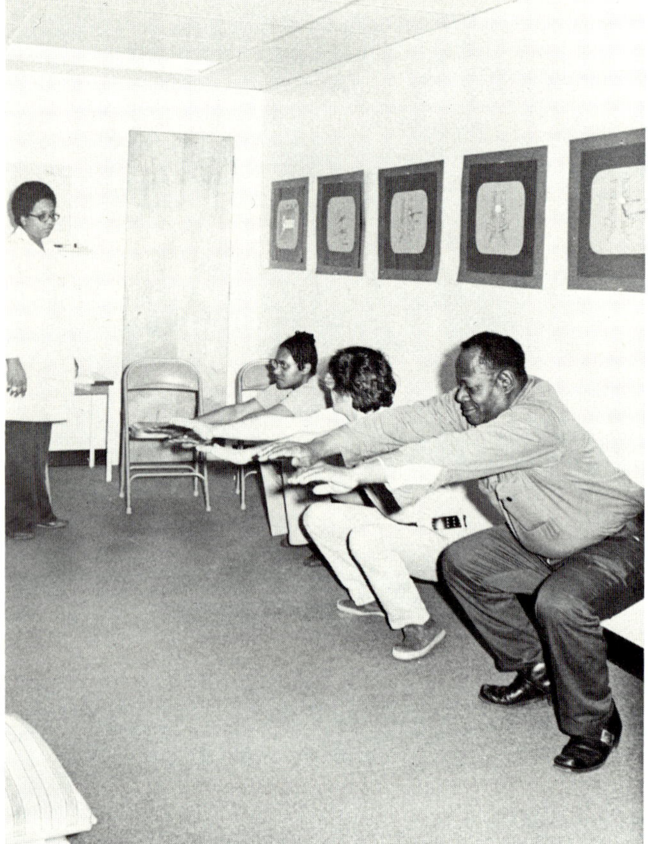

Figure 11-15. Clinic assistant demonstrating back care exercises.

(a) The diagnosis of diabetes mellitus has been established by either (i) or (ii) below:

(i) An abnormal glucose tolerance test by the criteria of Fajans and Conn (adjusted to serum values):

Fasting	$\geq$ 125 mg%
One hour	$\geq$ 185 mg%
Two hours	$\geq$ 140 mg%

Both one- and two-hour values must be at or above these levels.

(ii) Any one of the following "decompensation" criteria of O'Sullivan and Mahan:

(*a*) Fasting blood glucose level $\geq$ 140 mg%, *or*

(*b*) Postprandial blood glucose level $\geq$ 205 mg% (defined as a value within five hours of an unspecified meal), *or*

(*c*) Postprandial blood glucose level $\geq$ 340 mg% (defined as a value within three hours of ingestion of 100 gm. of glucose).

(*3*) *Clinic operation.* (a) *Intake visit.* At the first visit, the clinic assistant measures the patient's height and weight. She tests his urine for sugar and for protein; if the urine shows 3+ to 4+ sugar, she tests the urine for acetone also.

If the patient is a new diabetic, the clinic assistant teaches him how to test his urine for sugar. If he is on insulin, she teaches him how to test for acetone also. She then gives the patient an intake questionnaire to complete.

The nurse practitioner then sees the patient, explains her role in his care, and describes the clinic procedures. She tells him what to expect in terms of educational assessment, instruction, nutritionist input, and other services. She reviews the intake questionnaire and patient's medical record. She performs a limited physical assessment including fundoscopy, blood pressure measurement, and examination of the feet. On the basis of her findings she sets up an initial treatment program and interprets it to the patient.

To the patient with newly diagnosed diabetes, she gives a very brief review of the disease to allay his anxiety and obtain his cooperation in the treatment process. She gives him instructions regarding the care of the feet. If the patient is to be started on insulin, the nurse teaches him the basic steps and arranges further visits for additional teaching. If the patient is already on insulin, the nurse may either review the technique or defer to future visits as indicated. She then orders any necessary laboratory tests and refers him for a nutritionist appointment and a return appointment according to the clinic protocol.

After the patient's visit the nurse presents her findings to the physician consultant and discusses further management plans. If circumstances warrant, she may do so while the patient is in the clinic. (See Figure 11-16.)

(b) *Educational assessment and planning.* An educational assessment appointment with the nutritionist is made between the intake visit and the first followup visit. The nutritionist identifies each patient's needs and chooses an educational program to fit them. The program may consist of a scheduled group session or an individualized educational intervention including audiovisual materials, programmed instruction, printed materials, and books. She then outlines a basic nutrition and diet plan to the patient, gives him appropriate written materials, and refers him for future nutrition appointments as indicated.

(c) *Followup visits.* At each followup visit the clinic assistant checks the patient's weight, his blood pressure, and his urine for glucose and protein, and for acetone if indicated; she then gives him a symptom questionnaire to complete. The nurse practitioner reviews the questionnaire, the home urine sugar test results, and any laboratory data obtained since the previous visit. She examines the patient's feet and legs, with specific attention to athlete's foot, infection, ingrown toenails, ulcers, corns, lack of pulses or vibration sense, and signs of venous or arterial insufficiency. She then discusses with the patient his diet prescription, his home urine testing schedule, his medications, and future visits. Each patient is usually seen monthly in the first three months, then as often as necessary, but at least every six months.

(d) *Diabetes classes.* All patients enrolled in the diabetes clinic are referred to a two-hour diabetes class. Spouses are encouraged to attend.

During the first hour of the class a nutritionist briefly describes the nature of diabetes and the role of diet in its management. During the second hour a nurse practitioner discusses the medical implications of diabetes and the use of insulin and oral hypoglycemic agents.

The objectives of the classes are as follows:

(i) To provide the patient with basic information regarding the nature of diabetes and its complications.

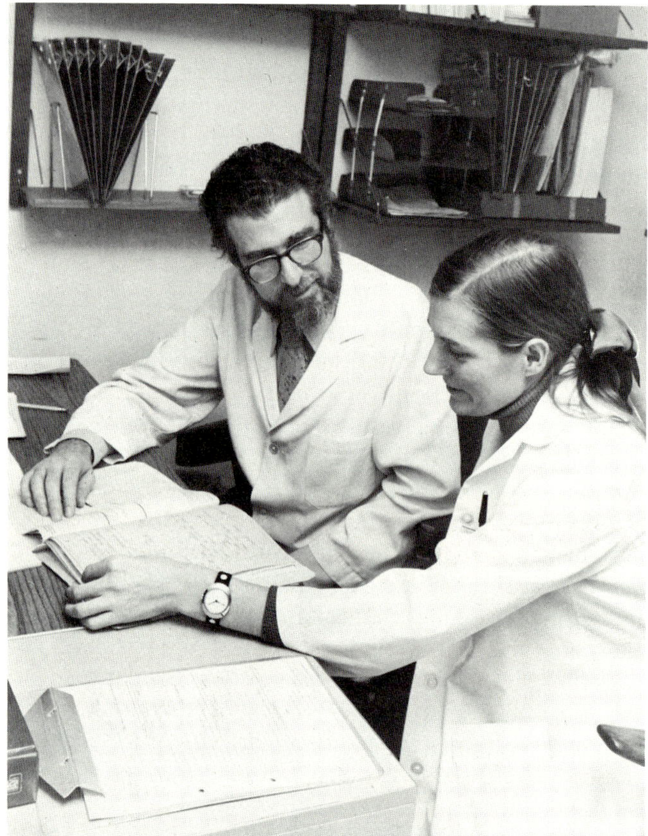

Figure 11-16.   Nurse practitioner discussing findings with physician consultant.

(ii) To instruct the patient in the methods and procedures used in the management of diabetes.

(iii) To alert the patient to the importance of good disease control in the prevention of acute and chronic complications.

(iv) To help the patient understand the relationship of diet and exercise to diabetes control, and to assist him in adopting eating patterns that will lead to optimum control of his disease.

(v) To teach the patient basic hygienic techniques for skin, foot, and dental care.

These educational objectives are further stressed during all followup visits to the diabetes clinic.

d.   Preventive maintenance hyperlipidemia clinic

(1) *Objectives.* The clinic's objectives are (a) to confirm the diagnosis and establish the type of hyperlipoproteinemia, distinguishing between primary and secondary hyperlipoproteinemia, and (b) to attempt normalization of serum lipoprotein levels and modify other risk factors predisposing to cardiovascular disease.

(2) *Referral criteria.* To qualify for referral from MHTS, patients should fulfill the following criteria:

(a) Age $\leq$ 30 years with cholesterol $\geq$ 240 mg%.
    Age 31–40 years with cholesterol $\geq$ 260 mg%.
    Age 41–60 years with cholesterol $\geq$ 280 mg%.
    Age 61–70 years with cholesterol $\geq$ 350 mg%.
or
(b) Age $\leq$ 40 years with triglycerides $\geq$ 175 mg%.
    Age 41–60 years with triglycerides $\geq$ 200 mg%.
    Age 61–70 years with triglycerides $\geq$ 250 mg%.

(c) After age 70, regardless of cholesterol or triglyceride elevation, patients will not qualify for the hyperlipidemia clinic.

(3) *Clinic operation.* (a) *Intake visit.* This is a group session, led by a trained vocational nurse, for five patients and their families. The purpose is to explain to them the nature of hyperlipidemia, to discuss aspects of the preventive approach to cardiovascular disease, to orient them to the clinic's program, and to describe followup plans (see Figure 11-17). A three-day food record and a diet questionnaire are given to each patient to be completed before his visit with the nutritionist.

(b) *First followup visit.* At this visit a cardiovascular examination is performed by the nurse practitioner and reviewed by the physician consultant. On the basis of all available information (interview, laboratory data, physical examination, and chart review) a comprehensive individualized program of risk factor modification is developed for each patient. This consists of specific treatment for:

(i) Hyperlipoproteinemia. A modified fat, low cholesterol diet is prescribed for Type II disease, or a modified fat, low carbohydrate diet for Type IV disease. The diet is supplemented later by drug therapy if deemed necessary.

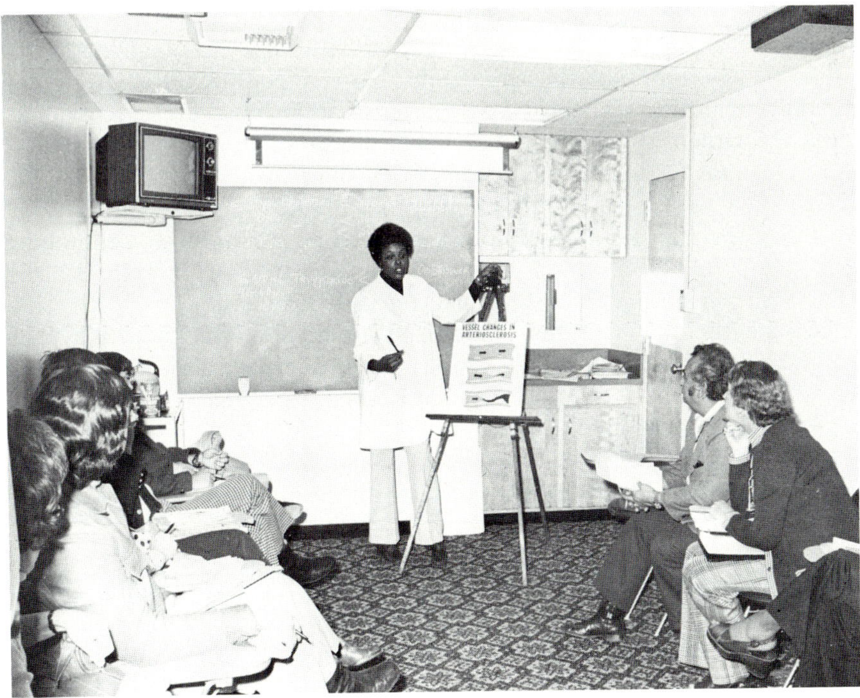

Figure 11-17. Hyperlipidemia class.

(ii) Obesity. A reducing diet is prescribed at one of four caloric levels and, optionally, the patient is referred to the weight control clinic.

(iii) Hypertension. A treatment program is instituted similar to the one used in the hypertension clinic.

(iv) Physical inactivity. A defined program of sports or exercise is recommended, geared to individual preference but adjusted to a specific caloric expenditure level.

(v) Cigarette smoking. Referral is made to the stop smoking clinic.

(c) *Nutritionist visit*. The nutritionist reviews the three-day food record and the diet questionnaire and supplements them with a detailed nutritional history. She then prescribes a diet according to the type of hyperlipoproteinemia present. She hands out appropriate printed dietary instructions and recipes and asks the patient to return for further nutrition counseling as needed.

(d) *Subsequent followup visits*. Three or four followup visits per year are planned for each patient to reinforce recommendations made for his risk factor reduction, to evaluate the efficacy of these recommendations, and to initiate drug therapy if indicated.

e. Preventive maintenance hypertension clinic

(1) *Objectives*. The clinic's objectives are (a) to confirm the diagnosis, establish the etiology, and grade the severity of disease in patients with suspected hypertension, and (b) to assume long-term management of patients with recently discovered, or already established, hypertension.

(2) *Referral criteria*. MHTS patients may be referred (a) for diagnosis: any patient with an initial diastolic BP level of 90 mm Hg or higher at any age; (b) for followup: any patient with sustained BP elevation as defined in (a), or previously diagnosed hypertension of any duration, on or off treatment.

(3) *Clinic operation*. (a) *Patient evaluation*. (i) *Confirmation of hypertension*. (*a*) Baseline blood pressure measurements. Three blood pressure determinations are used in confirming a diagnosis of hypertension: the blood pressure reading that initiated the patient's referral to the hypertension clinic and two casual blood pressure readings taken in the clinic one week apart. At the first baseline visit the clinic assistant sees eight to ten patients in a group, orients them to the clinic plans, measures their blood pressure, and schedules them for a second baseline visit in one week (see Figure 11-18). Known hypertensives skip the second baseline visit and instead are scheduled for an intake visit.

Before the second visit, the clinic assistant reviews the patient's chart to ascertain the results of laboratory work done in the past in order to determine which additional tests need to be ordered and to get the most current blood pressure reading.

At the second baseline visit, the clinic assistant, following a protocol based on blood pressure level and presence or absence of cardiovascular complications (see Figure 11-19), takes one or more of the following actions: (*1*) Instructs the patient to return in six to 12 months for further blood pressure evaluation, (*2*) refers the patient for portable blood pressure determinations, as described below, (*3*) orders laboratory work, (*4*) schedules the patient for an intake visit, (*5*) consults with the nurse practitioner or the physician or both.

The intake visit with a nurse practitioner is scheduled two to four weeks following the second baseline visit (the first baseline visit for known hypertensives).

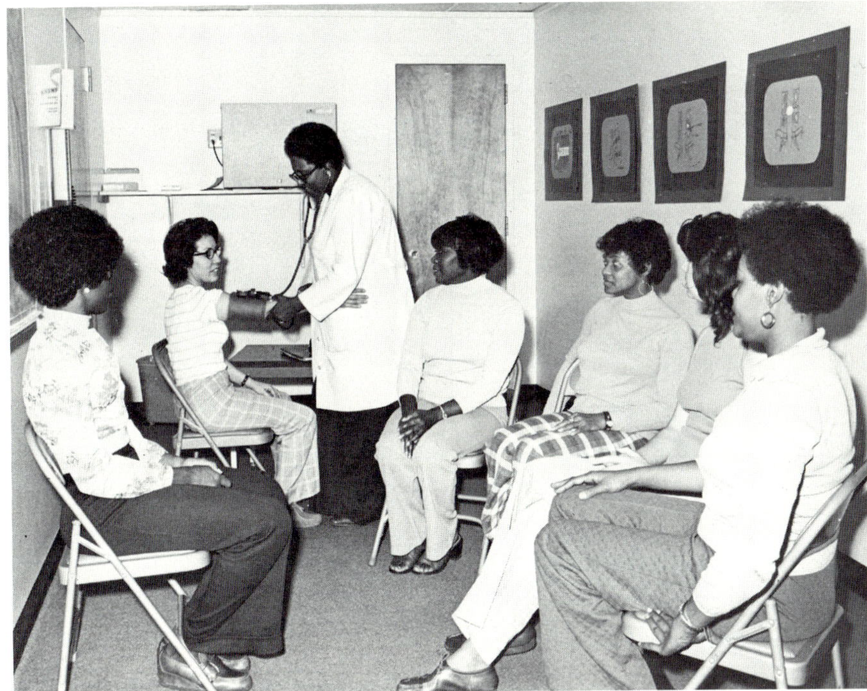

Figure 11-18.   Clinic assistant taking baseline blood pressures in a group.

(*b*) Portable blood pressure determinations (portometry). Patients whose casual blood pressure values seem inconsistent with their general clinical condition may have their home blood pressure measured with a portometer. This consists of a special blood pressure cuff connected to a portable tape recorder (see Figure 11-20). The patients wear the portometer on two successive normal working days and are asked to raise the cuff pressure above a certain level every 30 minutes, while awake. The blood pressure is recorded automatically on magnetic tape and later printed out in graph form. The multiple readings are reported to the hypertension clinic staff. If portometry is not available, manual home blood pressure measurements may be used instead.

(ii) *Diagnostic workup*. This is limited to patients with sustained hypertension only. The standard protocol calls for (*a*) cardiovascular examination by the nurse practitioner, and (*b*) a test "package" consisting of a complete blood count, urinalysis, serum sodium, potassium, creatinine and uric acid, two-hour postprandial blood glucose, chest x-ray, and electrocardiogram. Under certain circumstances, upon physician recommendation, 24-hour urinary vanillyl mandelic acid, urine culture, and intravenous urogram also are obtained.

(b) *Patient management*. (i) *Intake visit*. At this visit the nurse reviews the patient's chart, obtains a detailed history, does a complete cardiovascular examination, and records her findings. She then presents her findings to the physician consultant and suggests a management plan based on the clinic protocol.

The physician may see the patient at this point, check the nurse's findings, and briefly describe to the patient the diagnosis and treatment of hypertension. Alternately, the physician may be satisfied with the nurse's presentation, discuss the management plan with her, and allow her to proceed according to the protocol.

	1	2	3	4	5	6	7	8	9	10	11	12	13	14	15	16	17	18
On birth control (BC) pills?	—	—	Y	Y	Y	Y	Y	Y	Y	Y	Y	Y	N	N	N	N	N	—
Hypertensive prior to starting BC pills?*	—	—	N	N	N	N	N	Y	Y	Y	Y	Y	—	—	—	—	—	—
CV complications†	N	Y	N	Y	N	Y	—	N	Y	N	Y	—	N	Y	N	Y	—	—
BP group (first BP)	0	0	0	0	1–2	1–2	1–2	0	0	1–2	1–2	1–2	0	0	1–2	1–2	1–2	—
BP group (second BP)	0	0	1	1	0	0	1	1	1	0	0	1	1	1	0	0	1	2
Refer to family planning clinic; stop BC pills			X	X	X	X	X											
Return for observation (obs.)	12 mo.		6 mo.		6 mo.			6 mo.		6 mo.			6 mo.		6 mo.			
Go to module 4 (portometer availability)				X		X			X		X			X		X		
Return for intake in 2–4 weeks							X					X					X	
Order intake lab tests							X					X					X	
Consult with RMD or SMD		X																X

*It will be assumed patient was not hypertensive if he does not know.
†CV complications—cardiac enlargement by x-ray, and/or left ventricular hypertrophy by ECG, and/or serum creatinine $\geq$ 1.5 mg%

Figure 11-19. Second blood pressure decision module.

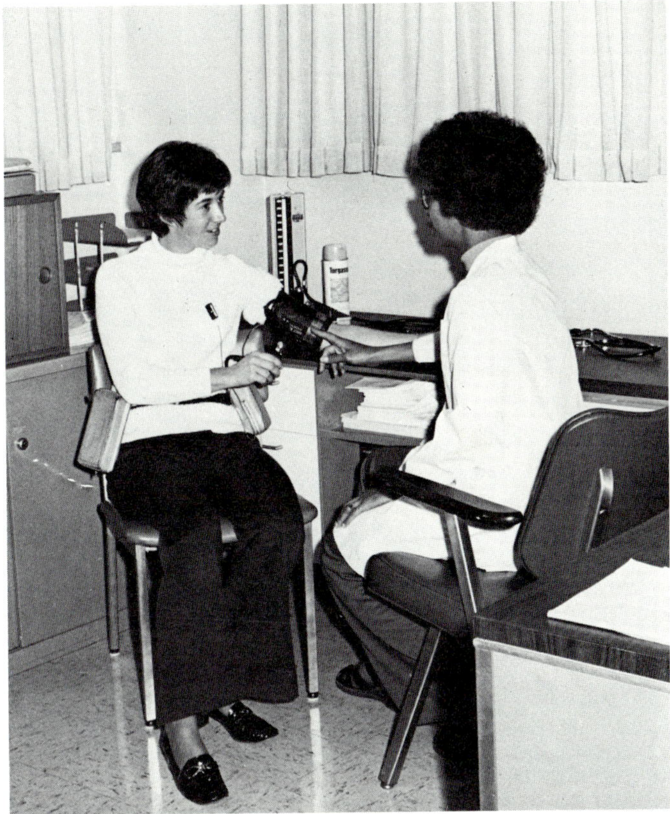

Figure 11-20. Portometry demonstration.

The nurse then outlines to the patient the proposed treatment, including diet, exercise, medications, and cessation of smoking. She answers questions and allays patient anxiety. She reviews the diet and makes necessary changes, such as potassium supplements, salt reduction, and weight control. She teaches the patient as needed, giving him moral support and encouragement to continue with the treatment. She then arranges for followup care.

(ii) *Followup visits.* Patients are seen at intervals of one week to six months depending on the severity of their disease and the mode of treatment. At each visit the nurse practitioner interviews the patient regarding the presence of cardiovascular symptoms or side effects of therapy. She checks his blood pressure and does a limited physical examination as needed. Ordinarily, she checks the blood pressure in the right arm in the sitting position; she checks it immediately after standing and after two minutes of exercise if the patient is taking a drug that may produce postural hypotension, such as guanethedine. She orders certain laboratory tests periodically, according to the protocol or as indicated. She changes the type or dosage of medication per protocol, or with the consent of the physician consultant.

Between followup visits the nurse reviews laboratory and x-ray results and patient telephone messages; she acts upon them per protocol, or brings them to the physician consultant's attention, and implements advised changes by contacting the patients.

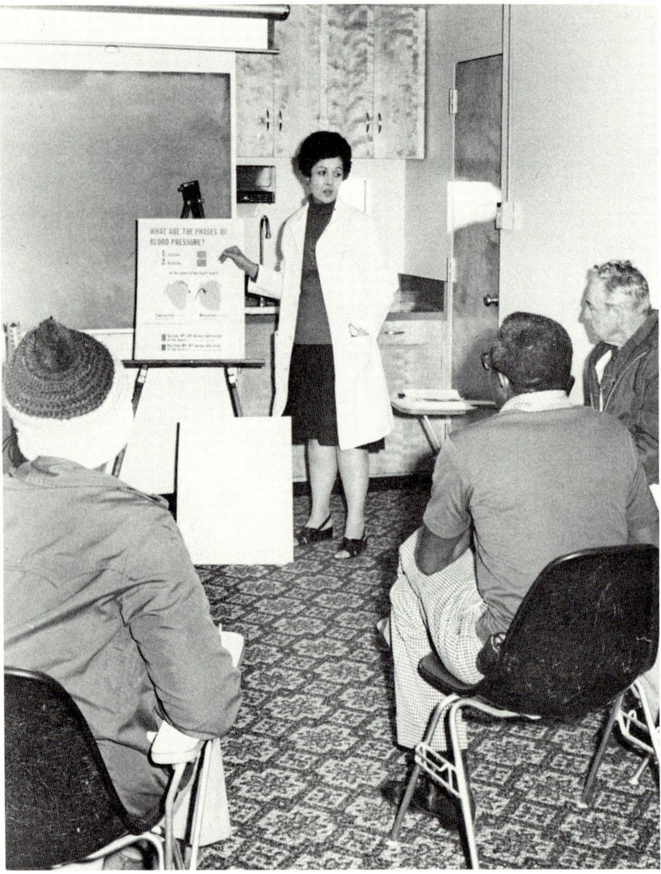

Figure 11-21. Hypertension class.

(iii) *Hypertension classes.* Every patient under care in the hypertension clinic attends a hypertension class as part of his treatment plan. The class is taught by a nurse practitioner once a week and lasts an hour. It is an informational group session to which spouses are invited. (See Figure 11-21). Its objectives are as follows:

(*a*) To introduce the patient to the circulatory system, including the functions of the heart and arteries.

(*b*) To enable the patient to differentiate between systolic and diastolic blood pressure in order to be able to interpret his blood pressure readings.

(*c*) To encourage acceptance of hypertension as a controllable but not curable disease.

(*d*) To explain the value of blood pressure control in the prevention of cardiovascular complications.

(*e*) To familiarize the patient with the measures necessary for control of his blood pressure.

(*f*) To help the patient identify risk factors that may influence his disease.

(*g*) To promote an understanding of the importance of regular followup.

(*h*) To orient the patient to the hypertension clinic and the roles of the nurse practitioner and physician consultant.

In order to achieve these objectives, a combination of didactic methods, group process techniques, and teaching aids are use. The class is only an introduction to patient education, which then proceeds on a one-to-one basis during each followup visit to the hypertension clinic.

f. Preventive maintenance respiratory clinic

(1) *Objectives*. (a) To provide an initial assessment to patients with chronic obstructive pulmonary disease or bronchial asthma and establish a baseline of disability.

(b) To instruct patients in the recognition of the early symptoms and signs of respiratory decompensation.

(c) To offer specific training in the home management of chronic bronchopulmonary disease so that patients and families can cope more effectively with it.

(d) To provide postinstruction patient assessment and maintain continuing surveillance and support.

(2) *Referral criteria*. Any patient who has deficient respiratory function from either chronic obstructive pulmonary disease or chronic bronchial asthma may be referred from MHTS or by physicians.

(3) *Clinic operation*. (a) *Intake visit*. Each patient has an initial assessment performed by a nurse practitioner, consisting of a relevant history and physical examination and the following baseline studies: chest x-ray, electrocardiogram, spirometry, sputum for cytology, tuberculin test, and arterial blood gases. The results are reviewed with the physician consultant, who may want to corroborate significant findings. The patient is then referred to the respiratory classes or for individual instruction, depending on his needs.

(b) *Respiratory classes*. Six 90-minute classes are held weekly for groups of six to eight patients (see Figure 11-22). A nurse practitioner is the predominant

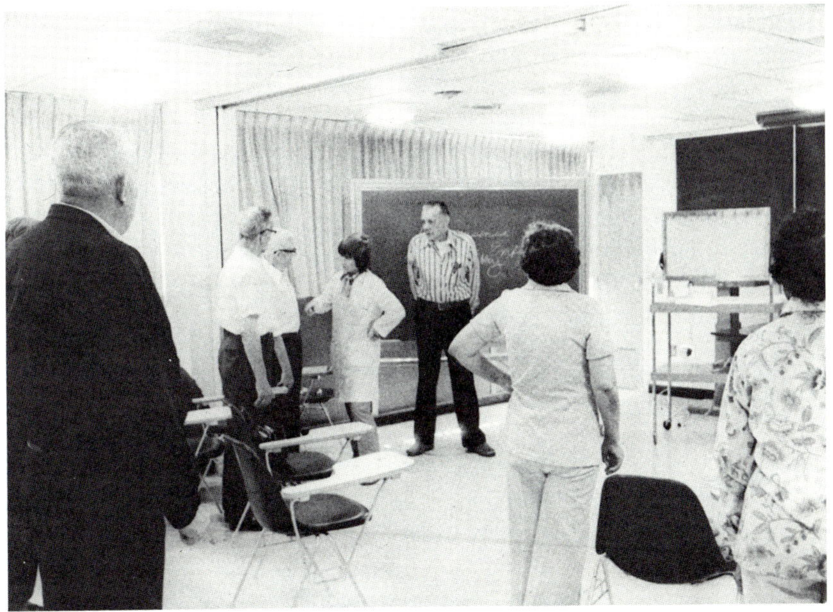

Figure 11-22.   Respiratory class.

instructor; she gives an overview of the classes and their rationale, teaches breathing and relaxation techniques and postural drainage, discusses the psychological implications of obstructive pulmonary disease and methods of coping, provides tips to prevent acute episodes, and describes the types and dispensation of respiratory medications. The physician consultant leads one session devoted to the pathophysiology of respiratory disease. A respiratory therapist is present at another session to demonstrate the use of home respiratory equipment and review the role of inhalants and positive pressure breathing in treatment.

(c) *Followup visits*. Following the series of classes, each patient is reassessed as to his physical status and progress, and plans are made for periodic followup and individual instruction as needed. If he is still smoking, he is referred to the stop smoking clinic. He is also alerted to symptoms and signs for which he should contact the nurse practitioner for advice or an interim visit.

g.   Preventive maintenance special kidney clinic

(1) *Objectives*. The clinic's objectives are (a) to evaluate patients with bacteriuria, hematuria, proteinuria, and elevated serum creatinine discovered through MHTS, (b) to maintain patients with asymptomatic bacteriuria and normal urinary tract under surveillance, (c) to treat and follow patients with bacteriuria who are symptomatic or have anatomic or functional urinary tract abnormalities, and (d) to complete the diagnostic workup of patients with other renal abnormalities and refer them to their physicians for appropriate management.

(2) *Referral criteria*. Patients may be referred from MHTS with one or more of the following abnormalities:

(a) Significant bacteriuria: (1) single urine culture with 100,000 or more bacterial colonies/ml, in a patient with urinary symptoms; (2) two consecutive urine cultures with 100,000 or more colonies/ml of the same organism, in an asymptomatic patient.

(b) Proteinuria: 1+ or more in two consecutive urine specimens.

(c) Hematuria: three red cells or more per high-power field in two consecutive urine specimens.

(d) Creatinemia: serum creatinine 1.4 mg% or greater.

(3) *Clinic operation*. (a) *Patient evaluation*. (i) Bacteriuria workup. A questionnaire is administered to determine past and present history or symptoms of urinary tract disease. Three consecutive urine cultures, microscopic urine examination, creatinine clearance, and intravenous urogram are obtained; 24-hour urine protein, 18-hour urine osmolality, and residual urine are measured. Voiding cystourethrogram, renal scan, or more complex tests are added if indicated.

(ii) Proteinuria workup. A questionnaire is administered and a urinalysis performed routinely. If the first morning urine specimen analysis is abnormal, Bence-Jones protein test, sickle cell preparation, 24-hour urine protein, urine culture, creatinine clearance, 18-hour urine osmolality, and intravenous urogram are also done.

(iii) Hematuria workup. A questionnaire, urinalysis, 24-hour urine protein, urine culture, sickle cell preparation, creatinine clearance, and 18-hour osmolality are the initial procedures, followed by serum protein electrophoresis, intravenous urogram, renal scan, cystoscopy, and arteriography where indicated.

(iv) Creatinemia workup. Urinalysis and urine culture, 24-hour urine protein, creatinine clearance, and 18-hour urine osmolality are performed routinely. Sickle cell preparation, serum protein electrophoresis, and intravenous urogram are added if necessary.

(b) *Patient management.* (i) Patients with bacteriuria, symptomatic or associated with urinary tract abnormalities, are treated according to a standard protocol and monitored at appropriate intervals.

(ii) Patients with asymptomatic bacteriuria are observed and treated only when indicated by a special protocol.

(iii) Patients with urinary abnormalities other than bacteriuria are referred to their physicians in the Department of Medicine after completion of evaluation.

h.   Preventive maintenance stop smoking clinic

(1) *Objective.* The clinic's objective is to enable groups of patients to permanently stop smoking.

(2) *Referral criteria.* Patients may be MHTS-, physician-, or self-referred, as long as they: (a) desire to stop smoking, and (b) are willing to join a group.

(3) *Clinic operation.* The clinic is operated by a coordinator, a former stop smoking clinic graduate, assisted by one or more group leaders. The coordinator is responsible for the development and implementation of program content, the proper functioning of group leaders, and overall clinic operations. The clinic schedule consists of an individual session followed by fifteen 90-minute group meetings held twice a week during the first month, then once a week. Both daytime and evening groups are available. Each group is limited to 12 persons.

(a) *Intake visit.* This is an individual interview during which the group leader discusses the patient's concerns about his smoking, explains what the clinic can offer him, and reviews the dates, times, and content of clinic meetings with him. The patient's motivation to quit smoking is assessed and reinforced and the mutual expectations of patient and clinic are established. The patient then makes an informed decision to join the clinic or not to. If he decides to join, he registers, pays the fee, and is enrolled in a group. If he decides not to, the interview is terminated, but the patient has the option to return at a later date.

(b) *Group meetings.* Through group discussion, patients are provided with information and counseling about preparing to quit, what to do after the last cigarette, how to deal with craving, long-range problems of "staying clean," health aspects of smoking, becoming a nonsmoker, exercise, and proper nutrition. The program introduces concepts from the following areas: addictive theory, self-actualization, assertive training, self-awareness.

(c) *Maintenance program.* Maintenance-group meetings are held once a week for clinic graduates who wish to maintain their status as ex-smokers. The program is used either as immediate reinforcement upon completion of the 12-week clinic sessions, or as long-range reinforcement, "where you go when you feel yourself heading for trouble,"—trouble being a cigarette. Some meetings are conducted with no staff member present, in order to provide a greater number of leadership opportunities for maintenance-group members.

(4) *Group leader training.* Potential group leaders are successful graduates of the stop smoking clinic. They have been positive and helpful group members and have shown interest in and concern for fellow group members. They also display an understanding of the smoking problem and an interest in the subject of smoking cessation. Potential group leaders possess sufficient ego strength to sustain themselves and to become models for others.

Group leader training consists of familiarizing trainees with smoking behavior information, group leadership techniques, and the stop smoking clinic model. During the initial training period, the trainee serves as an apprentice to the group leader (usually the clinic coordinator). The group leader reviews each group meeting with the trainee, sharing concerns about the group's problems and their possible solutions.

The second and long-range training period begins with the trainee's assuming group leadership. After each group meeting, the trainee group leader and clinic coordinator review the group's progress together. This training situation is prototypic of the continuing relationship between the group leader and clinic coordinator.

Group leader meetings are held once a week. During the meetings leaders share group experiences, introduce new materials and ideas and make reports on recently published smoking cessation articles.

Training is an ongoing learning experience for each group leader rather than a set procedure taking place on a set time schedule. After one year a group leader is able to conduct a group effectively and be in control of all situations that might arise within it.

(5) *Evaluation*. Patients are contracted by phone six months and one year after the date prescribed by the clinic to quit smoking. Each patient's smoking status is recorded for each month that has elapsed since the patient's last contact with the clinic. Smoking is defined as any tobacco consumed on a regular basis.

i.   Preventive maintenance weight control clinic

(1) *Objective*. The clinic's objective is to provide overweight patients with a method of weight loss and control using a group approach coupled with individual nutrition counseling.

(2) *Referral criteria*. To be eligible for the clinic, MHTS patients have to (a) weigh at least 20 percent over ideal weight for their height and frame as determined by the Metropolitan Life Insurance Company tables, and (b) have a definite desire to lose weight and a willingness to participate in a group program.

(3) *Clinic operation*. The clinic program consists of an orientation session with a group leader followed by a series of 12 weekly group meetings of 90 minutes duration. The groups, composed of about 20 members, are conducted by a nutritionist, who coordinates the program, and by group leaders. The latter are previous program enrollees who have lost weight successfully and who have participated in a special training program. An internist is actively involved in the program as a resource person.

(a) *Intake visit*. When a patient desires to enroll in the clinic program, he is given an appointment for a conference with a group leader. The conference is an orientation session for a small group of about six interested persons. Each is requested to complete a nutrition history questionnaire, which asks for information relating to the patient's past experiences with dieting, his reasons for overeating, his current eating and exercise habits, and any medical problems he may have. The group leader then briefly describes the design and content of the program, the group leader's expectations of each prospective member, and the fees involved. If the patient decides to join a group, he is requested to pay the fee covering the 12-week program and is given the date and time of the first group meeting.

(b) *Individualized diet preparation*. After the group leader has interviewed each prospective group member, she delivers the completed nutrition history questionnaires and the corresponding records to the nutritionist, who uses them to develop each person's eating plan. This is a personalized diet that takes into consideration food and cultural preferences, life style, methods of cooking, and any medical restrictions of the patient. The diet is patterned after the American Diabetes and American Dietetic Associations' Food Exchange System, which is a flexible program listing a variety of foods.

(c) *Group meetings.* A multifaceted approach is used in these meetings, both in subject matter (diet, exercise, nutrition education, behavior modification, self awareness) and methodology (group discussions, question and answer periods, nutritionist and physician presentations). The underlying philosophy stresses the setting of realistic goals and attitudes, the acceptance of individual responsibility, and the provision of alternate methods of dealing with emotions.

When a patient has completed the basic 12-week program, he has the option of attending on-going biweekly alumni group sessions. The format for these sessions is planned according to the needs of the group members. Mutual support based on openness and sharing continues to be encouraged in these sessions.

(4) *Group leader training.* The instruction program includes basic education in nutrition, as well as reading assignments that cover the etiology of obesity, group leadership concepts, behavior modification techniques, and other topics. Much of this material has been compiled in a group leader's training manual developed by a group leader with the assistance of the nutritionist. Other materials developed for group leaders include a reference book containing the latest journal reprints in obesity research, behavior modification, group dynamics, and related subjects. An increasing number of low-calorie, low-cost, easily prepared recipes that are also modified for low-cholesterol, low-sodium, ulcer, vegetarian, and other special diets are continuously developed and collected. These aid the group leader in suggesting even more flexible meal plans for the group members.

Instruction is followed by on-the-job experience. This starts with group co-leadership by the trainee and the nutritionist; then the trainee acts as a group leader with the nutritionist as an observer; and finally the trainee assumes full leadership.

11. Outcomes

a. Referral/arrival ratios.   The referral/arrival ratio is the ratio of the number of patients referred from MHTS to a preventive maintenance clinic and the number who actually arrive in the clinic. The ratio, an outcome of an interaction of factors related to patient perceptions, staff behavior, and system operation, serves as a rough index of the "acceptance" of a preventive maintenance program by patients and providers.

Referral/arrival ratios have been measured for most preventive maintenance clinics since their inception and are presented in Table 11-3. To be counted as an arrival, a patient must have kept his appointment within six months of his MHTS visit.

For a more detailed evaluation of referral outcomes an analysis was done of the behavior pattern of patients with elevated blood pressure referred from MHTS to the hypertension clinic (see Figure 11-23). Of 182 patients referred during the period August—October 1973, 106 showed up in the clinic for their first baseline

Table 11-3. Referrals and Arrivals from MHTS to Preventive Maintenance Clinics

	Third Quarter, 1974			Fourth Quarter, 1974		
	No. Ref.	No. Arriv.	Ratio	No. Ref.	No. Arriv.	Ratio
Arthritis	130	65	0.50	45	18	0.40
Diabetes	54	39	0.72	32	19	0.60
Hyperlipidemia	24	17	0.71	150	91	0.61
Hypertension	324	208	0.64	267	169	0.63

	First Quarter, 1975			Second Quarter, 1975		
	No. Ref.	No. Arriv.	Ratio	No. Ref.	No. Arriv.	Ratio
Arthritis	42	17	0.40	67	43	0.64
Diabetes	54	41	0.76	34	26	0.76
Hyperlipidemia	155	69	0.45	126	69	0.55
Hypertension	213	135	0.63	261	170	0.65

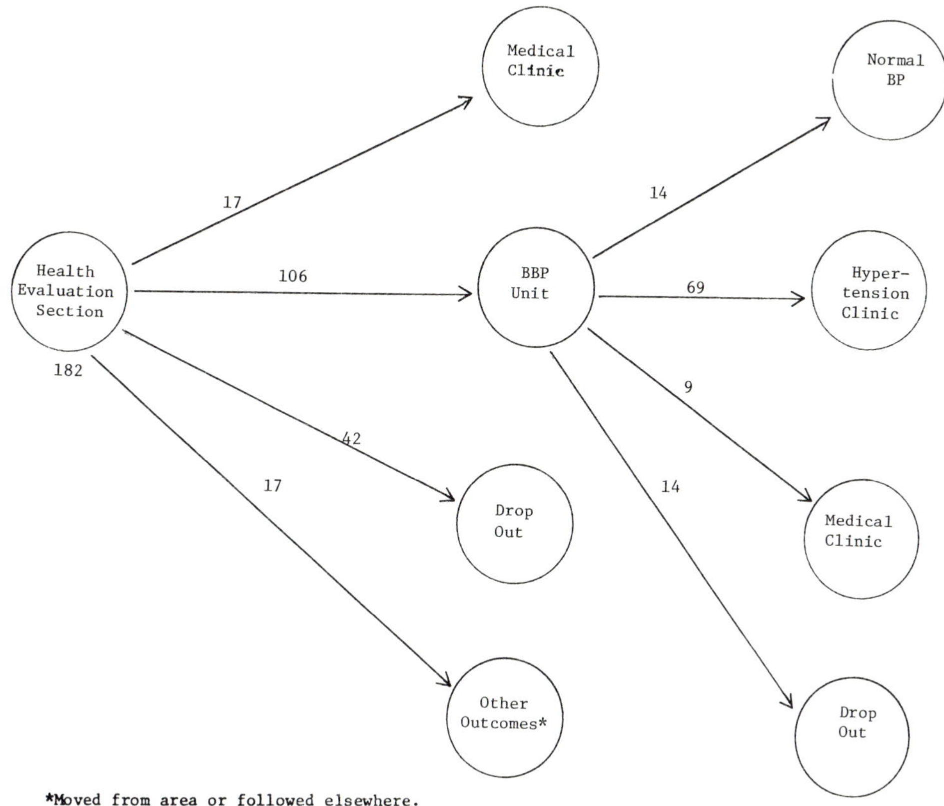

*Moved from area or followed elsewhere.

Figure 11-23.   Referrals to hypertension clinic from health evaluation section.

blood pressure measurement. Of the 92 patients with confirmed hypertension, 69 continued followup treatment in the clinic; 26 patients returned to their physicians for followup care; and 14 patients were found on reexamination to be normotensive. The large majority of patients with confirmed hypertension did, therefore, receive preventive maintenance care.

b.   Patient satisfaction.   To assess patient satisfaction, a questionnaire was handed out by the receptionists to all patients visiting the preventive maintenance clinics between May 28 and July 6, 1973. During that period 138 respondents had an appointment in the hypertension clinic and 102 in the diabetes clinic.

Patients expressed overwhelming satisfaction with their visits in answering questions on how they felt about the competence of the nurse, the attention paid to them and to their concerns, the explanation of the results of their examination, and the advice they were given. Of the hypertension clinic patients 94 percent said they were "very satisfied" and 5 percent "fairly satisfied" on a five-point scale ("very satisfied," "fairly satisfied," "neither satisfied or dissatisfied," "fairly dissatisfied," and "very dissatisfied"). Of the Diabetes Clinic patients 87 percent said they were "very satisfied" and 7 percent "fairly satisfied."

If given a choice, 84 percent of the patients with high blood pressure said they would prefer to receive most of their followup care from a nurse practitioner in the hypertension clinic, 11 percent said they would prefer followup care from a doctor, and 5 percent did not respond. Of the diabetic patients, 71 percent said they would prefer to receive most of their followup care from a nurse practitioner in the diabetes clinic, 18 percent said they would prefer followup care from a doctor, and 11 percent did not respond.

When patients were asked if they had received all of the information about their health problem that they wanted, 74 percent of the hypertension clinic patients and 77 percent of the diabetes clinic patients said they had.

c. Disease outcome.   In the absence of long-term observations on morbidity and mortality, intermediate results have been obtained to evaluate disease outcome. In the hypertension clinic, for example, blood pressure control has been used as an outcome index. Table 11-4 shows the mean diastolic blood pressure for a group of 123 patients at their entry into the hypertension clinic and during their second year of followup in the clinic, which was chosen as a more stable period of blood pressure control than the first year. The results indicate that a significant reduction in blood pressure occurred in patients under care in the hypertension clinic.

Patients enrolled in the stop smoking clinic were telephoned by an interviewer at the end of one year regarding their smoking behavior. Table 11-5 shows that almost one-half said they had not smoked any tobacco on a "regular basis" for one year.

d. Productivity.   To stay viable, a preventive maintenance program has to be cost-effective. A measure of such is the productivity of personnel employed, which depends not only on an individual's performance but also on the operational framework within which he works. In any new program time must be allowed to train personnel to reach their maximum capabilities and to establish a system that

Table 11-4. Comparison of Blood Pressure on Entry into Hypertension Clinic and During Second Year Following Entry ($N = 123$)

	On Entry	During Second Year
Mean diastolic blood pressure (mm Hg)	98.54	90.55
Standard error of the mean	0.83	0.84
Mean diastolic blood pressure reduction (mm Hg)		7.99
Standard error of the mean		0.86

Table 11-5. Telephone Evaluation of Stop Smoking Clinic Patients One Year Following Enrollment

		Smoking Status					
		Not Smoking		Smoking		Unknown	
Year of Enrollment	Total Number	No.	%	No.	%	No.	%
1973	135	65	48	58	43	12	9
1974	155	71	46	77	50	7	5

operates at an optimal level. Factors that affect mature system productivity include facility design, types and distribution of personnel, task assignments, and patient flow. Figure 11-24 shows, in graphic form, the parameters used to measure productivity, as applied to the arthritis clinic. These parameters are defined below:

(1) *Number of patients seen:* the number of new and return-visit appointments kept by patients, per month, as recorded in the arthritis clinic daily appointment schedules.

(2) *Total nurse time in clinic:* the number of days per month of nurse time devoted to all activities of the clinic, including seeing patients, consulting with

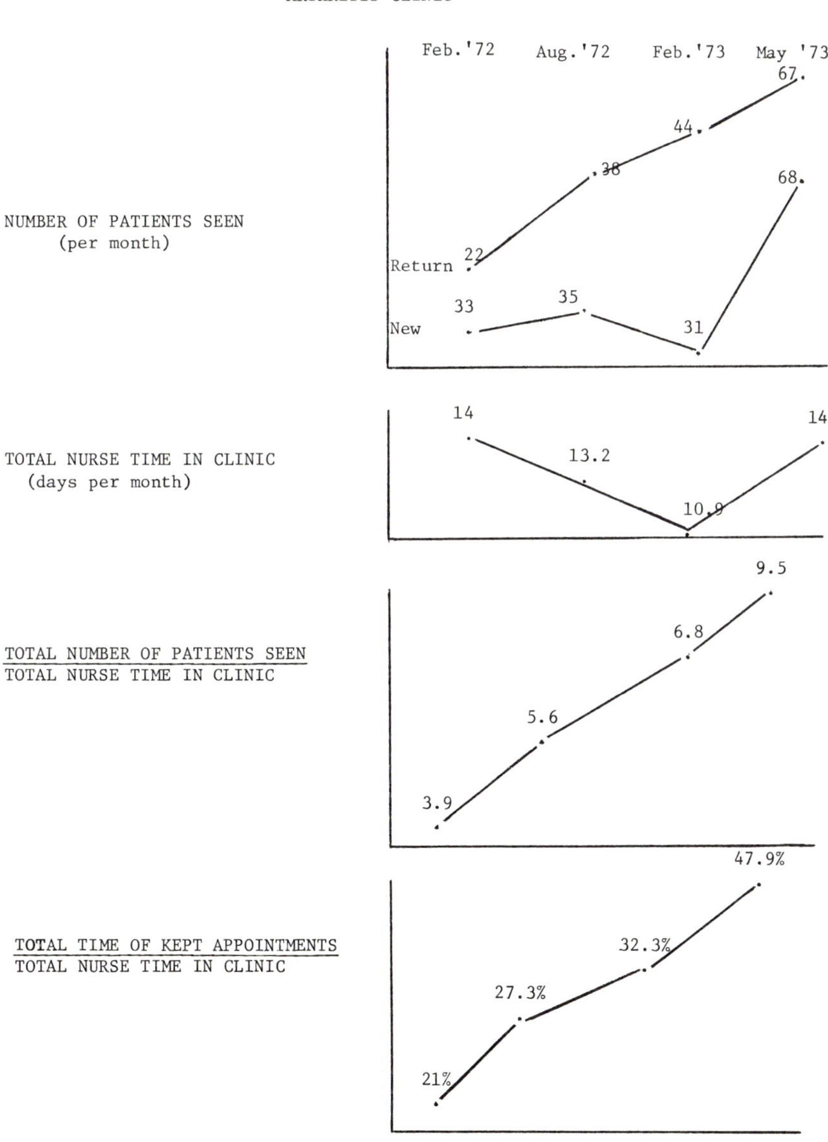

Figure 11-24. Graphs showing parameters used to measure productivity as applied to the arthritis clinic.

physicians, telephoning patients, reviewing patient charts, documenting patient care events, compiling statistics, etc. Each nurse submits a monthly activity report that shows the number of clinic hours she has worked in a particular clinic. The nurse time devoted to the arthritis clinic in a month is obtained by adding the hours spent by all nurses in the clinic during that month. The number of nurse days per month is then derived, seven and a half hours being equivalent to one day.

(3) *Total number of patients seen per total nurse time in clinic:* the number of patients seen per nurse per day in the arthritis clinic. This statistic, an indication of clinic throughput, depends on allocation of nurse time to various activities within the clinic.

(4) *Total time of kept appointments per total nurse time in clinic:* the proportion of the nurse practitioner's total time devoted to the arthritis clinic that is spent seeing patients. This statistic, a measure of clinic productivity, ideally would approach 100 percent.

It is apparent from Figure 11-24 that the productivity of the arthritis clinic was quite low at its inception. The following factors were thought to contribute to this situation:

(a) The number of patients who were referred to the arthritis clinic, and who actually arrived in the clinic, was much smaller than anticipated; consequently, the clinic schedules were often sparsely filled.

(b) There were many cancellations, owing possibly to ambiguities in the referral process or to patient reservations about a new and untried mode of service.

(c) The institution of innovative and complex appointment scheduling procedures for the clinics caused many incorrect appointments, probably contributing to the high no-show rate.

(d) Much nurse time was spent in documenting clinic activities both for patient care and for research purposes.

(e) Insufficient delegation of responsibilities to the nurse support staff (clinic assistants, licensed vocational nurses, and receptionists) resulted in ineffective teamwork. New roles proved difficult to assume. Nurse practitioners found themselves overburdened as they attempted to handle all details of clinic operation in addition to their new assignments for primary patient care, but they resisted transferring tasks to others. The nurse support staff found it a big adjustment to begin taking directions from nurse practitioners after a tradition of taking orders from doctors, who carried the weight of undisputed authority.

(f) The apprehension aroused by their new roles, coupled with incomplete treatment protocols, led the nurse practitioners to seek physician advice more frequently than had been expected.

As the above problems became evident, appropriate solutions were sought and implemented. It was gratifying to see the subsequent improvement in productivity. This continues to be monitored on a quarterly basis; trends are closely analyzed and serve as a basis for operational changes. Table 11-6 depicts the trends observed in the number of patients seen per nurse day in the preventive maintenance clinics in 1974 and 1975.

e. Utilization. In order to calculate the cost of care in the preventive maintenance clinics, total annual resource utilization was obtained by medical record review of patients enrolled in the diabetes and hypertension clinics. The review

Table 11-6.   Patients Seen Per Nurse Day

Clinics	Quarters, 1974				Quarters, 1975			
	1st	2nd*	3rd	4th	1st	2nd	3rd	4th
Arthritis	11.9	13.7	12.2	13.2	11.8	13.7	12.2	11.1
Back care†	19.1	26.4	13.5	20.4	22.1	15.6	21.3	18.7
Baseline blood pressure†	17.5	22.9	19.0	25.0	24.5	25.5	25.5	24.4
Diabetes	10.7	10.9	10.5	12.8	12.6	14.4	11.9	13.0
Hypertension/ hyperlipidemia	14.2	12.8	14.6	17.0	17.2	16.3	13.2	13.3
Special kidney	8.9	8.2	7.7	7.4	11.0	10.7	12.4	10.1

*Includes only the months of April and May.
†Vocational nurse or clinic assistant.

included visits to physicians and paramedical personnel as well as tests performed. It was limited to the second twelve months following entry of patients into the clinics in order to obtain a relatively stable group of patients who had remained under care of the clinics for at least two years. The data presented in Table 11-7 show that the visitation rate of patients with diabetes and hypertension is approximately twice the national average, approximately four physician visits per year, for the general population. This rate is not inordinate, considering the chronicity of the conditions involved and the level of treatment and surveillance required.

Table 11-7.   Use of Services Per Patient in Diabetes and Hypertension Clinics for Second 12-Month Period Following Entry*

	Diabetes Clinic ($N = 33$)	Hypertension Clinic ($N = 123$)
Visits		
Physician visits—medical clinic	1.88	2.11
Physician visits—other clinics	1.66	1.80
Nurse Practitioner visits—diabetes or hypertension clinic	3.00	4.30
Other paramedical visits	1.18	0.64
Total all visits	7.72	8.85
Tests		
MHTS	0.33	0.49
Laboratory tests	8.64	9.22
X-rays	5.73	2.62
Special procedures	1.55	0.54
Total tests	16.25	12.87

* All service utilization figures have been corrected for age and sex.

Table 11-8. Unit Costs for Health Services Used by Patients

(a) Physician Services

| | Direct Costs: | | | | | Indirect Costs: | |
| | Salaries and Wages Including Benefits | | | | | | |
	Physician	Support Personnel	Sub-Total	Non-Payroll	Total	Overhead and Plant Operation	Total Unit Cost
Medical appt:							
new and new return							
(30 min)	$12.43	$7.00	$19.43	$0.71	$20.14	$8.38	$28.53
return (15 min)	6.22	3.98	10.20	0.36	10.56	4.19	14.75
MHTS followup							
(15 min)	6.22	3.98	10.20	0.36	10.56	4.19	14.75
Medical nonappt.							
(10 min)	3.03	2.03	5.06	0.22	5.28	2.79	8.07
Gynecology appt.							
(15 min)	6.41	3.36	9.77	0.60	10.37	4.19	14.56
Gynecology nonappt.							
(10 min)	4.28	1.99	5.19	0.40	5.59	2.79	9.46
Specialty clinic							
appt. (15 min)	6.35	4.76	11.11	0.80	11.91	4.49	16.40
Specialty clinic non-							
appt. (10 min)	4.08	3.06	7.14	0.52	7.66	2.88	10.54

Table 11-8. (Continued)

(b) Nurse Practitioner Services

	Nurse	Physician	Support Personnel	Non-Payroll	Total	Overhead and Plant Operation	Total Unit Cost
Health evaluation (30 min)	$4.30	$2.95	$1.45	$1.18	$9.88	$1.29	$11.17
Hypertension clinic (15 min)	3.19	1.76	2.39	0.76	8.10	3.44	11.54
Other preventive maintenance clinics (15 min)	3.51	1.93	2.64	0.84	8.92	3.78	12.70
Other health center	3.37	0.00	2.52	0.79	6.68	3.60	10.28

(c) Other Services

							Total Unit Cost
(1) Multiphasic testing (MHTS)							$17.46
(2) Clinical laboratory tests							1.66
(3) Radiology diagnostic films							4.10
(4) Special procedures							5.66

f. Costs. Unit costs were developed for each outpatient service at the Kaiser-Permanente Medical Center in Oakland for a six-month period, January 1 to June 30, 1973. For physician and nurse practitioner visits these costs included, for each visit, personnel incomes, fringe benefits, supplies, equipment amortization, plant operation, and overhead. Personnel costs per visit were derived from actual time worked and the number of patients scheduled within that time. The unit cost for laboratory tests was the average cost per test for all laboratory tests provided to these patients. Similarly, the unit cost for special procedures, such as electrocardiogram, was the average cost for all such procedures performed on the patients. The unit cost per x-ray was derived from the total costs for diagnostic radiology services divided by the number of x-ray films taken. The MHTS costs have been reported previously.[43,44] These unit costs, detailed in Table 11-8, were used to calculate the annual cost of health maintenance of diabetic and hypertensive patients as revealed in Table 11-9.

The annual cost of health maintenance for a well/well patient has been reported to be $67.17.[4,42] The incremental cost of diabetic care can be inferred to be $168.06 − 67.17 = $100.89 per year, and of hypertensive care $148.21 − 67.17 = $81.04 per year.

E. CONCLUSION

The Kaiser-Permanente experience in health maintenance described above is only a small step in the direction of a truly comprehensive health care system. It is evident, however, that such an effort can be undertaken at a reasonable cost. But "more than money is needed to stop the public from smoking, drinking, eating too

Table 11-9. Cost of Services Per Patient in Diabetes and Hypertension Clinics for Second 12-month Period Following Entry

	Diabetes Clinic ($N = 33$)	Hypertension Clinic ($N = 123$)
Visits		
Physician visits—medical clinic	$ 24.92	$ 26.72
Physician visits—other clinics	24.63	26.83
Nurse practitioner visits—diabetes or hypertension clinic	54.72	49.62
Other paramedical visits	15.47	7.37
Total all visits	$119.74	$110.54
Tests		
MHTS	$ 5.76	$ 8.56
Laboratory tests	10.30	15.31
X-rays	23.49	10.14
Special procedures	8.77	3.66
Total tests	$ 48.32	$ 37.67
Grand total	$168.06	$148.21

much, and driving too fast."[30] Promoting and maintaining the public's health requires commitment from all concerned: from government, from health industry, and, most importantly, from each and every individual. Health education programs and alternative methods of health maintenance are important ingredients in stimulating individuals to assume responsibility for the quality of life they seek. Health care providers, and especially physicians, can and should assume a more active and catalytic role in this process.

REFERENCES

1. *Provisional Guidelines for Automated Multiphasic Health Testing and Services,* Vol. 1, *Planning Principles.* Report No. PB 195 654, National Technical Information Service, Springfield, Va., 1970.

2. World Health Organization. Constitution. Geneva: W.H.O., 1960.

3. Terris, M. "Approaches to an Epidemiology of Health." *Am. J. Pub. Health* 65(1975):1037–1045.

4. Richart, R. "Monitoring Performance in a New Medical Care Delivery System." *Proceedings of an International Conference on Health Technology Systems,* M. F. Collen, ed. Potomac, Md.: Operations Research Society of America, 1974.

5. Breslow, L. "Consumer-Defined Goals for the Health Care Systems of the 1980's." In *Technology and Health Care Systems in the 1980's,* M. F. Collen, ed. DHEW Publication No. (HSM) 73-3016. Rockville, Md., 1973.

6. Peacock, P. B., Colman, A. C., and Lutius, T. "Preventive Health Care Strategies for Health Maintenance Organizations." *Prev. Med.* 4(1975):183–225.

7. McLeod, G. K., and Prussin, J. A. "The Continuing Evolution of Health Maintenance Organizations." *N. Eng. J. Med.* 288(1973):439–443.

8. Hilleboe, H. H., and Larimore, G. C. "Preventive Medicine." *Principles of Prevention in the Occurrence and Progress of Disease.* Philadelphia: W. B. Saunders Co., 1965.

9. Fuchs, V. R. *Who Shall Live?* New York: Basic Books, 1974.

10. White, L. S. "How to Improve the Public's Health." *N. Eng. J. Med.* 293(1975):773–774.

11. National Conference on Preventive Medicine. "Theory and Application of Preventive Medicine in Personal Health Services." Preliminary Report. May 1975.

12. Veterans Administration Cooperative Study Group on Antihypertensive Agents. "Effects of Treatment on Morbidity in Hypertension. I. Results in Patients with Diastolic Blood Pressures Averaging 115 through 119 mm Hg." *JAMA* 202(1967):1028–1034.

13. Veterans Administration Cooperative Study Group on Antihypertensive Agents. "Effects of Treatment on Morbidity in Hypertension. II. Results in Patients with Diastolic Blood Pressures Averaging 90 through 114 mm Hg." *JAMA* 213(1970):1143–1152.

14. Breslow, L. "Early Case Finding, Treatment and Mortality from Cervix and Breast Cancer." *Prev. Med.* 1(1972):141–152.

15. Randall, K. J. "Cancer Screening by Cytology." *The Lancet* 4(1974):1303–1304.

16. Shapiro, S., Strax, P., Venet, L., and Venet, W. "Changes in 5-Year Breast Cancer Mortality in a Breast Cancer Screening Program." In *Seventh National Cancer Proceedings.* Philadelphia: J. B. Lippincott Co., 1972.

17. Still, J. W. "Adult Preventive Medicine: The Fourth Phase in the Evolution of Medicine." *J. Amer. Geriatr. Soc.* 16(1968):395–407.

18. Chidel, M. R., and Whitesie, J. D. "A Hypertension Clinic. Four Years' Experience in a Provincial Hospital." *Practitioner* 202(1969):542–548.

19. Miller, L. V., and Goldstein, J. "More Efficient Care of Diabetic Patients in a County Hospital Setting." *N. Eng. J. Med.* 286(1972):1388–1391.

20. Wang, M. K. "A Health Maintenance Service for Chronically Ill Patients." *Am. J. Pub. Health* 60(1970):713–721.

21. Gordon, D. W. "Health Maintenance Service: Ambulatory Patient Care in the General Medical Clinic." *Med. Care* 12(1974):648–658.

22. Runyon, J. W., et al. "A Program for the Care of Patients with Chronic Diseases." *JAMA* 211(1970):476–479.

23. Bullough, B. "The Source of Ambulatory Health Services as It Relates to Preventive Care." *Am. J. Pub. Health* 64(1974):582–590.

24. Roger, M. W., et al. "A Family Health Care Center—An Ongoing Student Endeavor." *Am. J. Pub. Health* 62(1972):199–204.

25. Benjamin, R. R., and Shapiro, S. "Counseling as Preventive Medicine." *Hospitals* 47(1973):105–108.

26. La Dou, J., Sherwood, J. N., and Hughes, L. "Health Hazard Appraisal in Patient Counseling." *West. J. Med.* 122(1975):177–180.

27. Lalonde, M. *A New Perspective on the Health of Canadians.* Ministry of National Health and Welfare, Ottawa, 1974.

28. Milio, N. "A Framework for Prevention: Changing Health—Damaging to Health—Generating Life Patterns." *Am. J. Pub. Health* 66(1976):435–439.

29. Simmons, J. J. "Complex Issues Facing Health Education." Editorial. *Am. J. Pub. Health* 66(1976):429–430.

30. Davis, A. E. "On Oracles, Education and the Public Weal." *J.A.M.A.* 235(1976):2845–2846.

31. Nordyke, R. "Definition and Goals of Primary Care." In *Advances in Primary Care,* M. C. Kallstrom and S. R. Yarnall, ed. Seattle: Medical Computer Services Association, 1974.

32. Lewis, C. C., and Resnick, B. A. "Nurse Clinics and Progressive Ambulatory Patient Care." *New Eng. J. Med.* 277(1967):1236–1241.

33. Beloff, J. S., and Karper, M. "The Health Team Model and Medical Care Utilization." *J.A.M.A.* 219(1972):359–366.

34. Collen, F. B., Madero, B., and Soghikian, K. "Kaiser-Permanente Experiment in Ambulatory Care." *Am. J. Nurs.* 71(1971):1371–1374.

35. Sox, H. C., Sox, C. H., and Tompkins, R. K. "The Training of Physician's Assistants. The Use of a Clinical Algorithm System for Patient Care, Audit of Performance and Education." *N. Eng. J. Med.* 288(1973):818–824.

36. Komaroff, A. L., et al. "Protocols for Physician Assistants. Management of Diabetes and Hypertension." *New Eng. J. Med.* 290(1974):307–312.

37. Phillips, D. F. "Protocols for Patient Care." *Hospitals* 49(1975):85–88.

38. *Design and Use of Protocols.* M. Kallstrom and S. Yarnell, ed. Seattle: Medical Computer Services Association, 1975.

39. Glen, J. K., and Goldman, J. "Task Delegation of Physician Extenders—Some Comparisons." *Am. J. Pub. Health* 66(1976):64–66.

40. *The Kaiser-Permanente Medical Care Program: A Symposium.* A. R. Somers, ed. New York: The Commonwealth Fund, 1971.

41. Garfield, S. R. "A New Medical Care Delivery System." *Sci. Amer.* 222(1970):15–23.

42. Garfield, S. R., et al. "Evaluation of an Ambulatory Medical Care Delivery System." *New Eng. J. Med.* 294(1976):426–431.

43. Collen, M. F., Kidd, P. H., Feldman, R., and Cutler, J. L. "Cost Analysis of a Multiphasic Screening Program." *New Eng. J. Med.* 280(1969):1043–1045.

44. Collen, M. F., Feldman, R., Siegelaub, A. B., and Crawford, D. "Dollar Cost per Positive Test for Automated Multiphasic Screening." *New Eng. J. Med.* 283(1970):459–463.

CHAPTER TWELVE

Health Education as an Adjunct to MHTS

F. Bobbie Collen

A. Introduction
B. Objectives
C. Educational Component Within the Health Testing Area
D. The Educational Component Associated with Health Testing
E. Summary and Conclusions

A. INTRODUCTION

Since, in the field of medical care, the initial step is usually taken by an individual seeking the resolution to some health problem, or reassurance regarding his health status, it has been generally assumed that the seeker's motivation would lead him to comply with the consequent advice, care, or treatment prescribed.[1] This compliance however, has been found lacking in the patient's responsive behavior in follow-up care.[2,3] Increasingly, a need has been recognized for an educational component that can motivate the patient into active participation in behalf of his own health maintenance.[3,4]

It is generally agreed that the education of persons to, about, within, and in relation to periodic health examinations is a commendable activity.[5] It seems logical that the process of health status determination would render an individual more receptive to communications about disease, and the factors influential in its arrest and control, and also about health and the practices most suitable to its promotion and maintenance.[6]

Traditionally, the concept of patient education has been regarded as a function of the doctor-patient relationship in the daily delivery of medical care.[7] This highly prized confidential relationship, conducted through dialogue, has long been taken for granted by the medical provider in the belief that it is serving as an educational tool.[8] The possibility of ineffective communication due to inappropriateness of terminology, the patient's level of understanding,[9] or his reluctance to request clarification for fear of appearing stupid, has seldom been recognized.[10] Or if it has, the result is a frustrating situation for the physician who, under pressures of work and time, is prevented from ascertaining positively that the patient has completely comprehended his communication and is in a position to follow his instructions, or that perhaps the patient's anxiety level has risen to block his full understanding.[11]

A resolution to this state of affairs is surfacing in the current medical care field. Rapidly increasing knowledge and new and more sophisticated technology,[12] diffusion of confusing and sometimes inaccurate data by the mass media in advertising innumerable health products and medications,[13] and the growing overwhelming demand for health services including periodic health examinations[14] are causing medical providers to turn for assistance to trained paramedical personnel and to printed and audiovisual materials that can effectively perform needed educational tasks.[15,16] While there is no guarantee that communications on health behavior and practices will lead to desirable action,[17] such efforts at a time when people are themselves voluntarily seeking information would seem to hold promise.[18]

In pursuit of this line of reasoning,[19] a decision was made in 1967 to add an educational component to the automated multiphasic health testing program at the Kaiser-Permanente facility in Oakland, California.[20] The educational adjunct, in 1969, took the form of a health education center, which functioned both within and in association with the Multiphasic Health Testing Services (MHTS).[21] It utilized paramedical personnel,[22] counseling,[23] group discussion methods,[24] exhibits,[25] and printed and audiovisual materials in the form of films, tapes (audio and video), and displays, all housed in a specialized library.[26]

Some 130,000 persons from the environs of the Oakland facility are serviced through individual, family unit, union, academic, and other groups, under a variety of health plan arrangements. This community is primarily a working population ranging from lower class to upper middle class. Among the comprehensive services offered (comprising emergency, hospital, outpatient clinics, home care, and ancillary departments such as x-ray, laboratory, and pharmacy), the availability of periodic health evaluations through a multiphasic program has attracted growing numbers of people.[28] Their contact with the health testing service is a voluntary one, stemming from either physician referral or self-selection.[29] Once an individual has undergone the multiphasic testing experience, he is likely to return for repeated visits at will.[30] Research examinations of matched study and control groups have revealed a significant cost benefit to periodic health evaluations, especially for middle-aged men.[31,35] Thus a unique opportunity arises for this population of patients to be educated to and within their health testing experience, especially for those to whom this is an initial exposure. Further opportunities for education follow as the patient is referred to the preventive maintenance clinics for ambulatory care attention[32] and to the health care services, such as the library,[26] exhibits,[25] counseling,[23] group discussions and open forums.[24] Figure 12–1 demonstrates the possible flow available for delivery of the educational component in the various MHTS settings.

B. OBJECTIVES

The AMHTS Advisory Committee to the National Center for Health Services Research and Development,[27] which advocated health testing service as a part of patient management, recommended health education as an effective tool in guiding the patient to good self-care, through (1) being informed about the kinds of tests and their importance and (2) being provided with general health education and counseling on preventive medical measures. It appeared that this education could be well delivered by trained paramedical personnel, comprising nurse practitioners, nurses, health educators, health counselors, etc., under the overall supervision of the managing physician.[22] Accordingly, the objectives of the educational adjunct to this MHTS were established to focus upon the following:

1. Objectives for Patients

a. Within the MHTS setting

(1) Acquainting the incoming examinee with the automated MHTS program.
(2) Providing helpful explanations of the purposes of each of the tests.
(3) Impressing upon the examinee the value and importance of individual responsibility in health maintenance and preventive medicine.

b. In association with the testing service

(1) Offering a convenient physical resource for in-depth health information.
(2) Providing counseling services on referral from the testing area for those in need of further information, clarification, reassurance, orientation of family members, etc.
(3) Organizing and conducting educational forums, such as classes, discussion

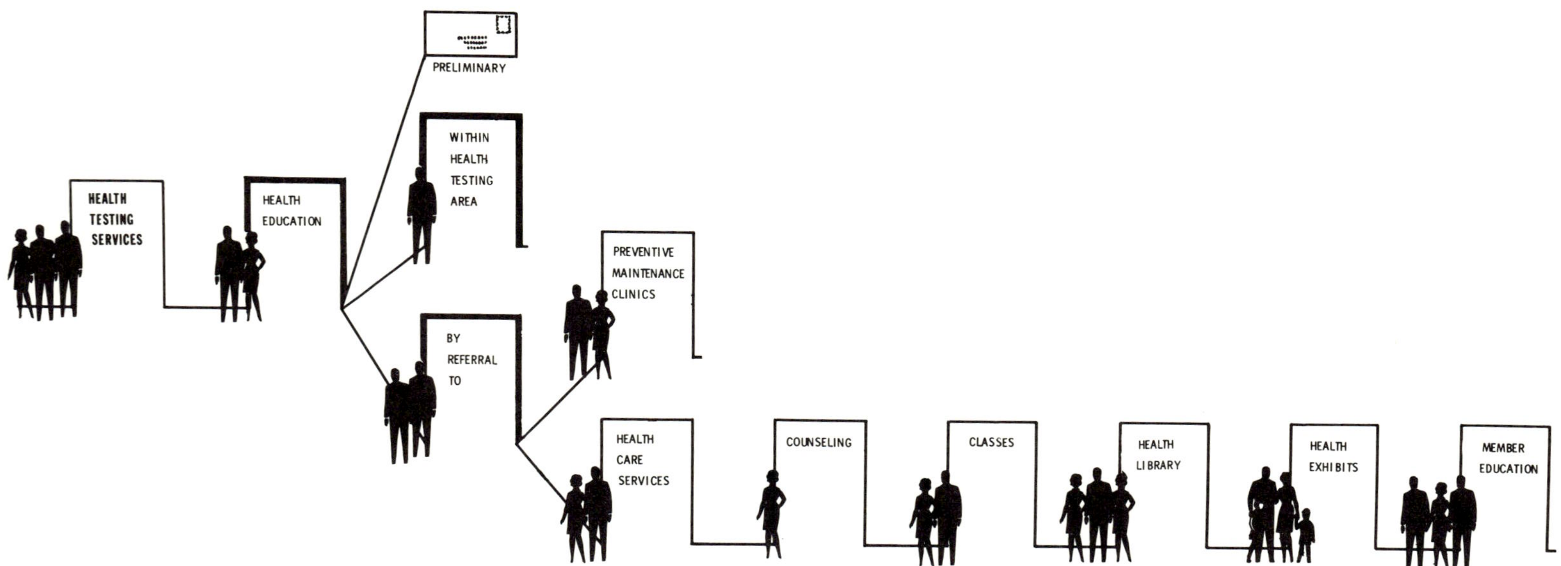

Figure 12-1. Patient flow into educational settings.

groups, and meetings, that would enhance the knowledge of the involved and interested persons.

2. Objectives for Staff

(1) Orienting the performing professional and paramedical staff to the concept, objectives, and methodology of health education.

(2) Providing consultative assistance in this area as needed.

(3) Providing a physical setting for reference for the health testing staff, and one to which they could refer patients for specialized information.

(4) Serving as a similar resource to hospital and clinic staff at the Oakland and other Kaiser-Permanente Medical Centers, for their own edification or as referral for patients.

3. Objectives for the General Community

(1) Offering a portion of the adjunctive educational setting—exhibits, library, and meeting forums—as a free resource to the health plan membership and to the community at large.

(2) Providing community schools, youth and adult, and other organizations with a specialized educational resource in the area of health care knowledge.

(3) Serving as a model to institutions in the United States and other countries interested in developing this approach to its actualization in their particular settings.

(4) Serving as a training ground for students and volunteers interested in actively participating in the health field.

C. EDUCATIONAL COMPONENT WITHIN THE HEALTH TESTING AREA

When the potential of integrating an educational component into the automated health testing service was recognized, a team effort was organized to acquaint medical care providers with it and to develop appropriate physical settings and materials.

Attention was first given to improving the orientation of incoming examinees to the MHTS program. For this purpose an illustrated leaflet was prepared, which could be mailed to each prospective patient along with confirmation of the forthcoming appointment. This pamphlet was expected to serve several functions: (1) informing the patient as to what procedures he might expect to be performed upon his person, and the amount of time to allow (so as to allay any anticipatory anxieties); (2) explaining the purpose of each major procedure, with the help of clearly captioned illustrations (so as to forestall confusion or misunderstanding); (3) informing the patient how to prepare for parts of the program, including dietary instructions for the blood and urine tests; (4) reassuring the patient of the confidentiality of the test results and their availability not to the patient, but to the physician or nurse practitioner for discussion with him; and (5) affirming the value of a periodic health examination both to the examinee and the provider of care.

Upon registration, the new examinee was invited to watch a slide program in the entry waiting room (Figure 12-2). This offered those unfamiliar with the multiphasic testing experience, or those who may have failed to read or fully

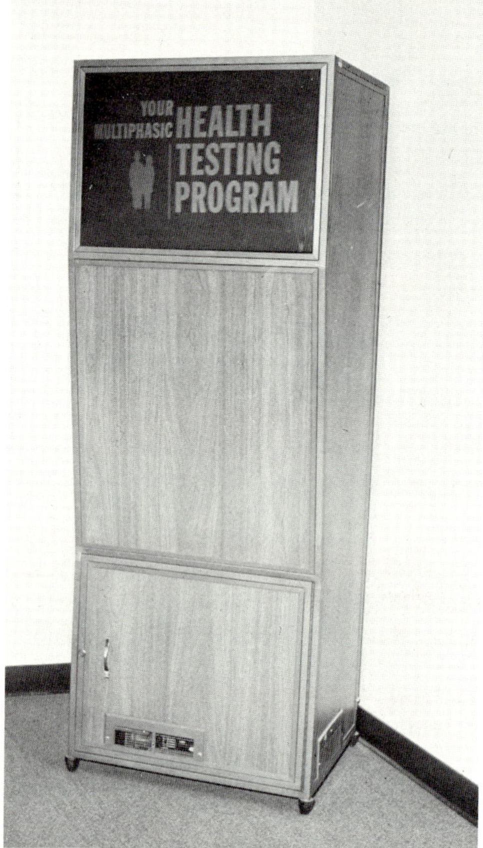

Figure 12-2.   Entry room orientation slide program.

understand the mailed brochure, a preview of what would transpire at each testing station. The step-by-step progression of the slides through the anticipated encounters was aimed at making him feel comfortable in the setting. Although other forms of visual and audiovisual media were considered, the simple slide program was selected as most appropriate. The MHTS is a dynamic process with periodic inclusion, experimentation, or discontinuance of new tests and equipment, and the flexibility of slides permitted insertion, deletion, or change in the visual program in the most economical fashion. Presentation could thus be kept up to date and relevant to the expected experience of the viewer.

Informational communication was provided by signs, wall displays, and pamphlets in a number of locations:

(1) In the entry waiting room: displays were mounted on three of the four walls. On one wall was a three-dimensional panel showing four "Steps to Health": "Learn About Health," "Keep Fit," "Health Testing," and "Use Health Care Services." On two other walls were labeled photographs illustrating activities available for each step at the Oakland facility (Figure 12-3).

(2) In the dressing booths: each of the booths in the men's and women's dressing areas was fitted with an instructional panel regarding the required extent of

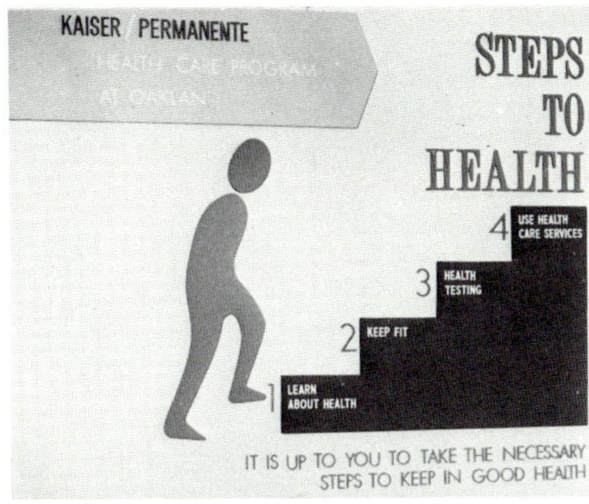

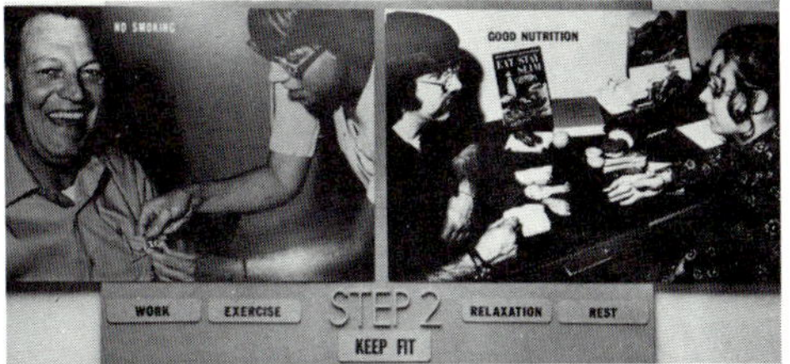

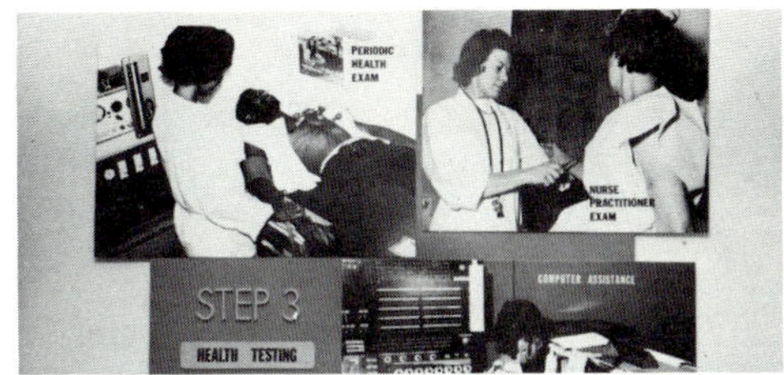

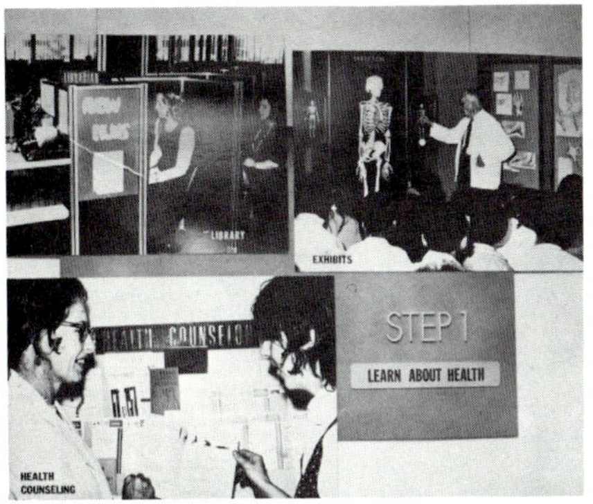

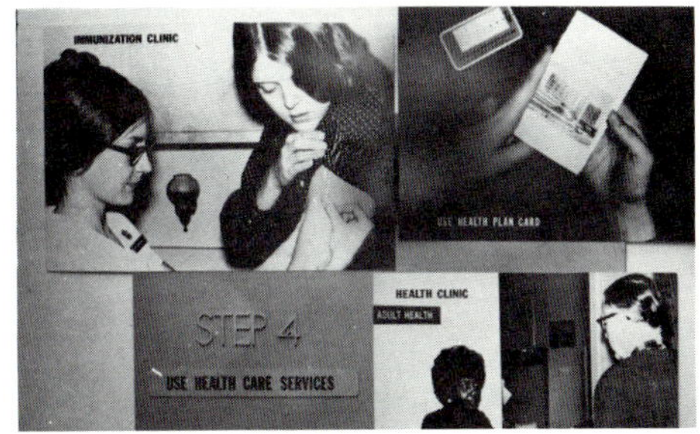

Figure 12-3. Entry room and steps-to-health and wall displays.

disrobing, the handling of valuables, the procedure for putting on the paper gown, and where to proceed next. These instructions helped eliminate confusion and embarrassment for the examinee.

(3) At the electrocardiograph test stations: two similar three-dimensional displays, one for each sex's waiting area, provided fundamental information on the risk factors in heart disease. The figure of a normally proportioned human body (male in the men's area and female in the women's) showed an obese outline superimposed; listings were given of the risk factors to be avoided for preventing heart disease and of the location and availability of services to assist the patient having this problem (Figure 12-4).

(4) At the anthropometry station: an explanatory panel (Figure 12-5) pointed up the importance of balanced diet and regular exercise for the maintenance of proper physical size and weight, and their value in minimizing medical problems through the pursuit of physical well-being.

(5) At the chest x-ray station: an explanatory panel emphasized the value of chest x-rays for disease detection, and the preventive role of good health habits, such as abstention from smoking (Figure 12-6).

(6) At the breast x-ray/mammography station: besides a panel explaining the need for and value of breast x-rays (Figure 12-7), a wall display illustrated the procedure for breast self-examination (Figure 12-8) and invited the examinee to

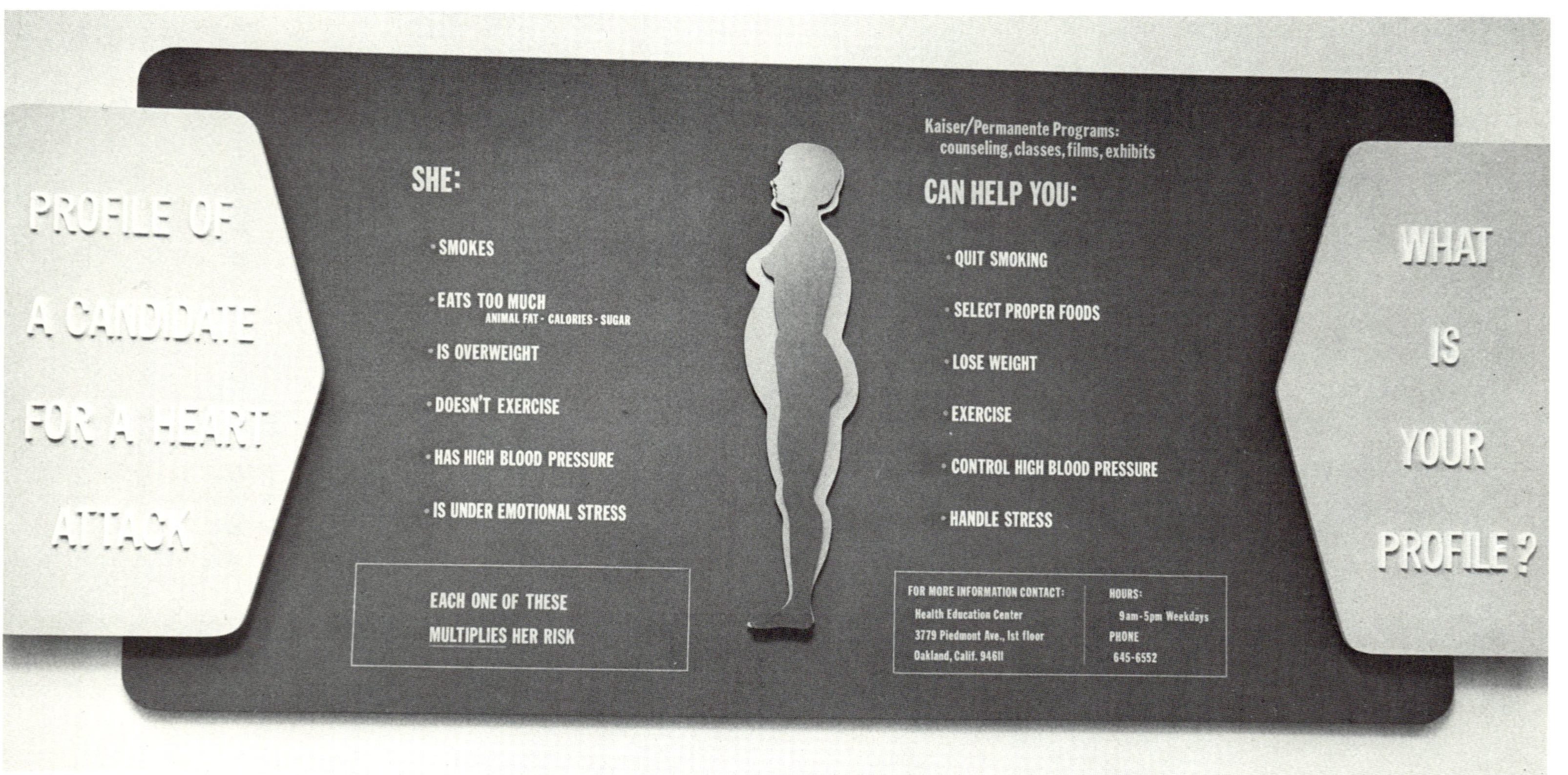

Figure 12-4. Risk factors in heart disease.

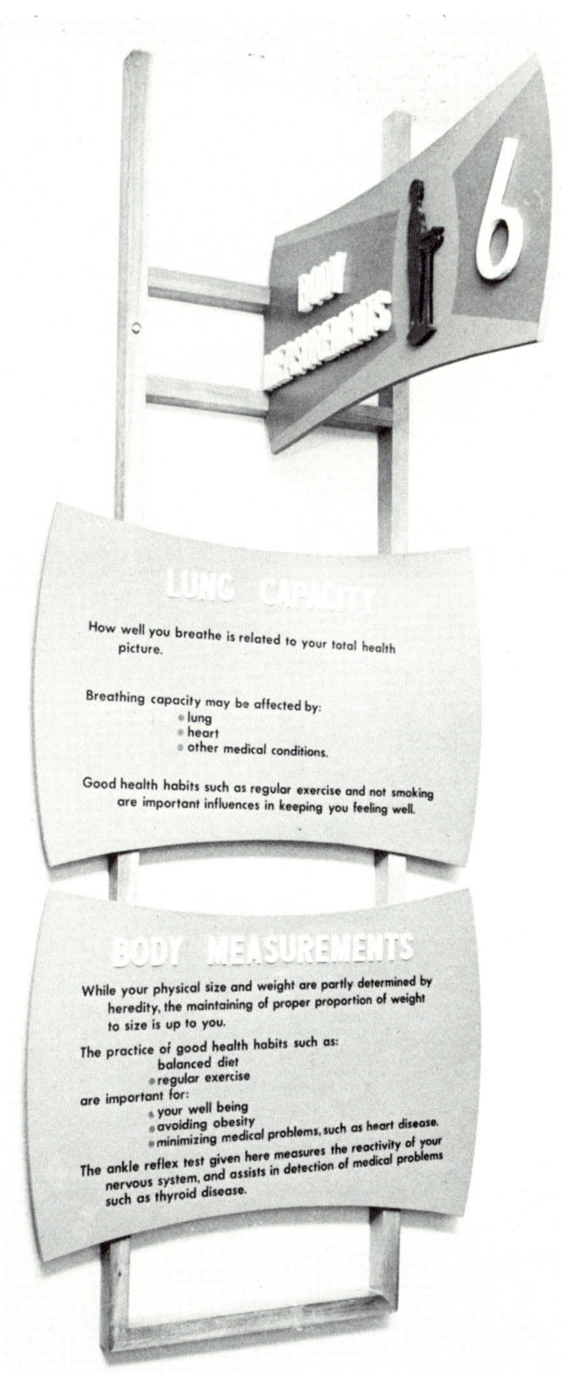

Figure 12-5. Body measurement and spirometry panels.

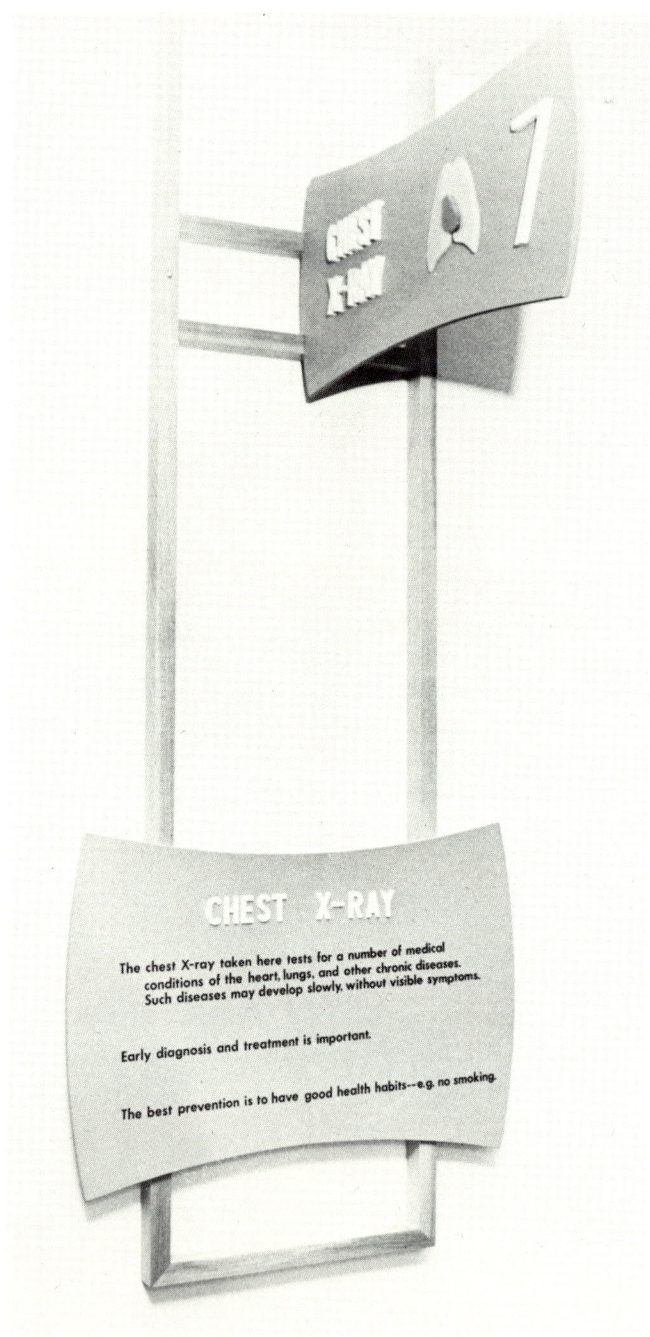

Figure 12-6. Chest x-ray panel.

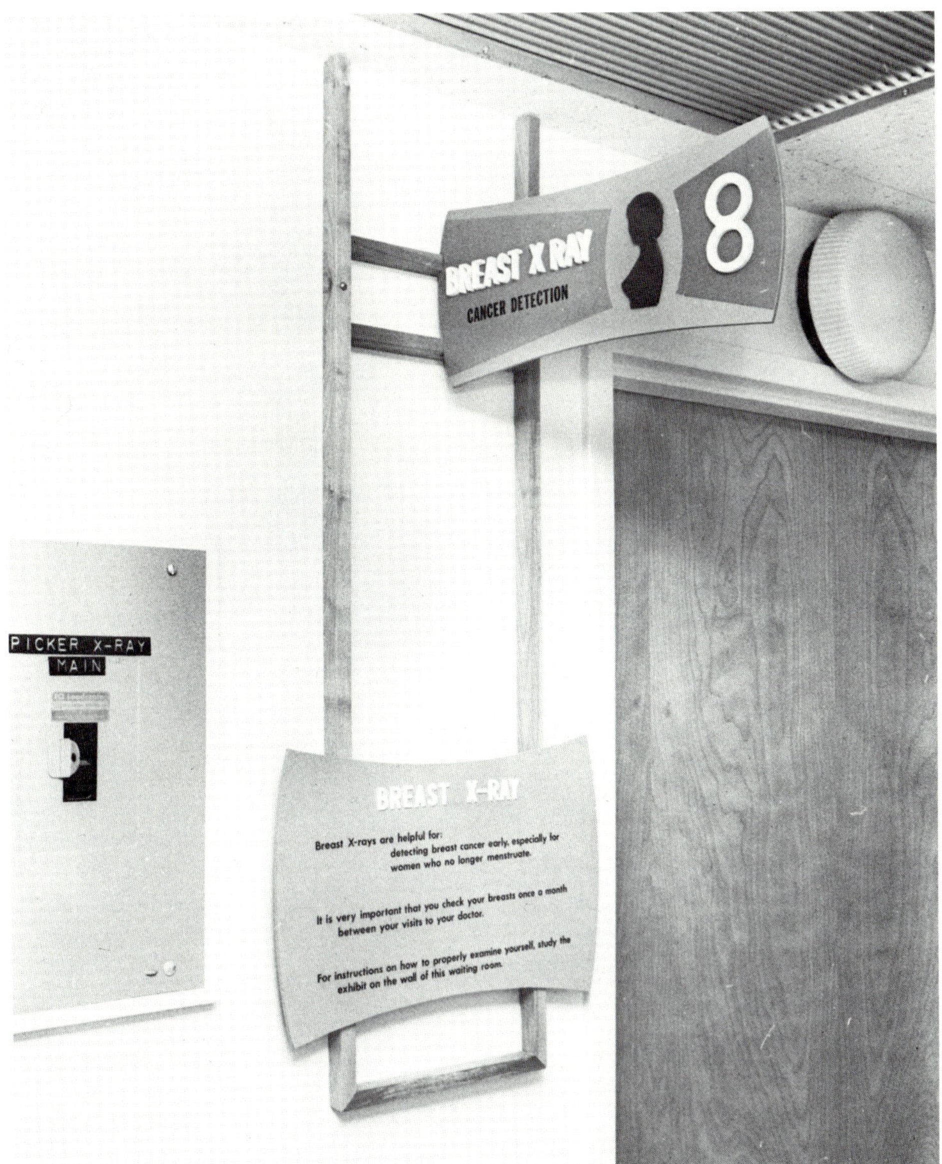

Figure 12-7. Breast x-ray panel.

view a film on this subject in the patient health library of the health education center.

(7) At the lung testing room: a panel explained the function and value of the test for ventilatory capacity of the lungs (Figure 12-5).

(8) For the eye station: two panels explained (a) the importance of vision testing and good eye care, and (b) the tonometry test for glaucoma and the value of its early detection (Figure 12-9).

(9) For the hearing station: (a) a wall display on the problem of noise pollution

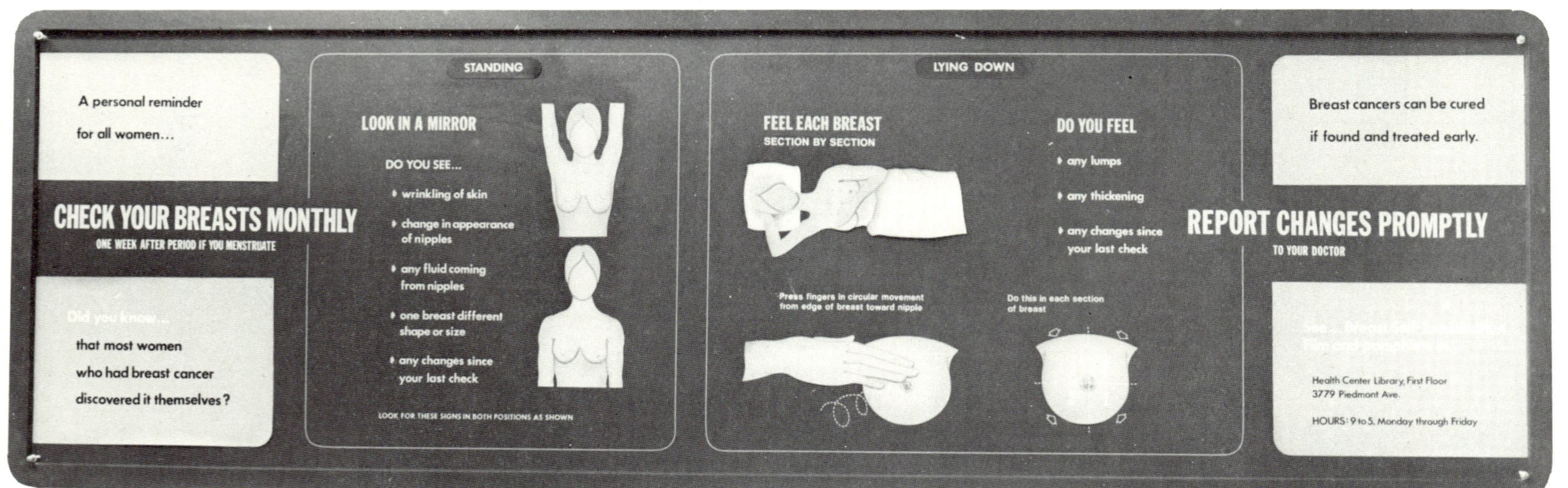

Figure 12-8. Breast self-examination display.

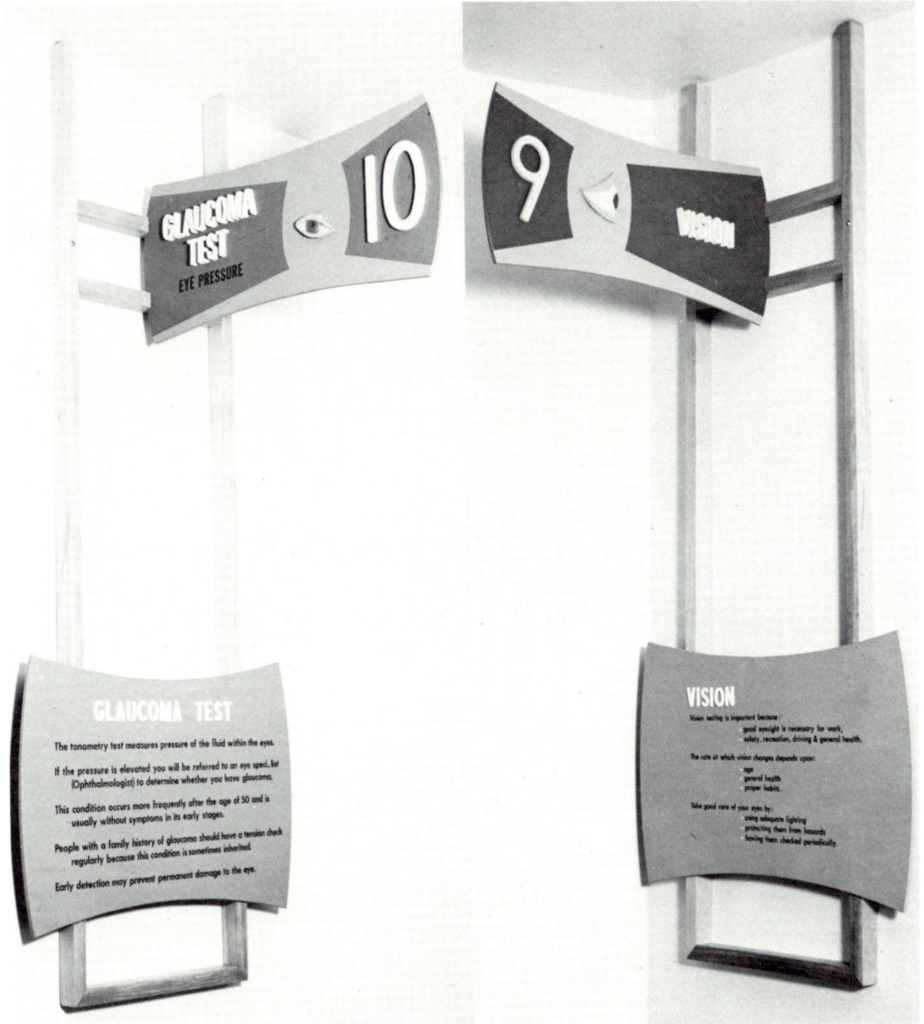

Figure 12-9.   Vision testing and tonometry panels.

depicted noise levels and how to avoid hearing loss (Figure 12-10), and (b) specific instructions in each hearing test booth guided the patient taking the hearing test.

(10) At the history questionnaire area: in each private booth, where the patient was to sort a deck of questionnaire cards, wall posters gave clear instructions for handling the card box.

(11) In the physical examination waiting room: for those patients desiring a physical examination immediately following their battery of tests, a second waiting room handled registration for a visit with a nurse practitioner. Here two separate slide programs were on sequential display, one describing the health care services available in the health education center, the second dealing with the prevention of health hazards related to smoking, drinking alcoholic beverages, and the misuse of drugs. Wall photographs also acquainted the viewers with some

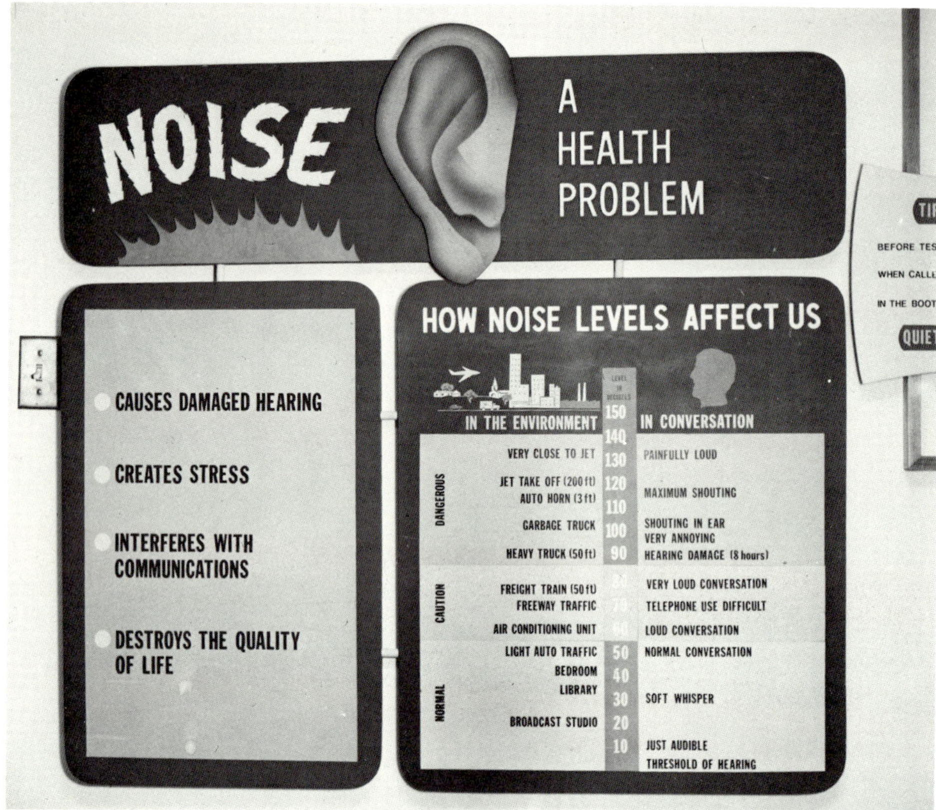

Figure 12-10. Noise pollution wall display.

of the ongoing health care services mentioned in the slide program, such as family planning, nutrition counseling, etc.

(12) In the physical examination area: during the physical examination, patients were encouraged to voice concerns relating to minor as well as major problems, and explanations were given through interactive verbal dialogue. On the basis of the questions asked, a series of succinct "Suggestions to Patients" (Figure 12-11) was developed, reviewed for accuracy by physician consultants, and distributed by the staff as needed for take-home reinforcement of given information and advice. In addition, pamphlets that had been developed for use in the patient health library were made conveniently available. These pamphlets related to a variety of minor discomforts and health problems (e.g., menopause, hiatus hernia) (Figure 12-12) and to current educational programs (e.g., stop smoking, weight control, etc.) (Figure 12-13).

(13) The triage referral process: all multiphasic examinees were informed on how to use the medical care system effectively for making future appointments. For those over the age of forty the value of and instructions for making appointments for a sigmoidoscopy examination for detection of cancer of the colon was outlined. Ill patients were directed immediately to the clinics for treatment by the physician. Persons with early asymptomatic or chronic disease were referred to the preventive maintenance clinics to receive primary care, which included for-

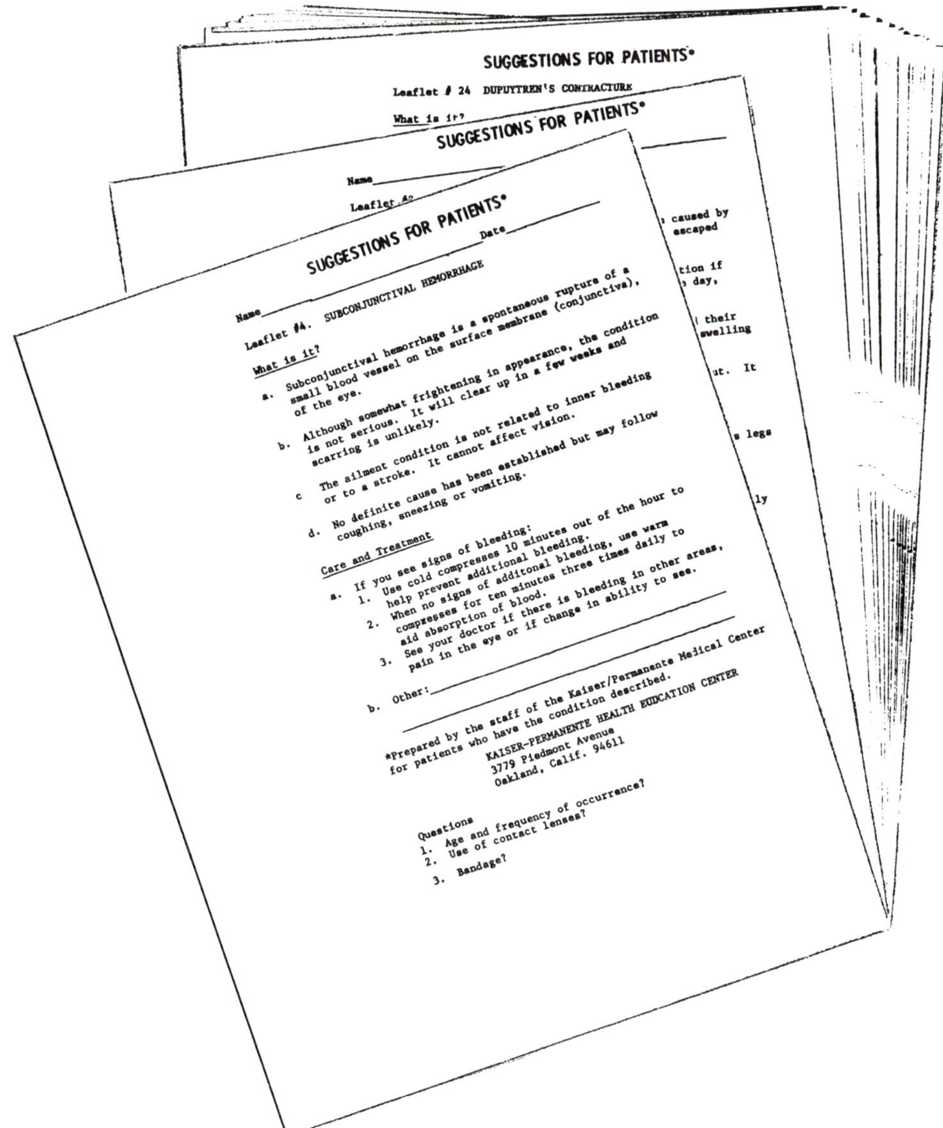

Figure 12-11.   Health suggestions to patients.

malized educational aspects.[32] To those in whom nothing abnormal had been discovered during the testing program, brochures describing the patient health library and exhibits (Figure 12-14) were presented, with the verbal recommendation to avail themselves of this specialized resource for health information.

During the weekly staff meetings of the nurse practitioners and supervising physicians, the exchange of experiences and consultation regarding problem situations[22] also included the handling of the health educational program. The escorting of patients to the library and exhibit sections was discussed, but the difficulties associated with the use of volunteers, and the lack of funds for paid

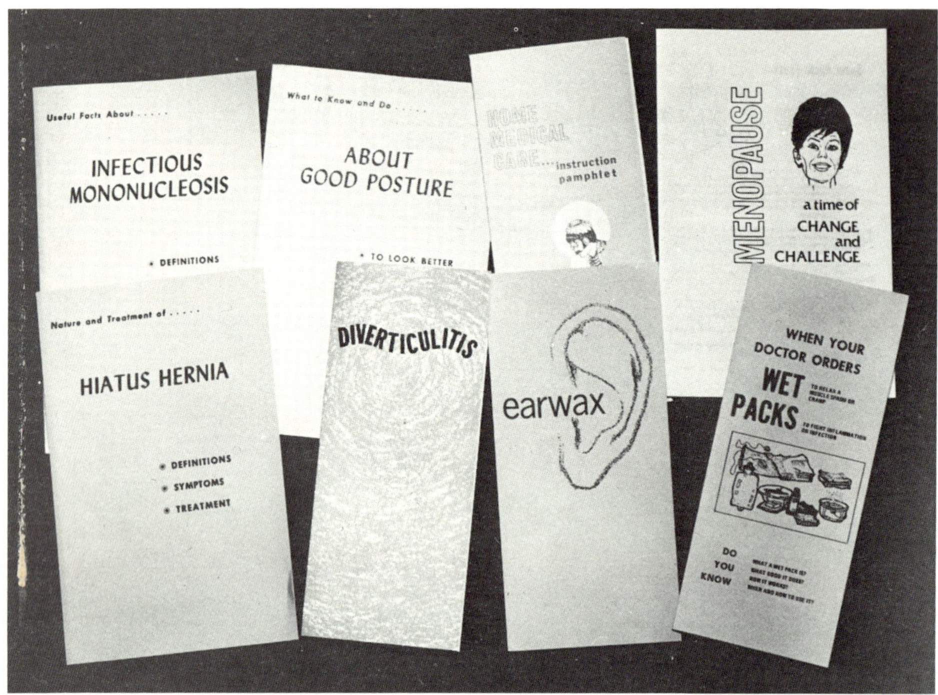

Figure 12-12.   Educational pamphlets on health problems.

workers, precluded its actualization. Because the testing experience lasted two to three hours (with an additional half-hour for the physical examination), it was thought perhaps to be too much to expect an individual, especially if he is working, to take further time to pursue a referral to an educational setting. The viewing of film programs in preventive medical care (for example, on the nature of diabetes, hypertension, urinary infections, or the care and prevention of poison oak, the common cold, etc.) within the physical testing area might yield more

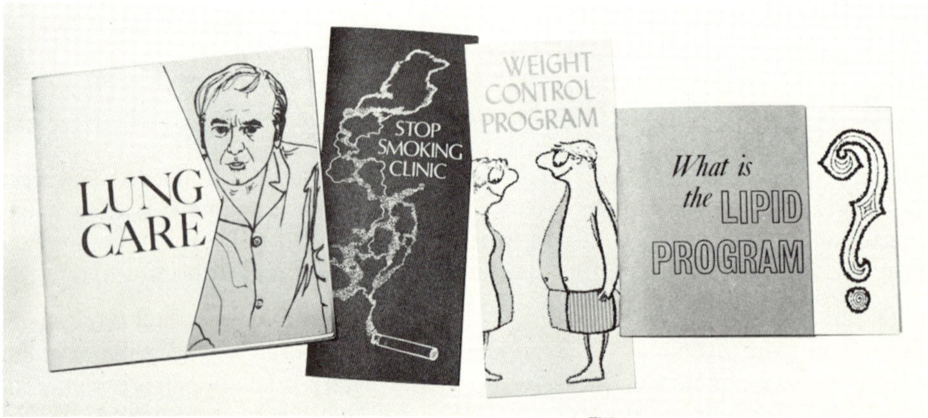

Figure 12-13.   Informational pamphlets on group educational programs.

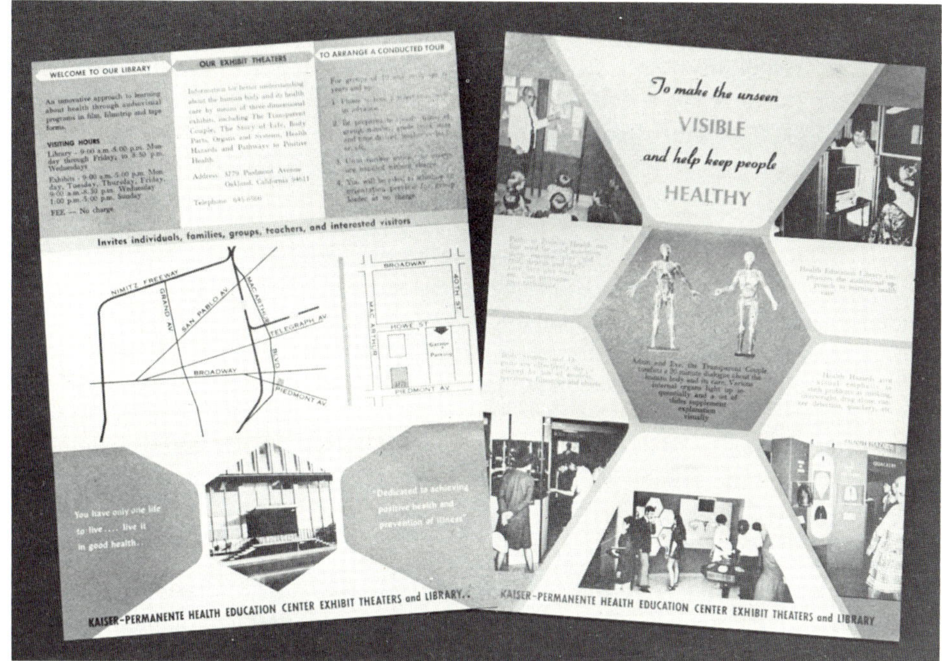

Figure 12-14. Brochure on library and exhibits.

fruitful results, but since this, too, would require extra time, the experiment was not undertaken at the MHTS in Oakland.

Responses to a survey on satisfaction with the MHTS experience, conducted just before the educational components were added, revealed a high degree of patient satisfaction with services rendered.[33] A similar survey on the educational features yielded numerous favorable remarks, but these were not tabulated.

D. THE EDUCATIONAL COMPONENT ASSOCIATED WITH HEALTH TESTING

Fulfillment of the second objective laid down by the AMHTS Advisory Committee Guidelines report[27] (that for patient health education to serve effectively as an adjunct to a multiphasic screening program and to physician services, it must also "provide general health education and counseling regarding preventive medical measures") was undertaken through the planning and development of a health care services division. Within its scope were included:

(1) General and specialized counseling for health, pregnancy termination, nutrition, community resources, etc.

(2) A health library for specialized printed materials and audiovisual programs in a variety of formats.

(3) A health exhibits area, including three-dimensional models, wall displays, charts, electronic equipment, etc.

(4) A conveniently located sales shop for health-related materials.

(5) Classes, discussion groups, and meeting forums.

Because of this educational component's value for all patients and the community at large over and above the MHTS population, it was regarded as a set of services in association with rather than an integral part of the multiphasic program. Referral to these services was thus open to all physicians, other professional and resource staff, other institutions, and self-selection.

1. Counseling

Early in the operation of the nurse practitioner facet of the multiphasic program, and of the patient health library, the need was recognized for counseling services pertaining to educational assessment, clarification of instructions, in-depth explanation of the nature of conditions and of the kinds of educational services available, nonmedical information, other referral resources, and emotional and empathic support for those evidencing such need. A health counselor was used experimentally in both the library and the multiphasic settings. Finally a separate area by the library was restructured to serve as a specialized counseling facility (Figure 12-15).

The objectives of this service were to:

(1) Provide individuals with health education appropriate to discovered needs.
(2) Promote the concept of preventive health behavior and health maintenance.
(3) Clarify and facilitate the medical care processes.

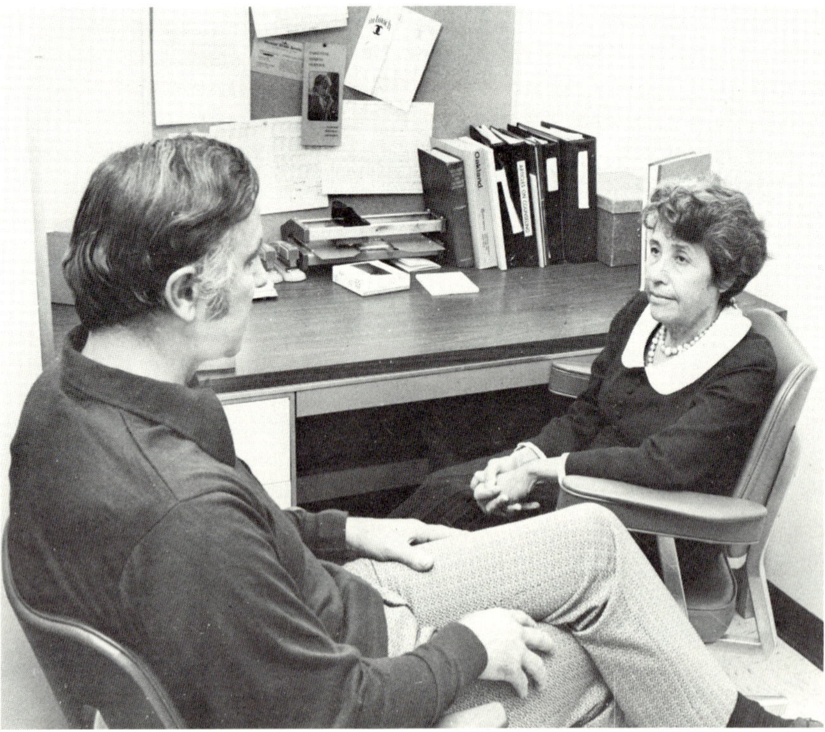

Figure 12-15.   Health counseling services.

(4) Counsel patients in need of a listening ear, and give emotional support where appropriate.

(5) Conduct specialized pregnancy and pregnancy termination counseling.

(6) Foster the patient's acceptance of new roles and systems in health care.

(7) Orient the patient to the multiple resources available at the Oakland facility and the community at large, and where appropriate help him reach these resources.

To promote achievement of these goals, in-service training of paramedical professionals was provided under the supervision of an administrator and physician director. Health educators, nurse practitioners, the librarian, and other staff attended communication sessions for group learning and exchange of experiences in health education and counseling techniques. These personnel served on an on-call rotational basis in order to accumulate ongoing experience with this activity. Coordination, including scheduling, supervision, and record-keeping, was handled by a health educator in collaboration with the librarian. The clientele comprised patients referred by physicians and nurse practitioners in the multiphasic program and also by clinicians, nurses, nutritionists, the librarian, and other staff personnel from the medical center. Individuals could also be seen on self-referral.

The services were available on both an appointment and a drop-in basis. A reference library for the staff and materials for distribution by them comprised educational, organizational, and community directory resources and other aids. Close collaboration was quickly established with the social service department and the medical and nursing staffs. The program pertaining to pregnancy and abortion counseling was considered a good area for the training of volunteers under the "gatekeeper"[34] concept. A continuing on-the-job training program was developed and conducted by a health educator for volunteers with qualifying backgrounds. This included a work study program for college students, which functioned during a two school-year period.

Course content emphasized education in interviewing and counseling techniques. Because of the high turnover of the volunteer group, at considerable expense to the administration, the decision was made to substitute a clinical assistant; this move proved successful.

Examination of the records showed that on average, health counseling was provided to approximately 75 individuals each month. This figure was exclusive of the nutritional services, which are discussed in another chapter.[35] Of the various referrals made by the nurse practitioners in the MHTS physical examination section, the greatest proportion was to the health counseling service.

The majority of problems disclosed by the counselees related to marital difficulties, which accounted for 22 percent of all visits. Others included requests for information about specific diseases, sexual problems, depression, parent-child friction, tension headaches, work difficulties, abortion counseling, physical incapacities, and bereavement grief. Analysis of recorded referrals revealed 43 percent to be by nurse practitioners, 30 percent by physicians, 9 percent by other health personnel, and 18 percent on self-referral (Figure 12-16). Evaluation of this service in 1973 determined that each visit cost $15.85. Efforts to reduce this expense included the scheduling of patients by appointment, and replacement of

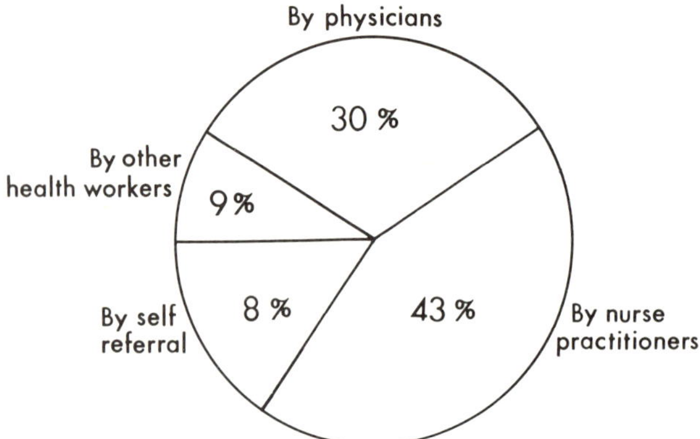

Figure 12-16.   Origin of referrals to health counseling service.

nurse practitioners by a trained clinic assistant for the active pregnancy and abortion counseling portion.[23]

2. Patient Health Library

For much of the educational component in the delivery of medical care, especially in its preventive aspects, printed and audiovisual materials could be used effectively; for this purpose the planners agreed upon developing a lay health library. While articles in the literature had described an increasing use of such instructional aids by physicians in private practice[36,37] and the use of a structured fee-charging pilot course in a health care setting to teach persons self-help in the fashion of a paramedic,[38] the use of a library as an adjunct to health testing and in association with it had no known forerunner.

Objectives outlined for the library included the provision of:

(1) A centralized referral service that would complement and reinforce the educational component in MHTS and the general medical care delivered by physicians and care providers in the Oakland setting and elsewhere.

(2) A health education resource to the community at large.

(3) Authentic and accurate information for improved comprehension of the nature and management of specific disease entities and of health-related problems.

(4) Clarification and correction of any health misconceptions.

(5) Facilitation of self-help where applicable to health care and maintenance.

(6) A materials resource for staff members for in-service education, research and other assistance.

(7) A training ground in health-related education for students and volunteers.

It was hoped that successful operation of such a library would have potential value for (a) saving physician, nurse, and health staff time from repetitious explanations and instructions, (b) improving the quality of the medical provider-patient relationship through clearer understanding of and more meaningful insights into disease conditions, (c) serving as an avenue for improving patient satisfaction with supportive services, and (d) reducing ultimate costs of health care through more optimal utilization of health professional services.

A preliminary survey of the Oakland physicians had revealed one-third to be supportive of the concept and potential of a specialized library for education of their patients, one-third neutral, and one-third either in disagreement or disinterested in this approach. A survey of 1,287 randomly selected health plan members similarly showed one-third who actively expressed intent to avail themselves of such a learning center. With no specific prototype to serve as a model, the construction of this area was conceived as a unique design, emphasizing the use of audiovisual media. Two thousand square feet of allocated space included 24 viewing booths arranged in a central square (Figure 12-17), within which were the staff and their working equipment, and surrounding which were storage areas, shelves for books and printed materials, several study carrels, a comfortable reading area, and pamphlet racks. A small projection room for group viewing occupied one rear corner, and a closed-circuit television watching area for six persons the other. The remainder of the space was separated out for an audiovisual workshop and repair room and a small classroom. Each booth (Figure 12-18) was equipped with a swivel and side chair, a cart for an audiovisual projector (or record player for tapes), two sets of headphones, a light-buzzer system to signal for assistance, and a pad and pencil for note-taking. The projectors were equipped with rear-view screens that enabled the visitors to view programs in a variety of formats, including 16 mm film, super-8 and standard-8 mm motion picture, film strips with sound cassette, and slide carousel.

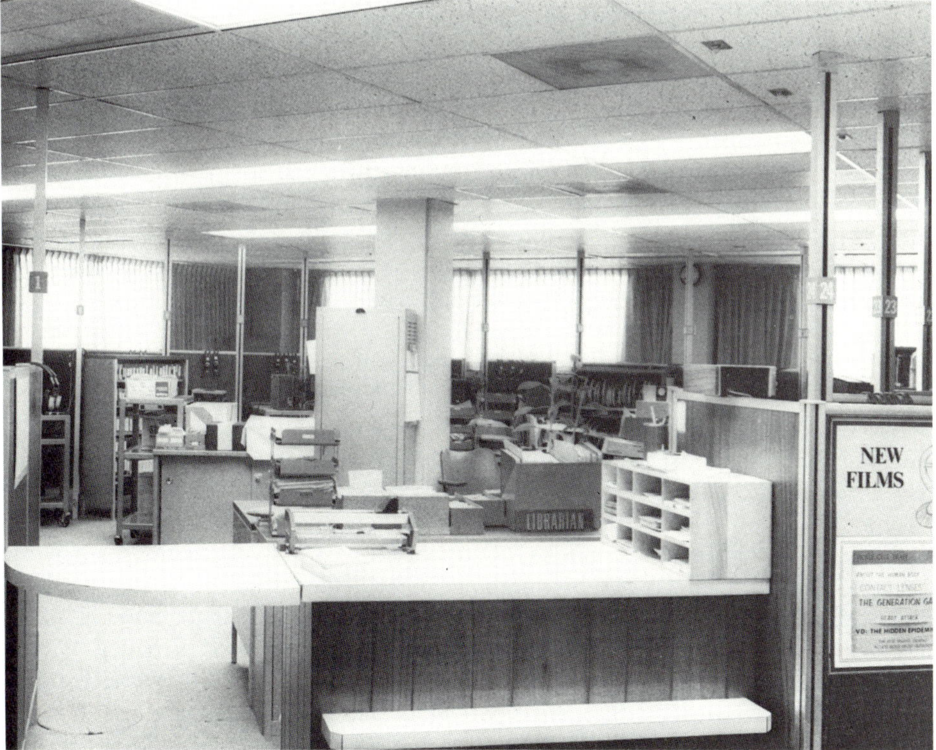

Figure 12-17. Patient health library.

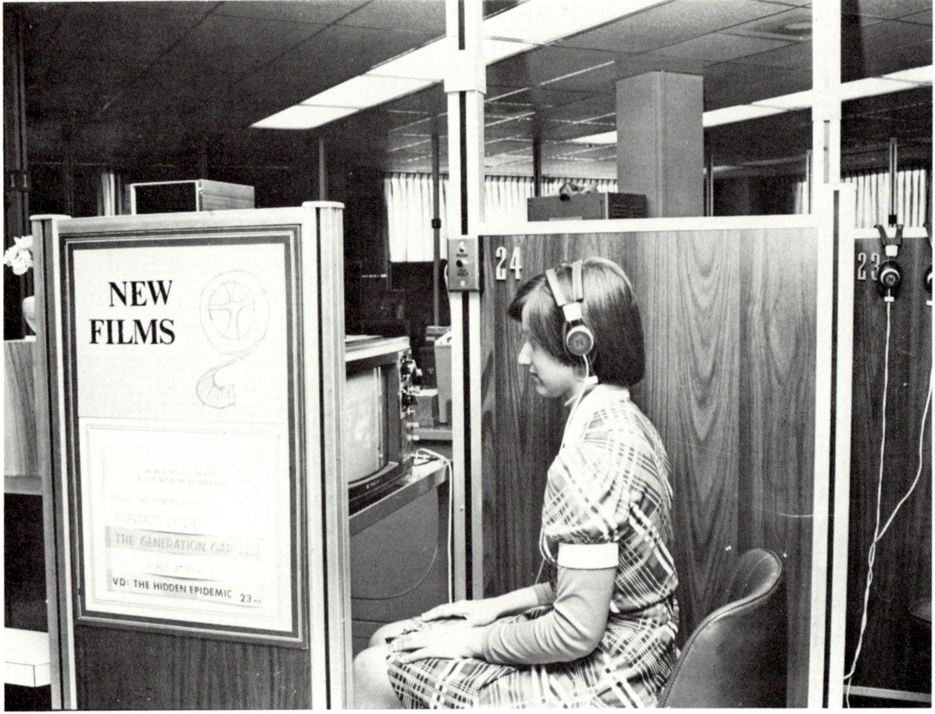

Figure 12-18.   Patient in a library booth.

The search for, preview, and acquisition of suitable programs and materials was a continuing endeavor. Each acquisition required preview and consensus. The programs accumulated pertained to both health and disease with emphasis on prevention, and included newborn and infant care, the child at each stage of growth and development, preadolescence, the teen years, family life education, family planning, prenatal care, immunizations, nutrition and weight control, acute and chronic conditions, etc. Increasing awareness of personal responsibility was encouraged by the promotion of materials dealing with physical fitness, body mechanics and good posture, the physical, mental, social, and emotional components of well-being, and others. Pamphlets to reinforce the audiovisual programs were available for free distribution (Figure 12-19). Many of these had been developed in-house (Figure 12-14). Addresses of sources where others could be obtained at nominal cost were prominently displayed. From a meager beginning in July 1969, to the end of December 1974, the inventory grew to 290 pieces of software (177 titles), 360 books, and 190 pamphlets. A large variety of reference readings, including articles, books, dictionaries and encyclopedias, also were available. A list of film programs, updated periodically, told the visitor what he could see (Figure 12-20), and folders listing equipment, book titles, and pamphlet inventory and samples were readied for distribution to interested provider visitors and institutions. The staff library of resource references also was an active and growing service that the paramedical personnel (nurse educators and group leaders) found increasingly useful.

In 1975, the library was staffed by a librarian, a library assistant, and a small

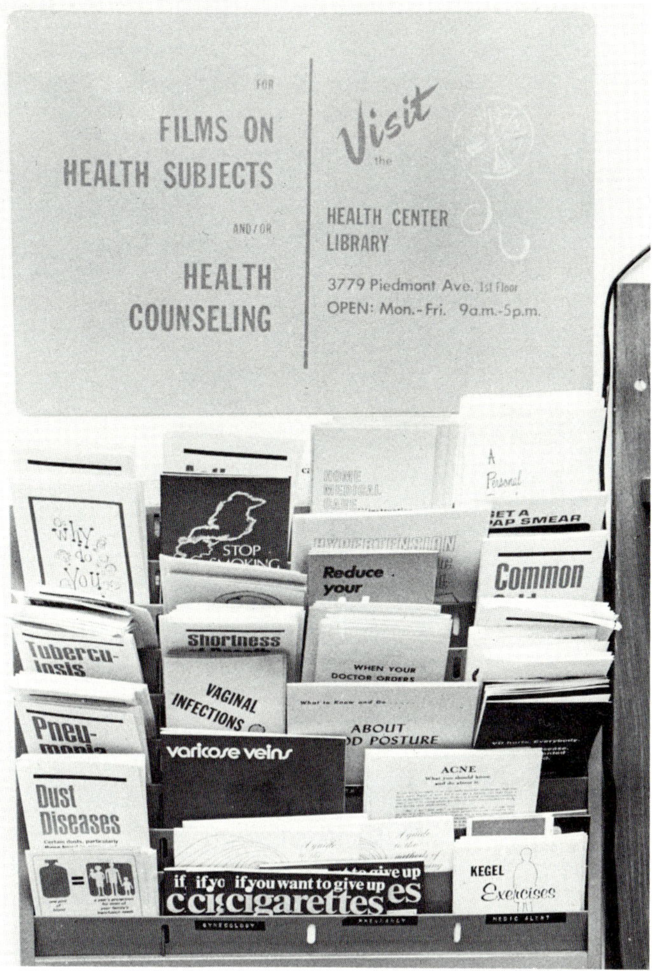

Figure 12-19.   Pamphlets as reinforcement for film subjects.

number of volunteers. Equipment maintenance and in-house development were under the direction of the audiovisual supervisor, who had one assistant. Hours were 9:00 A.M. to 5:00 P.M., Monday through Friday, Wednesday evening to 8:30, and Sunday afternoon from 1:00 to 5:00. Access to the library was free. Referrals could be from any of the staff physicians, nurse practitioners, nurses, or allied health workers from any of the Kaiser-Permanente facilities or any teacher from the community or schools, or one could be self-referred.

Patient and visitor flow was simple and direct. Each individual registered at the counter, where a library record form was filled out. If he requested an audiovisual program, he was directed to a booth, where use of the headphone and call button was demonstrated. After he had seen the program, when the patient signaled the library worker, he was given appropriate printed material, answers to his questions, and information and pamphlets on ongoing group educational programs (Figure 12-21). He then moved on to his next library activity (another film, reading, resource information, referral to health counselor, etc.) or departed.

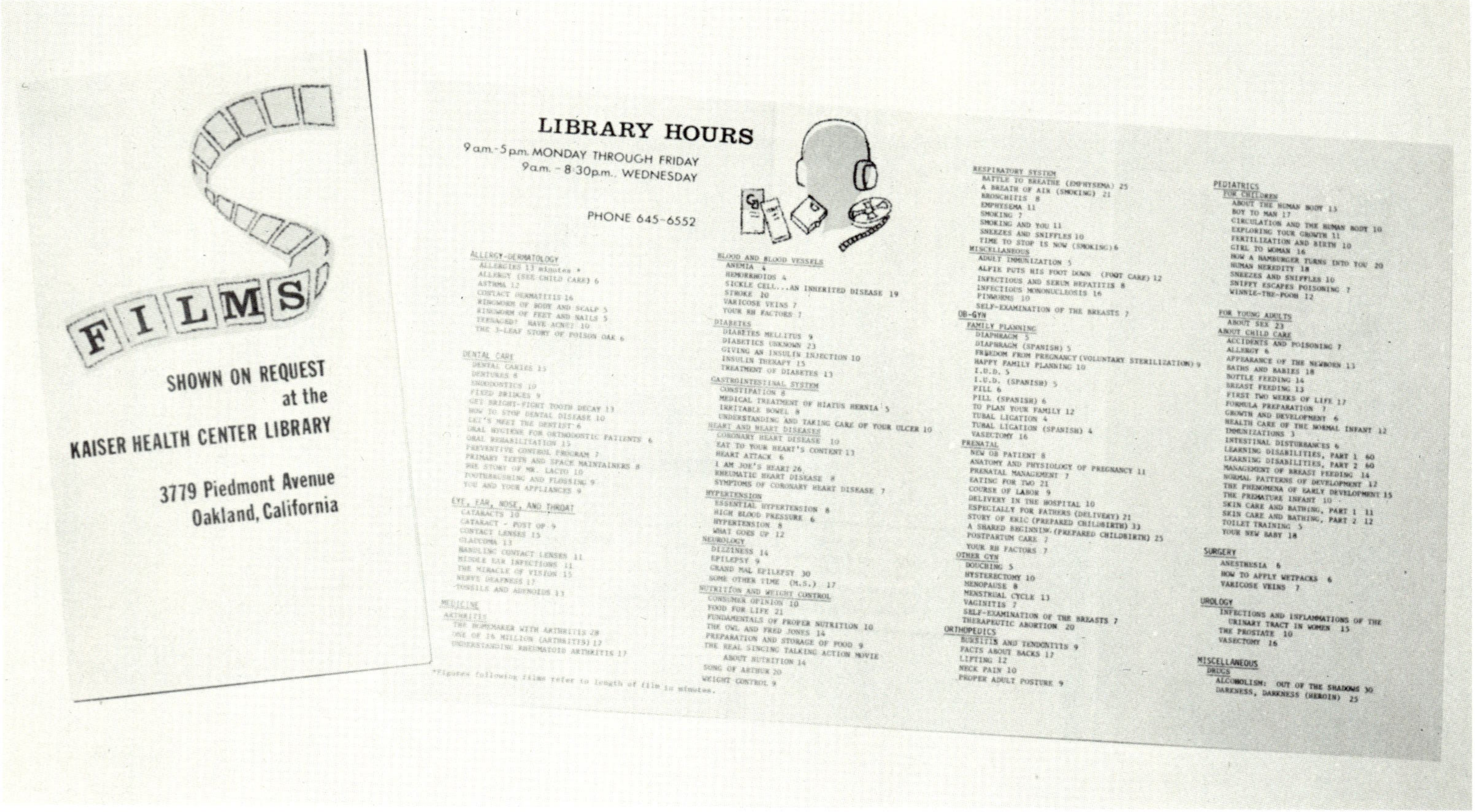
FILMS

SHOWN ON REQUEST at the KAISER HEALTH CENTER LIBRARY

3779 Piedmont Avenue
Oakland, California

LIBRARY HOURS

9 a.m.-5 p.m. MONDAY THROUGH FRIDAY
9 a.m. - 8:30 p.m., WEDNESDAY

PHONE 645-6552

ALLERGY-DERMATOLOGY
ALLERGIES 13 minutes *
ALLERGY (SEE CHILD CARE) 6
ASTHMA 12
CONTACT DERMATITIS 16
RINGWORM OF BODY AND SCALP 5
RINGWORM OF FEET AND NAILS 5
TEENAGED? HAVE ACNE? 10
THE 3-LEAF STORY OF POISON OAK 6

DENTAL CARE
DENTAL CARIES 15
DENTURES 8
ENDODONTICS 10
FIXED BRIDGES 9
GET BRIGHT-FIGHT TOOTH DECAY 13
HOW TO STOP DENTAL DISEASE 10
LET'S MEET THE DENTIST 6
ORAL HYGIENE FOR ORTHODONTIC PATIENTS 6
ORAL REHABILITATION 15
PREVENTIVE CONTROL PROGRAM 7
PRIMARY TEETH AND SPACE MAINTAINERS 8
THE STORY OF MR. LACTO 10
TOOTHBRUSHING AND FLOSSING 9
YOU AND YOUR APPLIANCES 9

EYE, EAR, NOSE, AND THROAT
CATARACTS 10
CATARACT - POST OP 9
CONTACT LENSES 15
GLAUCOMA 13
HANDLING CONTACT LENSES 11
MIDDLE EAR INFECTIONS 11
THE MIRACLE OF VISION 15
NERVE DEAFNESS 17
TONSILS AND ADENOIDS 13

MEDICINE
ARTHRITIS
THE HOMEMAKER WITH ARTHRITIS 28
ONE OF 16 MILLION (ARTHRITIS) 17
UNDERSTANDING RHEUMATOID ARTHRITIS 17

BLOOD AND BLOOD VESSELS
ANEMIA 4
HEMORRHOIDS 4
SICKLE CELL...AN INHERITED DISEASE 19
STROKE 10
VARICOSE VEINS 7
YOUR RH FACTORS 7

DIABETES
DIABETES MELLITUS 9
DIABETICS UNKNOWN 23
GIVING AN INSULIN INJECTION 10
INSULIN THERAPY 15
TREATMENT OF DIABETES 13

GASTROINTESTINAL SYSTEM
CONSTIPATION 8
MEDICAL TREATMENT OF HIATUS HERNIA 5
IRRITABLE BOWEL 8
UNDERSTANDING AND TAKING CARE OF YOUR ULCER 10

HEART AND HEART DISEASES
CORONARY HEART DISEASE 10
EAT TO YOUR HEART'S CONTENT 13
HEART ATTACK 6
I AM JOE'S HEART 26
RHEUMATIC HEART DISEASE 8
SYMPTOMS OF CORONARY HEART DISEASE 7

HYPERTENSION
ESSENTIAL HYPERTENSION 8
HIGH BLOOD PRESSURE 6
HYPERTENSION 8
WHAT GOES UP 12

NEUROLOGY
DIZZINESS 14
EPILEPSY 9
GRAND MAL EPILEPSY 30
SOME OTHER TIME (M.S.) 17

NUTRITION AND WEIGHT CONTROL
CONSUMER OPINION 10
FOOD FOR LIFE 21
FUNDAMENTALS OF PROPER NUTRITION 10
THE OWL AND FRED JONES 14
PREPARATION AND STORAGE OF FOOD 9
THE REAL SINGING TALKING ACTION MOVIE ABOUT NUTRITION 14
SONG OF ARTHUR 20
WEIGHT CONTROL 9

RESPIRATORY SYSTEM
BATTLE TO BREATHE (EMPHYSEMA) 25
A BREATH OF AIR (SMOKING) 21
BRONCHITIS 8
EMPHYSEMA 11
SMOKING 7
SMOKING AND YOU 11
SNEEZES AND SNIFFLES 10
TIME TO STOP IS NOW (SMOKING) 6

MISCELLANEOUS
ADULT IMMUNIZATION 5
ALFIE PUTS HIS FOOT DOWN (FOOT CARE) 12
INFECTIOUS AND SERUM HEPATITIS 8
INFECTIOUS MONONUCLEOSIS 16
PINWORMS 10
SELF-EXAMINATION OF THE BREASTS 7

OB-GYN
FAMILY PLANNING
DIAPHRAGM 5
DIAPHRAGM (SPANISH) 5
FREEDOM FROM PREGNANCY (VOLUNTARY STERILIZATION) 9
HAPPY FAMILY PLANNING 10
I.U.D. 5
I.U.D. (SPANISH) 5
PILL 6
PILL (SPANISH) 6
TO PLAN YOUR FAMILY 12
TUBAL LIGATION 4
TUBAL LIGATION (SPANISH) 4
VASECTOMY 16

PRENATAL
NEW OB PATIENT 8
ANATOMY AND PHYSIOLOGY OF PREGNANCY 11
PRENATAL MANAGEMENT 7
EATING FOR TWO 21
COURSE OF LABOR 9
DELIVERY IN THE HOSPITAL 10
ESPECIALLY FOR FATHERS (DELIVERY) 21
STORY OF ERIC (PREPARED CHILDBIRTH) 33
A SHARED BEGINNING (PREPARED CHILDBIRTH) 25
POSTPARTUM CARE 7
YOUR RH FACTORS 7

OTHER GYN
DOUCHING 5
HYSTERECTOMY 10
MENOPAUSE 8
MENSTRUAL CYCLE 13
VAGINITIS 7
SELF-EXAMINATION OF THE BREASTS 7
THERAPEUTIC ABORTION 20

ORTHOPEDICS
BURSITIS AND TENDONITIS 9
FACTS ABOUT BACKS 17
LIFTING 12
NECK PAIN 10
PROPER ADULT POSTURE 9

PEDIATRICS
FOR CHILDREN
ABOUT THE HUMAN BODY 13
BOY TO MAN 17
CIRCULATION AND THE HUMAN BODY 10
EXPLORING YOUR GROWTH 11
FERTILIZATION AND BIRTH 10
GIRL TO WOMAN 16
HOW A HAMBURGER TURNS INTO YOU 20
HUMAN HEREDITY 18
SNEEZES AND SNIFFLES 10
SNIFFY ESCAPES POISONING 7
WINNIE-THE-POOH 12

FOR YOUNG ADULTS
ABOUT SEX 23

ABOUT CHILD CARE
ACCIDENTS AND POISONING 7
ALLERGY 6
APPEARANCE OF THE NEWBORN 13
BATHS AND BABIES 18
BOTTLE FEEDING 14
BREAST FEEDING 13
FIRST TWO WEEKS OF LIFE 17
FORMULA PREPARATION 7
GROWTH AND DEVELOPMENT 6
HEALTH CARE OF THE NORMAL INFANT 12
IMMUNIZATIONS 3
INTESTINAL DISTURBANCES 6
LEARNING DISABILITIES, PART 1 60
LEARNING DISABILITIES, PART 2 60
MANAGEMENT OF BREAST FEEDING 14
NORMAL PATTERNS OF DEVELOPMENT 12
THE PHENOMENA OF EARLY DEVELOPMENT 15
THE PREMATURE INFANT 10
SKIN CARE AND BATHING, PART 1 11
SKIN CARE AND BATHING, PART 2 12
TOILET TRAINING 5
YOUR NEW BABY 18

SURGERY
ANESTHESIA 6
HOW TO APPLY WETPACKS 6
VARICOSE VEINS 7

UROLOGY
INFECTIONS AND INFLAMMATIONS OF THE URINARY TRACT IN WOMEN 15
THE PROSTATE 10
VASECTOMY 16

MISCELLANEOUS
DRUGS
ALCOHOLISM: OUT OF THE SHADOWS 30
DARKNESS, DARKNESS (HEROIN) 25

*Figures following films refer to length of film in minutes.

Figure 12-20. Health library film list.

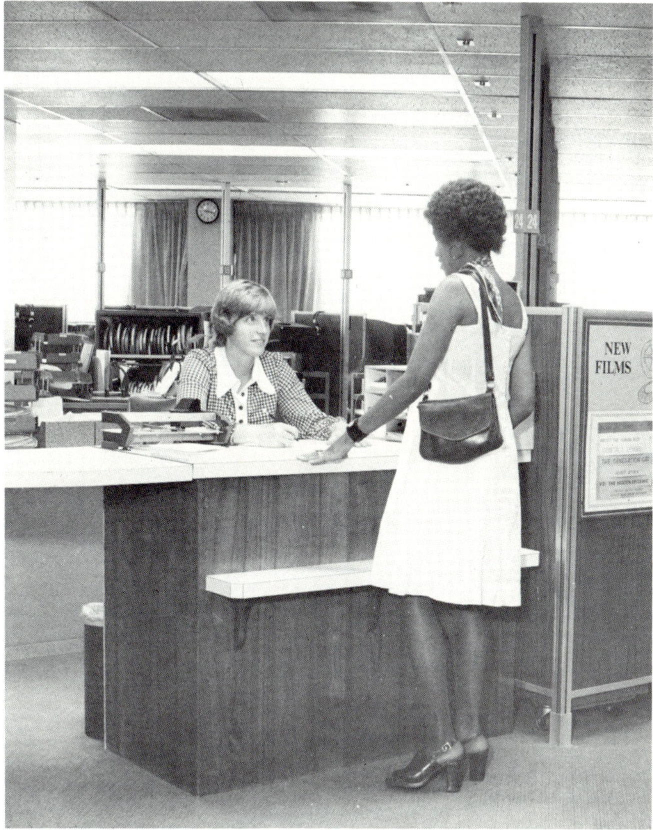

Figure 12-21.   Assistance to a library visitor.

Data gathered on library utilization included personal statistics (sex, birth date, medical record number, referral source, or, if self-referred, whether a first or repeat visit, etc.) and materials used during the visit. After keypunching for statistical computation by the computer, the records of those who were health plan members were sent for insertion in the patient's chart. The physician was thus kept apprised of compliance with his referral to the library, what educational materials were used, and what, if any, other resource referrals were made.

Beginning orientation of provider staff to the library facility took the form of noon meetings for physicians and invitational guided tours for administrative and employee personnel. House staff were acquainted with the setting shortly after their internship experience began each year. For the community, open-house events were conducted, and notices of programs (Figure 12-22) were posted in public areas. Periodic news coverage was maintained in both the house and membership bulletins.

Adoption of the library service as an adjunctive arm of the health care delivery system was a gradual process. From a beginning count of 82 persons in its first month of operation, July 1969, steady growth reached an attendance peak of 1,012 visitors during one month in July–December 1973. Figure 12-23 illustrates the

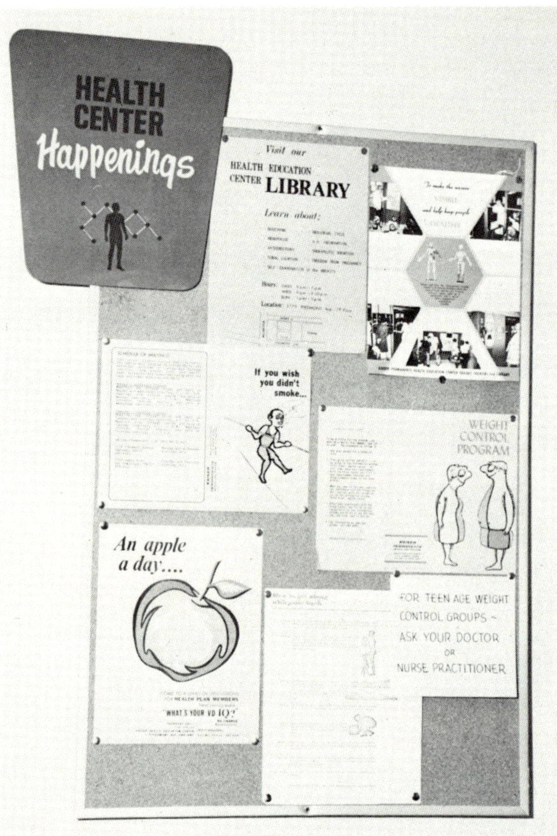

Figure 12-22. Bulletin board program notices.

utilization of the library in six-month increments, giving attendance figures and film showings to individuals.

Examination of attendance records to determine viewer characteristics (Figure 12-24) disclosed that women users outnumbered men by a wide margin. One reason might be the very active referrals made to the library by the family planning and prenatal services. A large majority of the visitors were discovered to belong to the younger age categories and to have rather high academic standing, with an impressive proportion having college or postgraduate education. This finding served to corroborate the documentation of other studies[39] that the better educated avail themselves more readily of educational opportunities, and pointed up the need for some effort to reach those of lower educational achievement, who could profit at least as much as the library users.

Referrals by medical providers confirmed the finding in the original preliminary survey of physicians, 31 percent of whom had expressed interest, and 25 to 32 percent of whom were actually making referrals. An additional 14 to 24 percent of referrals from the nursing and other health worker staff brought the total referrals from professional sources to approximately one-half of the library attendees (Figure 12-25). Having been once exposed to this setting, approximately 35 to 40 percent made return visits.

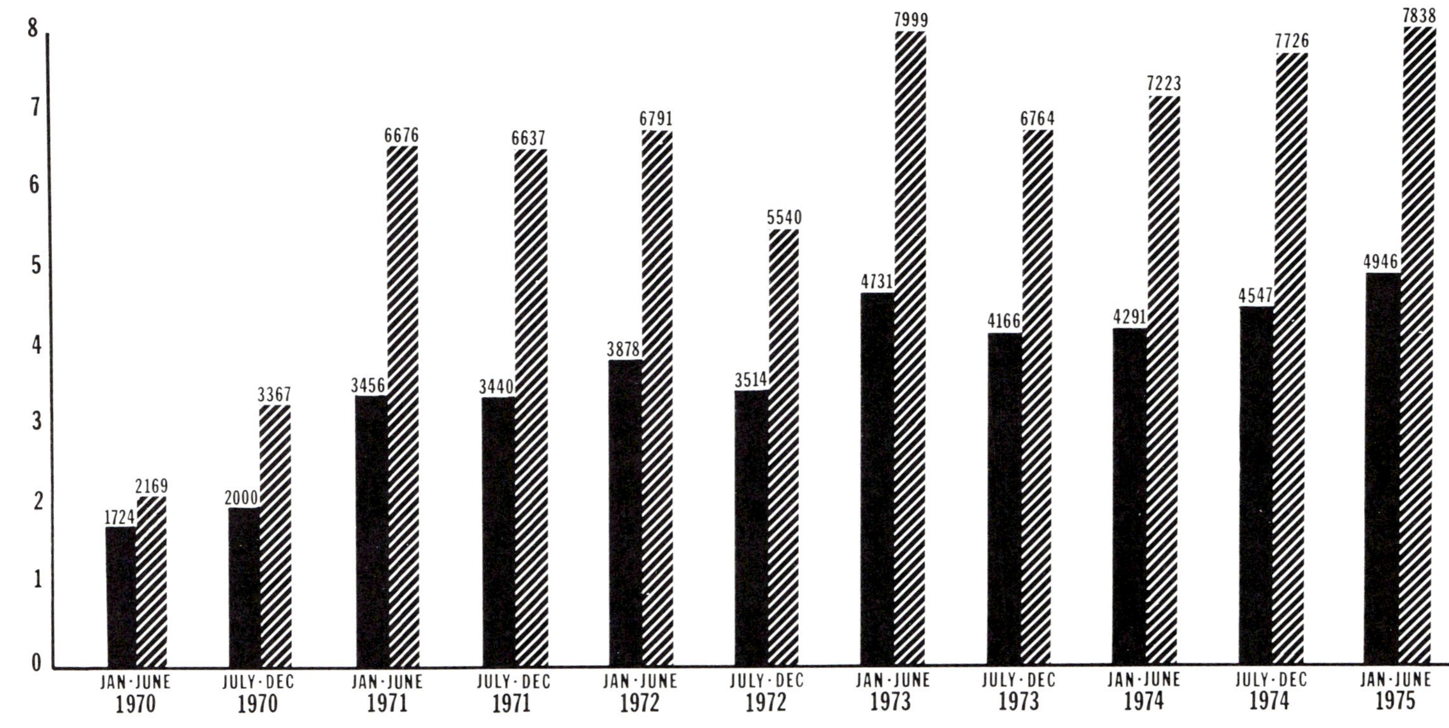

Figure 12-23. Library utilization by attendance and film showings.

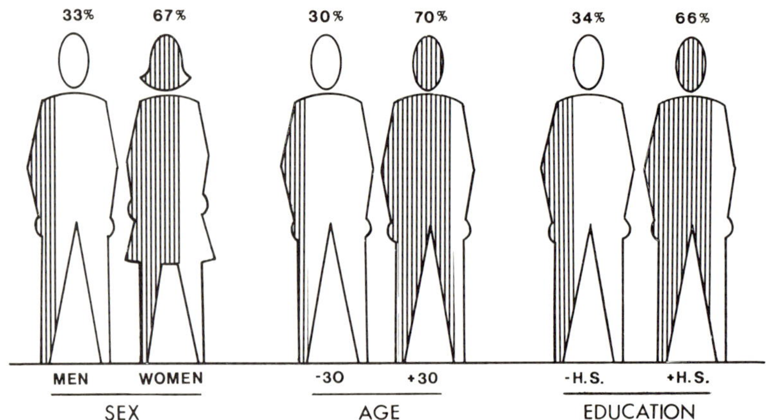

Figure 12-24. Library visitor characteristics.

Questionnaire responses showed a high degree of patient/visitor satisfaction with the library concept and the services rendered (Figure 12-26). Viewed as a complement to health care, the great majority of users felt it was both helpful and necessary and perceived the quality of materials available as good to excellent. In these terms the library did seem to be fulfilling its purpose of serving as an educational resource and information center that could help guide patients through a complex health care system and add to their health knowledge. Inclusive of referrals, repeat visits, and film usage by classes and clinics, the numbers exposed to library film programs rose to some 800 persons monthly. However, a breakdown analysis showed that inadequate use of this referral center was made by other than the prenatal and family planning clinics of the medical center.[36] The number of persons that could be conveniently served in the library was projected at 50 to 60 per day. In 1975, based on a 48-hour work, double the number of referrals could be easily accommodated. The enlistment of more active referral support from physicians and provider staff, while recognized as essential to the

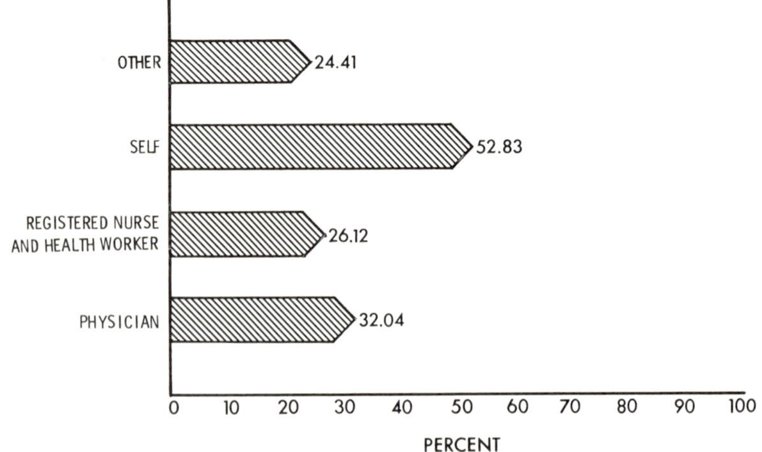

Figure 12-25. Source of referrals to patient health library.

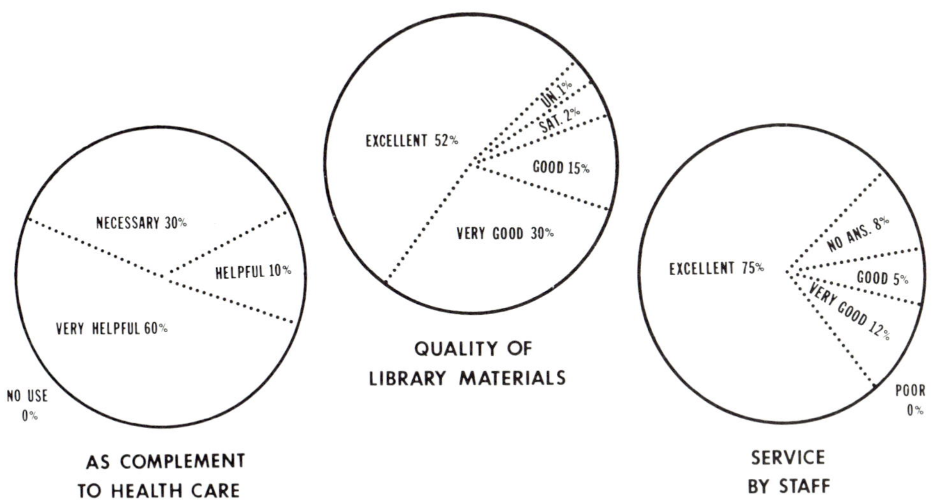

Figure 12-26. Library user's reactions.

successful library operation, was extremely difficult to achieve for a number of valid reasons. Among these were (1) the newness and unfamiliarity of this concept, (2) the neglect in the education of physicians and other care personnel of the value of such a service, and its consequent omission as a resource from their traditional armament of prescriptive choices, (3) its uniqueness and unproven status, (4) the time, effort, and cost of in-depth in-service education through contacts, reports, and whatever other approaches might make and keep the library actively visible.

Examination of developmental and purchase records revealed starting costs (including building of furniture and equipment, installation of hardware, and acquisition of software materials) to be close to $22,000. Monthly operating costs, including staffing, amounted to under $3,000. On this basis, the cost per visitor was figured at $3,85, without assigning any cost to persons participating in classes or clinics where library materials were used. Since service could be provided without additional expense to a far larger number of visitors, this unit cost could easily be reduced. Successful operation of the library at or near its potential thus called for finding ways to increase patient arrivals after referral, and for more active public relations promotion. Present efforts toward improving staff relations and library awareness include quarterly reports, periodic distribution of updated listings of materials, requests for preview assistance, attempts to involve the physicians in consultations, open-house events for house staff, talks to the various individual divisions of the center, and requests for suggestions and lists of materials needed by the providers for patient education. Special referral forms to some of the clinics (e.g. diabetes, hypertension, etc.) have been developed and distributed. Miscellaneous services not covered by the hospital medical library also are handled, such as patient education article files, search, and interlibrary loans. In 1975, over 20,000 pamphlets were made available to the clinics for distribution to patients. Gradually these efforts have brought results, such as the long-term loan of film programs for patient orientation in the surgery clinic examining rooms, the hospital post-partum room, and the medical and pediatric clinic waiting rooms.

The library, like any new idea, had to overcome the usual resistance to change, which required a tremendous and persistent tenacity. From the vision and initial actualization of a concept to its acceptance and utilization as a promising and effective resource the gap remains wide indeed. With the establishment in 1971 of a national Presidential Committee to determine the needs of the American people for education to health, and to develop appropriate programs and avenues, recognition of a health library as a valuable approach might encourage the providers to better utilize it as a resource, and with effective promotion sanctioned by their authoritative positions, lay persons would more willingly avail themselves of the educational opportunities such a library offers. Over time, it is hoped the value of the patient health library and its increased utilization, which reduces its cost, will permit it to serve its intended function and fulfill the objectives for which it was established, both as an adjunct to the multiphasic program and in service to all patients, care providers, and the community.

3. Exhibits

In accordance with the ancient adage that a picture is worth a thousand words, the role of exhibits as an effective communication medium in general education of the lay public has long been accepted.[40] Their lure in the health field has been evident in world fairs, specifically developed health fairs sponsored by medical societies and other organizations,[41] and halls of health in museums of science and industry in major cities.[42] Separate health museums, utilizing multimedia approaches, have been established at Cleveland, Hinsdale, Ashville, Dallas, Fort Worth, Kansas City, Portland, Los Angeles, New York, Washington, and elsewhere.[43] Within a medical care setting Lankenau Hospital in Philadelphia and Reading Hospital in Reading, Pennsylvania,[44] have long used three-dimensional educational devices for improving understanding of disease conditions.

In conformance with the objective "to provide general health education . . . regarding preventive medical measures,"[27] the value of incorporating exhibits into the health education center, which was to be established as a pilot at the Oakland facility, was immediately recognized. In fact, its potential merit as an educational resource for persons involved in comprehensive ambulatory care, and for members of the general community, determined the administrative decision to open access to this arena free of charge to all.

Plans for the allocated 2,000 square feet of space (Figure 12-27) centered around developing exhibits that would concentrate upon making important aspects of normal health visible, and would emphasize positive approaches regarding how to minimize health hazard risks. Hence the focus would be on "care for health" rather than treatment of illness alone.[25]

The objectives established were to:

(1) Provide a physical facility that would offer Kaiser Foundation Health Plan members an exposure to a visible educational area dealing with positive health.

(2) Develop exhibits that could (a) stimulate awareness of and interest in identifying with personal health, (b) disseminate accurate health information, (c) clarify misconceptions and increase understandings about health, (d) place a high value on health maintenance and protection by the individual, (e) supplement other avenues of health education, and (f) be presented in lively enough fashion so

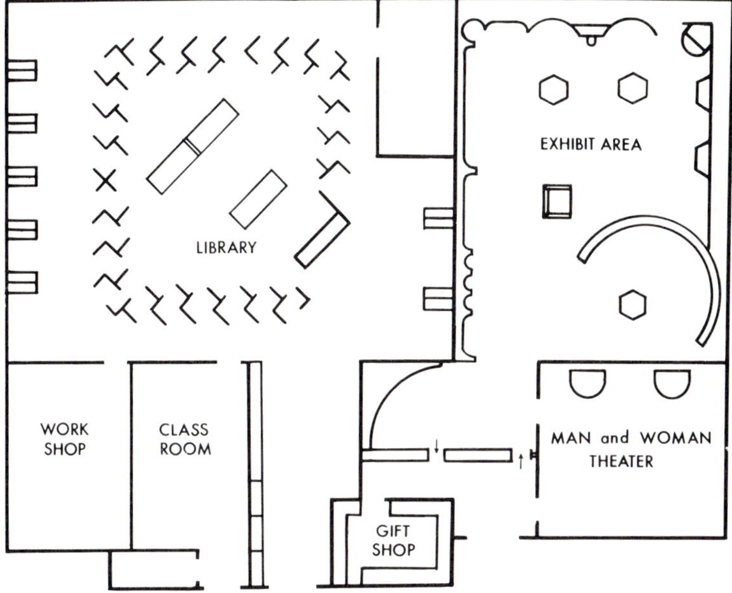

Figure 12-27.   Floor plan of educational areas.

as to encourage repeated visits and to motivate visitors to recommend their viewing to relatives and friends.

(3) Serve as a referral source for physicians, nurses, and other health workers, educators, etc.

(4) Provide opportunities for in-service education of allied health personnel, such as student nurses, aides, and volunteers.

(5) Serve the community at large as a resource for authentic health information.

These objectives were to be accomplished by:

(1) Developing exhibits that, through appropriateness of information, effective visual, auditory, and printed formats, and simplicity of language and presentation would offer outstanding appeal to the viewer.

(2) Providing for interactive participation so as to involve the individual directly in the learning process.

(3) Encouraging active responses through guided tours, questionnaires, suggestion box, and the like.

(4) Keeping the exhibits dynamic, updated, and in continuously good working order.

Under the overall theme "You have only one life to live—live it in good health," selected exhibits were purchased or created, developed, and constructed on site. The space allowed was divided into three areas:

(1) A small sales shop. Here the visitor could buy health-related materials such as books (on care of the back, care of the feet, the human body, infant care, learning disabilities, etc.), models of body parts and organs, body care sundries, and so on (Figure 12-28).

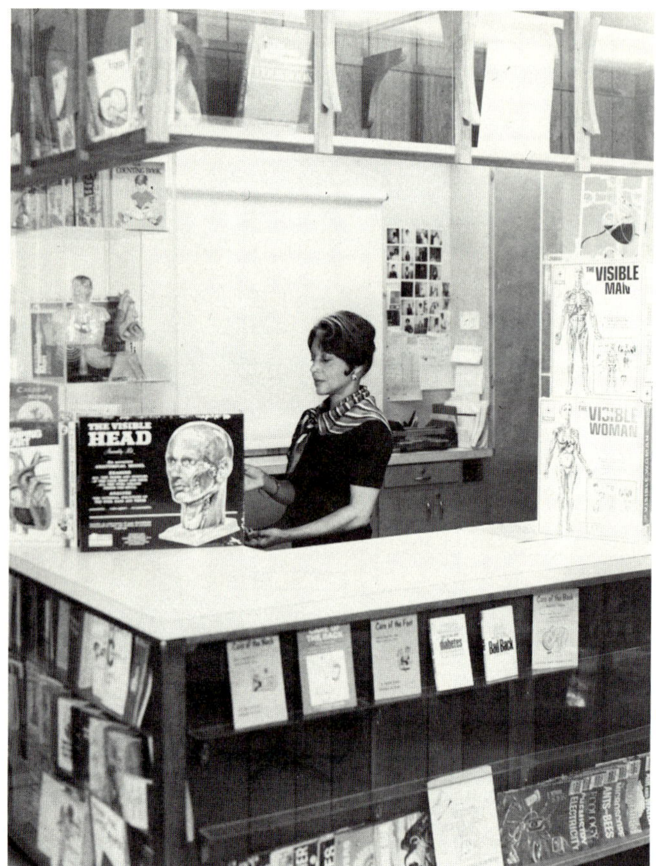

Figure 12-28. Health-related sales shop.

(2) The dialogue theater. Two life-size transparent figures, named Adam and Eve (Figure 12-29), were purchased and placed in a specially constructed 36-seat theater setting. As they slowly revolved under black ultraviolet light, they conducted a 20-minute dialogue about their anatomy, physiology, and body care, during which time their various accurately simulated internal organs were illuminated in sequential synchronization to their talk. In accompaniment, a set of colored illustrative slides was projected on a screen between them, to enhance the presentation into an effective multimedia experience. When not in performance, these figures could be inspected from a large window in the exhibits area.

(3) The exhibits area. Selected exhibits on display included:

(a) Human Reproduction. This exhibit had two major portions, "The Story of Life" and "Family Planning." The first (Figure 12-30) began with observation of the transparent couple and proceeded to life-sized three-dimensional models of the male and female reproductive systems. "How Life Begins" was a panel containing an enlarged model of the uterus within which sequentially lighted eggs moved through the ovaries, fallopian tubes, and uterus to demonstrate fertilization of the ovum, cell division, and implantation. "Stages of Pregnancy" was a hexagonal component containing fetal models, the sequential lighting of which

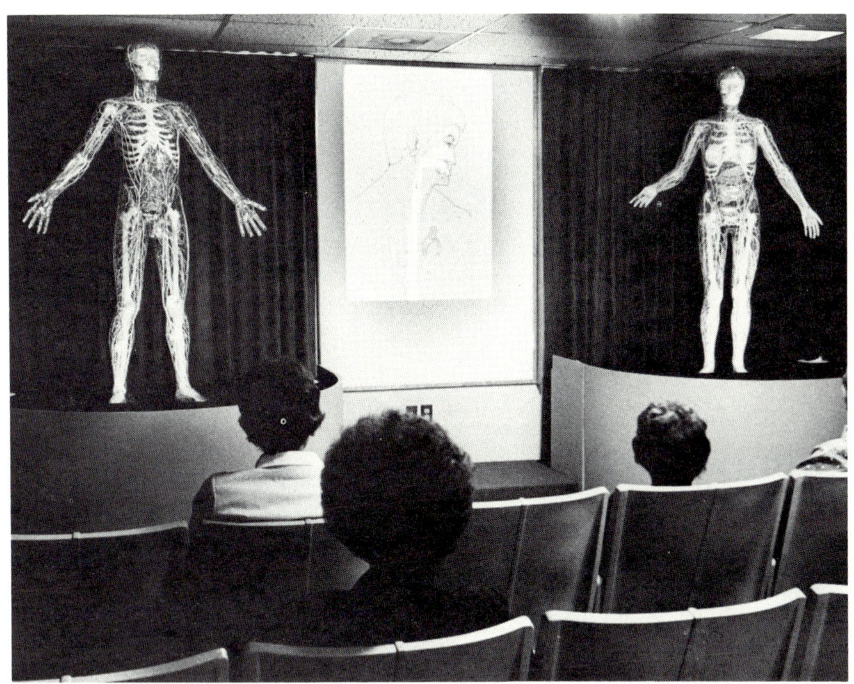

Figure 12-29. The transparent couple.

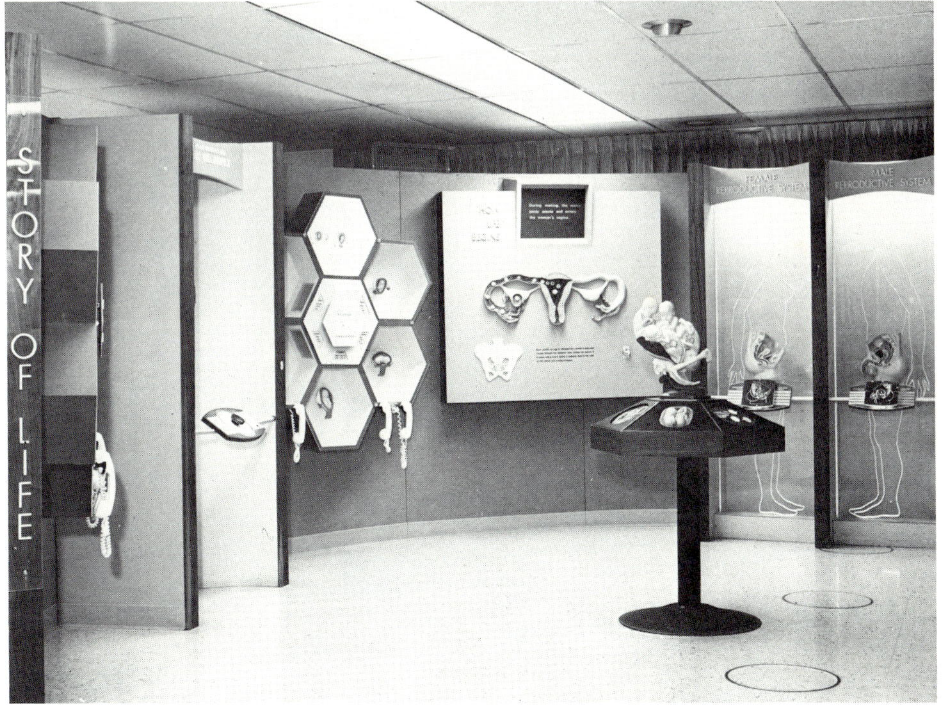

Figure 12-30. "Story of Life" exhibit.

was synchronized to a narrative tape. A model of a pregnant woman demonstrated fetal development in utero. "Stages of Labor," a hexagonal display case, held realistically painted models with an audiotape describing a single, normal delivery, a pedestal pertaining to multiple births, illustrated graphic transparencies on identical and fraternal twins, and a three-dimensional model of quintuplets positioned inside the pelvic girdle.

In the family planning portion (Figure 12-31), messages on the advantages of having a planned child and the problems attendant to population explosion were depicted against a sequentially lighted pictorial background. Information on suitable acceptable contraceptive methods was placed on a drum that could be manipulated by the viewer.

(b) Body Development (Figure 12-32). Exhibits here included displays on body systems, a series of silent filmstrips in separate projectors, a thin-man chart, body organs (preserved and colored specimens embedded in plastic), a skeleton with lighted side panels for front- and rear-view bone classifications, a participatory exhibit on proper body mechanics, and models of the hand, foot, cells, skin, eye, ear, and body senses (Figure 12-33).

(c) The Healthy Heart (Figure 12-34). In addition to animated chart information on the heart and circulatory system, the visitor was provided with a participatory

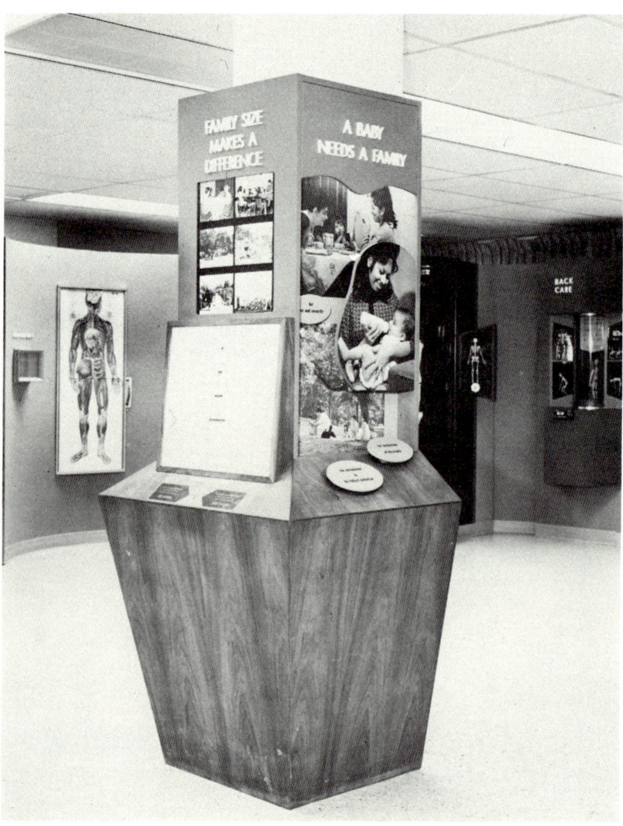

Figure 12-31.   Family planning exhibit.

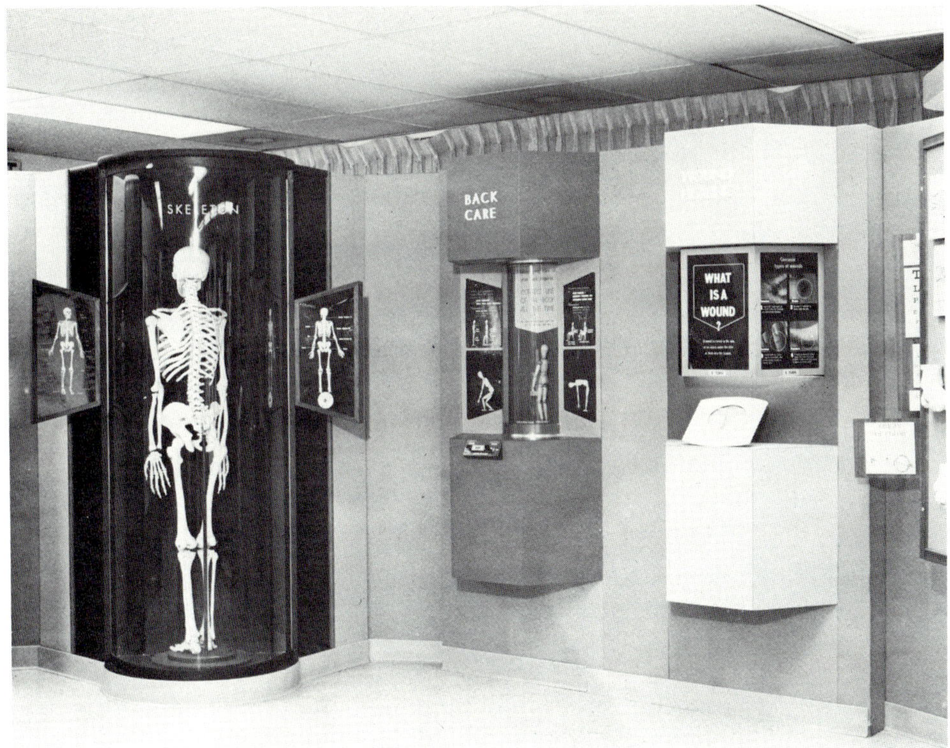

Figure 12-32.   Body care and development exhibit.

opportunity to see his own heart beat via a simulated model, and to check his own pulse rate before and after exercise.

(d) Health Hazards (Figures 12-35, 12-36). Selected exhibits with participatory features, using mirrors and charts, pertained to the problems of overweight and malnutrition. A cigarette-smoking display contained two preserved lungs, one of a smoker and the other of a nonsmoker, and charts. Information on medical quackery utilized actual fraudulent devices. A panel on cancer detection listed the seven warning signals. A filmstrip program gave information on venereal disease. A lighted panel, which the viewer controlled, gave information on the effect of drugs and drug abuse on the brain.

(e) Pathways to Positive Health (Figure 12-37). This area accentuated health protection and maintenance by attending to nutritional needs, dental hygiene, and the physical, mental, emotional, and social aspects of good health. The ease and low cost of safeguarding a home for children was also visually displayed (Figure 12-38). An "Ask the Juke Box" exhibit (Figure 12-39) let the visitor play taped health messages on commonly asked questions regarding health and disease. A suggestion box requested comments to guide future modifications and developments.

Attendance records, kept since the opening of the exhibit theaters on Thanksgiving Day, 1969, showed an average monthly attendance of about one thousand. Promotional and publicity activities were minimal; attraction to this service depended chiefly on the distribution of a descriptive brochure (Figure

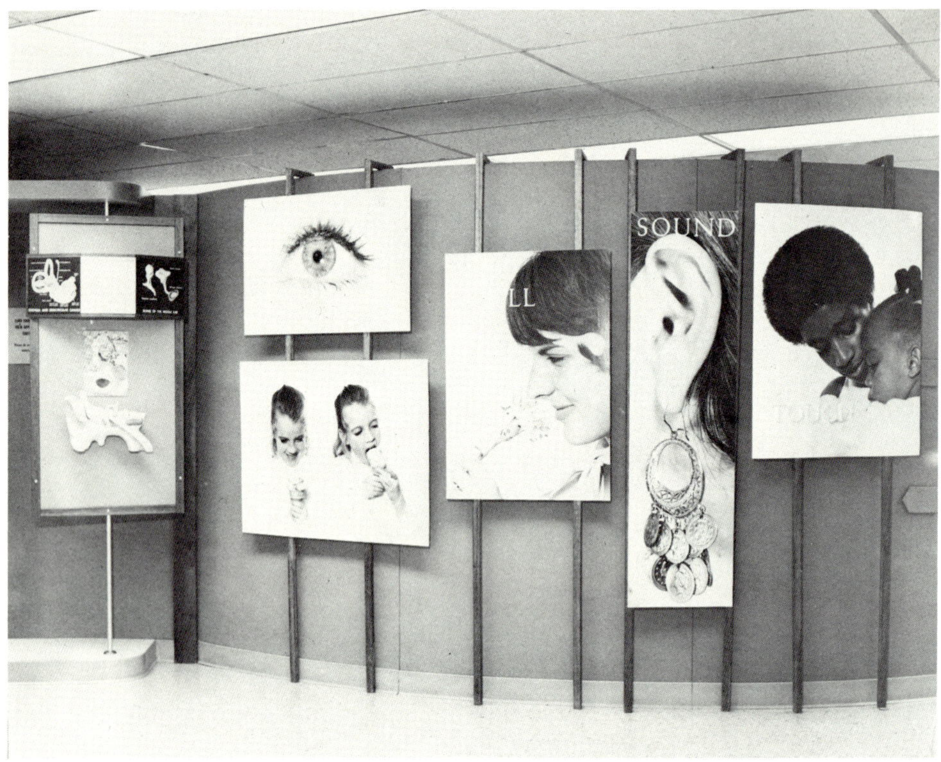

Figure 12-33.   Five senses display.

12–14), referrals from the multiphasic program and other medical and health providers, and word of mouth. As awareness of the exhibit theaters spread to the public, the need for providing conducted tours became evident, and a volunteer tour guide or docent program was developed. A training program was provided for interested persons having some subject-matter background, a handbook manual was prepared, and an orientation guidebook was printed for teachers and leaders of incoming groups. Advance bookings included a preview orientation of the group leader and the completion of records giving specific information on the group, their number, needs, and requests. Every effort was made to provide one tour guide for every fifteen students in the group, with the expectation that there were sufficient accompanying adults to forestall any disciplinary problems. To enhance the educational experience of the visitors, some form of feedback report was occasionally requested. The originality and ingenuity of some of the responses led to the posting of these on a "Feedback Board" to permit sharing with newer visitors. Examination of the record forms revealed consistent bookings by teachers of classes, especially in the middle grades, from schools in the surrounding communities. Instructors of students in the allied health field and the community colleges also had been sending in their students. While sources of referrals from the medical center provider staff were not specifically recorded, supplies of brochures were made available to the various clinics and especially the multiphasic program. Occasional spot checking disclosed visits by family members of

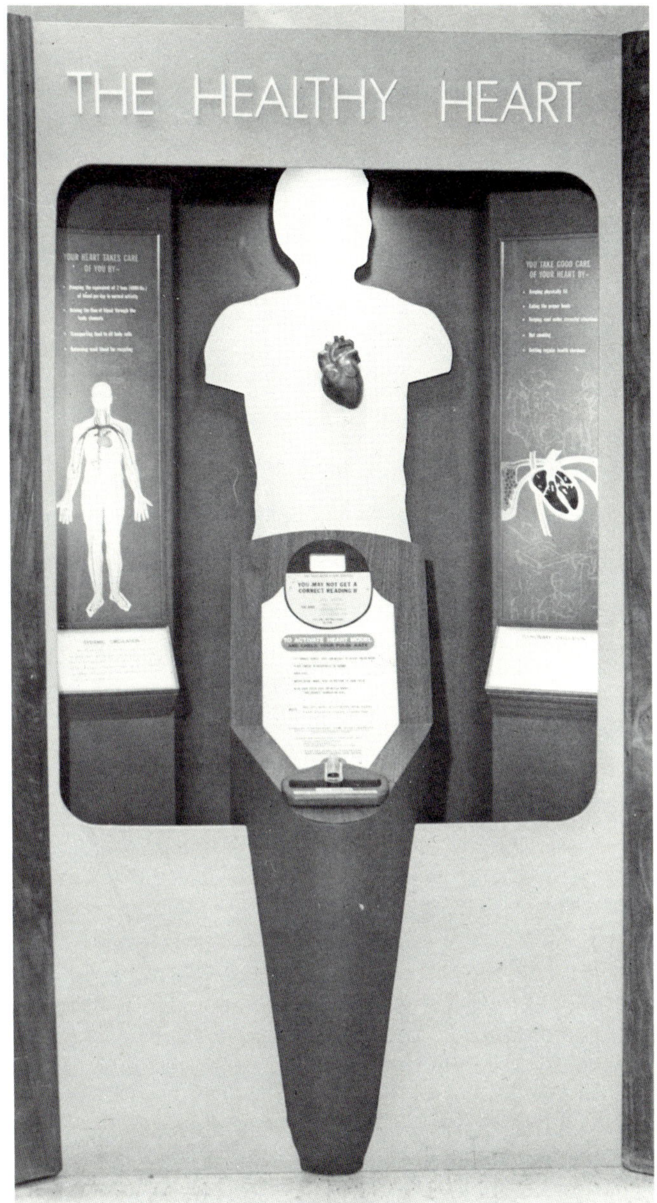

Figure 12-34.   Healthy heart exhibit.

a patient with a recent heart attack, a father discussing ''The Story of Life'' with a son of puberty age, or a mother in similar exchange with a young daughter, a visually handicapped youngster being helped to feel an anatomical model, some youths engaged in working the panels pertaining to drug abuse, venereal disease, and smoking, or an elderly couple at the ''Ask the Jukebox'' machine.

A small evaluative study was conducted to determine the characteristics of

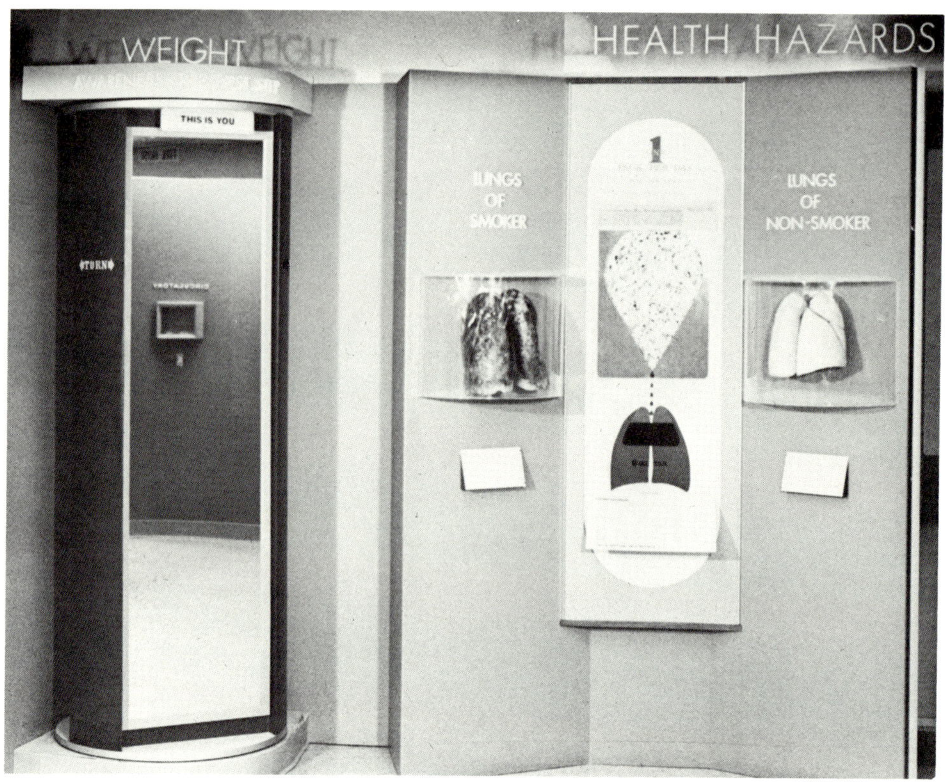

Figure 12-35. Health hazards: smoking and weight problems.

visitors attracted to the exhibits (Figure 12-40). Responses from 238 viewers revealed about two-thirds to be under 30; over 70 percent were women; 46 percent had some education beyond high school; approximately two-thirds were non-Kaiser Health Plan members; and one out of five visitors was nonwhite. Of this sample, 95 percent expressed interest in returning for a repeat visit, and 99 percent would recommend it to others.

A registration log drew voluntary signatures and addresses of viewers from all states of the Union and all parts of the world, including Canada, Europe, Asia, Australia, South America, Africa, and India. Numerous requests regarding these displays and exhibits have been made, and the intent to emulate many of them has been expressed. At least one similar hall of exhibits patterned after this model has been developed locally.

For the first five years of existence the costs of exhibit construction, installation, and purchases totaled in excess of $30,000. Annual expenses for maintenance, repairs, and updating, including staffing, amounted to approximately $40,000. Calculated for the year 1973, which saw a visitor attendance of 9,500 persons, the cost per visitor was $4.30.

Even more than for the health library, utilization of the exhibit theaters fell far short of its potential goal. Of the average of 51 visitors per day (on a 48-hour week) only 12 were members of the health plan and 39 were from the general public. The number of persons who could easily be accommodated was well over 300 per day.

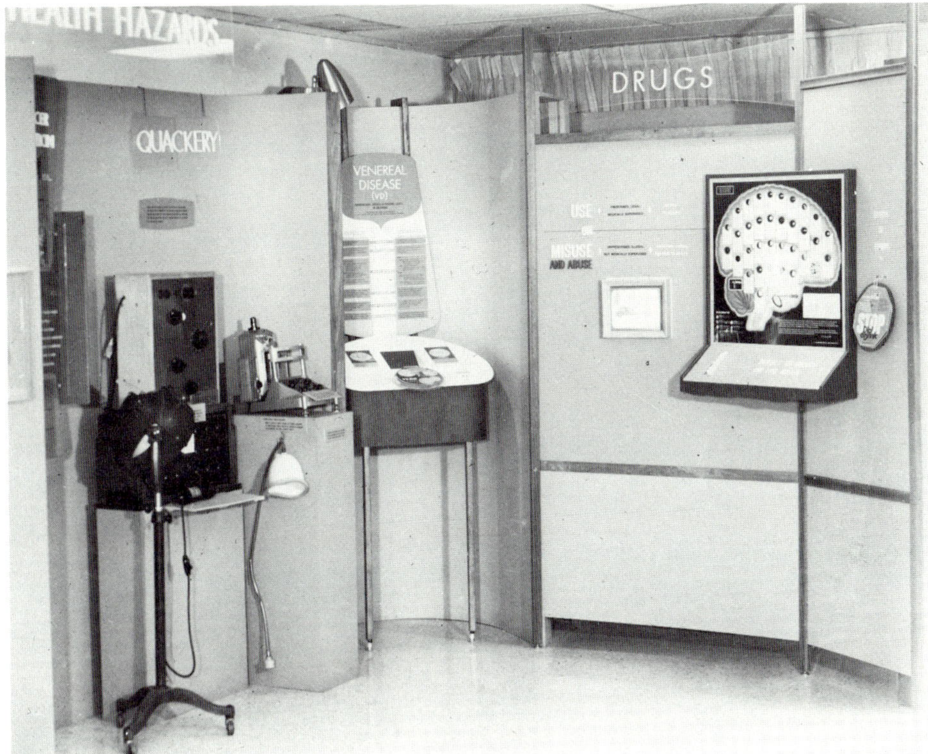

Figure 12-36.   Health hazards: drug abuse, VD and quackery.

Thus the present numbers could be multiplied sixfold if the rate of referrals from medical care providers could be increased. All of the problems and limitations discussed for the library pertain to the exhibits as well. Recognition of the exhibits as a valuable tool for lay education to health[46] must somehow be expressed not only through lip service but by specific referrals and encouragement of patient arrivals as well. With effective promotion by those in positions of authority and leadership, there is no doubt that exhibits and displays can serve a useful function in helping persons of all ages to become a better informed, alerted populace and in guiding them toward gaining meaningful insights into their individual responsible role in health maintenance and protection.

4.   Educational Forums

The educational components developed for the several preventive maintenance clinics (diabetes, hypertension, family planning, lipid, back care, etc.) as complementary to inpatient education for coronary sufferers and their families and for those with respiratory conditions and health concerns are reported in Chapter Eleven. The need remained for formalized member education, as expressed in the 1,287 responses to a preliminary survey conducted before the establishment of the health education center. On the basis of the ranked order of potential subject-matter areas, monthly evening sessions were planned, invitational letters mailed,

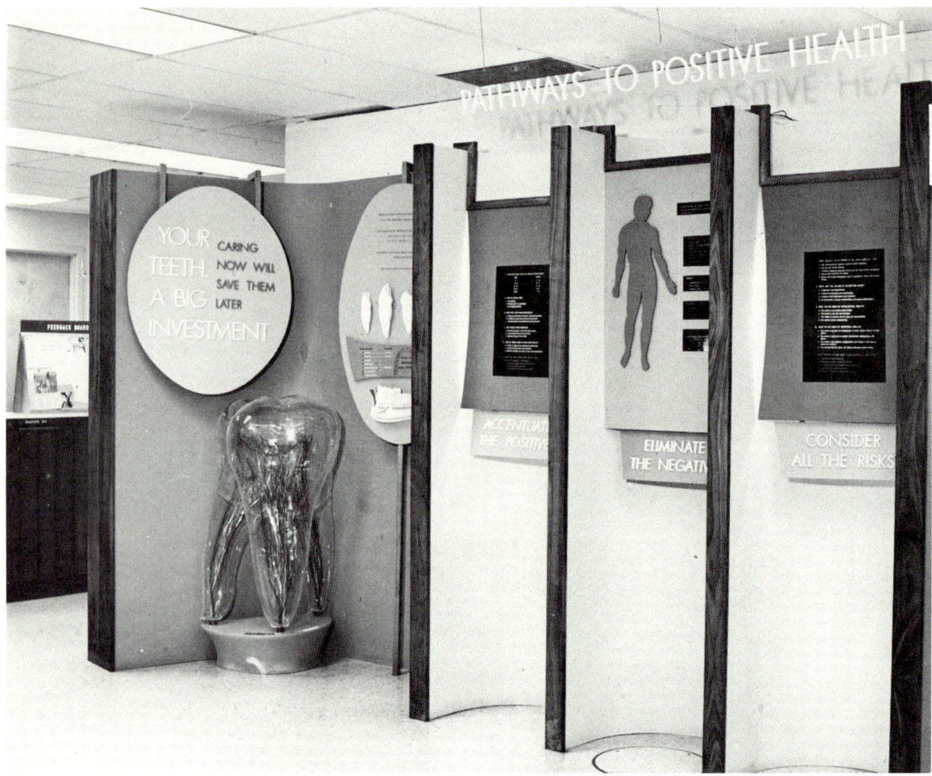

Figure 12-37. Pathways to positive health.

and attractive posters (Figure 12–22) attached to bulletin boards in the library, halls, and clinic areas. Since the program's inception in 1970, educational topics have included allergies, cancer, heart trouble, hypertension, mental illness, nutrition, sickle cell anemia, back problems, and others (Figure 12–41). Reaction sheets and questionnaires have been periodically distributed in an effort to improve attendance by treating relevant subjects of interest. A repeat interest survey, conducted in the summer of 1974, formed the basis for scheduled meetings on human sexuality and learning disabilities and repeat sessions on some already conducted, such as hypertension, mental health and tensions, and nutrition and disease control. Working relationships established with the member relations department of the health plan and with the public relations division permitted collaboration for provision of regular publicity in the organization bulletins and community newsprint media. Use of the meeting room for such community groups as the Diabetes Association and Consumers Cooperative Association helped promote considerable good will and cooperation. Erratic attendance figures stemmed not only from the competition of television programs, and the reluctance of people to leave their homes at night, but also from the physical setting, which did not enjoy a fine reputation as a safe neighborhood. Satisfaction with the quality of meetings, as expressed by those who attended, was very high. Costs to the administration were reduced because publicity expenses were ab-

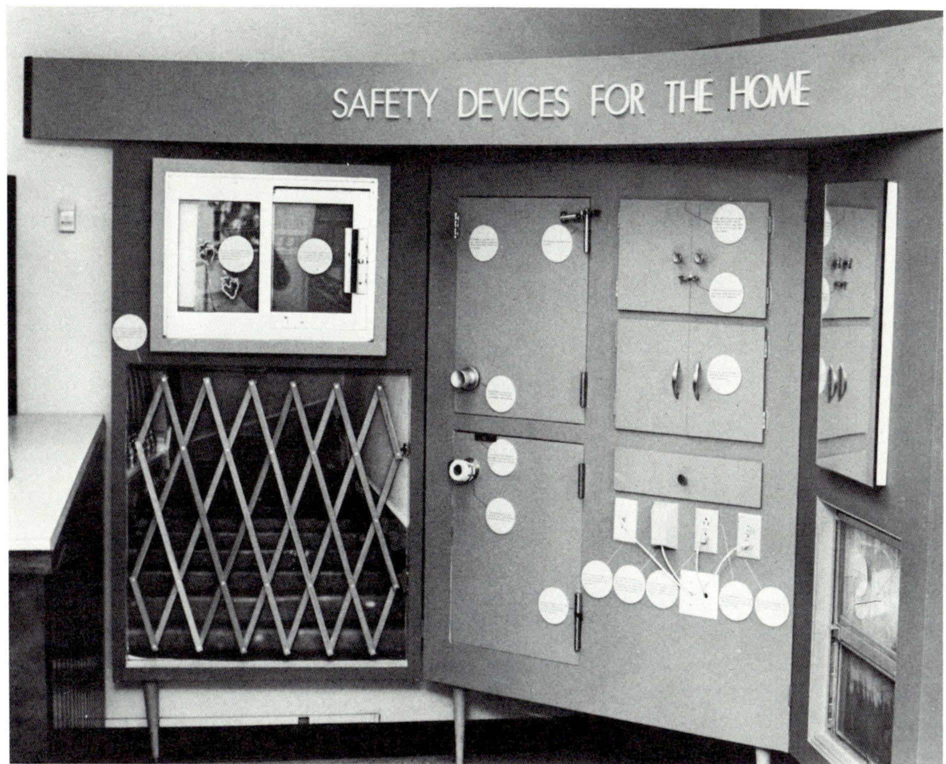

Figure 12-38.   Safety in the home exhibit.

sorbed by the Kaiser-Permanente public relations department, and guest speakers contributed their time. The program was deemed to be of especial value to those who can best improve their inadequate knowledge of health care by hearing and questioning an authority in a medical care setting. Since "human health is too precious a gift to disregard, and disease costs too high to be afforded, even by the richest societies,"[47] such a focus provided by health education meetings could well serve to bring individuals in earlier for good quality medical and health care, with emphasis upon preventive measures. This kind of education of the public can well be directed to teaching persons how to decrease their need for and dependence on remedial treatment by making it feasible to "change the focus from complaint response to health maintenance . . . and under health surveillance to bring significant symptoms promptly to medical attention."[28] As reported in the literature, knowledge regarding illness and health "like almost any other subject is distributed through the public in a J curve; many persons have a vague idea of some information items. . . . Health knowledge can be affected by time, the parade of events,"[10] and by such variables as age, sex, level of education, depth of attention, etc. The promise of educational forums, where relevant subjects are dealt with by reliable authorities, and which focus on prevention and the individual's role in health maintenance, is that of assisting in the redirection of demand for services by an alerted and more knowledgeable patient population.

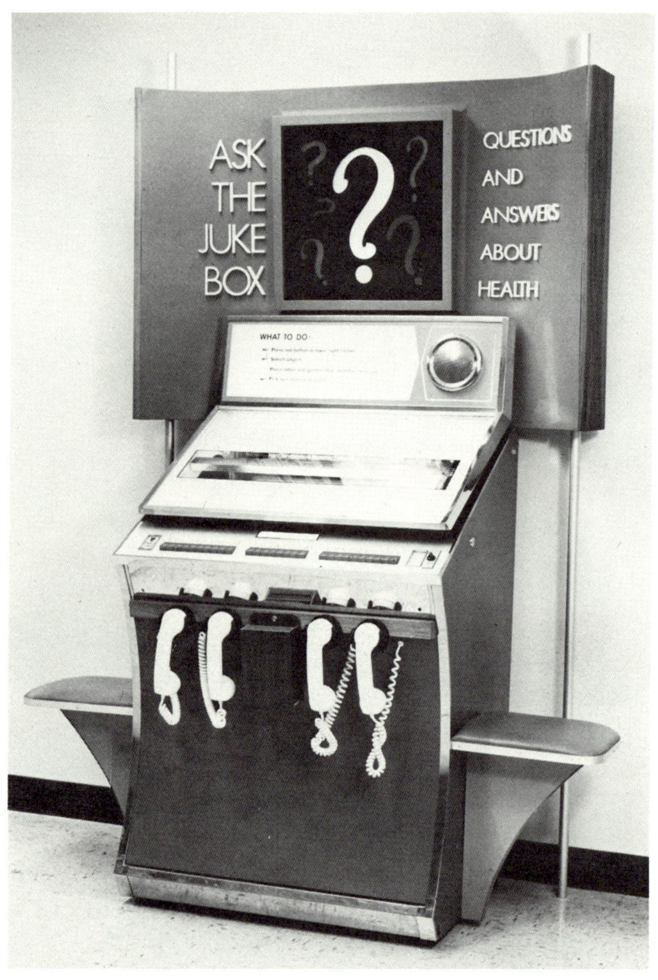

Figure 12-39. ''Ask the Jukebox'' exhibit.

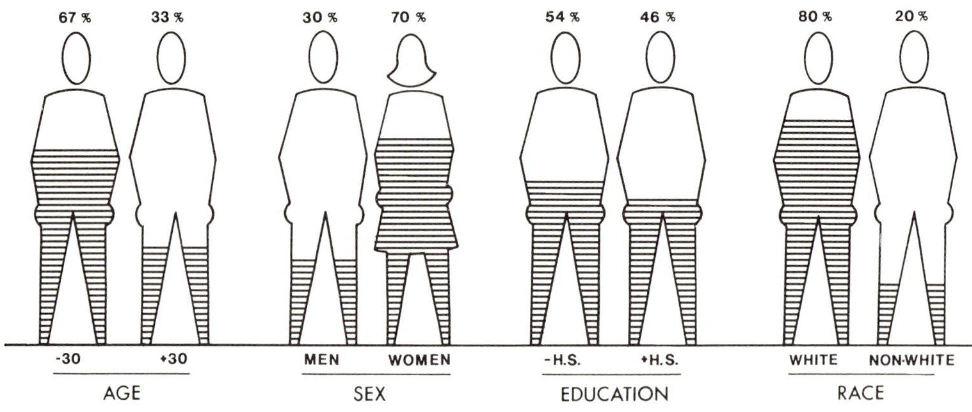

Figure 12-40. Exhibit viewer characteristics.

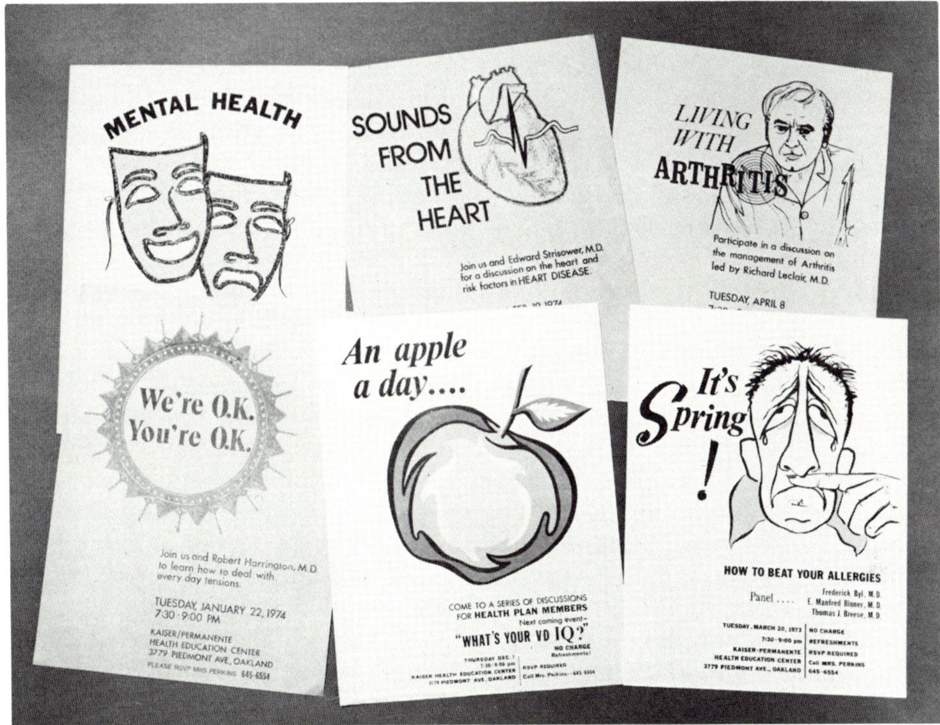

Figure 12-41. Member education meeting posters.

E. SUMMARY AND CONCLUSIONS

The planning, development, and establishment at the Kaiser-Permanente Medical Center in Oakland, California, of a formalized educational component within and in association with the automated multiphasic health testing service has been a pioneering effort with no known forerunner to serve as a model. This chapter has described its various parts and discussed their operation, costs, potential value, strengths, and limitations. Evaluation of some portions has been undertaken and patient acceptance and satisfaction explored. It is readily admitted, as several studies have indicated, that impressive discrepancies exist between the high standards of medical and good health care offered, and the actual responsive behavior of people.[48,49] Attention to health practices is doubtless related to opportune learning situations and the level of people's anxieties. It is well known that "most people organize their defenses when they first perceive symptoms that threaten their health . . . nearly everyone delays taking action for at least a short time. This period of delay permits adaptation to the threat and realignment of defenses for coping with it."[50] Also the wide range of individual differences in characteristics such as genetic constitution, intelligence, coping with stress situations, prior experiences, and general behavior patterns[51] must be taken into account. Thus the challenge for organized educational opportunities lies not only in making these available but also in reaching out to interest and arouse persons at an early time, in developing interactive relationships during and after the delivery of health care, and in discovering methods for motivating individuals to assume an active participatory role in their own health care for optimum well-being.[57]

Much remains to be done. Concerted efforts need to be made by providers to recognize the conflict between professionally determined medical and health needs and the way individuals perceive them, in order to minimize potential frustration and ease access to available services.[52] There should be much closer coordination between all divisions of the comprehensive care delivered at the hospital, the outpatient clinics, the ancillary services, the multiphasic program, the health education center, the home, and community institutions and media to provide human beings with a continuous health care spectrum. The establishment of a National Center for Health Education with Dr. Robert L. Johnson as President was a step in the right direction.[53]

The question has been asked: "How much better care of their health is taken by those who are better informed about health and disease than by those who are less informed?"[16] An approach to the answer has been sought through the components herein described (including interactive dialogue, counseling, group methods, classes, clubs, exhibits, displays, teaching aids, printed materials, and audiovisual programs housed in a specialized library accompanying and associated with a health testing process to discover present and potential health needs), which provide one way of "automatically elevating preventive medicine to equal status with sick care, a new first in medical history."[54] By serving this broadly based educational function, which holds promise for redirecting the focus from illness to health care,[55] such endeavor may become a model for others to emulate and improve upon, for it can be designed to fulfill the qualification requirements outlined by the national Department of Health, Education and Welfare for a health maintenance organization[56] and to fit any care setting.

REFERENCES

1. Suchman, E. A. "Health Orientation and Medical Care." *Am. J. Pub. Health* 6(1966):47–105.

2. Davis, M. S. "Variations in Patients' Compliance with Doctors' Orders." *J. Med. Education* 41(1966):1037–1048.

3. Rosenberg, S. G. "A Case for Patient Education." *Hospital Formulary Management* 6(1971):14–17.

4. American Public Health Association. "A Model for Planning Patient Education." Report of the Committee on Educational Tasks in Chronic Illness, APHA, Public Health Education Section, October 1970.

5. Simonds, S. K. "Validation, Acceptance and Utilization of Patient Education in the Total Health Care System." Paper presented at Conference in Health Education of the American Hospital Association, Chicago, October 1969.

6. Feldman, J. *The Dissemination of Health Information.* Chicago: Aldine Press, 1966.

7. Freeman, H. E., et al. "Patient-Practitioner Relationships." In *Handbook of Medical Sociology,* pp. 273–295. Englewood Cliffs, N. J.: Prentice-Hall, Inc., 1963.

8. Bloom, S. *The Doctor and His Patient.* New York: Russell Sage Foundation, 1963.

9. Seligman, A. W., et al. "Level of Medical Information among Clinic Patients." *J. Chron. Dis.* 6(1957):497–509.

10. Wade, S. E. "Trends in Public Knowledge about Health and Illness." *Am. J. Pub. Health* 60(1970):485–491.

11. Pratt, L., Seligam, A., and Reader, G. "Physicians' Views on the Level of Information among Patients." *Am. J. Pub. Health,* 47(1957):1277–1283.

12. Etzweiler, D. D. "Current Status in Patient Education," *J.A.M.A.* 220(1972):583.

13. Steiner, G. A. *The People Look at Television.* New York: Knopf, 1963.

14. Brodsky, P. N., and Sagen, O. K. "Motivations Toward Health Examinations." *Am. J. Pub. Health,* 49(1959):514–527.

15. Chez, R. A. "Teaching Resources for Patient Education." *Medical Times* 97(1969):168–174.

16. Editorial: "Better Ways to Instruct Patients." *Physician's Management Journal,* 1969, pp. 82–93.

17. Suchman, E. A. "Social Patterns of Illness and Medical Care." *J. Health and Human Behavior* 6(1965):2–16.

18. Swinehart, J. W. "Voluntary Exposure to Health Communications." *Am. J. Pub. Health,* 58(1968):1265–1275.

19. Garfield, S. R. "A New Medical Care Delivery System." *Scient. Amer.* 222(1970):15–23.

20. Collen, M. F. "The Multitest Laboratory in Health Care of the Future." *Hosp.* 41(1967).

21. Collen, F. B., et al. "The Educational Adjunct to Multiphasic Health Testing." *Prev. Med.* 2(1973):247–260.

22. Taller, S. L., and Feldman, R. "The Training and Utilization of Nurse Practitioners in Adult Health Appraisal." *Med. Care* 12(1974):40–48.

23. Soghikian, K. "Evaluation of Health Counseling Programs in Health Education." Kaiser-Permanente Health Education Center, Oakland, Annual Progress Report (1974), 4, Appendix 6.

24. Ross, H., Collen, F. B., and Soghikian, K. "Health Education Discussion Groups for Worried-Well Patients." Kaiser-Permanente Health Education Center, Oakland, California, 1972. Unpublished.

25. Collen, F. B., and Soghikian, K. "Health Exhibits Accentuate the Positive." *Hosp.* 48(March 16, 1974).

26. Collen, F. B., and Soghikian, K. "The Patient Health Library: A New Medical Care Resource." *Health Services Report,* U.S. D.H.E.W., 89(1974):236–243.

27. Collen, M. F., et al. "Provisional Guidelines for Automated Health Testing and Services," Vols. 1 and 2, pp. 4–5, 17–18, 81. Washington, D. C.: U.S. D.H.E.W. 1970.

28. Breslow, L. "An Historical Review of Multiphasic Screening." *Prev. Med.* 2(1973):176–196.

29. Collen, M. F. "Periodic Health Examination Using an Automated Multitest Laboratory." *J.A.M.A.* 195(1966):830–833.

30. Cutler, J. L., et al. "Multiphasic Checkup Evaluation Study: Methods and Population." *Prev. Med.* 2(1973):197–206.

31. Collen, M. F., et al. "Multiphasic Checkup Evaluation Study; Preliminary Cost Benefit Analysis for Middle-aged Men." *Prev. Med.* 2(1973):236–246.

32. Collen, F. B., Madero, B., and Soghikian, K. "Kaiser-Permanente Experiment in Ambulatory Care." *Am. J. Nurs.* 71(1971):1371–1374.

33. Soghikian, K., and Collen, F. B. "Acceptance of Multiphasic Screening Examinations by Patients." *Bull. N.Y. Acad. Med.* 45(1969):1366–1375.

34. Robinson, D. "Gatekeeper." *Fam. Health* 4(1972):72–74.

35. Ramcharan, S. R., et al. "Multiphasic Checkup Evaluation Study. 2. Disability and Chronic Disease After Seven Years of Multiphasic Health Checkups." *Prev. Med.* 2(1973):207–220.

36. Gay, J. R. "Education and Instruction of Patients in Private Practice." *J.A.M.A.* 167(1968):1616–1618.

37. Cox, C. J. "Time-Saver for MDs." *Med. Econ.,* September 18, 1967, pp. 101–104.

38. Busek, L. C. "Where Patients Are Their Own Paramedics." *Med. Econ.* 49(1972):115.

39. Young, M. A. C. *Health Education Monographs,* 23–28. New York: Society of Pub. Health Educ., 1968.

40. Hovland, C. L., et al. *Communication and Persuasion.* New Haven: Yal Univ. Press. 1957.

41. Derryberry, M. "Notes on Exhibits as a Health Education Medium." *U.S.P.H.S. Public Health Monographs,* 8. Washington, D.C., 1953.

42. Gebhart, B. "From Exhibits and Health Fairs to Health Museums." *The Executive,* November 1961.

43. Gebhart, B. "Health Exhibits—The Cleveland Health Museum." *Can. J. Pub. Health,* February 1960. Also, brochures from the various museums of science and industry.

44. Reports from Lankenau and Reading Hospitals.

45. Beeston, J. J. "Educating the Public: A Multi-Media Approach." *Ann. N. Y. Acad. Sci.* 142:493–496.

46. Riehle, H. "Educational Exhibits—Right On!" *Audiovisual Instruction* 16(1971):47.

47. Editorial. *Prev. Med.* 2(1973):1.

48. Kasl, S. V., and Cobb, S. "Health Behavior and Sick Role Behavior, Parts I and II." *J.A.M.A.,* 12(1966):246–266, 531–541.

49. Plaut, T. F. "Psycho-social Forces of Public Health Problems." *Internat. J. Health Educ.* 9(1966):38.

50. Bard, M. "Price of Survival for Cancer Victims." *Trans-Action* 3(1966):3.

51. Graham, S. "Sociological Aspects of Health and Illness." Chapter 9 in Faris, R. E., *Handbook of Medical Sociology,* pp. 310–348. Skokie, Ill.: Rand McNally & Co., 1964.

52. Hockbaum, G. M. "An Apple a Day: Does Fear Keep the Patient Away?" *Trans-Action,* November-December 1965.

53. Merwin, Donald J. *National Center for Health Education News Bulletin,* May 1976.

54. Garfield, S. R. "The Computer and Health Care Systems." In Collen, M. F., et al., *Hospital Computer Systems,* p. 29. New York: John Wiley & Sons, 1974.

55. Shapiro, I. "HMOs and Health Education." *Am. J. Pub. Health* 65(1975):5.

56. Report of the Task Force on Consumer Health Education. "Toward a National Policy of Health Promotion and Consumer Health Education." A working paper, National Conference on Preventive Medicine, June 1975.

57. Davies, N. E. "On Oracles, Education and the Public Weal." *J.A.M.A.* 235(1976):2845–2846.

CHAPTER THIRTEEN

Mental Health Component of Multiphasic Health Testing Services

Robert L. Harrington

A. INTRODUCTION

Many authors have summarized the advantages of integrating mental health and medical care, and a number of deterrents to this union have been noted.[1] This chapter avoids this entire stance. It is assumed that the advantages of mental health input into medical care should no longer be weighed; the issue is not *if*, but *how* mental health can be comprehensively integrated into medical care. In this chapter, an evolving integration of mental health into the medical care delivery system will be presented, using multiphasic health testing as the point of entry.

B. BASIC REQUIREMENTS OF MHTS

Before discussing the integration of the mental health component (MHC)* into the multiphasic health testing service (MHTS), it is worthwhile to examine the basic tenets of MHTS:

There exists a data set of information about an individual that is extremely useful to the medical decision maker (MDM).†

This information can be gathered from a large number of individuals by a specialized service prior to the MDM visit.

This prior knowledge increases the comprehensiveness, efficiency, and effectiveness of the MDM's evaluation.

Clearly, the basic objective of MHTS is to collect useful data for the MDM. In general screening, the information and measurements are expected to provide a valid, comprehensive profile for a specific individual. This profile is expected to either reassure the MDM of the absence of a condition or to alert him to the existence of an abnormality that deserves further consideration.

It is apparent that the major role of the MHTS is communications: collecting, correlating, and formatting information for the MDM. To be effective, the questionnaires and the measurements must apply to the examinee, the purpose of the examination, and the needs of the MDM. The complexity of these variables makes it difficult for multiphasic health testing to be considered as an essential component in medical care. This lack of a "universal multiphasic," the ultimate health test that will fit all situations, should not deter the development of multiple comprehensive tests to meet variable situations. The alternative of distilling multiphasic questionnaires and extracting the lowest common denominator in order to have a single test is not a valid strategy. When this is done, the examinee and the MDM find the questionnaires lack clarity and pertinence; the examinee fails to take

The statistics cited were supported in part by NIMH Grant #MH24109: Systems Approach to Mental Health Care in an HMO Model.

---

* The mental health component (MHC) is broadly defined to encompass the subjective qualities of the health care transaction. It summarizes acquired personal information, psychosocial data, and previous medical care behavior and includes any factors that affect the patient-provider relationship.

† The medical decision maker (MDM) is defined as a health professional who recommends a course of action for the patient. This person is designated by the health care system to have access to medical information, and to prescribe treatment or health care advice. The MDM may be a physician, nurse, social worker, psychologist, or any other paramedical provider.

the evaluation seriously and the MDM tends to revert to a traditional health examination.

An important consideration in multiphasic health testing is the eventual use of the information by the MDM. Often this information pertains solely to MDM/patient interaction at the time of a physical examination. The MDM correlates the test data with both the physical examination and supplemental questions. The outcomes are:

(1) *Direct action.*   The treatment is initiated, a concern is resolved, advice is given, etc.

(2) *Observation.*   The decision is made to observe the patient or the test results for change over a period of time.

(3) *Disregard.*   The decision is made to dismiss a symptom or a test result because of additional information, lack of supporting data, etc.

(4) *Information referral.*   Retesting, second-level testing, or an opinion is requested for the examining MDM's consideration.

(5) *Treatment referral.*   Specific evaluation or treatment is solicited without further consideration by the examining MDM.

The requirements of these five outcomes must be planned for by MHTS if the evaluation is to be considered useful by the MDM.

C. PROBLEMS OF INTRODUCING THE MENTAL HEALTH COMPONENT (MHC)

Attempts to add MHC to MHTS recall the original difficulties faced by multiphasic theoreticians, plus several additional problems unique to this situation:

(1) The appropriateness of mental health questions to *each* individual and the specification of the purpose of the mental health examination continue to be problems for screening broad populations.

(2) Mental health screening lacks general tests that evaluate accurately and generate precise reports.

(3) The MDM has highly variable requirements for mental health data. Compounding this problem is a wide variation in the MDM's ability to interpret MHC results, ask supplemental questions, and substantiate data by examination.

(4) Few MDMs have the time and the diverse skills required to intervene in mental health areas. Therefore, referral resources must be available, and the testing must aid in the referral triage procedure. The testing does not have to specify a diagnosis, but it should indicate the area of the problem.

The difficulties of adding the MHC to an MHTS can be simplified by narrowly defining the purpose, the population, and the needs of the MDM. The MHTS can adopt mental health programs from operating multiphasic systems that assess psychosomatic potentials, catalogue psychological symptoms, aid in defining psychiatric disorders, etc.[2] It is suspected that stand-alone, fee-for-service MHTS would benefit from this approach, since they can offer the MDM several choices of MHC, thereby tailoring the evaluation to MDM needs and practice style.[3]

Expanding the MHC beyond specific, limited tasks greatly complicates the application. In prepaid group practice situations where MHTS is under the jurisdiction of the medical care delivery system, the advantages may warrant this effort, yet the complexities of the medical care delivery system may inhibit the integration of expanded mental health services. As will become evident in this chapter, it is not possible to deliver universally accepted health testing that will address the diverse needs of all populations and all MDMs. (Even the current computerized, branching questionnaires and sophisticated test-ordering protocols fail to achieve comprehensive testing.) Therefore, operational MHTS tend to focus on general health issues or may narrow their scope to "mini-phasic" evaluations that evaluate specific issues, e.g., cardiovascular screening, preoperative physicals, etc.

This chapter will not describe a definitive MHC-MHTS linkage; it will outline a pragmatic, evolving health appraisal system being implemented at a new Kaiser-Permanente facility in San Jose, California. Although this design is primarily for an "in-house" MHTS within a prepaid group practice, a significant portion is transferable to other health testing services.[3]

D. CONCEPTUAL LINKAGE

The fundamental starting place for MHC-MHTS linkage is the collection of useful data for the MDM. Attempts to implement this seemingly straight-forward objective identify more difficulties. Mental health has lagged behind the advances of MHTS primarily because the mental health profession evaluates complex, individualized data without precise, general tests. Often the format of the results fails to be a medically useful profile. Compounding this difficulty is the unfortunate separation of psyche and soma that occurs in both the thinking and professional alignments of medical care personnel. MHC must make the decision tasks of the medical provider easier, save him time, conserve costs, or all three. Too often, attempts at integrating MHC have had the opposite results. The MDM is presented with clinical ambiguities, asked to perform the time-consuming role of a mental health professional, or charged the cost of an elaborate mental health screening procedure that is unrelated to medical decision making.

If the MHC-MHTS linkage is to be used to achieve integration of mental health with general medical care delivery, it can neither limit its scope to symptoms of anxiety and depression, nor be content with somatization or psychopathology. It must address the needs of the MDM in providing health care and sick care delivery. The MDM should be presented with a more complete set of data, formatted to achieve the desired integration of mental health and medical care delivery. To accomplish this, the MHC must address these issues:

(1) *Health concerns.*   Are there "hidden agendas"? What *are* the reason(s) for the MHTS evaluation? (Frequently, reassurable concerns slip past the MDM because the underlying reason for the visit was not elicited.)

(2) *Symptoms.*   Symptoms are generally well covered in standard MHTS, yet the meaning of the symptom to the examinee is overlooked. What does that symptom mean to this person?

(3) *Symptom-concern interactions.*   What interactions occur between his physical symptoms and health-related concerns or current problems-in-living?

(4) *Predictions of medical care behavior.*   What factors in this individual bring him to medical attention? Will he adhere to treatment regimens? Will he establish a therapeutic MDM-patient relationship?

(5) *Psychosocial problems.* What life events are occurring or anticipated by the patient? Are any of his life roles weakened?

(6) *Strengths.* What is his capacity for adaptive and coping behavior? What are his strong life roles?

(7) *Psychopathology.*   Does this individual have symptoms that warrant a psychiatric evaluation?

(8) *Prevention.* Is there significant psychosocial risk and impaired coping behavior to warrant intervention?

(9) *Referral.*   Recommend possible courses of action to the MDM regarding aberrant medical behavior and inappropriate medical concerns, and list available resources.

(10) *Information.*   Provide information to the examinee regarding MHC-MHTS evaluation, risk-taking behavior, and community sources of aid.

(11) *Health profile.*   Provide a summary document that will assist multiple providers in maintaining a consistent approach and treatment orientation between multiphasic health testing evaluations.

The MHC is faced with a formidable task in this broad, ambitious new role. It cannot be simply considered the screening instrument for psychiatric referral; it is, instead, a catalyst for effective consumer-provider interaction and improved health-seeking behavior. No current psychological tests or tools will evaluate all of the above parameters. Even the most extensive psychiatric profiles provide limited information regarding medical care. A considerable amount of useful information for the MDM can be obtained, however, if mental health is directly involved in medical care and if access is gained to the individual's concerns, symptoms, past medical history, past medical behavior, current life events, and self-perceptions of life role performances.

The linking of MHTS and the mental health component is based upon the close articulation of a large number of separate variables. Foremost is the necessity to collect information regarding the individual's *self-perceptions* and his previous *behavior* in the medical setting. This is a crucial point. MHC must include information regarding past medical utilization and not limit its data to a set of mental health questionnaires.

Important data are lost if only self-perceptions are used, since incongruities between self-perception and behavior may escape detection. Since past medical care behavior is a function of both the individual's behavior and the medical system's behavior, the MHTS must have intimate knowledge of the user's medical system. For example, it would be unwarranted to consider the failure to establish a physician-patient relationship as a risk factor if the medical system hampered patient reentry to the same physician.

Therefore, in order to incorporate an individual's behavior within the medical care system as a mental health component, the medical system must accurately reflect the consumer-provider interactions. That is, the behavior of the medical care system must be a known constant before deviations in consumer-initiated utilization can be identified.

E. INCENTIVES, BEHAVIOR, AND MENTAL HEALTH COMPONENT (MHC)

Before proceeding with the strategy of implementing MHC-MHTS linkage, we must discuss why the MHTS should address the complexities of medical care behavior.

First, self-perceptions when correlated with known medical behavior provide a powerful, predictive instrument that is useful for medical decisions. There also is considerable pressure on the medical care system to move into preventive programs that are directly related to behavior and life style.[4] In the last two decades, the major causes of morbidity and mortality have been greatly influenced by personal actions and styles of living. Thus, if the individual would actively participate in self-preservation behavior, the demands on the medical care system would be significantly reduced and the level of health in the population would rise.

Health maintenance organizations are being encouraged by both legislation and prepayment incentives to enter preventive care.[5] There are financial rewards for successful prevention under prepayment. (This assumes, of course, that prepayment funding is allowed to remain competitive with fee-for-service.) For prepayment to be the sole incentive, the costs of identifying risk factors and providing some type of effective intervention must be less than the cost of the anticipated medical outcome, or the procedure must be perceived as beneficial and warranting the additional cost by either the MDM or the patient. Even though the prevention incentive of prepayment is difficult to cost-account, it will encourage prepaid group practices to attempt some innovative programs.

Unfortunately, consumer prevention incentives are less apparent. They rely on the belief that awareness and self-preservation factors are sufficient motivation to change behavior. This is naive. Cigarette smoking, obesity, drunken driving, and other known risk-taking behaviors occur in spite of extensive awareness campaigns.

Regardless of whether or not there are adequate provider and consumer incentives, health care systems are being asked to apply prevention to behavior. Clearly, the most financially rewarding starting point in a prepaid group practice is in discouraging behavior that leads to inappropriate medical utilization. If this behavior could be decreased in a manner acceptable to the provider and beneficial to the consumer, the prepaid financial reward would be significant. Next would be consumer behavior to which the individual is already motivated (e.g., he requests to stop smoking). Finally, it would be ethically and financially useful to screen for psychosocial risk factors that are suspect as antecedents for both emotional and physical illness,[6] because of the possibility of reducing the degree of morbidity and the cost of treatment.

The emphasis on behavior has heightened the necessity of combining psychological approaches with the diagnostic and therapeutic tools of modern medical science.[7] The purpose of this chapter is not to reiterate the arguments for a comprehensive health care delivery system, nor is it to describe the difficulties inherent in such a comprehensive care system. Instead, a practical starting point will be described from which a total health care program can evolve—a system approach—integrating emotional health and physical health into a comprehensive health care delivery system.

F. INVESTIGATION OF MHC LINKAGE

A particularly useful classification system for studying medical behavior was reported by Garfield.[8] The medical decision maker divides patients into two groups based on whether or not significant abnormalities were discovered after multiphasic health testing and physical examination. The patient's perception of being either well or sick is used to complete the classification. (See also Chapters Two, Eleven, and Fifteen.) This results in four distinct health status groups:

(1) *Well.* The MDM has not discovered a significant abnormality and the patient reports feeling well. Essentially the patient asks: "I feel well, am I?"

(2) *Asymptomatic/Sick.* The MDM has discovered a significant abnormality in a patient who feels well (e.g., anemia or hypertension).

(3) *Sick.* The MDM concurs with this patient, since significant abnormalities are associated with the patient's symptoms of not feeling well. (Self-limiting illnesses are excluded.)

(4) *Symptomatic/well.* The MDM does not find a significant abnormality, although the patient perceives himself as sick. This is the "worried-well" in the Garfield classification.

Preliminary investigation of these four health status groups reveals that patient perception is a strong predictor of medical behavior. The symptomatic/well person (worried-well) utilizes outpatient services at the same rate as the sick patient. This is *twice* as often as those individuals who perceive themselves as being well. Interestingly, this behavior is not modified by the person's being told that he is well following the multiphasic health testing and the MDM physical examination.

The symptomatic/well individual has a significantly higher number of visits, tests, prescriptions, and problems-in-living than a matched group who perceive themselves as well. It is a mistake to consider the symptomatic/well to be a psychiatric patient, since he does not meet the criteria of psychopathology.* At present, the symptomatic/well represent a distinct group of individuals who behave differently in a large prepaid group practice. For example, they do not maintain continuity of care by establishing a doctor-patient relationship. It is not known whether this is a phenomenon of the symptomatic/well patient or whether this is a subtle rejection by the examining physicians.

Medical behavior is somewhat artificially divided into health behavior and illness behavior. Health behavior can be considered as action taken by the individual to avoid becoming ill or to detect disease before the development of symptoms.[10] Illness behavior consists of actions that occur when an individual considers himself ill (usually associated with symptoms) and he is seeking both confirmation (diagnosis) and treatment.

The symptomatic/well demonstrate that—at least in prepaid group practice— the division between health and illness behavior is not distinct. The

---

*For the purposes of this chapter, *psychopathology* is defined as evidence of a psychiatric symptom(s) of a magnitude that prevents the individual from functioning in a significant life role (marriage, work, family, etc.); i.e., the person is failing to perform or is on the verge of failure in a previously established role. In contrast, *problems-in-living* are difficulties of psychosocial nature that do not prevent role performance, but may hinder performance or satisfaction.

symptomatic/well utilize sick care services as if they were seeking diagnosis and treatment; yet, upon thorough examination, the MDM is unable to arrive at a diagnosis. Characteristically, the symptomatic/well are *not* reassured by the lack of a diagnosis. Instead, they continue to make repeated inappropriate visits to sick care services. In the process, they have multiple laboratory tests, many x-ray procedures, and receive more prescriptions for symptomatic relief than other health status categories.

The proportion of symptomatic/well patients has been measured at 6 percent[9] and 11.6 percent[11] when using MHTS as the entry point. (It should be mentioned that MHTS is the logical entry point, because the assignment of health status categories does not refer to self-limited illness, such as upper respiratory tract infections. Arriving at health status categories based on the presence or absence of a diagnosis in outpatient clinics is not always possible, because the physician may write an impression or a descriptive diagnosis.) These measured percentages are considered to be lower than the actual proportion of symptomatic/well in a prepaid population, because another suspected characteristic of this group is a tendency to avoid entry into clinics that have time delays for appointments, e.g., MHTS.

As previously mentioned, one of the problems in integrating mental health into a multiphasic health testing program is the distinction between emotional illness and factors that may or may not be prodromal indications of emotional illness. This distinction is critical. A systematic approach is not possible if psychiatric illness is haphazardly classified with psychosocial problems-in-living.

Although it is well known in psychiatric circles that many individuals will visit a physician shortly before psychiatric decompensation, they do not choose MHTS as their point of contact. A preliminary review of 2,300 adults examined by MHTS revealed that less than 1 percent had symptoms requiring psychiatric intervention.[9] The impression in this study was that prepsychiatric patients tended to use urgent care areas rather than scheduled visitations such as MHTS. The patients who were referred for psychiatric intervention were those with primarily chronic problems. Acute psychiatric decompensation occurred in a negligible percentage of individuals who had scheduled their MHTS appointments before the onset of their psychiatric symptoms.

Our preliminary findings indicate that it is extremely useful to identify the proportion of the patients with problems-in-living. In a one-year retrospective medical record review, these individuals show increased medical utilization (physician visits, laboratory tests, prescriptions, etc.), two or three times that of the patient who does not report a problem-in-living. This increase stems from both the patient and the physicians. The patient increases the number of self-generated visits. The physicians respond by ordering tests to rule out disease and by writing prescriptions for symptom relief. Therefore, not only are patients with problems-in-living at higher levels of psychosocial risk, but they have increased contact with the medical care delivery system.

It is the opinion of the author that mental health efforts should be directed at this 20 percent proportion of the population using MHTS who report problems-in-living. Indications in this study[9] and by others[6] suggest that this segment of the population with problems-in-living are more vulnerable to disease in the near future. At this time, the results of selected early interventions are still under investigation, and it is not yet known whether illness risk can be reduced by intervention programs. Yet, because these people are high medical utilizers of outpatient services, there is a significant financial incentive for a prepaid system to explore interventions directed at psychosocial problems as an alternative to self-generated appointments in the medical system.

Another reason for directing the thrust of mental health towards those with problems-in-living is that they are still capable of adaptive and coping behavior. This allows for a wider range of interventions that are educational in nature. In addition, these individuals are already aware of their impaired performance or reduced level of role satisfaction, and they acknowledge such problems once the subject is discussed with them.

In contrast, less than 1 percent of the MHTS examinees have psychopathological symptoms that require therapeutic interventions available only in a psychiatric setting. These patients are readily identified at MHTS and, with few exceptions, they accept psychiatric referral and have high arrival rates at the psychiatric clinic.

The relationship between social stress and psychiatric symptoms such as depression has been reported.[12] Patients with unexplained, self-initiated medical visitations should be carefully evaluated. In our investigation, problems-in-living and unexplained increased medical utilization occurred in the same population. We suspect that a proportion of this same population are vulnerable to physical or emotional illness at a later date. This correlation of increased medical visits and problems-in-living is suspected to be a prodromal condition for patients who arrive at psychiatric outpatient services.[3] In a random selection of new patients that voluntarily applied for psychiatric outpatient appointments, over 30 percent were symptomatic/well patients in the year before their first psychiatric visit.[9]

Life stress and psychiatric disorders have been studied by a number of investigators in several populations.[13-15] In general, these investigations have demonstrated an increase in symptomatology with life stress. It is logical that a similar relationship exists between life stress and symptomatology that would precipitate medical visitation.

To date, very little attention has been given to self-initiated medical visitation as a predictor for eventual utilization of health facilities. The author believes that if preventive health programs are to be effective, they should be applied to this population with problems-in-living and increased medical visitation. If the mental health component has a direct role in the detection of patients at risk in the medical setting, then innovative intervention programs can be provided at the health education/medical interface. To do so requires that MHTS take a direct role in the entire medical care delivery system.

Goals in this mental health application are extremely different from those in the psychiatric clinic (although there is a similarity to certain types of short-term crisis therapies). Intervention by health education for patients with problems-in-living is not the same as psychotherapy for those with psychopathological symptoms. Health education intervention is immediately directed at greater self-sufficiency, improved performance, and increased role satisfaction. The community, rather than the psychiatric clinic, should be considered as a resource for these health education programs; and, except for those instances where community resources are unavailable in a particular area, the health educational program should not try to directly provide that intervention.

MHTS is the logical entry point for mental health testing for several reasons. First, the patient is not acutely ill, and so he does not object to a thorough examination. Second, he is expecting a comprehensive evaluation and has set aside the necessary time. Third, the acceptance of psychosocial testing is greater if it is combined with all health issues. Of even greater importance is the finding that counseling regarding problems-in-living is considered by patients as a welcome and significant part of comprehensive testing.[3]

G. IMPLEMENTING STRATEGIC ELEMENTS

In this evolving approach of linking MHC-MHTS with the total medical care system, seven distinct steps can be described: (1) the identification and analysis of formal and informal entry systems, (2) a legible medical record of prior care, (3) psychosocial questionnaires, (4) a summary psychosocial vignette, (5) trained nurse practitioner/physician teams, (6) a broad spectrum health education program, and (7) a patient tracking system.

1. Identification and Analysis of Formal and Informal Entry Systems

Most group practice settings provide the potential patient with information regarding the eventual utilization of the medical group. Obviously this information is necessary for orderly entry. Even a well-informed patient has difficulty in determining the urgency and appropriateness of his appointment. Unfortunately, when inappropriate self-entry regularly occurs, the medical care system responds by creating more elaborate entry methods. For example, a favored approach with subspecialty clinics is to disallow self-referral by the patient and to insist that the person be referred by another physician. Essentially, this adds another turn to the "medical maze."

Over time, dissatisfied low-utilizing persons will have an adverse effect on a health insurance program, since they will self-select a more responsive medical care system. Conversely, it is our impression that families with one or more high medical utilizers (regardless of whether they are considered to be chronically ill) tend to remain as members of a health plan. With time, the high utilizer learns to run the "medical maze" and is an expert on informal entry.

In response to complex entry systems, the patients may develop informal entry systems by overstating their symptoms to the appointment clerk, relying on patient assistance personnel to help them achieve preferential entry, or asking a hostile spouse to intimidate the system. Commonly, the utilization of emergency services or urgent care clinics increases because the patient "gives up" on attempting to understand the appointment system. Informal entry poses two basic problems: First, the conscientious patient (generally a low medical utilizer) becomes discouraged, since informal entry makes queues longer. Second, providers are less certain of the referral source and consequently are less able to plan for appropriate staffiing to render needed services.

Knowledge of both formal and informal systems is extremely useful if medical behavior is to be satisfactorily evaluated. For example, patient adherence to medical advice cannot be rated for effectiveness if the average member cannot follow the recommended complex entry path. Informal entry systems will exist, but they are prevalent in systems with long queues or complex entry protocols.

2. A Legible Medical Record of Prior Care

In traditional health testing, very little attention is given to the past performance of the individual in the medical care setting. If medical behavior is to be used to detect incongruities between an individual's self-perceptions and his health status, this information must be available in a legible format (see Fig. 13-1). The information need not be exhaustive or all-inclusive; its purpose is simply to allow tracking of medical behavior in those individuals who do not have a complicated medical problem.

It should be mentioned that complex medical problems, such as diabetes, are not followed in this fashion, since their medical records do not lend themselves to simple abstracting. The "sick" health status group in most populations is approximately 10 to 15 percent. As a group, they tend to be appropriate utilizers, they return to the same physician or department, and they do not tend to self-enter. It has been our impression that the sick category is most effectively tracked by the traditional medical record. The remaining 85 to 90 percent can be monitored by a relatively simple data system with only 12 to 18 months of medical visitation information online.

In our research project, 18 months of visitation was selected, because it would coincide with the psychosocial questionnaires and an online computer system. When the computer file is full, visits beyond one year are converted to "hard copy" printouts and filed in the chart. This procedure alleviates the problem of electronically storing increasingly large amounts of clinical data.

Figure 13-1 is a display of a visit section from the MHTS profile. The information was gathered by a chart abstractor for use by the nurse practitioner (MDM). Upon review and physical examination, the nurse practitioner will add to or delete from the profile. This document will remain in the medical record for future reference by MDMs who encounter this individual.

3. Psychosocial Questionnaires

In order to achieve a cost-efficient, systematic evaluation of an individual, considerable effort has been made to acquire the history by self-administered questionnaires. Besides questions that deal with symptoms, past medical history, and family history, information is needed about past and anticipated life events plus self-perceptions of role performances. (See Figure 13-2.)

In distinguishing patients requiring psychiatric referral from those suffering problems-in-living, these instruments have been selected to provide clear behavioral definitions of the type of problem being faced by patients, rather than resorting to scales whose output is aimed at psychopathology. Assessment has been limited to instruments that are likely to provide medical decision makers with highly usable, easily read indicators that will effectively augment the diag-

18-Month Visit History (Last Six Visits Displayed)

Total Visits (in last 18 months) 14			Self-Generated 12		Failure to Keep Appt's. 4	Anticipated Visits 13
Clinic	Date	Complaint	Diagnosis		Treatment	Refer/Return
Emergency room	9/26/74	Headache	Migraine		Demerol 50 mg Phenergan 50 mg	None
Medical drop-in	10/5/74	Flu	None		Verification of treatment	None
Nurse practitioner	11/6/74	Backache	Low back strain		Valium 5 mg #50 1 Tid & hs	Return PRN
Medical drop-in	12/12/74	Diarrhea	Viral GI synd.		Lomotil #10 Verif. of treat.	None
Medical drop-in	1/8/75	Cough/cong.	URI		Culpac-Neg. Dimacol #14	URI Program Health Ed.
Multiphasic	1/19/75	Testing	Problem list updated		Routine lab	Return 18 months

PROBLEM LIST

1. Migraine headaches
2. Overweight
3. Marital difficulties
4. No primary provider
5. Absenteeism requires verification of treatment

ACTIVITY

1. Partial control—ergotamine
2. Uncontrolled—diet prescribed
3. Referral—intervention program
4. Assigned RN/MD team
5. Instruction given

Figure 13-1. An example of a past visit history summary.

HEALTH CARE APPLICATIONS
KAISER-PERMANENTE MEDICAL OFFICES - San Jose

<table>
<tr><td>DATE:</td></tr>
<tr><td>NAME:</td></tr>
<tr><td>BIRTHDATE:</td></tr>
<tr><td>M. R. NUMBER</td></tr>
<tr><td>DO NOT WRITE IN THIS SPACE</td></tr>
</table>

I. SCHEDULE OF RECENT AND ANTICIPATED EXPERIENCES

These yellow forms are only for Evaluation of your total health status, and will not become a part of your medical record.

If any of these life events have happened to you in the last 12 months, check a box in the Column headed "Past".

If you anticipate that the event may happen to you in the next 12 months, check a box in the Column headed "Future".

(CHECK ALL ITEMS THAT APPLY)

	PAST		FUTURE		
1.	☐	100	☐	—	Death of spouse
2.	☐	73	☐	—	Divorce
3.	☐	65	☐	—	Marital separation
4.	☐	63	☐	—	Jail term
5.	☐	63	☐	—	Death of close family member (except spouse)
6.	☐	53	☐	—	Major personal injury or illness
7.	☐	50	☐	—	Marriage
8.	☐	47	☐	—	Fired at work
9.	☐	45	☐	—	Marital reconcilation
10.	☐	45	☐	—	Retirement
11.	☐	44	☐	—	Change in health of family member (not self)
12.	☐	40	☐	—	Pregnancy
13.	☐	39	☐	—	Sex difficulties
14.	☐	39	☐	—	Gain of new family member
15.	☐	39	☐	—	Business readjustment
16.	☐	38	☐	—	Change in financial state
17.	☐	37	☐	—	Death of close friend
18.	☐	36	☐	—	Change to different occupation
19.	☐	35	☐	—	Change in number of arguments with spouse
20.	☐	31	☐	—	Mortgage over $10,000
21.	☐	30	☐	—	Foreclosure of mortgage or loan
22.	☐	29	☐	—	Change in responsibilities at work
23.	☐	29	☐	—	Son or daughter leaving home
24.	☐	29	☐	—	Trouble with in-laws
25.	☐	28	☐	—	Outstanding personal achievement
26.	☐	26	☐	—	Spouse begin or stop work
27.	☐	26	☐	—	Begin or end school
28.	☐	25	☐	—	Change in living conditions
29.	☐	24	☐	—	Change in personal habits (self or family.)
30.	☐	23	☐	—	Trouble with boss
31.	☐	20	☐	—	Change in work hours or conditions
32.	☐	20	☐	—	Change in residence
33.	☐	20	☐	—	Change in schools
34.	☐	19	☐	—	Change in recreation
35.	☐	19	☐	—	Change in church activities
36.	☐	18	☐	—	Change in social activities
37.	☐	17	☐	—	Mortgage or loan less than $10,000
38.	☐	16	☐	—	Change in sleeping habits
39.	☐	15	☐	—	Change in number of family get-togethers
40.	☐	13	☐	—	Change in eating habits
41.	☐	13	☐	—	Vacation
42.	☐	12	☐	—	Christmas
43.	☐	11	☐	—	Minor violations of the law

After Dr. Thomas Holmes' Schedule of Recent and Anticipated Experiences

G1075

OVER

Figure 13-2a. Psychosocial questionnaires for mental health component.

II. **ASSESSMENT OF CURRENT LIFE CONDITIONS**

Check the boxes in Column headed "Self" for the items that best describe your situation.

Check the boxes in the Column headed "Spouse" for the items that best describe your spouse's situation.

(CHECK ALL ITEMS THAT APPLY)

	SELF	SPOUSE		
1.	☐	☐	—	Often sick
2.	☐	☐	—	Can't sleep
3.	☐	☐	—	Worry a lot
4.	☐	☐	—	Argue a lot
5.	☐	☐	—	Weigh too much
6.	☐	☐	—	Smoke too much
7.	☐	☐	—	Drink too much
8.	☐	☐	—	Lose self in work
9.	☐	☐	—	Careful with money
10.	☐	☐	—	Away from home a lot
11.	☐	☐	—	Uptight a lot of the time
12.	☐	☐	—	Too concerned about money
13.	☐	☐	—	Satisfied with way of life
14.	☐	☐	—	Have to take too many pills
15.	☐	☐	—	Have to visit doctors often
16.	☐	☐	—	Family most important asset
17.	☐	☐	—	Often disappointed by others
18.	☐	☐	—	Find relaxation with friends
19.	☐	☐	—	Find peace of mind being alone
20.	☐	☐	—	Often seek advice from others
21.	☐	☐	—	Don't take advice given by others
22.	☐	☐	—	More sensitive to pain than most people
23.	☐	☐	—	Church is a stabilizing influence in life

24. When I am troubled it is usually about (specify most frequent concerns, e.g., health, marriage, family, finances, job, etc.)

____

____

What I do first about my trouble is ________________________

____

If that doesn't work I next ____________________________

____

When all else fails I ________________________________

____

KAISER-PERMANENTE MEDICAL OFFICES - San Jose — -2- — *OVER*

Figure 13-2b.

III. **SCHEDULE OF SOCIAL FUNCTIONING**

Please answer *each* question according to the way you feel today.

Circle Y to indicate YES (Y)   Circle P to indicate PERHAPS (P)   Circle N to indicate NO (N)

If you are not sure how you feel, answer PERHAPS (P).

SECTION 1 — WORK

THIS SECTION HAS TWO PARTS. IF BOTH ARE IMPORTANT TO YOUR
PRESENT SITUATION, ANSWER BOTH.

PART A — EMPLOYED ☐ *(CHECK IF MORE IMPORTANT THAN PART B)*

1. Do you like the work you are doing? . . . . Y P N
2. On the whole, do you like the people you work with? . . . . Y P N
3. Do you feel you are in the right kind of work? . . . . Y P N
4. Do you have any really satisfying hobbies or interests outside work? . . . . . Y P N
5. Do you have enough opportunity for getting ahead in your work? . . . . . . Y P N

PART B — HOUSEWIFE — HOMEMAKER ☐ *(CHECK IF MORE IMPORTANT THAN PART A)*

6. Do you like being a housewife - homemaker? . . . . Y P N
7. Do you have enough daily social contacts? . . . . Y P N
8. Does your work give you enough satisfaction? . . . . Y P N
9. Do you have any satisfactory hobbies or interests, apart from work? . . . . . Y P N
10. Are you content to remain a housewife - homemaker? . . . . Y P N

SECTION 2 — FINANCE

THIS SECTION ALSO HAS TWO PARTS. IF BOTH ARE IMPORTANT TO
YOUR PRESENT SITUATION, ANSWER BOTH.

PART A — EMPLOYED ☐ *(CHECK IF MORE IMPORTANT THAN PART B)*

11. Do you live more comfortably than you did two years ago? . . . . Y P N
12. Are you able to save? . . . . Y P N
13. Do you feel at ease about spending? . . . . Y P N
14. Are you reasonably secure financially? . . . . Y P N
15. Do you *feel* financially secure? . . . . Y P N

PART B — HOUSEWIFE — HOMEMAKER ☐ *(CHECK IF MORE IMPORTANT THAN PART A)*

16. Can you manage on your housekeeping money without a lot of anxiety? . . . . Y P N
17. Do you have any income, other than housekeeping money? . . . . Y P N
18. Do you feel at ease about spending? . . . . Y P N
19. Generally speaking, does being a housewife satisfy you? . . . . Y P N
20. Do you feel financially secure? . . . . Y P N

Figure 13-2c.

III. **SOCIAL FUNCTIONING** (continued)

PLEASE ANSWER ALL THE QUESTIONS IN THE REMAINING SECTIONS

SECTION 3 – FRIENDS

21. Do you have a close friend in whom you can confide? . . . . Y P N
22. Outside of your family, do you feel there are people who really care about you? Y P N
23. Do you enjoy making acquaintances? . . . . Y P N
24. Would you want your friends to turn to you with their problems? . . . . . Y P N
25. Do you enjoy entertaining or treating people? . . . . Y P N

SECTION 4 – FAMILY LIFE

26. Are you interested in your spouse's hobbies and/or activities? . . . . Y P N
27. Do you discuss your money, work or other problems with your spouse? . . . . Y P N
28. Do you enjoy family life? . . . . Y P N
29. Do you feel your spouse understands you? . . . . Y P N
30. Do you feel that you understand your spouse? . . . . Y P N

SECTION 5 – PERSONAL LIFE

31. Are you really satisfied with your marriage? . . . . Y P N
32. Do you feel that your spouse really cares about you? . . . . Y P N
33. Does sex bring you much enjoyment in your marriage? . . . . Y P N
34. Do you like to be with children? . . . . Y P N
35. Can you relax? . . . . Y P N

SECTION 6 – ENERGY

36. Do you feel overworked? . . . . Y P N
37. Do you feel too tired to work? . . . . Y P N
38. Do you find that your mind is underactive? . . . . Y P N
39. Do you feel too tired to enjoy life? . . . . Y P N
40. Do you feel frustrated because you are prevented from doing things properly? . Y P N

SECTION 7 – HEALTH

41. Do you have frequent headaches? . . . . Y P N
42. Do you suffer from aches and pains? . . . . Y P N
43. Is sex an unwelcome activity in your life? . . . . Y P N
44. Are you concerned about your health? . . . . Y P N
45. Is your imagination painful to you? . . . . Y P N

KAISER-PERMANENTE MEDICAL OFFICES - San Jose –4–

Figure 13-2d.

PLEASE ANSWER ALL THE QUESTIONS IN THE REMAINING SECTIONS

SECTION 8 — PERSONAL INFLUENCE

46. Do you often feel disappointed by people you trust? . . . . Y   P   N
47. Do you often find that people like being hurtful to you? . . . . Y   P   N
48. Do you feel that circumstances are often against you? . . . . Y   P   N
49. Do you find that people are often against you? . . . . Y   P   N
50. Would you like to have more power and influence? . . . . Y   P   N

SECTION 9 — MOOD

51. Are you at times very depressed? . . . . Y   P   N
52. Do you often feel vaguely insecure? . . . . Y   P   N
53. Do you feel overly guilty at times? . . . . Y   P   N
54. Do you ever wish you were dead? . . . . Y   P   N
55. Do you find that people are often unappreciative of your efforts? . . . . . . Y   P   N

SECTION 10 — HABITS

56. Are you inclined to drink too much? . . . . Y   P   N
57. Do you take drugs or medicines to help you relax? . . . . Y   P   N
58. Do you tend to get overactive or overexcited? . . . . Y   P   N
59. Do you tend to eat too much or too little? . . . . Y   P   N
60. Do you often do things that cause trouble for yourself or for others? . . . . . Y   P   N

Figure 13-2e.

429

III. **SOCIAL FUNCTIONING** (continued)

SECTION II — OUTLOOK ON LIFE

> THIS SECTION ASKS YOU TO RATE YOUR RESPONSES ALONG THE
> SCALE GIVEN BELOW. THE SCALE RANGES FROM ONE TO TWENTY.
> A RATING OF ONE INDICATES THAT YOUR RESPONSE IS "NOT AT
> ALL", AND A RATING OF TWENTY INDICATES THAT YOUR RES-
> PONSE IS "COMPLETELY". THE SCALE ALLOWS YOU TO RATE
> YOUR RESPONSE ANYWHERE THAT YOU FEEL IT BELONGS BE-
> TWEEN THESE TWO EXTREMES.

61. Have you achieved your ambition in life?

NOT AT ALL   **CIRCLE ONE**   **COMPLETELY**

1 2 3 4 5 6 7 8 9 10 11 12 13 14 15 16 17 18 19 20

62. Do you feel hopeful for the future?

NOT AT ALL   **CIRCLE ONE**   **COMPLETELY**

1 2 3 4 5 6 7 8 9 10 11 12 13 14 15 16 17 18 19 20

63. Do you feel that your life has meaning?

NOT AT ALL   **CIRCLE ONE**   **COMPLETELY**

1 2 3 4 5 6 7 8 9 10 11 12 13 14 15 16 17 18 19 20

64. Has life given you enough scope for self expression?

NOT AT ALL   **CIRCLE ONE**   **COMPLETELY**

1 2 3 4 5 6 7 8 9 10 11 12 13 14 15 16 17 18 19 20

65. When you look back, do you feel that life was worth the struggle?

NOT AT ALL   **CIRCLE ONE**   **COMPLETELY**

1 2 3 4 5 6 7 8 9 10 11 12 13 14 15 16 17 18 19 20

Figure 13-2f.

430

nostic treatment process as well as provide predictions regarding the likelihood of future medical care. The Holmes* and the Heimler† scales were chosen for gathering the required psychosocial information because they provide data that are readily interpreted by both the patient and the MDM. During our evaluation of these instruments, many of our patients expressed surprise regarding the amount of change that occurred in their lives and their role performances from the very act of answering the questionnaires. With this degree of awareness, it is relatively easy for the medical decision maker (MDM) to counsel the patient on psychosocial topics. Equally important, the MDM can readily interpret these questionnaires. The MDM feels comfortable in producing the questionnaire and reviewing the responses with the patient, since neither scale requires complicated analyses to serve this function.

The importance of this review by the MDM in the presence of the patient cannot be overstated. During this interaction the trained MDM can determine whether or not the reported information is accurate, assess the patient's ability to cope, and judge whether a referral for further evaluation is warranted.

In contrast, sophisticated psychological instruments such as the computerized Minnesota Multiphasic Personality Inventory (MMPI) are difficult to interpret to the patient in the same fashion. The author believes that these more advanced scales are useful in the hands of a trained psychological counsellor for a second-level evaluation.

Preliminary analyses of the psychosocial questionnaire (Figure 13-2) indicate that psychosocial data are extremely useful when combined with past behavior in the medical system.[9] The important point is not the use of these particular instruments; instead, it is the concept that the MDM has readily available information that allows a better understanding of the patient. The health status category, past and anticipated experiences, current life conditions, social functioning, past medical history, recent symptoms, and past medical behavior combine to form a powerful data base. This information, together with the results of multiphasic health testing, the physical examination, and the interaction with the patient, gives the MDM the opportunity to arrive at medical and mental health decisions.

4. A Summary Psychosocial Vignette

As previously discussed, the display format is important in the integration of mental health components and medical care. In noncomputerized systems, all questionnaires must be manually reviewed. This presents some difficulties because of the inability to suppress noninformative responses. Also, correlations of answers from separate sections are not highlighted for the MDM's attention.

Our complete report contains demographic data about the patient and the family, an 18-month review of medical care, interval medical history, past medical history, reason for MHTS, laboratory results of MHTS, the Holmes Scale, Assessment of Life Conditions, and the Heimler Scale. With this system, any item can be correlated with any other item or with a group of items. This capability

---

* After Dr. Thomas Holmes' Schedule of Recent and Anticipated Experiences.
† After the Heimler Scale of Social Functioning, Copyright, Eugene Heimler, 1967.

allows considerable flexibility, since correlations can be made between any items regardless of whether they are suppressed on the format.

5. Trained Nurse Practitioner/Physician Teams

In many instances the MDM using the MHC-MHTS report will be a physician. In our implementation we employ nurse practitioners under close supervision by a physician. Regardless, if MHC data are added to multiphasic data, the staff must be trained to add counseling on psychosocial factors after the physical examination.

Our experience has shown that the following factors are essential if this procedure is to be effective:

(a) The counseling should be provided, if at all possible, by the health professional who gives the physical examination. This allows the rapport of the physical examination to carry over into the counseling process.

(b) Detailed information regarding psychosocial referral to community resources should be available in written handouts to conserve time. For example, brochures should be available for each community program that describe it in greater detail and inform the patient how to enter it.

(c) If continuity of care is present, incentives exist for both the patient and the MDM, whose expectation should be that they will meet again in the course of continuing health care. They may agree that they will meet again for a multiphasic examination when required, or that the patient will return to the same MDM for medical reasons between multiphasic examinations.

Patient compliance with counseling is higher when this ongoing relationship is present. In addition, the MDM is more effective in counseling when other aspects of care revert back to his practice. For example, if the patient has some unrealistic expectations regarding fever and a high visit record for viral illnesses, it is a direct benefit to the MDM to discuss this concern. In fact, the MDM will reduce visits on his own schedule if his counseling is effective. In addition, MDMs prefer some type of followup in order to evaluate the effectiveness of their counseling efforts.

(d) The addition of a backup counselor is necessary for the MDM, at least for the first year of operation. In our project this individual is a psychiatric social worker who is thoroughly familiar with the entire medical system and the multiphasic environment. Initially, over 40 percent of all patients received counseling from him in the presence of the MDM. By the end of the year this volume was reduced to less than 5 percent as the MDMs became proficient.

It is important that the backup counselor not be deeply embued with traditional psychiatry, or he will tend to revert to psychiatric intake interviews. He must have the ability to assess the entire situation and take advantage of existing coping or adaptive behavior of the patient.

In a fully trained staff, the backup counselor primarily serves to aid the MDM in unusual situations, usually in the examination room with the MDM present. For certain problems, such as psychiatric referral or complicated community referral, the backup counselor will take the patient to an office in order to conserve the MDM's time and to avoid interfering with his schedule.

In the San Jose system, the backup counselor serves additional roles as Director of Health Education and as a member of the MHTS staff. This provides the necessary feedback loops to our own intervention resources and the multiphasic data collection.

6. Broad-Spectrum Health Education Program

A broad array of health education programs have been developed, into which patients identified as having problems-in-living can be channeled. In keeping with distinctions between those requiring psychiatric referral and the larger group with problems-in-living, these programs have been carefully designed to provide members with direct assistance in learning skills to make better adjustments in their own daily lives.

The content in each of the health education programs was generated from identified groupings of patients having problems in parent-child relationships, job instability, marital dysfunction, etc. The difficulty in effecting a favorable adjustment in these significant life roles is well known to psychotherapists. These programs are not considered by the MDM (nor presented to the patient) as a quick solution to the problem; rather, they are designed to create awareness, understanding, and opportunity for the patient. Using a combination of lectures, class discussion, and rehearsal of more adaptive behaviors, they attempt to assist patients to resume normal functioning of vital life roles, primarily by helping them learn new and more effective ways of living and by prompting specific behavioral changes in their life styles. Each program is open-ended; other resources and advanced courses are offered to provide for continued growth and expanded opportunities.

For example, those with problems of obesity are not only helped to become aware of the medical and physical problems associated with obesity, but are encouraged to develop programs of weight control that will generalize to their daily functioning out of class. For those experiencing problems in maintaining effective parent-child relationships, specific training is provided in developing strategies that can increase their effectiveness and satisfaction with their individual family interactions. Armed with written programs for bringing about desired changes in behavior, parents learn to track not only the responses of their children, but their own as well, so that needed adjustments can be made in their child-management styles.

Several features have been incorporated in these programs to insure their success in improving personal adjustment. First, program titles have been written so that potential trainees need not regard themselves as failures or abnormal in order to enroll. These programs are not restricted to referred patients. Since they are open to the community, individuals select themselves to attend. Patients may also take family members or friends if they desire.

A second feature is brevity: most of these programs run no more than six weekly meetings. Third, all programs emphasize correct changes in behavior, giving relatively minor attention to simply imparting information or increasing awareness. Fourth, the programs are designed to maximize the effects of group support for changing behavior. Whatever the reason for referral, trainees need not feel isolated or unique. Given this basic condition for acceptance, group members help each other in their efforts to change and provide needed motivation during the sometimes difficult first steps to finding alternatives.

A fifth advantage is cost. As these programs are conducted through a local community college, our patients are responsible only for the nominal $3 registration fee. A sixth advantage lies in the provision of followup support by physician-nurse practitioner teams as members return for regularly scheduled appointments. Being aware that their enrollment in these programs was both initiated and monitored by the medical staff, members are more likely to implement their newly learned skills than if participation were independent of their overall medical care.

Evaluation of the effectiveness of these programs is continuing, and added measurements of specific behavioral changes are being installed. The desired outcome is not only improved member well-being, but a reduction in otherwise inappropriate use of the medical care delivery system.

7. A Patient Tracking System

In this application of MHC-MHTS, patient behavior must be carefully monitored, since inappropriate medical behavior is being used to alert the medical care system to a potential problem. In most medical systems inappropriate behavior will come to the attention of an MDM in the course of providing medical care between multiphasic evaluations. The medical chart, if it is to reflect patient behavior and continuity of care, must inform the MDM of all interactions between the patient and the medical system.

Specifically, the medical record should include items such as (1) failure to keep appointments, (2) late cancellations, (3) telephone advice, (4) patient-initiated visits, (5) medical system-generated visits, (6) failure to arrive at referral sites, (7) compliance with prescriptions, laboratory tests, etc., (8) failure to establish a primary care provider relationship, (9) failure to return as directed, (10) statements regarding member satisfaction, (11) informal entry routes.

The MDM needs this additional information in order to assess patient behavior at each visit. Essentially, short documentations are required of every patient-medical system encounter. Too often, important information is not charted and inappropriate behavior by the member escapes the attention of the provider.

H. SUMMARY

The linkage of the mental health component to multiphasic health testing as described herein requires a change in perspective. Mental health is asked to apply its expertise to serve patients experiencing problems-in-living and to assist the medical care delivery system with inappropriate medical utilizers. This requires that mental health interventions operate at two levels. The first is a broad, general approach that involves altering the medical care delivery system to detect, counsel, and refer problems-in-living. The second involves maintaining the traditional psychiatric service to treat those patients with symptoms of psychopathological intensity.

This separation is essential, since the number of patients with problems-in-living is greater than the capabilities of the most progressive psychiatric service. Yet, in terms of total need and medical costs, the patient with problems-in-living and inappropriate medical utilization (symptomatic/well) is unique. The symptomatic/well patient receives more tests, more symptomatic drugs, and more radiation than his ill counterpart.

There are indications that the symptomatic/well are at high risk for illness, accident, and psychiatric visitation. It should not be construed that these patients are psychiatrically or psychosomatically disturbed. They are not. They may become physically or emotionally ill or both, if you choose to make this distinction between psyche and soma.

It is not known whether early intervention with the symptomatic/well will reduce potential illness or even inappropriate medical utilization. Clearly, here is a group of patients that can readily be identified with a moderate modification of the medical care delivery system. Their high medical costs, without perceivable benefits, provide a substantial incentive for a prepaid medical system to develop innovative approaches. A satisfactory solution has the potential to reduce medical costs, improve care, and increase medical accessibility by substantial factors.

Alterations in the medical care delivery system not only can serve in the detection of the symptomatic/well, but also can be used to measure the effectiveness of interventions by observable behavioral outcomes. It is important that mental health document its activity in credible terms. We can no longer profess to provide early intervention and prevention without cost-accounting the impact of these services on the entire medical care delivery system.

REFERENCES

1. APHA—Position Paper: *Mental Health and Comprehensive Health Services Programs,* APHA Mental Health Task Force, 1975.

2. Gordon, R. E. "Psychiatric Screening Through Multiphasic Health Testing." *Am. J. Psychiatry* 128(1971):51–55.

3. Harrington, R. L. "The Delivery of Comprehensive Health Care" (unpublished).

4. Knowles, J. H., President of the Rockefeller Foundation, 1975 Address to the Rockefeller Foundation.

5. DHEW/PHS: *Forward Plan for Health FY 1977–81,* June 1975.

6. Holmes, T. H. and Masuda, M. "Life Change and Illness Susceptibility." In *Stressful Life Events: Their Nature and Effects,* pp. 45–72. New York: Wiley-Interscience, 1974.

7. Frank, J. Symposium at Albert Einstein College of Medicine, 1975.

8. Garfield, S. R. "The Delivery of Medical Care." *Sci. Am.* 222(1970):15–23.

9. Harrington, R. L. "Systems Approach to Mental Health Care in a HMO Model." NIMH Grant #MH24109. In progress.

10. Douglass, C. "A Social-Psychological View of Health Behavior for Health Services Research." *Health Serv. Res.* 6(1971):6–14.

11. Garfield, S., Collen, M., Feldman, R., et al. "Evaluation of an Ambulatory Medical-Care Delivery System." *N. Engl. J. Med.* 294(1976):426–431.

12. Ilfeld, F. W., Jr. "Current Social Stressors and Depression." APA Annual Meeting, 1976.

13. Uhlenhuth, E., Lipman, R., Balter, M., and Stein, M. "Symptom Intensity and Life Stress in the City." *Arch. Gen. Psychiatry* 31(1974):759–764.

14. Markush, R., and Favero, R. "Epidemiologic Assessment of Stressful Life Events, Depressed Mood, and Psychophysiological Symptoms—A Preliminary Report. In Dohrenwend, B. S., and Dohrenwend, B. P., eds., *Stressful Life Events.* New York: John Wiley & Sons, 1974.

15. Dohrenwend, B. P. "Social Status, Stress, and Psychological Symptoms." *Am. J. Public Health* 57(1967):625–632.

CHAPTER FOURTEEN

MHTS for Children

Henry R. Shinefield and Constance M. Allen

A.   CONCEPTS AND OBJECTIVES

The idea of well-child physical examinations or regular checkups is firmly established in pediatric practice. Beginning with well-baby examinations, continuing through school and camp checkups, to college and preemployment examinations, parents and children have become accustomed to repeated physical examinations during times of good health.

During these examinations the pediatrician advises and counsels children and families in good nutrition, normal development, and behavior, while also educating patients in matters of general health. But the underlying purpose of frequent examinations is to confirm good health and to seek and treat diseases and abnormal conditions. Optimal treatment or care may justify sophisticated tests in early detection of disease. Such tests need not be limited to traditional laboratory methods of examining blood and urine. On the contrary, the addition of questionnaires, observations, and measurements in a multiphasic format can yield a broader evaluation of the patient's health status than would otherwise be available.

Federal legislation enacted in 1967[1] required "early and periodic screening and diagnosis of individuals who were eligible for Medicaid and who were under 21 years of age to ascertain their physical and mental defects." Although some details in carrying out the law remain to be defined and clarified, a pediatric multiphasic health testing services (MHTS) program can be structured to satisfy this requirement. In California, for example, implementation of this federal law is proceeding with testing of children who are beginning school; a currently operating multiphasic program has demonstrated that these four- and five-year-old children can be tested in an economical manner.[2]

B.   SPECIAL TEST PHASES

Although a variety of procedures are suitable for multiphasic testing of children, recommendations for scheduling of tests and frequency of testing are diverse.[3,4] An example of such a scheme is shown in Table 14-1. Although some of these tests are often done as part of routine physical examinations, others would not ordinarily be included because they are too lengthy, would involve special skills, or might be too costly on an individual basis. For example, measurements such as height, weight, and blood pressure are commonly made. The administration of a developmental assessment, however, may require an examiner who is skilled in such procedures. Similarly, a psychosocial evaluation is both lengthy and expensive if done individually.

Some of the tests listed are true screening tests; others, such as some of the questionnaires, are tools by which information is collected. Medical and family histories are traditionally obtained by the doctor's questioning the parents and recording the information. Questionnaires can certainly satisfy this need. If parents complete such questionnaires at their leisure, the histories can also be made more extensive, yielding more information without increasing time spent by the physician.

As shown in Table 14-1, parent and child participate in pediatric multiphasic examinations, with the content of the test panel varying according to the child's age. The parents' contribution to the examination is largely through questionnaires. For infants, such questions may seek information about family structure and medical history, pregnancy history, and expectations of parents. For older children the emphasis would be on social interaction with peers, school performance, and behavior. Examples of questionnaires are shown in Figures 14-1 and 14-2. These forms, which are used in testing of school-age children, combine information about the medical history with information used for psychosocial evaluation.

Tests administered to the child also illustrate the variation in the tests at different ages. For example, testing for certain inborn errors of metabolism may be done in neonates; if normal, these tests need not be repeated. Other conditions that may develop over time require repeated testing, such as measuring hemoglobin in seeking anemia, or culturing urine in detecting bacteriuria. Some tests may need to be done only in specific at-risk groups, such as lead levels in certain geographic areas.

The psychosocial evaluation is based on information derived both from parental questionnaires and from testing of the child. Emotional problems can be subtle in their development and not become manifest until school performance or peer relationships are markedly affected. This phase attempts to detect these problems in their earlier states. The parent is questioned about various aspects of the child's behavior (see the questionnaires illustrated). Results of age-specific tests of the child are then combined with questionnaire findings, and a score identifies patients with current psychosocial problems that may affect future development.[5]

C. SPECIAL REQUIREMENTS

Multiphasic examinations are generally conducted in a testing area attended by the patients. Nurse's aides administer the tests or procedures. In the newborn and infant, testing may more appropriately be done on an individual basis; that is, rather than the parents attending a specific location, the various tests and procedures may be administered in the usual clinical setting or examination room. The underlying concept is unchanged: the replication of a group of standardized procedures, uniformly performed and recorded.

As children approach school age, multiphasic examinations can be administered in a testing area in the more conventional manner. However, there are unique features determined by age.

First, children are tested in groups of three or four, escorted through the various phases by a nurse's aide. In this way, the children assist and learn from each other, and their individual anxieties are reduced. Second, the sequence of the tests is specifically arranged so that psychosocial tests (the first phase) are temporally separated from the fearsome blood drawing for laboratory tests (the last phase); this arrangement permits optimal performance of the psychological tests. Third, "play" aspects of tests and visual evidence for the child of his test performance are emphasized whenever possible. Last, the willingness and ability of the child to cooperate is always considered, and is in fact a major determinant in the choice of tests.

Table 14-1. Pediatric Multiphasic Test Panels According to Age

TESTS AND PROCEDURES	Newborn	1 Month	3 Months	6 Months	12 Months	2–3 Years	4–6 Years	8–10 Years	12–14 Years
Child									
Musculo-skeletal	Length, height, weight ——————————————————————————————→								
Cardiovascular	Temperature, heart rate					Triceps skinfold ————→			
						Blood pressure ————→			
						Pulse ————→			
									Exercise tol.
Genito-urinary	Time of first urine dipstick				Dipstick ————→				
					Culture ————→				
					BUN ————→				
Gastrointestinal	Time of first meconium								
CNS and special senses	Head circumference ——————————→								
	Ant. fontanelle diam. ————————→								
	Transillumination					Vision ————————————————→			
	Hearing			Hearing ————————————→					
	Vision								
Metabolic-endocrine	PKU		Aminoacid Chrom.						
	Thyroid function					Thyroid function ————→			
	Aminoacid Chromatography (urine)					Choles-terol ————————→			
	Blood glucose								
Hematology	Hemogram				Hemogram ——————————————————————→				
	Blood group				Hemoglobin Electro-phoresis				
	G6PD								

Infections   VDRL   Tuberculin ———————————————————————————————→
                                                                                                           Rebella   VDRL
                                                                                                           titer
Psychosocial   Observation of   Develop-   ———————————→ Visual-motor   Human figure
                    maternal-infant   mental   Human figure   drawing
                    interaction   exam   drawing   Self-admin.
                                                                                             Peabody picture } ————→ questionnaire
                                                                                             vocabulary
                                                                                             Columbia
                                                                                             mental
                                                                                             maturity
                                                                                             WRAT

Parent
questionnaire   Family background   Parental   ———————————————————————→ Behavior
                                          attitudes   inventory
                    Parents attitudes   and per-
                                          ception
                    Family history   of baby
                                          Nutrition ——→
                                          Interval
                                          history   ———→

KAISER-PERMANENTE MEDICAL CENTER

**PEDIATRIC MULTIPHASIC
HISTORY QUESTIONNAIRE**

This form is to help your doctor give better health care. It is completely confidential and will be part of the medical record. These pages contain questions concerning your child's health, and other questions which will provide information necessary for your doctor to understand better your child's medical and physical condition.

IMPRINT AREA
(FOR OFFICE USE ONLY)

Child's Name: _______________________________

Questions answered by: Mother ☐ 120-1

Father ☐ 120-2

Legal Guardian ☐ 120-3

Adoptive Parent ☐ 120-4

If your child has had a multiphasic examination before, check ☐ 121 and go to question 21 (next page)

YOUR CHILD'S HEALTH HISTORY

YES   **NO**

1. Is your child generally in good health? ☐ 122 ☐

2. Has your child been seen by a doctor within the past 12 months? ☐ 123 ☐

3. Does your child have any health problems now? ☐ 124 ☐

4. Has your child ever had a serious illness? ☐ 125 ☐

5. Has your child had any of these operations?
   Tonsillectomy ☐ 126 ☐
   Circumcision ☐ 127 ☐
   Appendectomy ☐ 128 ☐
   Hernia repair ☐ 129 ☐
   Any other ☐ 130 ☐

6. Has your child ever:
   Had a serious injury? ☐ 131 ☐
   Broken a bone? ☐ 132 ☐
   Been knocked out or unconscious? ☐ 133 ☐
   Had any other accidents? ☐ 134 ☐

7. Has your child ever swallowed anything harmful? ☐ 135 ☐

8. Has your child ever been hospitalized for an illness or injury not already mentioned?   **YES**   **NO**   ☐ 136 ☐

9. Has a doctor ever said your child is allergic? ☐ 137 ☐
   Has your child ever had allergy testing? ☐ 138 ☐
   Does your child have a lot of trouble with frequent colds, coughs, runny nose? ☐ 139 ☐

10. Has your child ever had:
    Repeated ear infections? ☐ 140 ☐
    Bladder or kidney infection? ☐ 141 ☐
    Asthma? ☐ 142 ☐
    Allergic skin rash? ☐ 143 ☐
    Allergic reaction to food? ☐ 144 ☐
    Allergic reaction to medicine? ☐ 145 ☐
    Convulsions? ☐ 146 ☐
    Red or 10 day measles? ☐ 147 ☐
    3 day or German measles (Rubella)? ☐ 148 ☐
    Chicken pox? ☐ 149 ☐
    Mumps? ☐ 150 ☐

PREGNANCY HISTORY

11. At what time during your pregnancy did you FIRST see a doctor?
    First 3 months ☐ 151-1
    Middle 3 months ☐ 151-2
    Last 3 months ☐ 151-3

12. When you were pregnant did you take any of these medicines?   **YES**   **NO**
    Vitamins ☐ 152 ☐
    Iron ☐ 153 ☐
    Aspirin ☐ 154 ☐
    For nausea or vomiting relief ☐ 155 ☐
    Sleeping medicine ☐ 156 ☐
    Any others ☐ 157 ☐

13. Did you have any of these illnesses during your pregnancy?   **YES**   **NO**
    Bleeding during first 3 months ☐ 158 ☐
    Bleeding during last 3 months ☐ 159 ☐
    Severe vomiting or nausea ☐ 160 ☐
    High blood pressure ☐ 161 ☐
    Albumin or protein in urine ☐ 162 ☐
    Any serious disease ☐ 163 ☐
    Any x-rays ☐ 164 ☐

14. While you were pregnant were you: **YES**   **NO**
    More easily upset? ☐ 165 ☐
    Unhappy or blue for days at a time? ☐ 166 ☐
    Kept in bed because of severe vomiting or nausea? ☐ 167 ☐

15. Looking back at your pregnancy, was it:
    A happy time? ☐ 168-1 ☐
    An unhappy time? ☐ 168-2 ☐
    No different than usual? ☐ 168-3 ☐

07045 (REV. 10-75)

Figure 14-1a.   Basic four-page Pediatric Multiphasic History Questionnaire.

442

16. Did you have any of these difficulties with
the baby's birth?

	YES	NO
Labor longer than 24 hours	☐ 169 ☐
Labor less than 2 hours	☐ 170 ☐
Bleeding during labor	☐ 171 ☐
Caesarian section	☐ 172 ☐
Forceps delivery	☐ 173 ☐
Born feet first (breech)	☐ 174 ☐

17. Did you have any of these problems after
your baby was born?

Infection	☐ 175 ☐
Bleeding	☐ 176 ☐
Feeling depressed or "blue"	☐ 177 ☐
Any others	☐ 178 ☐

18. Did your child have any of these problems
at birth?

Premature	☐ 220 ☐
Postmature or overdue (over 3 weeks)	☐ 221 ☐
Rh factor	☐ 222 ☐
Jaundice or yellow color	☐ 223 ☐
Difficulty in taking first breath	☐ 224 ☐
Difficulty with breathing during first few days	☐ 225 ☐
Blood transfusion	☐ 226 ☐
Any others	☐ 227 ☐

19. How much did your child weigh at birth?

______ POUNDS ______ OUNCES
228-29 230-31

20. What type of food did you give your child
MOST often? (check only one)

Canned or evaporated milk formula	☐ 232-1
Prepared formula such as Similac	☐ 232-2
Special formula such as soybean	☐ 232-3
Breast milk	☐ 232-4
If breast milk did you breast feed:	
Less than 1 month	☐ 233-1
1-6 months	☐ 233-2
More than 6 months	☐ 233-3

Were there any difficulties with breast feeding   YES ☐ 234 ☐ NO

YOUR CHILD'S RECENT HISTORY

21. Does your child have any difficulties in:

Reading?	☐ 235 ☐
Spelling?	☐ 236 ☐
Arithmetic?	☐ 237 ☐
Speech?	☐ 238 ☐
Writing?	☐ 239 ☐

22. Does your child's teacher indicate any
discipline or behavior problems?   ☐ 240 ☐

23. Did your child go to nursery school?   ☐ 241 ☐

24. Does your child have his/her own room?   ☐ 242 ☐

25. Is your child naturally right handed?   ☐ 243 ☐

26. Is your child a twin?   ☐ 244 ☐
If yes, are they identical?   ☐ 245 ☐

27. If your child is a girl has she started to
have her monthly menstrual periods?   ☐ 246 ☐
If yes, started at what age? ______ years
247-48

28. How many hours a day does your child
watch TV?

Less than 1 hour	☐ 249-1
1-3 hours	☐ 249-2
3-5 hours	☐ 249-3
more than 5 hours	☐ 249-4

29. Does your child:

	YES	NO
Seem normally active?	☐ 250 ☐
Seem physically awkward or clumsy?	☐ 251 ☐
Have any physical problem which bothers him?	☐ 252 ☐
Seem satisfied with his/her looks?	☐ 253 ☐
Often complain of feeling sick or tired for no known reason?	☐ 254 ☐
Seem much more or much less active than other children his age?	☐ 255 ☐
Have a problem of bowel or bladder control?	☐ 256 ☐

30. Has any professional worker ever said your
child has this:

	YES	NO
Learning or reading problem?	☐ 257 ☐
Serious emotional or behavior problem?	☐ 258 ☐
Speech problem?	☐ 259 ☐
Mental retardation?	☐ 260 ☐
Addiction to drugs or alcohol?	☐ 261 ☐
Brain injury?	☐ 262 ☐

31. Has your child been treated during the past
year for:

	YES	NO
Learning or reading problem?	☐ 263 ☐
Serious emotional or behavior problem?	☐ 264 ☐
Speech problem?	☐ 265 ☐
Mental retardation?	☐ 266 ☐
Addiction to drugs or alcohol?	☐ 267 ☐
Brain injury?	☐ 268 ☐

Figure 14-1b.

		YES	NO

32. Does your child usually:

	YES		NO
Seem alert and interested in the world around him?	☐	269	☐
Seem to understand what's going on around him?	☐	270	☐
Seem able to concentrate his attention?	☐	271	☐
Make good use of toys, equipment and materials?	☐	272	☐
Seem immature in his interests?	☐	273	☐
Seem to lack interest in the world around him?	☐	274	☐

33. Does your child usually:

	YES		NO
Seem to understand when you talk to him?	☐	275	☐
Tell the truth?	☐	276	☐
Have a good sense of humor?	☐	277	☐
Seem in touch with the world (not lost in his own thoughts)?	☐	278	☐
Make sense when he talks (not seem confused or mixed up)?	☐	279	☐
Seem to have trouble understanding when you talk to him?	☐	280	☐

34. Does your child usually:

	YES		NO
Get along well with other children his own age?	☐	320	☐
Get along fairly well in the family?	☐	321	☐
Try to be like you or other adults?	☐	322	☐
Do what he is asked without question?	☐	323	☐
Get treated badly by any member of the family?	☐	324	☐
Have some trouble getting along with children his own age?	☐	325	☐

35. Does your child usually:

	YES		NO
Want to do things for himself whenever he can?	☐	326	☐
Keep on trying when something is hard to do?	☐	327	☐
Complete his jobs on his own?	☐	328	☐
Seem self-confident and happy?	☐	329	☐
Have reasonable self control?	☐	330	☐
Want things done for him that he could do himself?	☐	331	☐

36. Does your child:

	YES		NO
Often get into trouble when no one is watching?	☐	332	☐
Usually blame others for his troubles?	☐	333	☐
Often do things which are destructive or which hurt others or himself?	☐	334	☐
Often require severe punishment to make him behave?	☐	335	☐
Seem to be headed for trouble when he grows up?	☐	336	☐
Usually keep out of trouble when no one is watching him?	☐	337	☐

37. Do you want an appointment to talk with a counselor on our staff about your child's behavior, school, or social adjustment? ☐ 338 ☐

---

38. Do you feel that your child eats

too little?	☐	420-1
about right?	☐	420-2
too much?	☐	420-3

39. What kind of milk does your child USUALLY drink?

whole	☐	421-1
low fat	☐	421-2
non-fat (skim)	☐	421-3
other (such as soybean milk, etc.)	☐	421-4

40. How many large glasses of milk does your child drink a day? _______ glasses
422

41. What kind of salt does your family use?

plain	☐	423-1
Iodized	☐	423-2

42. Does your child usually:

	YES		NO
Take vitamins?	☐	424	☐
Eat breakfast?	☐	425	☐
Eat lunch?	☐	426	☐
Eat dinner?	☐	427	☐
Eat snacks between meals?	☐	428	☐

Figure 14-1c.

Please fill out the following table by checking the box that best answers the question: How often does your child eat this food? Check one, and only one box for each food listed.

FOODS	MORE THAN ONCE A DAY	ABOUT ONCE A DAY	ABOUT ONCE A WEEK	SELDOM OR NEVER	
Lettuce					429
Tomatoes					430
Cabbage					431
Greens or spinach					432
String beans					433
Sweet potatoes					434
Beets					435
Carrots					436
Peas					437
Fruit, canned					438
Fruit, fresh					439
Pineapple juice					440
Orange juice or grapefruit juice					441
Dry cereal					442
Bread					443
Rolls, muffins, or biscuits					444
Crackers					445
Cooked cereal					446
Grits					447
Rice					448

FOODS	MORE THAN ONCE A DAY	ABOUT ONCE A DAY	ABOUT ONCE A WEEK	SELDOM OR NEVER	
Spaghetti, macaroni, or noodles					449
Tortillas, corn					450
Tortillas, flour					451
Baked/dried beans					452
Meat					453
Poultry					454
Fish, shellfish, sea food					455
Lunch meat, cold cuts frankfurters, hotdogs					456
Liver					457
Eggs					458
Cheese					459
Cottage cheese					460
Peanut butter					461
Nuts					462
Butter or margarine					463
Ice cream, or ice milk					464
Custard, pudding					465
Cakes, cookies, pies, or candy					466
Potato chips, french fries, or snacks					467

Figure 14-1d.

KAISER
PERMANENTE
MEDICAL CENTER

FAMILY QUESTIONNAIRE

This form is to help your doctor give better health care. It is completely confidential and will be part of the Medical Record. Answers to these questions will give your doctor information about your family and home life. Please answer these questions carefully.

Form completed by: Mother ☐ 520-1

Father ☐ 520-2

Legal Guardian ☐ 520-3

Adoptive Parent ☐ 520-4

**IMPRINT AREA
FOR OFFICE USE ONLY**

1. **What is your marital status?**
(check one)

Married ☐ 521-1
Remarried ☐ 521-2
Never married ☐ 521-3
Divorced ☐ 521-4
Separated ☐ 521-5
Widowed ☐ 521-6

2. **How many children do you have?** _________ children
(522)

3. **What is your race or color?**
(check one)

White - Caucasian ☐ 523-1
Black - Negro ☐ 523-2
Yellow - Oriental ☐ 523-3
Other ☐ 523-4

4. **How far did you go in school?**
(circle highest grade completed)

Grade school: 1 2 3 4 5 6 7 8   524-25
High school: 9 10 11 12
College: 13 14 15 16 17+

5. **What is your wife's/husband's race or color?**
(check one)

White - Caucasian ☐ 526-1
Black - Negro ☐ 526-2
Yellow - Oriental ☐ 526-3
Other ☐ 526-4

6. **How far did he/she go in school?**
(circle highest grade completed)

Grade school: 1 2 3 4 5 6 7 8   527-28
High school: 9 10 11 12
College: 13 14 15 16 17+

7. **Does your family usually speak English at home?** YES ☐ 529 ☐ NO

8. **Do you have someone reliable to take care of your children when you need it?** ☐ 530 ☐

9. **Are your children cared for daily by someone outside the family?** ☐ 531 ☐

If YES, has it been the same person for the past year? ☐ 532 ☐

10. **Has any blood relative on either side of the family had:** YES   NO

Diabetes? ☐ 533 ☐
Convulsions or epilepsy? ☐ 534 ☐
Birth deformity? ☐ 535 ☐
Mental retardation? ☐ 536 ☐
Severe anemia? ☐ 537 ☐
Asthma, hay fever? ☐ 538 ☐
Bleeding tendency? ☐ 539 ☐
Addiction to drugs or alcohol? ☐ 540 ☐
Learning or reading problem? ☐ 541 ☐
Serious emotional or behavior problem? ☐ 542 ☐
Speech problem? ☐ 543 ☐

11. **During the past year, have any of the following occurred in your immediate family:** YES   NO

Family moved? ☐ 544 ☐
Pregnancy or childbirth? ☐ 545 ☐
Death, divorce, separation, loss of family member? ☐ 546 ☐
Marriage or reconciliation? ☐ 547 ☐
Serious injury or illness, problems with ageing relatives? ☐ 548 ☐
Loss of work, change of jobs, retirement? ☐ 549 ☐
Frequent or serious arguments or fights? ☐ 550 ☐
Money problems? ☐ 551 ☐
Sex problems? ☐ 552 ☐
Drug or drinking problems? ☐ 553 ☐
Serious trouble with the law? ☐ 554 ☐
Mental illness? ☐ 555 ☐
Some other serious problem or important change in family? ☐ 556 ☐

08047 (REV. 10-75)

Figure 14-2a.   Supplemental two-page Family Questionnaire.

446

12. **During the past year:**

YES   NO

Has anyone in your family been seriously upset, depressed or moody? . . . . □ 557 □
Have you been generally happy with your family's way of life? . . . . □ 558 □
Have you often felt lonely or cut off from other people or enjoyable activities? . . . . □ 559 □
Have you had serious marital problems? . . . . □ 560 □

13. **When you were growing up:**

Were you generally happy with the way you were raised? . . . . □ 561 □
Were you, or your husband/wife, often treated cruelly or beaten severly? . . . . □ 562 □
Did you, or your husband/wife, have serious problems in school? . . . . □ 563 □

14. **Do you usually (or very often):**

Feel you understand and get through to your children? . . . . □ 564 □
Agree with your husband/wife on how your children should be raised? (Does not apply □) . . . . □ 565 □
Enjoy taking care of your children? . . . . □ 566 □
Feel you are doing a good job of raising your children? . . . . □ 567 □
Feel able to manage your children when you are alone with them? . . . . □ 568 □
Lose your self control when any of your children really frustrates you? . . . . □ 569 □
Find yourself or your husband/wife angry and upset over any of your children? . . . . □ 570 □
Have someone you can turn to for advice when you have a problem with your children? . . . . . . □ 571 □

15. **Do you want an appointment to talk with a counselor on our staff about any problem in your family?** . . □ 572 □

Please complete the following for each child in the family having a multiphasic examination today.

NAME   MEDICAL RECORD NUMBER

Figure 14-2b.

The type of equipment to be used in the various test phases can be extremely varied. If sophisticated automated apparatus is available, it may easily lend itself to testing of older children without modification, but may not be usable for younger children. For example, if blood pressure is to be measured with automated equipment, the equipment may be suitable only for older children, unless the blood pressure cuff is changeable to accommodate the smaller child's arm. If size of the patients varies, and the equipment is not sufficiently adaptable, manual tests may prove to be more efficient.

Once blood specimens for laboratory testing are obtained, automated testing is commonly available. The difficulty here is in selecting appropriate panels for testing. Since the amount of blood obtainable from children often is limited, a choice must be made of which of the available tests will be most appropriate to growing children. Serum electrolytes and enzyme panels may be less useful than a simple hemogram, a thyroid function test, or a screen for rubella antibodies.

Computer processing of information obtained from testing, and particularly from questionnaires, is extremely useful. The computer programs can print the test values for percentiles according to age for ease of interpretation. The large body of information available from the questionnaires can also be more easily handled with computer programs. In addition to collecting and arranging historical information and presenting it in a simple and legible format, some of the questionnaires may have built-in redundant questions to serve as cross-checks for reliability; computer processing will avoid these redundancies in the report. The report may be presented in a manner that emphasizes possible abnormal findings.

Following completion of the report, examination by the pediatrician is essential. The multiphasic examination results must be interpreted, and appropriate followup of questionable or abnormal results must be instituted.

It is clear that the multiphasic screening examination for children is feasible and reasonable in cost. A second important question relates to the benefit of implementing such a program. Cost-benefit data are needed for supporting such widespread programs.[4] It is somewhat surprising that federal and state programs for screening have been mandated by law despite lack of such data.[6,7] Since by federal and state law we are embarking on screening programs throughout the United States, it is hoped that information can be collected to evaluate the usefulness of multiphasic health testing in health care delivery of children.

It should be emphasized that at a minimum, screening examinations must be part of a program that includes diagnosis and followup. This was emphasized more than 25 years ago by Mountin, who stated: "Granted that screening, or case findings, is the first step; unless, however, it is part of a program that makes provision for diagnosis, followup, and treatment, screening by itself loses much of its potential value."[8] An important contribution a screening program can make is to be instrumental in bringing an individual into an established medical care system.

REFERENCES

1. Federal Law: Social Security Act 1905 (a)4B 1967.
2. Allen, C. M., and Shinefield, H. R. "Pediatric Multiphasic Program." *Am. J. Dis. Child.* 118(1969):469–472.

3. Nelson, W. E., et al. *Textbook of Pediatrics*. 10th ed., pp. 208–213. V. C. Vaughan and R. J. McKay, eds. Philadelphia: W. B. Saunders Co., 1975.

4. North, A. F. "Screening in Child Health Care: Where Are We Now and Where Are We Going?" *Pediatrics* 54(1974):631–640.

5. Metz, J. R., Allen, C. M., Barr, G., and Shinefield, H. R. "A Pediatric Screening Examination for Psychosocial Problems" Pediatrics 58(1976):595–606.

6. "Early and Periodic Screening: Diagnosis and Treatment of Eligible Individuals under Age 21." Program Regulation Guide MSA-PRG-21, June 28, 1972, pp. 3–4.

7. California Assembly Bill 2068.

8. Mountin, J. W. "Multiple Screening and Specialized Programs." *Pub. Health Rep.* 65(1950):1359–1368.

CHAPTER FIFTEEN

MHTS as an Entry to Health Care

Sidney R. Garfield

A. **Introduction**
B. **The Concept**
C. **Evaluation of MHTS as a New Entry Mode**
D. **Implications of MHTS for the Future of Medicine**
E. **Conclusion**

A. INTRODUCTION

Throughout the evolution of the American free market system to its present status as a mixed free and regulated economy, society has constantly aspired to improve the welfare of mankind by what has been called a "Humanistic Bill of Rights." Those rights endeavor to assure access to an ever expanding list of necessities such as food, clothing, shelter, education, and benefits for such disadvantageous situations as disability and old age. It has appeared inevitable that access to medical care would be added to that list, since good health is essential to the fruition of most of those rights and certainly warrants a high priority as a necessity of life.[1]

Over the past half-century, a combination of new medical advances, increased demands, and accelerating costs have created enormous pressures in the United States for nationalizing medical care. Supporters of free enterprise in medicine have diligently sought alternative solutions to assure access to medical care, chiefly through vehicles such as Blue Cross-Blue Shield, health insurance, and prepaid health plans. Though those plans aspired to provide ready access to the sick by eliminating financial barriers, perversely they impaired the very access they were designed to assure, because of the markedly increased demand, inflationary costs, and maldistribution of physician services they inherently produced. In addition, what benefits they did provide contained large gaps in services for the poor and aged. In 1966, government intervention with Medicare and Medicaid to fill those gaps and equalize distribution served only to seriously aggravate the already existing impaired accessibility and inflationary costs, because of the great surge of demand the legislation produced. Thus, it has become apparent that the elimination of user fees is not a solution to improving care for the sick. A frustrating free-user, impaired-access paradox has negated much of the anticipated benefit.

The Kaiser-Permanente program has endeavored to achieve ready accessibility to medical care services by systemizing the delivery process and adding a highly organized, totally integrated medical and hospital delivery system to prepayment.[2] Despite the efficiency and comprehensiveness of that systemized delivery system, there has remained considerable impairment to access at the primary care level and a constant struggle to keep up with the free-user demand that prepayment produces—a demand that by consistently overloading its appointment systems causes untenable delays in access to its doctors. Efforts to improve access through special nonappointment "drop-in" clinics have generally proved unsatisfactory, owing to their queuing problems and the brevity and limitations of their services.

In striving to solve the free-user, impaired-access paradox and to improve our Kaiser-Permanente services, we have uncovered a basic defect in today's medical care delivery system that has heretofore passed unnoticed by the medical world. The recognition of that defect and the logic of its solution requires a clear insight into some special characteristics of medical care demand and supply of physician services. Those involve acceptance of the fact that the potential demand for medical care is not limited to sick people. Health is a spectrum consisting of well, worried-well, asymptomatic-sick, and sick states, with people constantly changing from one state to another, and with a great number of them uncertain and concerned about where they stand in that spectrum. Such uncertainty creates a tremendous potential demand for medical care, a demand that formerly was controlled by the price mechanism of the marketplace.

In the past, fees to users deterred most of the potential uncertainty demand (the well, worried-well, and asymptomatic-sick) and limited real demand primarily to the sick. Conversely, the elimination of user fees, as has occurred with expanding prepayment, health insurance, and other third-party payments in the United States, permitted a swing of demand to the well end of that spectrum, thereby converting most of the potential uncertainty demand into real demand.

Concurrently, on the supply side, our medical schools and physicians have concentrated through the years on teaching and practicing sick care techniques to match the demand of the sick under the fee-for-service system. The failure to recognize and adjust those traditional sick care techniques to the entry of uncertainty demand resulting from expanding free-to-user plans has created a serious mismatch in both the access capacity and care processes of the existing physician supply.

The concurrent existence of those two types of free-to-user demand (uncertainty and sick), which compete for traditional sick care physician services, has received little attention from medical planners, economists, and others; yet the mismatch it creates is a major reason for the resulting free-user, impaired-access, inflationary cost paradox[3]—a defect that historically has thwarted every attempt to improve medical care through the elimination of user fees.

B. The Concept

The elimination of user fees significantly alters the demand for medical care by flooding the delivery system with well, worried-well, and asymptomatic-sick. These people, who are uncertain and thereby concerned about their state of health, create a mismatch that impairs access to medical care, dissipates and wastes physician manpower, and results in inflationary costs.

The concept is that to correct the defects in the existing delivery system requires a design that better matches both the uncertainty demand and sick demand. This requires correcting both the mismatched work-up process and access capacity of the existing physician supply.

Sick care diagnosis is essentially a clue-directed, step-by-step search for patterns of illness, which can very efficiently be performed by the physician when clues are definite and his patient clearly ill. He can then readily focus on the problem and effectively serve the patient. With "uncertainty demand," clues are absent, vague, or misleading, requiring a different process, a meticulous checking out of all systems. This checking-out process can be very efficiently performed by paramedical services using protocols established by the physician.

Since the existing traditional delivery system enters patients exclusively through physician services, it was postulated that the new system design required two basic changes:

(1) A new method of entry, through a Multiphasic Health Testing Service (MHTS) utilizing multiphasic health testing and nurse practitioner physical examinations to separate that free-user demand into its basic health status groups: the well, worried-well, asymptomatic-sick, and sick.

(2) An adequate service to receive each of those groups: (1) a new health care service for the well and worried-well; (2) a new preventive maintenance service for the monitoring and surveillance of the asymptomatic-sick and high-prevalence chronic illnesses; and (3) the existing traditional sick care services, reserved for the sick.

Thus, the new medical care delivery system concept has four services, as diagrammed in Figure 15-1.

1. Multiphasic Health Testing Service (MHTS)

MHTS, the heart of the system, combines a detailed automated history with multiphasic panels of clinical and physiological laboratory tests, physical examinations by specially trained nurse practitioners working under the supervision of physicians, computerized information processing and data review.[4-6] Summaries of all significant findings, which become available while patients are still present in the health testing facility, permit online information for decisions with respect to

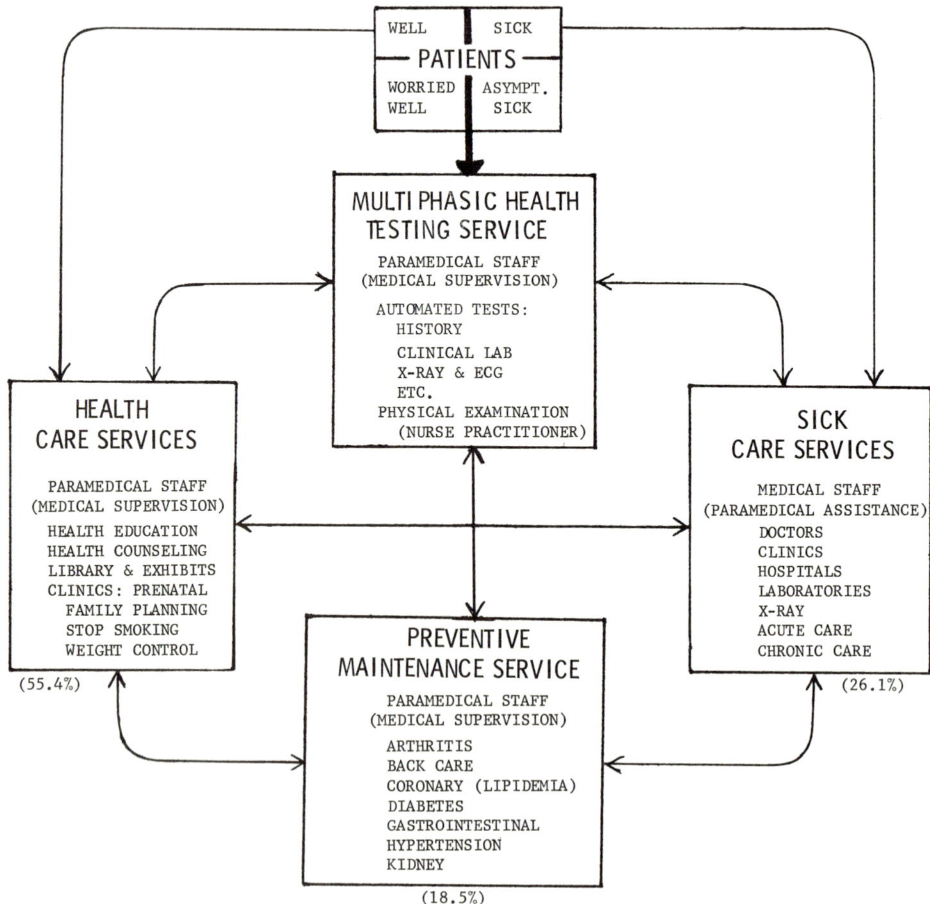

Figure 15-1. Conceptual model of MHTS as a new entry mode to a medical care delivery system.

required repeat or additional tests and/or referral of each patient to the appropriate services—health care, preventive maintenance, or sick care. In addition, each patient is informed of the optimal time to return for continued health monitoring services according to age, sex, health status, and predictive risks.

2. Health Care Service

This new service utilizes paramedical personnel, audiovisual techniques, movies, lectures, exhibits, and counseling.[7] This service is designed to provide health education for improving health and motivating people to stay well. Health care has been an elusive concept, chiefly because it has been buried in sick care and physicians have been too busy to care for well people. This separation of health care is a basic first step toward developing a new service to keep people well. To begin caring for well people is probably the real future of medicine. Such a service is also essential to keep well people from getting into sick care and using up scarce physician services.

3. Preventive Maintenance Service

This is a service for the monitoring and surveillance of asymptomatic and high-prevalence chronic illnesses (such as those listed in Figure 15-1). These services, when performed by specially trained nurses guided by manual and computerized protocols, and reporting physicians, can save a tremendous number of routine physician office visits.[8]

4. Sick Care Services

Sick care, with its high-level decisions on diagnosis, therapy, and complicated or rare illnesses, is clearly the realm of the physician, Here he becomes the manager of sick care; and relieved of the load of the well and worried-well and of much of the monitoring of chronic illness by the three other supporting services, the physician can now conserve his time for care of the sick for which he has been trained.

C. EVALUATION OF MHTS AS A NEW ENTRY MODE

An evaluation of MHTS as an entry mode for ambulatory medical care has been carried out and reported.[5,7] Since this new mode, described in B above, is to be compared with the "traditional medical system" in Kaiser-Permanente, a brief description of that system follows:

Kaiser-Permanente at Oakland serves approximately 130,000 Health Plan members, of whom about 100,000 are adults over 16 years of age.

Sick care services are provided by 14 specialty clinics: allergy, dermatology, emergency, medicine, neurology, ophthalmology, obstetrics-gynecology, orthopedics, otolaryngology, pediatrics, plastic surgery, psychiatry, surgery, and urology.

Traditionally in the Kaiser-Permanente Medical Care Program the entry mode for all new adult ambulatory patients of non-emergency type (i.e., primary care) is through physician appointments in the Department of Medicine, when not clearly definable as belonging to some other specialty.

Appointment clerks, guided by referral protocols, assign patients to appropriate clinics. In the medical department, an advice nurse assists the appointment clerks in determining referrals in questionable cases. Appointments are categorized into four general types: (1) new—the first time a patient sees a physician in the medical department; (2) new-return—a returning patient who has not seen his physician for a year or more; (3) return—a patient who is under care and has been seen by his physician in the past year; and (4) drop-in—a patient entering without a regular appointment.

New and new-return patients receive 30-minute appointments in the doctor's schedule to permit an initial comprehensive workup. Return patients are allocated 15-minute appointments, since presumably these patients have been worked up in previous visits and need only followup care. Drop-ins are handled as expeditiously as possible on a first-come, first-served basis.

1.   Objectives of MHTS as an Entry Mode

The major goals of this concept were to test and evaluate MHTS as a new entry mode to medical care, to use multiphasic testing and nurse practitioner physical examinations as a regulator so as to permit prompt access to health care and to sick care, and to make free-user demand manageable by a more effective use of appropriate resources.[5]

The objectives included:

(a) Providing prompt access to medical care, with the elimination of the queuing for physician services that has invariably accompanied free-user demand.

(b) Systemizing the new patient entry workup through MHTS plus nurse examinations so as to effectively separate the well from the sick with minimum involvement of the physician.

(c) Matching patient needs with appropriate resources: health care, preventive maintenance, and sick care.

(d) Conserving physician availability for care of the sick.

(e) Providing an effective program for total health care through a continuum of services; health care, preventive maintenance, sick care, and health evaluations periodically to update health status profiles.

(f) Developing that total health care system in a method satisfactory to both patients and staff.

(g) Determining whether these objectives can be accomplished in a cost-effective fashion.

2.   The Evaluation Study Design

A study design was constructed primarily to compare the medical care experiences of two basically similar groups of patients using (1) the Kaiser-Permanente "traditional medical system" (TMS) and (2) the new MHTS entry mode. In order to assure similarity, both groups of patients were subjected to the same series of eligibility criteria, establishing their need for a complete workup, since they or their medical problems were not previously known to their doctors. Then, they were randomly assigned by the appointment clerks to one or the other of these systems (TMS or MHTS) by the last digit of their medical record number. The same doctors provided services to both patient groups in order to assure comparable quality of care.

Figure 15-2 diagrams patient flow into both systems during the study period. A detailed description of the study evaluation is provided elsewhere.[8]

After 12 months of actual operation of the new system, a random sample of 4,369 charts of patients entering the traditional and new system were reviewed. Data abstracted from these charts were organized for analysis in accordance with: (1) entry mode—MHTS vs. TMS, and (2) health status group—the well, worried-well, asymptomatic-sick, and sick. This categorization helped to minimize bias due to possible differences in levels of illness in the compared groups.[8]

Data abstracted included the total recorded medical care resources used in the 12-month period by the patients in each group, including the entry visit, entry followup, health care (clinic) services, preventive maintenance, and (acute and chronic) sick care services.

Analysis based on these data, adjusted for age, sex, and health status differences, provided the basis for comparative utilization and cost analysis.

3. Evaluation Results

Table 15-1 shows that for the average ("standard") mix of patients, 568 entrants/1,000 were classified as being "well": they had no significant complaints and were confirmed by the professional staff to have no significant abnormalities; 116/1,000 were classified as being "worried-well": they had significant complaints

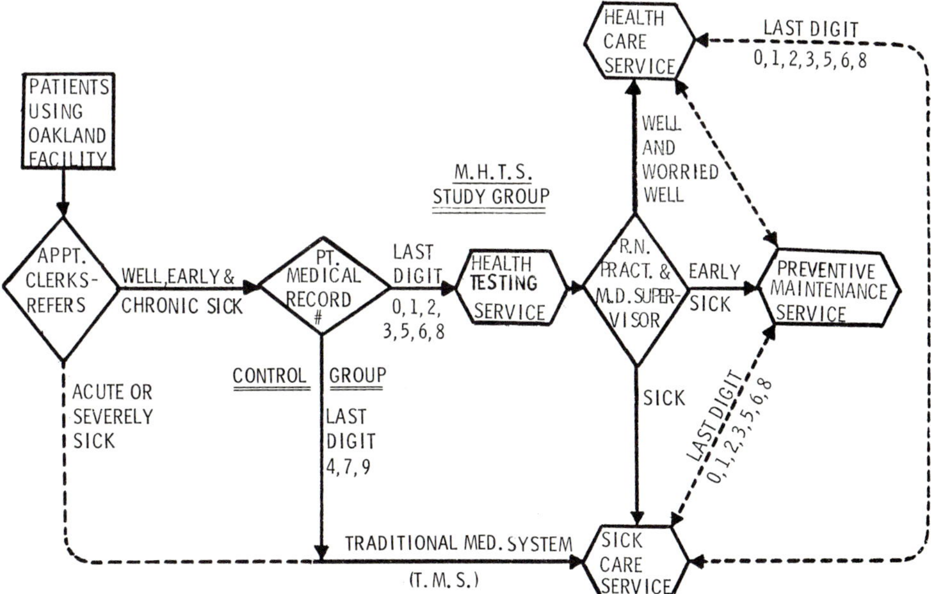

Figure 15-2.   Study-patient flow pattern for evaluation of MHTS as an entry mode to a medical care delivery system.

Table 15-1. Average Entry Mix by Health Status Group (HSG) for Any 1,000 New and New-Return* Patient (Pt) Entrants Seeking Medical Department Appointments (Age-Sex Adjusted)

Health Status Group	Number	Proportion	Pts/1,000 Entrants
Well	3,573	0.568	568
Worried-well	729	0.116	116
Asymptomatic-sick	247	0.039	39
Sick	1,736	0.277	277
All groups	6,285	1.000	1,000

*New-returns are patients who have not seen their physician within the previous 12 months and need a thorough workup.

but were found to have no significant abnormalities; 39/1,000 were classified as "asymptomatic-sick": they had no significant complaints but were found to have significant abnormalities; and 277/1,000 were classified "sick": they had significant complaints and were confirmed to have significant abnormalities.[5,8] It should be noted that 684 entrants (see Table 15-1, "well" and "worried-well") per thousand (more than two-thirds) were found by the health evaluation personnel to be well (no significant abnormalities). This supports our hypothesis that free care to users brings a large number of well and worried-well people into the delivery system.

Tables 15-2a and b, respectively, compare the physician hours and costs consumed in the entry workup for each 1,000 entrants in TMS vs. MHTS. These tables clearly show the new MHTS entry workup mode to be more effective in all respects, utilizing approximately one-third as many physician hours and consequently reducing physician costs 72 percent for the entry workup.

Tables 15-3a and b compare physician hours and costs in the medical department, including entry and followup care, for each 1,000 entrants in the TMS and MHTS systems for the 12-month period. Again MHTS proved to be more effective in both respects, achieving a 57 percent savings in physician hours and a 56 percent savings in doctor costs.

Tables 15-4a and b further compare the 12-month total utilization of physician hours and costs per 1,000 entrants in all clinical departments for TMS and MHTS. MHTS shows a significant saving over TMS, reducing physician hours by 43 percent and costs by 42 percent.

Table 15-5 compares the 12-month total resource utilization costs per 1,000 entrants in the two systems, including all physicians plus all supporting personnel including health care services, preventive maintenance services, nurse practitioners, overhead and fringe benefits, facilities costs, etc. MHTS saved $32,550 per 1,000 entrants or $32.55 per year per entrant over TMS.

Table 15-6, combining Tables 15-2, 15-3, 15-4, and 15-5, summarizes the comparative resource savings and cost effectiveness of MHTS over TMS. It demonstrates an overall reduction in total costs over the 12-month period of $32.55 per MHTS entrant, a 25 percent reduction over entry through TMS.

Table 15-7 demonstrates the markedly increased accessibility for new patient entry created by the new MHTS entry mode. As stated in the footnote of the table, the seven and ten days represent patient's options rather than true waiting

Tables 15-2. Comparison of Total Physician Hours and Costs in all Departments for *Entry Workup* Per 1,000 Entrants in TMS and MHTS, Proportioned by Health Status Groups (HSG) for 12 Months (Age-Sex Adjusted)

(a) Total Physician Hours for *Entry Workup*

	TMS Entry Mode			MHTS Entry Mode		
HSG	MD Hours /Pt/Year	Entrants /1,000	Total Hours	MD Hours /Pt/Year	Entrants /1,000	Total Hours
Well	0.68 ×	568	= 386	0.16 ×	568	= 91
Worried-well	0.77 ×	116	= 89	0.25 ×	116	= 29
Asymptomatic-sick	0.88 ×	39	= 34	0.27 ×	39	= 11
Sick	0.79 ×	277	= 218	0.36 ×	277	= 100
All patients	0.73 ×	1,000	= 727	0.23 ×	1,000	= 231

(b) Total Physician Cost for *Entry Workup*

	TMS Entry Mode			MHTS Entry Mode		
HSG	MD Visit $/Pt	Entrants /1,000	Total $	MD Visit $/Pt	Entrants /1,000	Total $
Well	36.25 ×	568	= 20,590	7.22 ×	568	= 4,101
Worried-well	41.89 ×	116	= 4,859	12.52 ×	116	= 1,452
Asymptomatic-sick	50.07 ×	39	= 1,953	13.11 ×	39	= 511
Sick	43.09 ×	277	= 11,936	18.30 ×	277	= 5,069
All patients	39.33 ×	1,000	= 39,338	11.13 ×	1,000	= 11,133

time, since appointments were available in two to three days, but patients generally preferred seven to ten days bookings.

Table 15-8 shows the results of a survey questionnaire administered to entrants into TMS and MHTS on the day of their examination. It was filled out immediately following the visit in the TMS medical department waiting room and in a special room provided in the MHTS physical examination area. Questionnaires were handed to patients willing to respond by the reception staff in TMS for four consecutive weeks, May 1 through June 1, 1973. There were 297 respondents who had 30-minute appointments in TMS. Questionnaires were distributed to 315 MHTS respondents during the period May 14 through May 25, 1973.

Respondents were mostly very satisfied with the service they received. As Table 15-8 reveals, no differences were found between TMS and MHTS patients in their satisfaction with the health evaluation or the competence of the person examining them. MHTS patients were significantly more satisfied than TMS patients with their length of wait for an appointment.

In addition to the data shown in Table 15-8, the acceptability of MHTS to patients was excellent.[4] Of those patients who fulfilled the criteria and were

Tables 15-3. Comparison of Total Physician Hours and Costs in the Medical Department Per 1,000 Entrants in TMS and MHTS Proportional Health Status Groups for 12 Months (Age-Sex Adjusted)

(a) Total Physician Scheduled Hours—Medical Department

	TMS Entry Mode			MHTS Entry Mode		
HSG	MD Hours /Pt/Year	Entrants /1,000	Total Hours	MD Hours /Pt/Year	Entrants /1,000	Total Hours
Well	0.87 ×	568 =	494.2	0.30 ×	568 =	170.4
Worried-well	1.13 ×	116 =	131.1	0.50 ×	116 =	58.0
Asymptomatic-sick	1.26 ×	39 =	49.1	0.45 ×	39 =	17.6
Sick	1.34 ×	277 =	371.2	0.72 ×	277 =	199.4
All patients	1.05 ×	1,000 =	1,045.6	0.45 ×	1,000 =	445.4

(b) Total Physician Costs—Medical Department

	TMS Entry Mode			MHTS Entry Mode		
HSG	MD Visit $/Pt/Year	Entrants /1,000	Total $	MD Visit $/Pt/Year	Entrants /1,000	Total $
Well	48.41 ×	568 =	27,497	16.63 ×	568 =	9,446
Worried-well	63.69 ×	116 =	7,388	27.95 ×	116 =	9,242
Asymptomatic-sick	73.88 ×	39 =	2,881	25.92 ×	39 =	1,011
Sick	76.42 ×	277 =	21,168	44.01 ×	277 =	12,191
All patients	58.93 ×	1,000 =	58,934	25.89 ×	1,000 =	25,890

offered the new MHTS, approximately 90 percent accepted. Satisfaction surveys showed that in the main, patients were very satisfied with either service they received, traditional doctor entry or MHTS. There was greater satisfaction with the earlier appointments available in MHTS. Most MHTS patients were pleased by the comprehensiveness and completeness of the total examination and the convenience of having it all done in one visit. Those who experienced MHTS expressed a clear preference for nurse practitioner physical examinations in the future.

In summary, the survey data showed MHTS was clearly acceptable to patients, and MHTS patients were generally as satisfied with the services received as were TMS patients. MHTS patients were significantly more satisfied with service availability and convenience. They stated strong preferences to return to MHTS services in the future.

Table 15-9 shows the results of a satisfaction survey of three staff groups made in the last quarter of the study: (1) 23 physicians (MDs) in the medical department and five physicians in obstetrics-gynecology (Ob-Gyn); (2) 23 nurses (RNs) from Medicine and 10 nurses in Ob-Gyn; and (3) eight nurse practitioners (NPs) plus 10

Tables 15-4. Comparison of Total Physician Hours and Costs in All Departments Per 1,000 Entrants in TMS and MHTS Proportioned for Health Status Groups for 12 Months (Age-Sex Adjusted)

(a) Per Total Scheduled Hours—All Departments

	TMS Entry Mode			MHTS Entry Mode		
HSG	MD Hours /Pt/Year	Entrants /1,000	Total Hours	MD Hours /Pt/Year	Entrants /1,000	Total Hours
Well	1.37	× 568	= 778.2	0.67	× 568	= 380.6
Worried-well	1.79	× 116	= 207.6	1.07	× 116	= 124.1
Asymptomatic-sick	1.67	× 39	= 65.1	0.85	× 39	= 33.2
Sick	2.11	× 277	= 584.5	1.45	× 277	= 401.6
All patients	1.64	× 1,000	= 1,635.4	0.94	× 1,000	= 939.5

(b) Per Total MD Costs—All Departments

	TMS Entry Mode			MHTS Entry Mode		
HSG	MD Visits $/Pt/yr	Entrants /1,000	Total Visit $	MD Visits $/Pt/yr	Entrants /1,000	Total Visit $
Well	77.90	× 568	= 44,247	37.98	× 568	= 21,573
Worried-well	102.40	× 116	= 11,878	62.47	× 116	= 7,247
Asymptomatic-sick	98.95	× 39	= 3,859	50.76	× 39	= 1,980
Sick	121.62	× 277	= 33,689	86.22	× 277	= 23,883
All patients	93.67	× 1,000	= 93,673	54.68	× 1,000	= 54,683

Table 15-5. Comparison of *Total Resource Cost* Per 1,000 Entrants in TMS and MHTS Proportioned by Health Status Groups for 12 Months (Age-Sex Adjusted)

	TMS Entry Mode			MHTS Entry Mode		
HSG	Total MD $ and All Other Costs/ Pt/Yr	Entrants /1,000	Total $	Total MD $ and All Other Costs/ Pt/Yr	Entrants /1,000	Total $
Well	108.90	× 568	= 61,855	74.60	× 568	= 42,373
Worried-well	145.30	× 116	= 16,855	107.42	× 116	= 12,461
Asymptomatic-sick	139.92	× 39	= 5,457	97.62	× 39	= 3,807
Sick	169.72	× 277	= 47,012	144.36	× 277	= 39,988
All patients	131,18	× 1,000	= 131,179	98,63	× 1,000	= 98,629

Table 15-6. Summary of Resource and Cost Effectiveness, Traditional Medical System (TMS) vs. Multiphasic Health Testing Service (MHTS) Entry Mode for 12 Months Per Standard 1,000 Entrants (Age-Sex Adjusted)

		TMS (per 1,000)	MHTS (per 1,000)	Diff. (TMS − MHTS)	Percent Reduction[†]
Entry and Entry Followup, MD (Entry workup) (See Table 15-2a and b)	Hours	727	231	496	68
	Costs	$39,338	$11,133	$28,205	72
Medical Department, MD (Includes entry and entry followup above plus	Hours	1,046	445	601	57
subsequent visits in 12 months) (See Table 15-3a and b)	Costs	$58,934	$25,890	$33,044	56
All Specialty Departments, MD (Includes Medical Department above and all	Hours	1,635	940	695*	43
other MD visits, 12 months) (See Table 15-4a and b)	Costs	$93,673	$54,683	$38,990	42
Total Resource Utilization (Includes all MDs above plus all supporting personnel, health care, preventive maintenance, nurse practitioners, overhead, facilities costs, etc.) (See Table 15-5)	Costs	$131,179	$98,629	$32,550	25

*Each entrant in MHTS saved 2.78 return visits ($\frac{695}{1,000} \times 4 = 2.78$ return visits).

[†]Percent reduction $= \dfrac{\text{TMS} - \text{MHTS}}{\text{TMS}} \times 100.$

Table 15-7. Comparison, TMS vs. MHTS, of Average Waits in Days for Entry Appointments for 1971 Baseline and for the Study Period

Entry Period	Average Wait in Days	
	TMS	MHTS
January 1971	36	—
January 1972	34	7*
January 1973	30	10*

*Patient option—MHTS appointments were available in two days. Some patients elected to enter later than the first available appointment, and figures shown represent the patients' option rather than actual offered waiting time.

support staff of the new MHTS. Staff members were asked to identify in what way (if any) the new entry system (MHTS) was of benefit or produced problems (1) to themselves and (2) to patients.

Every professional group listed more benefits from MHTS (e.g., MDs could see more patients; patients got earlier appointments) than problems (e.g., MDs lost contact with routine patients; patients were confused as to the MD's and the RN's role). One difference among the three staff groups was that while MDs and NPs saw an even balance of benefits for themselves and for their patients (25-28 and

Table 15-8. Patient Satisfaction Survey of Health Evaluations Provided by Traditional Medical System (TMS) and Multiphasic Health Testing Service (MHTS) Entry Mode

	How satisfied or dissatisfied were you with					
	1. The length of wait for this appointment?		2. The competence of the person who examined you?		3. This checkup?	
Answer	TMS ($N = 297$)*	MHTS ($N = 315$)	TMS ($N = 297$)	MHTS ($N = 315$)	TMS ($N = 297$)	MHTS ($N = 315$)
Very satisfied	45.1	71.7	79.5	85.7	74.0	81.4
Fairly satisfied	17.5	19.5	14.1	10.8	20.0	14.6
Neither	13.5	3.8	1.7	1.3	3.0	2.8
Fairly dissatisfied	12.4	1.9	0.0	0.3	0.6	0.6
Very dissatisfied	9.1	0.9	0.0	0.3	0.0	0.3
Don't know; no answer	2.4	2.2	4.7	1.6	2.4	0.3
	100.0%	100.0%	100.0%	100.0%	100.0%	100.0%

*N = number of respondents.

Table 15-9. Satisfaction Survey of Professional Staff Members as to Benefits and Problems from MHTS

	MDs ($N = 28$)*		TMS RNs ($N = 33$)		MHTS NPs and Aides ($N = 18$)	
	For Staff	For Patients	For Staff	For Patients	For Staff	For Patients
Benefits	25	28	17	29	16	17
Problems	14	13	10	9	11	9

*N = number of respondents.

16-17), the RNs saw almost twice as many benefits for their patients as for themselves (29-17).

Finally, staff members were asked with which medical care entry system in general they were more satisfied, and for what reasons. The physicians were equally divided in opinion: 43 percent preferred MHTS, 43 percent preferred TMS, and 14 percent did not answer or were not sure. Of the clinic nurses, 60 percent chose MHTS, 6 percent chose TMS, and 34 percent did not answer or were not sure. Of the nurse practitioners, 83 percent preferred MHTS, 6 percent preferred TMS, and 11 percent did not answer or were not sure.

4. Discussion of Evaluation Results

The effectiveness of this new MHTS entry mode in achieving its objectives can be judged from the following analyses of our studies:

a.   Accessibility effect.   The major objective of this new concept was to assure prompt access to medical care for free users of service. Traditionally, access is exclusively through the physician and therefore constrained by two variable physician-productivity functions: entrance capacity and return-followup sick care capacity. These two functions, entry and followup, traditionally performed by the same physician at the primary care level, tend to compete with each other for physician time. The more patients the physician enters, the more he must follow up; the more he follows up, the fewer he can enter. The pattern that evolves is an increasing followup load and decreasing entrance capacity through time. This seriously restricts new patient entry and inevitably results in severe queuing problems for service.

The new MHTS entry solved this problem by simply uncoupling the two functions—entry and followup—into separate services, so that the capacity of each could be optimized. The new method of entry through MHTS and nurse physical examinations has no followup services to provide, so it is open to full capacity for new patient workup and is readily expandable, whereas physician supply is not.

The positive effect of the new approach on access was clearly demonstrated. During the entire operational period of the evaluation, appointments were available for new patient workups within 24 to 48 hours, in contrast to four to six weeks of queuing in the traditional medical clinics (see Table 15-7).

b.   Systemization of the new patient entry workup. Through MHTS, consisting of multiphasic health testing plus nurse practitioner physical examinations and online information processing, the new entry mode achieved an efficiency of entry workup for new patients in one visit that could not possibly be equaled in the traditional physician-provided entry visit.

This effect was confirmed by the great amount of physician time conserved in the entry workup process by the MHTS approach compared to the TMS. Figure 15-3 shows the comparative amount of physician (MD) hours used for entry workups in the two modes.

c.   Matching patient needs with appropriate resources. The effectiveness of the MHTS in identifying patient needs and referring to appropriate resources is best demonstrated by the triage referrals that followed the comprehensive MHTS workup during the period of operation of the new entry mode. Figure 15-1 illustrates the referrals from MHTS to health care, preventive maintenance, and sick care during the stable period of the evaluation study, January 1973 to June 1973.

Entry through the MHTS therefore saved 100 percent of the entry visits to the medical department and referred only 8.9 percent to that department for specialty care. Of the remaining 91.1 percent, 17.2 percent of new patients who would ordinarily have had a duplicated entry visit to the medical department were expeditiously referred directly to indicated specialty clinics.

Only 26 percent (8.9 percent plus 17.2 percent) of all new patients entering

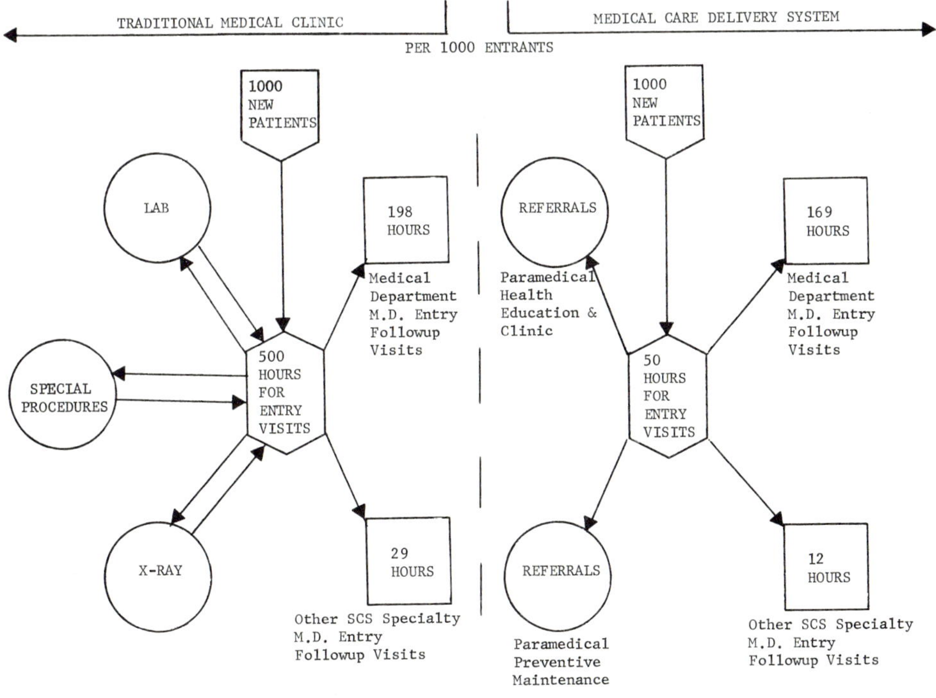

Figure 15-3. Comparative number of physician hours used for entry workups.

through MHTS actually needed to be referred to traditional physician services. The remaining 74 percent were referred to the new paramedical services in health care and preventive maintenance.

d.   Resource utilization and cost effectiveness of MHTS vs. TMS.   Comparative analysis of physician and other resource utilization, and of costs in the two systems, demonstrated MHTS to be definitely more efficient in physician and other resource utilization and to be more cost-effective.

Table 15-6 summarizes and compares doctor hours and costs of the two systems in a way that shows not only the cumulative 12-month total savings by MHTS, but also the analysis of those savings according to categories of care. First, it shows the total initial workup, i.e., entry and entry followup. Second, it presents the total medical department services provided in the 12 months. Third, it accumulates the total physician (MD) services, including specialty services; and last, it shows the total of all resources provided in the 12 months.

As Table 15-6 shows, most of MD hours and MD cost savings occurred in the initial entry workup. However, there was a total savings for the entire year in MD hours and costs as follows:

Total MD hours saved = 695 per 1,000, or .695 per entrant.
Total MD costs saved = $38,990 per 1,000, or $38.99 per entrant.

Adding all other resource costs resulted in a total saving of $32,550 per 1,000 entrants, or $32.55 per entrant for the year.

It is likely that this saving could be amplified by greater diversion of chronic illness monitoring to Preventive Maintenance. Also, adding more nurse practitioners (see Figure 15-4) would add considerable savings in MD costs.

e.   Physician accessibility for new patients and availability for return sick care.   Practically, the effects of MHTS on accessibility and availability could only be measured by comparison with the Oakland Medical Department physician schedules, since physician schedules, work styles, productivity of physicians, and comprehensiveness of workup varies in other settings.

At Oakland Kaiser-Permanente Medical Department, the physicians' schedules allot five appointments for new patient workups at 30 minutes each and 15 appointments for return visits at 15 minutes each. The MHTS evaluation study, using four nurse practitioners supervised by one physician, comprehensively worked up 55 new patients per day. In 1975, MHTS utilized multiphasic testing and nine nurses and one physician to work up 110 new patients per day.

Figure 15-4 shows the marked amplification of physician capacity for both new patient access and return visit availability produced by MHTS when employing four nurses and nine nurses.

D.   IMPLICATIONS OF MHTS FOR THE FUTURE OF MEDICINE

The principle of medical care as a "right" has generally been accepted in the United States; however, achieving that goal is unlikely in view of the current critically impaired accessibility to care. In fact, further overtaxing the already

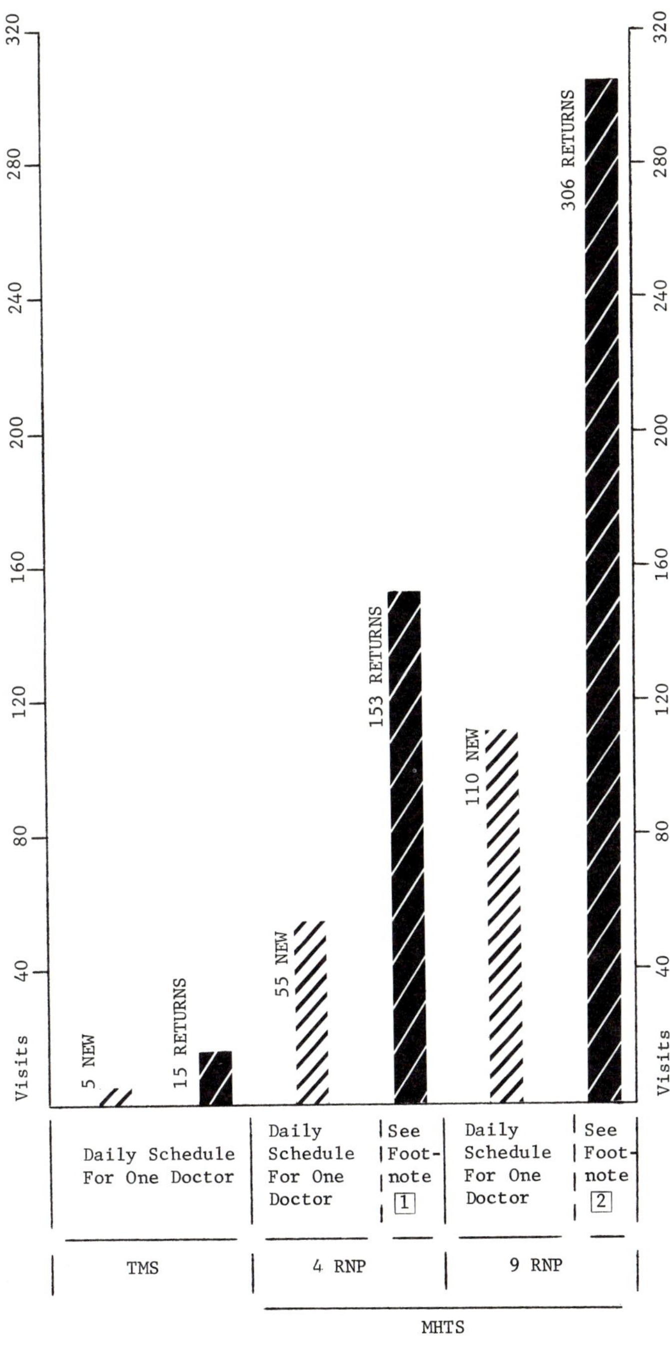

[1] Represents appointments made available in TMS by visits saved per Table 15-6 (55 × 2.78 = 152.9).

[2] Represents appointments made available in TMS by visits saved per Table 15-6 (110 × 2.78 = 305.8).

Figure 15-4. Comparison of physician schedule capacity for new and return patients in traditional (TMS) and MHTS systems using four and nine nurse practitioners (RNP).

overloaded delivery system can only reduce the accessibility and quality of care for the sick.

MHTS as an entry mode to a health care system helps resolve the problem of accessibility. The solution lies in the new method of entry through MHTS plus nurse practitioner physical examinations, which unlocks the physician from his traditional constraining position at the point of entry and conserves him for the sick care for which he has been trained. Entry workup and followup care by the same physician compete with each other for his time. The separation of entry from followup sick care is the key to increased capacity; their division into separate services permits the capacity of each to be optimized. MHTS, the new entry method, using automated equipment and paramedical staff supervised by a physician, greatly expands entrance capacity and is always open to new patients, since it has no followup sick care load. It is a thorough evaluative process, well suited to define patient needs. Followup sick care service, relieved of entry workups by MHTS, and further released from a considerable portion of the monitoring and surveillance of chronic illness by the new preventive maintenance service, develops a greatly expanded followup capacity for care of the sick.

This two-pronged expansion of entrance capacity and of followup sick care capacity greatly amplifies accessibility.

1.   Use of Paramedical Personnel

The three new divisions of this new delivery system, MHTS health evaluation, health care, and preventive maintenance, use existing types of paramedical personnel and so are relatively easily staffed and relatively inexpensive.

Though the system relies heavily on paramedical personnel, it uses them in a very selective way. The only special training required for MHTS is that of nurses to do physical examinations. (See Chapter Ten.) They are not taught to be substitute physicians and do not diagnose or treat patients. They merely record observations and measurements and, backed up by multiphasic testing, computer data processing, protocols with advice rules, and the supervising physician, they need only decide (as a team) whether the patient is well or sick and the appropriate resources to be used. Utilizing paramedical personnel with limited but specific skills requires that tasks be clearly defined and patient input be carefully systemized. The existing traditional delivery system with its heterogeneous entry mix is the antithesis of those requirements. This new MHTS entry to health care delivery with its clear division of referral services and its systemized patient input is the key to a safe and effective use of paramedical personnel.

2.   Transferability Opportunity

One of the exceptional features of this new concept is its ready transferability to almost any form of practice and almost any geographic area. It is, of course, admirably suited to prepaid group practice; however, it could be of equal value to medical society foundations and other types of health maintenance organizations (HMOs). Any group of physicians or solo physicians in private practice could adopt its principles; some already have. A small multiphasic health testing unit, such as a carrel type,[9] plus a few nurses trained in physical examinations will amplify many times almost any physician's capacity to provide entrance workups and consequently followup sick care.

Geographically, the three paramedical services, MHTS, health care, and preventive maintenance, supervised by a few physicians working in a neighborhood health clinic affiliated with a medical center, could bring high-quality health care into poverty areas rapidly and effectively.

E. CONCLUSION

In view of America's obvious commitment to comprehensive health services of high quality to every person, the importance of these research results and their potential benefits is self-evident. That goal can never be achieved without a delivery system that matches its patients' demands.

A medical care delivery system with MHTS, and with health care and preventive maintenance services supplementing sick care, promises to fulfill that need. It provides increased capacity, accessibility, appropriateness of services, comprehensiveness of care, continuity of both health care and sick care, and efficiency of resource utilization; and it is cost-effective. Its new services are relatively easily staffed, and it promises ready transferability and adaptability to most forms of practice and geographical areas.

This system design not only makes the free-user demand for care manageable, but makes the care itself more meaningful. It replaces the traditional fee-for-service patient regulator with a systemized MHTS health evaluation that refers patients according to their medical needs. The entrance of well people into the delivery system, in a fashion that refers them to appropriate health care services rather than discharges them to home, provides medicine with a great new opportunity—that of reversing its traditional preoccupation with sickness to a positive accentuation of health. This adds a new dimension to medical care that has been long overdue.

One can envision a new health care system of the future that will begin with a basic comprehensive MHTS health evaluation for each individual. The results of that evaluation will chart each individual's personal pathway through health care resources toward optimal health. Periodic updating of health evaluation profiles will monitor the homeostasis of vital body subsystems, and significant deviations will then trigger computerized warnings and corrective instructions. Health education will alert and advise measures to be taken against individual predictive risks, be they life style, hereditary, environmental, or age-sex linked through time.

Episodic acute illnesses may in large part be managed by programmed protocols and diagnosed against the background of each individual's updated health profile. Such individualized continuing health care would greatly reduce patient uncertainty and could, in large part, replace today's random entry demand with a smoother regulated use of appropriate resources that would not only be cost-effective but also could optimize the health of each individual throughout his lifetime.

It should be clear that this new medical care delivery system and this health care of the future could never be fully achieved without the large amount of individual information, cybernetic data feedback, protocols and advice rules, monitoring and surveillance that systemized MHTS health evaluation makes possible. Supplementing today's sick care services with this new system, and providing the accessibility it makes possible, can raise the quality and distribution of medicine in the United States to a level unparalleled in the world. Such is the great promise of this new delivery system for the medicine of the future.

ACKNOWLEDGMENT

The evaluation study reported in this chapter was performed under contract No. HSM 110-70-407 awarded by the National Center for Health Services Research, Health Resources Administration, Department of Health, Education, and Welfare. The final report to DHEW and the data tape files from this project are available from the National Technical Information Service (NTIS), PB 246 630.[8] This study was also supported in part by the Kaiser Foundation Research Institute and The Permanente Medical Group.

REFERENCES

1. Garfield, S. R. "Multiphasic Health Testing and Medical Care as a Right." *N. Eng. J. Med.* 283(1970):1087–1089.

2. Somers, A. R., ed. *The Kaiser-Permanente Medical Care Program.* New York: Commonwealth Fund, 1971.

3. Garfield, S. R. "The Delivery of Medical Care." *Scient. Amer.* 222(1970):15-23.

4. Feldman, R., Taller, S. L., Garfield, S. R., Richart, R. H., Collen, M. F., Cella, R., and Sender, A. J. "Forum: Allied Health Professionals." "Nurse Practitioner Multiphasic Health Checkups" *J. Preventive Med.* 2(1977).

5. Garfield, S. R., Collen, M. F., Feldman, R., Soghikian, K., Richart, R. H., and Duncan, J. H. "Evaluation of an Ambulatory Medical-Care Delivery System." *N. Eng. J. Med.* 294(1976):426–431.

6. Collen, M. F., Garfield, S. R., Richart, R. H., Duncan, J. H., and Feldman, R. "Cost Analyses of Three Health Evaluation Modes." *Arch. Int. Med.* 137(1977):73–79.

7. Collen, F. B., Madero, B., Soghikian, K., and Garfield, S. R. "Kaiser-Permanente Experiment in Ambulatory Care." *Am. J. Nurs.* 71(1971):1371–1374.

8. Collen, M. F., and Garfield, S. R. "New Medical Care Delivery System, Final Report, January 1975." National Technical Information Service (NTIS) PB 246 630.

9. Gilbert, F. "Multiphasic Screening Cut Down to Size." *Med. World News* 9(1968):60–61.

CHAPTER SIXTEEN

Specialized MHTS

Morris F. Collen

A. Introduction
B. MHTS for Industrial Practice
C. MHTS for Military Services
D. MHTS for Research Purposes
E. Uses of Mobile MHTS Units

A. INTRODUCTION

This chapter concerns itself with the application of multiphasic health testing services (MHTS) to special-purpose programs designed primarily to satisfy the objectives of the sponsoring organization and secondarily to serve the personal health of the patient. These types of MHTS are used mostly by industrial organizations and sometimes by the military for evaluating the physical fitness of their personnel. They are also well suited for special research studies on large populations. The specialized uses of mobile MHTS will also be considered.

B. MHTS FOR INDUSTRIAL PRACTICE

Health examinations have been widely provided in industry for many years, and furnishing periodic health examinations to executives has been a fringe benefit of many organizations. During the 1960s a Periodic Health Examination Group sponsored by the U.S. Public Health Service and consisting predominantly of medical directors of large industries was very active in studying and evaluating this practice.

Periodic health examinations are provided in accordance with the interest of the company administration in (1) evaluating and maintaining the health of both employee and management personnel, and (2) protecting its employees from work hazards to health. Such examinations are used for evaluation of prospective employees for acceptability of initial employment and initial job placement. They are also used for ongoing employee examinations and for determining requirements for replacement, disability evaluation, and rehabilitation of an already established worker. Large companies increasingly are using MHTS for these purposes.

Periodic executive health examinations provided by large organizations often employ personal physicians or occupational medical groups to furnish a specified test battery,[2,3] with a report going to the employee or a physician of his choice or both.

Occupational disease screening can also be used to detect shifts in group characteristics, especially for exposure to toxic environmental agents. Occupational health examinations generally are directed toward detecting and monitoring significant disorders, whether or not they are occupationally related. That is, in addition to pneumoconiosis and occupational dermatitis, such examinations usually screen for hypertension and diabetes. Furthermore, the relationship of occupational hazards to some conditions is very controversial. In some occupations (e.g., firefighting) coronary disease is considered to be an industrial condition covered by Workmen's Compensation; and foremen have been reported to have more peptic disease than craftsmen or executives.[4]

There is increasing concern in the United States with the low-grade health hazards present in the physical environment, which can affect large numbers of people over long periods of time. Especially in certain industries, workers can be exposed to significant concentrations of toxic chemicals, harmful physical agents (such as particulate dusts), and radiations (noise, heat, etc.).

The National Institute of Occupational Safety and Health (NIOSH) in the

Department of Health, Education and Welfare has the responsibility to protect the health of American workers by recommending standards and implementing laws banning or controlling hazards in their working environments.

The Occupational Safety and Health Agency (OSHA) in the Department of Labor was established to protect the workers' health by setting and enforcing standards that private industry was to meet or be fined for not meeting. Many employees will be required to have a periodic checkup to monitor them for early evidence of toxic effects of chemicals upon liver, kidney, lung, skin, etc.

NIOSH and OSHA are concerned about many environmental carcinogens. Arsenic, 4-aminobiphenyl, asbestos, auramine, benzene, benzidine, bis-(chloromethyl) ether, cadmium oxide, chromic acid, haematite, beta-naphthylamine, nickel, coal tar, and vinyl chloride are all occupational carcinogens proved to cause cancer in humans. Some of the suspected or almost-proved human carcinogens are aluminum, benzoyl chloride, chloroprene, wood dust, fibrous glass, radon daughters (free radiation in uranium mines), cutting-oil mists, aldrin and dieldrin (pesticides), and several anesthetics. At a recent review of environmental health, it was estimated that occupational factors account for more than 100,000 deaths per year in the United States.[5]

Large companies with their industrial medical departments continually adjust to NIOSH and OSHA requirements. A fully developed in-plant occupational health program will usually include preplacement examinations or screening, and periodic health appraisals or both.[6] Small organizations likely will contract with occupational medical groups for periodic health examinations of their employees.

In addition to a basic battery of MHTS tests (discussed in earlier chapters), industries that subject employees to excessive risk of lung cancer from airborne contaminants usually add sputum cytology to their occupational periodic health screening programs, with fiber-optic bronchoscopy followed at the first sign of metaplastic or neoplastic cells. Industries with excessive exposure to lead, mercury, or cadmium will add blood or urine tests for these metals. Employees with exposure to carbon tetrachloride, chloroform, fluorocarbons, etc., should receive additional liver function tests. And so each industry must customize its own examinations to its specific health hazards.

Occupational cancers develop sometimes simultaneously in multiple sites, so comprehensive multiphasic examinations are indicated. For example, asbestos workers have a high risk of developing carcinoma of the lung, gastrointestinal tract, and bladder, and also mesothelioma of the pleura and peritoneum; vinyl chloride produces cancer of the liver, brain, and lung;[7] coke-oven effluent produces lung and kidney cancer.[5]

1. Occupational Coding

The problem of coding occupations is a very great one. The U.S. Department of Labor's *Dictionary of Occupational Titles*[8] in its 1965 edition contained 21,741 separate occupations and listed a total of 35,550 defined occupational titles.

In response to the question on the medical questionnaire form, "What is your present occupation; what kind of work do you do now?" 2,542 consecutive patients recorded their occupation in their own words.[9] These occupations were then tallied and grouped. It was found that all occupations reported in this series of patients with a frequency of one to 1,000 or greater could be included in 170 occupational titles. Since an important objective of this program was to determine important health hazards to which patients are exposed, they were encouraged to report all of their occupational activities. It was apparent that a part-time job as a welder might be more significant as a health hazard than a full-time job as a cashier. Accordingly, without any attempt to avoid redundancy or overlapping, patients were asked to look over the list of occupations on the card shown in Figure 16-1 and to punch holes under all the occupations that most closely described their work. If they could not find their exact occupational title, they were asked to pick the ones they thought came closest.

The number of multiphasic occupations punched by a series of 1,820 consecutive patients is shown in Table 16-1. These are not multiple jobs, but multiple occupational titles or descriptions of all the patient's work activities.

The portable punch card shown in Figure 16-1 is a simple means of direct communication with the computer. The cards are prescored with a die, so that machine-readable holes are easily punched out by any stylus or pencil. Instead of

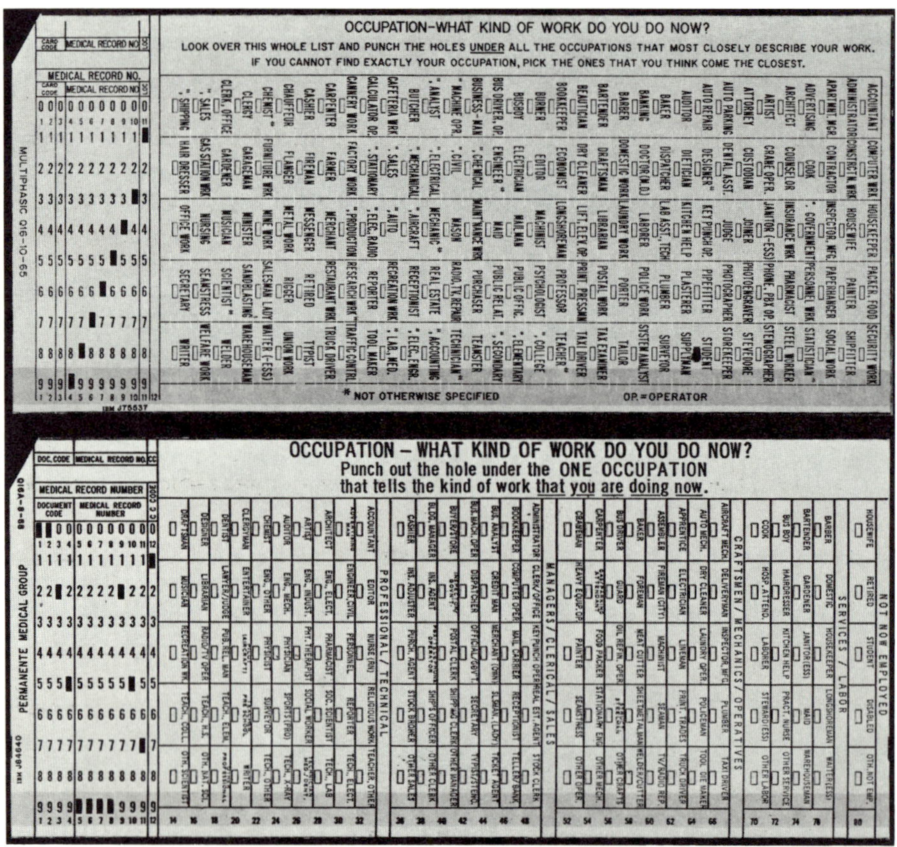

Figure 16-1. Occupational portable punch card for self-administration. Top card requests all occupational exposures for health hazards; bottom card is used for occupational classification.

Table 16-1.   Multiple Occupational Titles in 1,820 Consecutive MHTS Patients*

| No. of | Number | | | Percent | | |
Occupations	Total	Male	Female	Total	Male	Female
0–1	1,438	742	696	79	74.5	84.5
2	322	203	119	17.7	20.4	14.4
3	31	23	8	1.7	2.3	1
4	15	15	—	0.8	1.5	—
5	7	6	1	0.4	0.6	0.1
6	2	2	—	0.1	0.2	—
7	2	2	—	0.1	0.2	—
8	1	1	—	0.05	0.1	—
10	1	1	—	0.05	0.1	—
19	1	1	—	0.05	0.1	—
Totals	1,820	996	824	100	100	100

*Modified from Collen.[9]

checking the rectangle below the appropriate occupation, one merely punches out the rectangle, and the card is ready to be read by the computer's card-reading machine. (See also Figure 1-27.)

2.   Preemployment Examinations

Routine health examination of prospective employees is a prevailing custom in most large industries; the aim is to determine the individual's health status and physical fitness with reference to his capacity to do the job for which he is applying.

Preemployment health examinations in people under age 30 have a low yield rate of abnormalities, and since such age groups (especially women) have a high turnover rate, women under 30 who are not to be employed in potentially hazardous occupations are sometimes excluded from a preemployment examination.[10]

An MHTS can usually be modified readily to test for the specific conditions at occupational risk, such as color-blindness testing wherever color discrimination is a job requirement, baseline hearing acuity in noisy occupations, baseline chest x-ray in dusty environments, and baseline back x-rays for jobs requiring heavy lifting.

Preemployment urine screening tests are sometimes included in an attempt to detect users of heroin, cocaine, lysergic acid diethylamide (LSD), amphetamines, barbiturates, marihuana, and methadone. It is desirable to be particularly alert to make sure the urine sample is a valid one and that the prospective employee has given his informed consent for the MHTS examination to include the urine screening. Since preemployment examinations are only for the purpose of screening for employment, abnormal findings are not reported to any authorities; accordingly, no "damage" accrues to the applicant who has received such screening tests other than that he might not be hired.

It is difficult to develop a battery of tests that measure an individual's physical capacity to satisfy the physical demands of specific work tasks, such as those requiring large muscular efforts. Physical fitness can be divided into three major areas: medical fitness, organic function, and muscular performance. The first is estimated by conventional medical examination and represents the initial step in most evaluations for demanding physical tasks. The second measures the capacity to perform and recover from submaximal and maximal exercise; this is generally described as cardiorespiratory fitness. The last area, that of muscular performance, is described as the ability to perform certain acts requiring strength, balance, speed of limb movement, and coordination. Many approaches have been developed to attempt to accurately match individual physical capacity to job demands.[11]

A recently reported study[12] of 2,947 preplacement medical examinations of International Business Machine (IBM) employees included height, weight, blood pressure, pulse, urinalysis, hemoglobin, serologic test for syphilis, vision, audiometry, and chest x-ray. Physical examination was done by a physician. Cafeteria employees had a stool examination. Armed guards had a psychiatric evaluation. Employees over 40 had an electrocardiogram. Following the examination, the applicant was placed in one of three classifications: (1) acceptable without reservations for any type of employment; applicant has no limiting physical or emotional defects; (2) acceptable for limited type of employment; or (3) employment considered hazardous to self or others.

Kuh and Hanman in 1944 produced a manual for shipyard workers, *Physical Demands and Capacities Analysis*,[13] that was equally well suited for preplacement or replacement evaluation. The employee received a physical examination that could very readily have been provided by an MHTS; the data were used to determine whether the employee had the physical capacities to match the specific job demands. The approach of the Swedish military system to match conscriptees to military posts follows many of the principles developed by Hanman. (See C.)

3. Periodic Employee Examinations

Roberts,[14] as early as 1959, in a comprehensive review of the use of periodic employee examinations in industry, summarized the evolving practice of examining persons under age 30 every third year, between 30 and 40 every second year, and over 40 every year. Periodic employee examinations utilizing MHTS programs are now designed to satisfy the general objectives of a personal, preventive-medicine-oriented MHTS (as described in prior chapters), and a confidential doctor-patient relationship is usually maintained. They systematically screen also for the specific problems of occupational disease, including (a) cancers, (b) noncancerous conditions of the lungs (for example, asbestosis, silicosis, pneumoconiosis, and byssinosis), of the skin (contact dermatitis, chemical burns, etc.), of the central nervous system (neuritis, etc.), and of other target organs, and (c) the effect of physical factors (e.g., of chronic noise on hearing).

Health evaluations of employees are performed at appropriate intervals to determine whether the employee's health remains compatible with his job assignment and to detect any evidence of ill health that might be attributable to his employment. Certain employees and groups may require examinations more frequently than others as well as additional procedures and tests depending on their sex, age, physical condition, intercurrent illness, the nature of their work, and any special hazard involved. After age 40 or 45, it is customary in many industries to examine employees on or near their birthdays. Workers exposed to definite health hazards or whose work involves responsibility for the safety of others may have mandatory examinations even more frequently. Special health evaluation may be essential for certain job transfers, or on return to work after a specified number of days absent due to illness or injury. Some organizations also arrange a special examination at termination of employment or retirement.

In the United States, Europe, and Japan many large industries utilize MHTS to make periodic health examinations available to their employees. Such occupational MHTS usually include health questionnaires, height and weight measurements, chest x-ray and spirometry, electrocardiography and blood pressure test, visual testing with acuity and tonometry, and a battery of chemistry and hematology tests depending on the occupational hazards. Sometimes they include dental surveys, podiatric examinations for foot diseases, and gastrointestinal studies.

The Kaiser-Permanente Medical Care Program in Oakland, California, has routinely used its MHTS for preemployment examinations, in which case the examination findings are made available to the employer, and for periodic examinations of its employees, in which cases the results are confidential and available only to the patient's physician. Otherwise, the same MHTS facility is used, all examinees are commingled, and the examination process is identical.

Collings has described the New York Telephone Company's program in considerable detail.[1] This program services about 106,000 people and is offered on a voluntary basis to all employees with more than four years' service at a frequency based upon age: over 50 years, examined every year, 40 to 50 years, every two years, and under 40 years, every three years. Examinations are scheduled during regular working hours at its several geographical areas at permanent in-house facilities, supplemented by a mobile unit to reach remotely located employees. The battery of tests reported in 1972 included a self-administered health questionnaire, urinalysis, blood chemistry (including total protein, calcium, cholesterol, creatinine, glucose one hour after 75-gram glucose challenge dose, total bilirubin, urea nitrogen, uric acid, alkaline phosphatase, SGOT, LDH, and triglycerides), hematology (hemoglobin, red cell and white cell counts, hematocrit, and differential count when white cell count is abnormal), 12-lead electrocardiogram, 70 mm chest x-ray, vital measurements (temperature, pulse, height, weight, and blood pressure), audiometry, visual acuity and tonometry, spirometry, and arrangements for followup care. Since diagnosis and treatment are not provided by the company medical staff, arrangement for followup care is important. The costs of about $30 per MHTS examination as reported by Collings in 1972 indicate it to be a reasonably economic program.

Duffy, Medical Director for IBM,[15–17] initiated their MHTS in 1968. Examinations are available to all IBM employees in the United States and Canada, both in the field and at plant and laboratory locations. They processed almost 27,000 employees in the first 12 months, and 73 percent were found to have some defects. They provide only one examination between ages 40 and 59, a second at age 60, and a third at age 64. The entire examination takes 90 minutes and includes a self-administered optically scannable questionnaire, height and weight, urinalysis, blood chemistry (fasting glucose, urea nitrogen, total bilirubin, uric acid, cholesterol, triglycerides, SGOT, and LDH), hemoglobin and hematocrit, chest x-ray, electrocardiogram and blood pressure, visual acuity and audiometry.

All examination specimens and documents are sent to a central department in White Plains, N.Y., for analysis and interpretation. All data are entered and stored in a computer, and a computer-produced medical report is then sent back to the examination location. The medical report compares the current examination findings with those of prior examinations. A doctor or nurse reviews this report with the employee and urges the person to get treatment or further instructions from the family physician. A followup questionnaire is then sent to the employee to see if the patient saw his personal physician.

Exxon's corporate headquarters has a physical fitness laboratory to make available to employees an organized physical conditioning program. It subjects all eligible employees to a complete health evaluation, which provides medical clearance of presumably healthy people to participate in their exercise program. This examination includes a resting electrocardiogram (and an exercise ECG or treadmill test for all over 40), a self-administered medical history, body measurements, chest x-ray, spirometry, and clinical laboratory tests.[18]

Phillips Co. in the Netherlands, Belgium, and France offers its employees voluntary health checkups using an automated MHTS approach, including general medical and occupational health data. The program was initiated prior to 1960.[19]

Tokyo Shibaura Electric Co. Ltd. (Toshiba) established Japan's first MHTS in 1970[20] and uses several models, including mobile units. The central unit in Tokyo is an annex to a hospital and regularly processes an average of 30 examinees a day. Tests include blood, urine, and feces analyses; chest, abdominal, and gastrointestinal x-rays; height and weight; ECG and blood pressure; vision, ocular tension, and hearing; spirometry; retinal photography; medical and psychological questionnaires; and pelvic examination and cervical smear for women. Data processing is offline, and a computer data base provides comparisons of test data to prior examinations.

C. MILITARY MHTS

The use of automated multiphasic screening for the sorting out of inductees for the armed services would appear to be one of its most straightforward applications. Sweden uses a very advanced MHTS examination of military inductees. The U.S. Air Force has used the MHTS concept for periodic employee examinations but not for induction examinations. When cost data for the multiphasic examinations of a population with an average age of 46 years were compared with military physical examinations for a young healthy population, it was reported[21] that multiphasic testing is more expensive than the customary physician-oriented physical examinations. Systemizing the specific tests traditionally provided to draftees by using the multiphasic concept would be a more reasonable basis for comparison; it is difficult to see how a traditional physician labor-intensive operation can be more economical than a systemized paramedical-staffed technology-intensive program to provide the same tests.

Linroth, the Medical Director of the Armed Forces of Sweden, has developed advanced MHTS centers in Sweden that since 1969 have processed 60,000 conscripts each year.[22] He states that a national defense system based on the principle of universal conscription must possess adequate selection and drafting capabilities. Since 1969, Sweden has employed a new enrollment procedure for conscripts and a new MHTS test system for mass medical examination. What is innovative is the use of computer technology to match needs and resources. An analysis is made of the nation's needs, and when the resources have been examined and a data base of comprehensive personnel information established, a rational system of allocation has been used.

The 60,000 conscripts (the total resources) have to be allocated every year in varying numbers to about 2,000 categories of posts (the total needs). The many varied qualifications of the individual (medical, psychological, educational, and so on) have to be matched with the requirements of the different posts. Accordingly, a primary objective of the MHTS is to determine the physical capacity of each individual and match him to the demands of a specific job (e.g., radar operators will have different job demands than will infantry). Selection is therefore concerned with both health and capacity.

In order to obtain some idea of the requirements of the individual posts, there was first a job analysis (i.e., a work requirement analysis) for some 2,000 posts. The specifications for each post were collated, compared, evaluated in levels of requirement, and processed by computer. The results of practical field studies and investigations into the potential performance of conscripts in two or three important types of work provided a starting point from which reasonable levels of requirement were established for different variables in all posts.

By studying the performances of a representative group of the conscript population, it was possible to establish the mean values, the distribution, and the scatter of important variables. The levels of requirement could then be adjusted to fit the actual resources; that is, they could be evened out so that they corresponded in quantity and quality to the performances of the current population in various respects.

On the basis of clinical and military medical experience, guiding principles were established for each post's health requirements (acceptable degree of limitation of health).

Allocation means setting up the qualifications against the requirements so that each type of work is provided for, and actual resources are applied to satisfy as many needs as possible. Allocating the conscripts to their posts is done mainly by computer.

An analysis of the various posts has revealed a number of areas of performance and associated basic physical requirements to be of decisive importance in military life. Although performance will always depend on the total function of the organism, it is possible to state, with some degree of simplification, that each performance is conditioned by the function of certain organs and systems of organs. Those that primarily supply the requirements for performance are given in Figure 16-2.

The procedure for the military MHTS was drawn up with two factors in mind: the need for an accurate picture of the health of the individual, and the job performance requirements. After the examinations have been performed, the results are collated and evaluated, then expressed as a health and capacity profile,

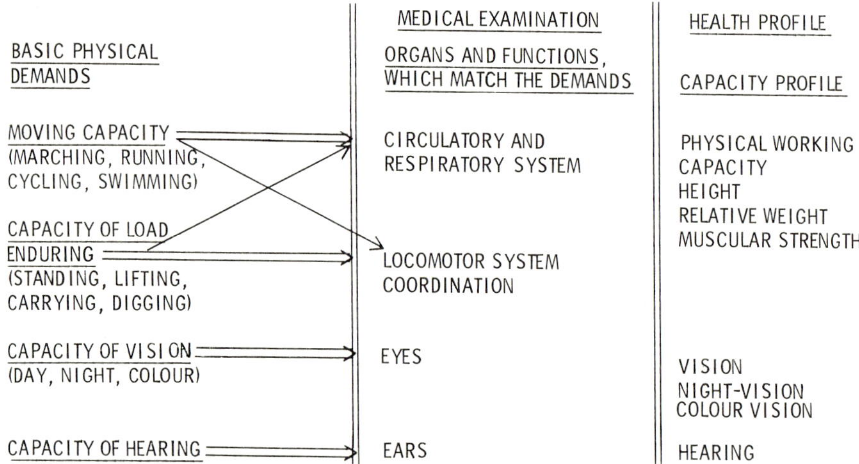

Figure 16-2. Physical demands, matching organ systems, medical examinations, and physical capacity profile. (Modified from Linroth[22].)

thus determining the individual conscript's qualifications and limitations for a certain post. Different examinations can provide information about one and the same organ or system of organs, but in different ways. By the use of different examinations that are complementary in various respects, an attempt is made to get a clear picture of the individual's prospects, free of errors and incorrect information.

The division of data into a health section and a capacity section proved useful to Linroth. Capacity is necessary for an individual to be able to meet the requirements of his work; data on capacity take into consideration the biological variation within the population, so that, for example, persons with above-average performance levels can be utilized in the best possible way. The health profile involves an evaluation of the functions in terms of limitations caused by illness or disablement, with respect to the requirements of the military post; that is to say, the degree of limitation of use is stated.

If a medical assessment is to be carried out for individual persons in a large population, certain norms must be followed. For health investigations, the principles followed are those of clinical medicine. The gradation of illness, defects, and disability is, however, made with due regard to military medical considerations. This uniform classification of disease within both civil and military medicine is naturally an advantage.

The assessment of capacity must relate the individual's results to the distribution of the variables (functions) within the current population. As there has hitherto been very little information about capacity factors, data have been collected during the last few years from representative material in the conscript population. The results provide information on mean values, scatter, distribution, and correlations for a large number of functions of the measurement of physical capacity.

In Sweden there are six enrollment centers. As a rule each center examines 100 men per day. The tests for each individual cover two days, which generally means that the examinees have to spend the night away from home.

The staff at each center consists of about 50 persons, 34 of whom are engaged in the medical examinations. Each team consists of eight doctors, five employed half-time and one full-time (the senior enrollment medical officer). Two doctors are conscripts. There are also three nurses and one optician, both categories employed half-time. The remaining 21 persons are conscripts trained as medical assistants.

The MHTS procedure takes the afternoon of one day and the morning of the next. A series of laboratory and other tests are carried out by paramedical staff, followed by the doctor's medical examinations, where he makes use of the preliminary test results and evaluates the overall function. The actual time needed for the MHTS is about 120 minutes. Secondary checks may be made on the second day or specialist examinations conducted at local hospitals or medical centers.

History questionnaires are dispatched to all conscripts about one month before they are due to report. Clinical laboratory tests include hematocrit and erythrocyte sedimentation rate, and urinalysis for albumin and sugar. X-ray examination of the chest is provided by a 10×10 cm. Odelca camera in two planes. Spirometry is included. The electrocardiogram is registered after 15 minutes' rest in a recumbent posture with the standard leads and five precordial leads. The blood pressure (systolic and diastolic) is also manually determined at this examination.

The vision is tested including color vision and night vision. The hearing test is carried out by tone audiometry with six frequencies.

Body measurements are important for the allocation of posts. Height and weight are the most important. Chest and waist measurements are also taken. The breadth of the femur condyle is also measured to indicate the size of the bone structure.

Determination of maximum isometric muscular contraction is carried out in standard positions for three groups of muscles (grip, elbow bending, and knee stretching).

Physical working capacity is measured using an ergometer bicycle. Since such work tests often take considerable time, a maximum test is at present used for the enrollment test; the examinee is required to work at a high constant load until he is exhausted. If his working time exceeds 12 minutes, the load is increased. Working capacity is defined as the maximum working intensity an individual is able to maintain for six minutes.

Physical examination is carried out by one doctor assisted by a conscript orderly. The doctor has an average of eight minutes in which to examine each individual. He also has at his disposal the history and the results of all the tests done previously.

Psychiatric examinations are carried out only for special reasons on about 15 percent of conscripts, taking from 20 to 50 minutes.

After his examination each conscript is given a written report containing the most important medical results and the normal values with which his results should be compared.

D. MHTS FOR RESEARCH PURPOSES

Multiphasic health testing is a useful tool for clinical, epidemiologic or health services types of research that involve large populations, since MHTS can provide large batteries of tests at low cost, and their data acquisition and processing techniques facilitate analyses of large volumes of data.

1. MHTS for Clinical Epidemiologic Studies

a. Walnut Creek contraceptive drug study.   A prospective study was carried out to determine the side effects of oral contraceptives by comparing the differences in health status between women who use the drugs and those who do not. Approximately 18,000 women within the Kaiser-Permanente Medical Care Program at Walnut Creek, California, were studied as to patterns of contraceptive use, effects of steroid contraceptive drugs on a generally free-living population, and population-based laboratory and clinical data of value for reference purposes.[23]
The MHTS included the following tests: health questionnaire including use of contraceptives, psychological questionnaire (MMPI), visual acuity, tonometry, hearing acuity, Achilles tendon reflex relaxation time, spirometry, blood pressure and pulse rate, 12-lead electrocardiogram, chest x-ray, body measurements, blood chemistry including one-hour glucose tolerance test, blood count, and ABO blood typing. In addition, specific tests pertinent to studying contraceptive drugs were included, such as urinalysis and urine culture, cervical smear for cancer, latex titer, protein electrophoresis, and thromboelastography.
Examination was repeated annually. Cross-sectional data analyses were done on women who had been using oral contraceptives, women who had discontinued using them, and women who had never used them before entry. The findings were divided into studies of socioeconomic and demographic factors related to fertility control, and physiologic studies of the effects of oral contraceptives on blood pressure, glucose tolerance, pulmonary ventilation, in vitro blood clotting activity, and psychologic depression.

b. Japanese-American stroke study.   An epidemiological study of cerebrovascular disease was conducted to obtain an overall assessment of stroke risk factors and an overall assessment of health of Japanese-Americans in California.[24] About 4,000 Japanese-Americans were examined in 1969–70 in the Kaiser-Permanente Oakland and San Francisco MHTS by examining 120 to 140 patients once a week for 35 weeks. In addition to the usual MHTS tests, special stations were added to include a detailed cardiovascular and nutritional history and neurological examination. Mammography was excluded. The examinations were conducted on separate days from those operated for the service of regular patients, but the research study benefited greatly from being able to use a well-tested, quality-controlled, efficient health testing operation.

2. MHTS for Health Services Research

a. Kaiser-Permanente multiphasic evaluation study.   A controlled long-term study to evaluate the efficiency of the periodic health examination utilizing MHTS has been conducted in the Kaiser-Permanente Oakland and San Francisco facilities since 1964.[25] A representative sample of about 5,000 persons aged 35 to 54 was selected in 1964, and they have been urged to undergo annual examinations. Approximately three-fourths of the original group were under surveillance after ten years. A comprehensive examination was provided, and the results of this study are described by Friedman in Chapter Eighteen.

b. Titograd MHTS study.   Titograd was selected as the site for a controlled six-year study of the effectiveness of health screening in Yugoslavia.[26] After a census of the city's population in 1969, 6,577 out of 13,150 individuals in the 30 to 49-year-old age group were assigned to the study group and the remainder to the control group. The study group received a comprehensive MHTS and followup care. Tests provided included anthropometry, chest x-ray, electrocardiogram, blood pressure, fundoscopy, spirometry, visual acuity, blood sedimentation rate, red and white cell counts, hemoglobin, blood urea nitrogen, latex fixation, glucose tolerance, serum cholesterol, serological test for syphilis, urinalysis, and cervical smear.

E. USES OF MOBILE MHTS UNITS

The MHTS concept is sufficiently flexible to allow its application to movable as well as stationary facilities. Mobile units were used as early as the 1930s for the screening of pulmonary tuberculosis, syphilis, and diabetes. With the advent of the multiphasic testing concept and improved technology, the current state of the art permits any individual, however remotely located, to receive a health evaluation comparable to that which he would receive at any large advanced MHTS center. Mobile MHTS units are used to deliver services to groups of individuals remotely located from any fixed MHTS center. Mobile units have been used in industry to provide examinations to remotely located employees.[27,28] The National Center for Health Statistics uses mobile units to conduct the National Health Examination Survey.

Mobile MHTS units are now available from several companies in the United States. They can be completely self-contained within a large van (see Garfield, Chapter Four), or they can consist of equipment that is transported in a smaller truck, unloaded, and set up as a temporary unit in the desired geographical location. Flow patterns of patients are generally less flexible in a mobile unit. Usually refrigerated blood specimens are transported to a central laboratory for analysis. Similarly, ECGs and x-rays usually are mailed for interpretation to physicians at a central location. MHTS personnel often live in local motels during the week and return to their homes for weekends. Travel and transportation costs for mobile units are very high. Referral followup arrangements to local physicians in the community are important, and a serious effort must be made to orient the local medical community to the mobile MHTS and obtain their cooperation so that their patients can receive its full benefits. A survey of mobile health units was published by the U.S. Army in 1974.[29]

A very successful mobile MHTS has been operated for the California Cannery Workers Union.[30,31] Each summer since 1967, while the seasonal employment is the highest, 21,000 cannery workers are examined in a mobile multiphasic unit, comprising three specially designed and equipped trailers (see Chapter Four, C). Multiphasic testing is repeated every year and includes the usual comprehensive battery of tests: health questionnaire, blood pressure and electrocardiogram, chest x-ray, spirometry, visual acuity and ocular tension, urinalysis, VDRL, serum glucose, urea nitrogen, uric acid, creatinine, total bilirubin, LDH, hematocrit, hemoglobin, breast examination, and cervical smear. Staff members were specifically trained to foster good relations with the cannery workers. The canneries are located in areas served by 14 county medical societies, involving more than 4,300 physicians. An active program of physician orientation was carried out and referral procedures devised with the help of the physicians. A vigorous campaign of worker education was carried out months before the mobile unit arrived.

The Tennessee Valley Authority (TVA) has also used MHTS mobile units for providing an occupational health program to about 25,000 employees scattered over 80,000 square miles in parts of seven states.[32] Remote area employees are scheduled for examination every two to three years. The MHTS tests include history, height, weight, vision and hearing tests, electrocardiogram, tonometry, chest x-ray, spirometry, urinalysis, serology, and blood specimens drawn for analysis in a central laboratory. In four permanent medical facilities a physician personally completes all periodic examinations. Patients in remote areas are tested in the mobile unit without being examined by a physician, but a doctor does review the MHTS report and decides on any necessary followup. The mobile health unit collects the medical data at the remote work site and transmits them to the central medical laboratory, where all blood specimens are analyzed, electrocardiograms are processed by computer, x-rays are interpreted by a radiologist, and data are eventually processed by computer, which provides a printout MHTS report that is sent to the appropriate area medical office.

REFERENCES

1. Collings, G. H., et al. "Multiphasic Health Screening in Industry." *J. Occup. Med.* 14(1972):434–496.

2. *Company Health Programs for Executives.* New York: National Industrial Conference Board, Inc., 1955.

3. Steiner, S. D. "Management Health Examinations Programs in General Motors." *J. Occup. Med.* 3(1961):424–428.

4. Dunn, J. P., and Cobb, J. "Frequency of Peptic Ulcer Among Executives, Craftsmen and Foremen." *J. Occup. Med.* 4(1962):343–348.

5. Nelson, N., et al. *Theory, Practice and Application of Prevention in Environmental Health.* Task Force II. National Conference on Preventive Medicine. Pp. 529–615, *Preventive Medicine USA* New York: PRODIST, 1976.

6. Howe, H. F. "Organization and Operation of an Occupational Health Program. Part 1." *J. Occup. Med.* 17(1975):360–400.

7. Berk, P. D., et al. "Vinyl Chloride Associated Liver Disease." *Ann. Int. Med.* 84(1976):717–731.

8. *Dictionary of Occupational Titles.* 3d ed. U.S. Department of Labor, 1965.

9. Collen, M. F. "Automated Multiphasic Screening and Occupational Data." *Arch. Environ. Health* 15(1967):280–284.

10. Rodman, M. H. "The Pre-employment Physical Examination; Recent Experience at Massachusetts Institute of Technology." *J. Occup. Med.* 7(1965):608–611.

11. Bernauer, E. M., and Bonanno, J. "Development of Physical Profiles for Specific Jobs." *J. Occup. Med.* 17(1975):27–33.

12. Schussler, T., Kaminer, A. J., Power, V. L., and Pompar, I. H. "The Preplacement Examination." *J. Occup. Med.* 17(1975):254–257.

13. Kuh, C., and Hanman, B. *Physical Demands and Capacity Analysis.* Oakland, Calif.: Permanente Foundation, 1944.

14. Roberts, N. J. "The Values and Limitations of Periodic Health Examinations." *J. Chron. Dis.* 9(1959):95–116.

15. Duffy, J. C. "Multiphasic Screening. A Dynamic Development in Medicine." *Arch. Environ. Health* 27(1973):267–268.

16. Hillyer, P. "Rx for Employees at 40: Preventive Medicine." IBM Employee Publication, *Think,* 1972:46–48.

17. Holcomb, F. W. "IBM's Health Screening Program and Medical Data System." *J. Occup. Med.* 15(1973):863–868.

18. Yaruote, P. M., McDonagh, T. J., Goldman, M. E., and Zuckerman, J. "Organization and Evaluation of a Physical Fitness Program in Industry." *J. Occup. Med.* 16(1974):589–598.

19. Beukers. H. R., et al. "Health Examinations is a Multinational Concern." *Proc. I.R.I.A.,* Toulouse, March 1973.

20. Yamaguchi, K. "The Toshiba Multiphasic Health Screening Centre." *Med. & Biol. Engng.* 9(1971):421–429; and Kobayashi, T. "Recent Progress in AMHT in Japan." In *Automated Multiphasic Health Testing.* New York: Engineering Foundation, 1971.

21. "Multiphasic Testing." In *Systems Analysis for a "New Generation" of Military Hospitals,* page 5.7. Arthur D. Little Co., April 1971. Available from NTIS.

22. Linroth, K. "Health Evaluation in Sweden for Special Reference to a Military Health and Capacity Investigation System for Personnel Selection." IHEA Conference, November 1974

23. Ramcharan, S., et al. *The Walnut Creek Contraceptive Drug Study,* Vol. 1. DHEW Pub. No. (NIH) 74-562, 1974.

24. Syme, S. L., et al. "Epidemiologic Studies of Coronary Heart Disease and Stroke in Japanese Men Living in Japan, Hawaii, and California." *Am. J. Epidem.* 102(1975):477–525.

25. Cutler, J. L., Ramcharan, S., Friedman, G., Dales, L., Collen, M., et al. "Multiphasic Checkup Evaluation Study 1–4." *Prev. Med.* 2(1973):197–246.

26. Thorner, R. M., Djordjevic, D., Vukmanovic, C., et al. "A Study to Evaluate the Effectiveness of Multiphasic Screening in Yugoslavia." *Prev. Med.* 2(1973):295–301.

27. Fitzpatrick, M. M., and Zaves, N. A. "Mobile Multiphasic Health Screening—Mediclinic." *J. Occup. Med.* 4(1962):343–348.

28. Robertson, L. T. "Periodic Examination in Industry by Mobile Equipment." *Arch. Indust. Health* 13(1956):250–252.

29. James, J. J., and Stuart, R. B. "Survey of Mobile Health Units." United States Army Health Services Command. Report HCSD-13, June 1974.

30. Yedidia, A., Bunow, M. A., and Muldavin, M. S. "Mobile Multiphasic Screening in an Industrial Setting: The California Cannery Workers' Program." *J. Occup. Med.* 11(1969):602–622,

31. Yedidia, A. "California Cannery Workers Program. Multiphasic Testing as an Introduction to Orderly Care." *Arch. Enrivon. Health* 27(1973):259–263.

32. Craig, J. L. "Automated Multiphasic Health Testing. The TVA Experience. *Arch. Environ. Health* 27(1973):264–266; and, "How to Organize and Operate a Regional Health Testing Facility." In *Automated Multiphasic Health Testing.* New York: Engineering Foundation, 1971.

CHAPTER SEVENTEEN

Systems Evaluation of MHTS

Morris F. Collen

A. Introduction
B. Historical Review of MHTS Systems Evaluation
C. Evaluation of Resources Used; Cost Analysis
D. Effectiveness of MHTS
E. Efficiency of MHTS
F. Cost Effectiveness of MHTS
G. Physicians' Acceptance of MHTS
H. Summary of MHTS Systems Evaluation

A. INTRODUCTION

The development and operation of large technological systems require great resource investments over long periods of time. As a result, it is essential to carefully evaluate the effectiveness of such systems in achieving their defined health care objectives (i.e., does the program work?) and their efficiency in the use of costly resources (i.e., how much does it cost?).

The evaluation of a system (or a program) is a formalized attempt to measure the extent to which it achieves its specified objectives. Since the objectives for each system participant may be different, formalized evaluation of a large system is usually very complex and expensive and sometimes can be a frustrating experience.

From the viewpoint of the patient, a multiphasic health testing service (MHTS) will be evaluated primarily in terms of the outcome from the health examination, and he will depend mainly upon his physician to evaluate its technical quality. The patient may evaluate the waiting time for an appointment, the time taken to complete the examination, his general satisfaction with the facility and the examination process, and the cost of the procedure. Most important to him is the ability of the MHTS to accurately determine his health status, identify his health care needs, and favorably affect any conditions that might result in disability, morbidity, and mortality. (See Chapter Eighteen.) Finally, the patient will have to decide: ''Is this health checkup worth it to me, and should I comply with all the advised referrals?''

From the viewpoint of the physician, an MHTS will be evaluated primarily for its effectiveness in detecting previously unknown disease in his patient and in providing useful measurements as to the changing status of known disease. He will also be concerned as to its availability for patient referral and its cost to the patient. He will be especially sensitive to the proportion of his patients for which he finds a clinically important abnormality that was overlooked by the MHTS (''false negatives''), since this type of error is most serious to the patient if a potentially disabling and correctable condition has been missed. Less serious, but of considerable concern to both the patient and physician, will be the proportion of patients who are reported to have abnormalities that cannot be confirmed (''false positives''), since this increases the costs of examination followup and generates unnecessary anxiety in the patients. The format and content of the MHTS report is critically evaluated by the physician, since it directly impacts the efficiency of his own patient care process. A report with the relevant test results organized in a manner consistent with his own patient examination process will conserve his time, whereas a report that appears disorganized and has missing data will delay his diagnostic evaluation and increase costs. (See also Chapter Two, F.)

From the medical facility administrator's viewpoint, an MHTS will be evaluated as to the expenses for each phase (i.e., personnel, supplies, and equipment) and the total operating costs; the prevalence of conditions identified; and the cost to identify a positive condition (cost per positive test). He will consider the cost effectiveness of installing alternative equipment or procedures and, in his reports to his policy maker, may evaluate the financial return on investment.

System evaluation from the viewpoint of the administrator is usually a dynamic process, in that evaluation information is usually used to modify and improve an ongoing system. Such evaluation models require that ongoing information on system performance is fed back to the administrator, who examines the achieved performance and output, compares them to the desired objectives, and acts accordingly.[1]

From the viewpoint of the health care system planner or policy maker, who is concerned with the total care of a defined population, an evaluation of the results projected for a specified or requested budget (a cost effectiveness analysis) is very critical. He will consider the costs not only of MHTS but of the followup care. He will compare the costs per 1,000 persons per year for providing health examinations to the costs of not providing health examinations. He will have to decide, for example: is it worth spending $2,000 to find one woman with breast cancer?

To attempt to satisfy all the above viewpoints, the evaluation process will need to examine all of the cells in the evaluation matrix shown in Table 17-1. This matrix should be applied to each of the MHTS phases and to the program as a whole, since for certain benefits (e.g., patient satisfaction and reassurance) the value of the whole system appears to be greater than the sum of its parts.

Cost analysis has been defined (by a DHEW committee organized to develop guidelines for cost analyses of automated multiphasic health testing[2]) as the determination of costs within an operational system, which may be presented as cost per test, cost per patient class, total cost of operation, etc. (See C.)

Cost effectiveness analysis has been defined [2,3] as a comparison of the economic efficiency of alternative systems having the same objective. This form of inter-program cost and effectiveness comparative analysis determines whether or not the output of one system requires fewer resources than another to obtain the desired degree of accomplishment; it can be done without putting monetary values on changes in health status or attempting to quantify "quality-of-life" effects. (See F.)

Administrators commonly evaluate the economic aspects of a project by estimating its profitability. A simple method for evaluating a capital investment proposal is the *payback* method, which is the investment divided by the projected annual savings, and which predicts the number of years necessary to pay back the investment. Another common method for estimating profitability is by the average *return on investment* (ROI) method; the total monetary gain (net profits or net savings) is divided by the number of years of projected investment life to obtain the average gain per year, which is then divided by the initial cost to provide an average return on investment. Grimaldi,[4] reporting a return on investment study for periodic health examinations of middle-management employees, found a greater return on investment for a group receiving examinations than for a control group who did not, owing to reduced medical expense claims in the examined group.

Cost benefit analysis is defined as an attempt to compare all the costs of an activity with all the potential benefits to be derived. The DHEW committee[2] required that all secondary costs and all benefits be defined and reduced to a common denominator, i.e., valued in monetary terms, so that the dollar value of the two could be compared. In cost benefit studies it is necessary to estimate the decrease in adverse consequences of the disease and in the costs of treatment (early and delayed) as a result of the findings of MHTS. Benefits not only include

Table 17-1. A Matrix for a Comprehensive Evaluation of an MHTS

	(A) System and Care Process (Examples of Criteria)	(B) Patient Process and Outcomes (Examples of Criteria)
(1) *Resources used* (system inputs)	Facility, equipment, personnel and supplies costs for each phase and for total MHTS.	Patient's total time for transportation and waiting, and for examination process. Patient's fees paid plus lost earnings.
(2) *Effectiveness* (system outputs)	Number of patients examined per day; yield rates; percent true positives, percent false positives; percent true negatives, percent false negatives. Physician acceptability.	Percent appropriate referrals to health maintenance for reassurance; to hypertension, diabetes, etc. for followup sick care and preventive maintenance. Patient satisfaction.
(3) *Efficiency* (3.1) Outputs/inputs	Number of tests/day/personnel; number of tests/day/equipment.	Number of patients detected/$000; percent arrivals/referrals.
(3.2) Inputs/outputs	Cost/patient; cost/positive test; cost/true positive test; cost/true negative test.	Total cost/well patient. Total cost/sick patient. Cost/breast cancer patient.
(4) *Cost Effectiveness* (4.1) New vs. existing system comparisons.	Compare costs of new procedure vs. existing procedure.	For an existing group of doctors determine the costs to "well" patients of replacing traditional examinations by MHTS.
(4.2) Alternate system comparisons	For same physicians, compare costs of process "A" vs. process "B"	For a specified health care service, compare costs for system "A" vs. "B".
(5) *Cost Benefit* (5.1) New vs. existing system comparisons	For an incremental expense, what added alternate benefits and services are possible?	Effect on patients' outcome (mortality, morbidity, disability) of an incremental expense to existing MHTS.
(5.2) Alternate system comparisons	For same expense, compare M.D. hours, number of patient visits, and services received for systems "A" vs. "B"	Effect on patients' outcome of a specified expense for alternate "A" (e.g., MHTS) vs. "B" (e.g., the traditional physician health examination.)

direct measurable changes in costs of real resources used as a result of the changes in morbidity and mortality, but require some estimates of the effects on the quality of life, i.e., better health, better mental status, years of extended happy life, etc.[5-7] For the individual in a general testing program, for example, direct monetary costs might include loss of income while the tests are being performed, loss of earnings due to early versus late hospitalization, and expenses to the individual and the family resulting from early versus late hospitalization. Furthermore, each individual balances the costs of compliance with referrals versus the costs of noncompliance.

Quantifiable measures of all relevant inputs and outputs to health care systems have been impossible to obtain. Thorner[8] suggested that determinations of incremental changes in health (as program objectives or outputs) and in health services (as inputs) could be the usual measures applied to evaluation of health care programs. Several attempts at cost benefit analyses of MHTS have been made[9-11] but they have not yielded useful results, owing to the complexity of the analyses and the difficulty in quantifying all the costs and benefits to the individual and to society if the test is done or is not done, is positive or negative, and so on.

Randomized clinical trials have been strongly advocated by Cochrane[3] as the best way to evaluate medical care programs including MHTS. Large-scale clinical trials involving MHTS versus no MHTS are very expensive; some require at least ten years to measure comparative benefits (see Chapter Eighteen, E); and it is difficult to maintain test conditions on large experimental and control groups for the required periods. The randomized clinical trial approach is essentially one form of cost benefit study. (Randomized clinical trials will be considered in Chapter Eighteen.)

As has been repeatedly emphasized, an MHTS should always be viewed as an integral part of some larger program or system (e.g., a health care delivery system, an industry, a military program, etc.). Thus, an MHTS, to be properly evaluated, must be studied to determine to what extent it achieves its defined objectives within the overall program. For example, within a health care delivery system, it is necessary first to define the objectives of the overall health care program and then identify the specific subobjectives of the MHTS. (See Chapters Two and Three.) Finally, it becomes necessary to measure the effectiveness with which each objective is achieved, and to identify the costs and other results of the MHTS program.

The general goal of a health care delivery system is usually to provide care of high quality at a cost its patients can afford and will support. The objectives of an MHTS must be in full agreement with that of its overall health care delivery environment. From the viewpoint of this chapter, these objectives generally will include improving the process of providing health care by:

(a) Increasing the efficiency of providing health checkups by conserving physician and patient time and by decreasing the costs of examinations, while increasing quality and comprehensiveness of the examinations, and maintaining good acceptability and support of both care providers and users.

(b) Providing an efficient entry mode to the health care delivery system.

(c) Determining the health status of the examinees, detecting early or asymptomatic disease, and monitoring the status of disease already known.

The evaluation of MHTS acceptability and effects on patients' outcomes will be considered in Chapter Eighteen.

B. HISTORICAL REVIEW OF MHTS SYSTEMS EVALUATION

Long before MHTS evolved as a system concept, the literature already evidenced some controversy as to the value of health examinations. (See also Chapters One and Eighteen.) In 1945, Kuh[12] reviewed the available publications and concluded that there was "no conclusive evidence that the periodic health examination is a practical means for improving the health or longevity of the masses." He suggested that health examinations were "practical only for selected groups and individuals" and advocated "early sickness consultation"—that is, promoting the early seeking of medical advice for illness so as to capitalize on the motivation created by the symptoms. Later, occupational health physicians led by Siegel[13] also encouraged early sickness consultation coupled with selected periodic mass screening programs for those diseases in which early detection had proved of value.

In 1959, Roberts[14] comprehensively reviewed the literature, because periodic health examinations were being increasingly advocated and undertaken, especially in industry. Citing the varying yield rates of abnormalities being reported from different patient groups, he emphasized the use of this important measure in evaluating an MHTS program. He also reviewed the few patient outcome studies available at that time and observed that the discovery of remediable conditions was not often followed up by successful treatment, even if effective treatment was available. He expressed concern over false negatives, noting that "most physicians have had the sad experience of seeing a patient die soon after an examination which revealed no threat to his life." Roberts supported the concept that health examinations have a positive benefit for the "worried-well" patient in that they are "very often able to allay a patient's anxiety about his health following an examination which reveals no justification for such anxiety." Roberts summarized the practice that was then being adopted by many: to examine persons under 30 years old every third year, those between 30 and 40 every second year, and only those 40 or over every year. He suggested that in between comprehensive health examinations, brief "multiphasic screening types of examinations" could be provided. Roberts further suggested that "one of the greatest yields from health examinations might be their patient educational value, even though this defied actual measurement."

In 1960, Burr[15] reported an evaluation of periodic health examinations in 1,458 company employees, of which 44 percent were found to have significant disease findings, and concluded that the savings to the company more than justified the cost of the examination program. In 1961, Clark, et al.[16] reported the yield rates from the first examination of 1,500 male executives aged 24 to 76 (average 45 years) and expressed surprise at the high proportion of false positives and false negatives and at the degree to which physicians disregarded abnormal test results in arriving at their diagnoses. Clark considered an abnormal test finding in the absence of a confirming followup clinical diagnosis to be a false positive, but recognized that with the passage of time and repeated examinations it might turn out to be a true positive test representing disease undetected by the examining physician. He also noted, since one of the objectives of "periodic health examinations is to preserve health, that negative test results, by demonstrating the absence of disease, have an important though unmeasurable value." Many reviews of yield rates of MHTS screening programs were published in the 1960s.[17,18]

In 1962, Wade et al.[19] presented one of the few health examination evaluation studies with a relatively long-term (seven-year) followup. They reported on 765 males in an industrial executive health program, in which examinations were provided by certified internists at specified intervals according to age of examinee, with some screening examinations in each of the intervening years. Wade reported that 37 percent of disease that produced disability was diagnosed at periodic health examinations before the onset of the disability; he concluded that "the major causes of death, cardiovascular disease and malignancies, were almost always diagnosed at 'periodic' examinations." He could not demonstrate that the course of any employee's disease was changed by virtue of early diagnosis.

David,[20] in 1961, advocated research in reducing the cost of examinations so as to make them equally available to all socioeconomic levels. He reported that data available from the National Health Survey indicated that family members 45 years of age and over, in families with incomes over $7,000 per year, averaged 70 visits per 100 persons per year for general checkups; families with incomes from $4,000 to $7,000 averaged 50 visits per 100 persons; families with incomes from $2,000 to $4,000 averaged 40; and for families with incomes under $2,000 it was 50, presumably because these services were available to the indigent in many areas of the country.

Spitzer[21] recently emphasized the epidemiologists' criterion of testing in health examinations for only those physical conditions or diseases whose natural outcome can be altered in a way that benefits the patient or society. He excluded benefits of palliation for incurable conditions and of reassurance for psychosomatic and psychosocial problems, which actually represent by far the most common problems for which patients seek primary medical care. Lave's task force[7] suggested that criteria applied to preventive care should equally be applied to acute care.

Forst[22] reported no significant differences in benefits from providing health examinations every year to 24- to 48-year old army aviator officers as compared to examinations every two to three years for other armed services officers. Although this was not exactly a controlled study, it supported the general contention that frequent health checkups for young adults were not cost-effective.

Although the Kaiser-Permanente Medical Care Program had been providing periodic health examinations as a contractual benefit to its subscribers since 1942, not until 1971 did Smillie[23] formulate a policy for Kaiser-Permanente on this issue. Based upon the evaluations reported in these chapters, he took the position that in the best interests of one's continued good health, every adult should have an initial complete health examination. "For repeat periodic health checkups after such an initial examination, in which everything was found to be normal, healthy robust young adults in their twenties can wait an interval of three years or more. If the physician finds something that requires more frequent attention, even though it may not be a severe threat to one's health, the physician should advise return visits as frequently as needed. For healthy young adults in their thirties, periodic health checkups at about two- to three-year intervals are recommended, after the initial checkup. If you are in your forties, an examination about every eighteen months to two years is recommended. If you are in your fifties, sixties, or older, your doctor can tell you how often to return. If everything was normal the last time and you feel healthy and full of zest, an annual checkup is recommended.'' This was a significant departure from the then current position of recommending annual health examinations for every one. In fact, Kaiser-Permanente physicians now actively discourage annual checkups for healthy adults under age 40 if an initial examination is negative; instead, they advise these young persons to seek care early when they notice any changes in well-being (i.e., early sickness consultation).

C. EVALUATION OF RESOURCES USED; COST ANALYSIS

An essential aspect of the evaluation of an MHTS involves identifying and measuring all resources used in the program—that is, all system inputs. The number of full-time equivalents of personnel used is a critical system input. Other resources allocated, such as space, equipment, and supplies, are also important to identify and measure. A cost analysis will determine expenses for facility space, equipment, personnel, and supplies.

For the health care delivery system or community within which the MHTS is located, the costs of all resources used should include estimates of the costs of getting the people to the MHTS and the costs of followup care from MHTS referrals.

An accurate, reliable cost analysis[2] requires establishing a ''cost center'' for the expense accounts of each phase or station of the MHTS. The cost center will identify and assign any expense (and revenue) item over a significantly long period (such as 12 months) to average out seasonal variations and peaks due to intermittent ordering customs (e.g., receiving a six-month supply of x-ray films on one day). It will identify and prevent MHTS costs from being charged to another program and separate out the costs of irrelevant activities. By distributing the costs over the number of examinations completed during the cost period, an estimate can be made of the average unit cost per examination. A useful way to study a program is to ask: what would it cost to transfer or replicate the MHTS?

A cost analysis of the Oakland Kaiser-Permanente MHTS for a full year in 1968 has been reported[24] and is compared to a half year in 1973 (see Table 17-2). Included were the physician costs for interpretations of electrocardiograms and x-rays. Not included were the costs for followup physician examinations (i.e., physical examinations, gynecological examinations with cervical smear, sigmoidoscopy, and followup examinations by any physician or allied health personnel) as arranged by the patient or the MHTS.

The total direct costs were made up of about 70 percent for salaries and wages (including fringe benefits), 21 percent for supplies, and 9 percent for equipment depreciation.

Indirect expenses were allocated to each phase and applied to salaries and wages to cover actual expense of services from other departments, such as accounting, payroll, personnel, and purchasing. Indirect costs also included plant

Table 17-2. Unit Costs of MHTS Phases, 1968 and 1973

Phase		1968*		1973†
1.	Mammography	1.34		0.84
	Mammography (per examinee)	(4.90)‡		(3.60)§
2.	Chest x-ray	0.46		1.07
3.	Electrocardiography	1.02		0.65
4.	Blood pressure	0.42		0.25
5.	Spirometry	0.31		0.49
6.	Visual acuity	0.29		0.42
7.	Tonometry	0.55		0.54
8.	Audiometry	0.25		0.44
9.	Clinical lab	4.49		4.58
10.	Questionnaire	0.37		1.12
11.	Anthropometry	0.46		0.41
12.	Other tests‖	1.43		—
13.	Reception, supervision, etc.	2.89		2.39
14.	Computer processing	2.00		1.46
		16.28		14.66
	Overhead	2.54		2.80
	Total direct and indirect costs	$18.82		$17.46

*September 1967–August 1968, for 47,404 examinees.
†January–June 1973, for 17,463 examinees.
‡For about 10,000 women, age 48 and older.
§For 3,689 women, age 48 and older.
‖Retinal photography and Achilles reflex test were included in 1968 but not in 1973.

operation, comprised of "equivalent costs of ownership" (depreciation, finance charges and interest expense) and "maintenance" (janitorial services, maintenance supplies, telephone, and utilities).

For this program, over the five-year period the total cost per MHTS examination for each patient has been held below $20 by (a) eliminating a few tests (item 12 in Table 17-2) not considered to be useful (e.g., retinal photography and Achilles reflex test) and transferring immunizations out to the "Health Center"; and (b) gradually increasing the volume of patients processed from about 100 to 180 per day.

Mammography was the single most expensive test. Cephalocaudal and lateral x-ray views of each breast were taken and interpreted by a radiologist, at a unit cost of $0.84 in 1973 (costs shared by all examinees). Since this test was given only to women age 48 or older, the actual expense per female examinee was $3.60.

Chest roentgenography included a single postero-anterior view recorded on 70 mm film and interpreted by a radiologist, at a unit cost of $1.07 in 1973.

The unit cost for a six-lead electrocardiogram, including interpretation by a cardiologist, was only $0.65 in 1973.

Sphygmomanometry was performed by automated instruments operated by technicians, at a cost of $0.25 (1973).

Respirometry (the one-second and total forced expiratory vital capacity) was measured by an automated spirometer, at a cost of $0.49 per test (1973).

Visual acuity for each eye was tested (with corrective lenses, if worn) by a modified Sloan wall chart. The number of letters (four or more) incorrectly read was equivalent to a visual acuity of 20/40 or less, a degree of impairment for which eye examinations were routinely recommended, at a unit cost of $0.42 (1973).

Ocular tension was measured (in both 1968 and 1973) by a registered nurse using a Schiotz tonometer, at a unit cost of $0.54 (1973).

Hearing acuity was tested at a unit cost of $0.44 (1973) with an automated audiometer, for six frequencies from 500 to 6,000 cycles per second, at sound intensities from 10 to 90 decibels.

The total cost of the clinical laboratory phase, including urine and blood tests and the administration of glucose solution for diabetes testing, was $4.58 (1973).

The general item identified in the table as "reception, supervision, etc." included six people (two registration receptionists, two appointment clerks, one nurse supervisor, and one relief nurse) at a unit cost of $2.39 per examinee in 1973.

In Table 17-2 the costs for data processing are shown to be $1.46 per multiphasic examination in 1973, including personnel, supplies, and equipment in the computer center as well as in the local "computer data-input room" in the multiphasic laboratory area. (An amount of $2.50 per examination allocated in prior years for the central staff for research purposes was excluded).

An overhead item of $2.54 (1968) and $2.80 (1973) was included to represent central administration costs.

It is to be emphasized that these unit costs in 1968 of $18.82 per multiphasic examination are related to the patient load of about 2,000 per month. In 1973, 3,000 patients were examined per month, and despite the five-year inflation factor, the unit cost per examination was essentially unchanged. If only 1,000 patients were examined monthly, the cost per patient would probably increase to $40–$50. (See Figure 17-1.)

D. EFFECTIVENESS OF MHTS

The degree of attainment of program objectives is usually defined as program effectiveness. Program effectiveness is thus the ratio of the attained objectives attributed to the program activity to the proposed or expected objectives.[25] The primary objective of MHTS is to economically provide a good-quality health evaluation (see Chapter Two, D)—that is, to determine the health status of the examinee, detect unknown disease, monitor the status of known disease, and reassure the well. Accordingly, evaluation of MHTS effectiveness should, as a minimum, determine the yield and referral rates, the effectiveness in detecting targeted asymptomatic disease, and the patients' satisfaction with the process.

If MHTS is to function as a successful participant in the health care system, some measure of physicians' acceptance of and satisfaction with the program should also be included in effectiveness evaluation.

It has been proposed that evaluations of screening programs should consider the effect of the MHTS on patient outcome.[27] However, patient outcome depends more upon effectiveness of therapy than upon effectiveness of disease detection. The ability to favorably alter the course of the condition should be a criterion for MHTS test selection (see Chapter Three) and is an important factor in MHTS cost

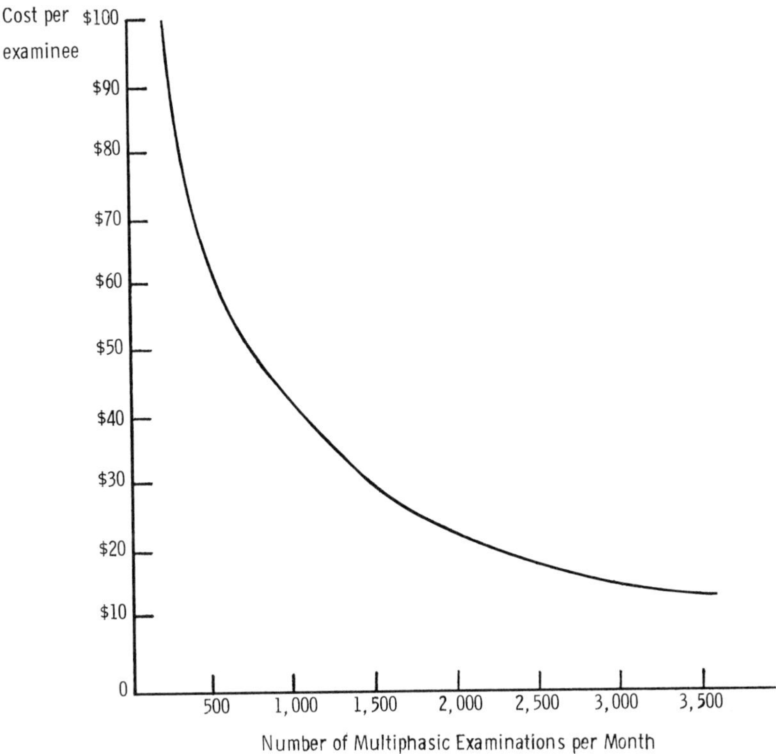

Figure 17-1. Relationship between MHTS cost per person and monthly volume.

benefit analysis, but it is essential that evaluation distinguish between (1) disease detection and diagnosis and (2) treatment and rehabilitation. For example, from the viewpoints of the patient, family, employer, and society there are clear benefits for planning purposes from effective early detection of an incurable disease, even though the treatment is not at all effective in altering the natural course of the disease.

1. Determination of Health Status of Examinees

An extensive literature has accumulated on health status indices. A useful and simple method of classifying MHTS examinees by their health status is that developed by Garfield[27] and Richart.[28] (See Chapter Two, C.) Such categorizing of patients can be done as soon as the MHTS data become available, so that the patient's history can be compared with the MHTS findings (including the final physical examination data). A patient is classified as "well" if he has no significant medical complaint or problem and if he has no clinically significant finding or abnormality on the MHTS examination. He is classified as "worried-well" if he has a significant medical complaint or problem but there are no clinically significant findings. A patient is "asymptomatic-sick" if he has no complaints but he is found to have a clinically significant finding (e.g., elevated blood pressure). A patient is "sick" if he has a significant complaint and the MHTS finds a significant abnormality.

Table 17-3.   Percent Distribution of 1916 MHTS Examinees by Health Status Groups, by Age and Sex

	Well	Asymp-tomatic-Sick	Worried-Well	Sick	Total
Males, Ages:					
15–24	3.8	1.3	1.9	0.5	2.9
25–44	21.0	19.9	9.6	6.4	17.6
45–64	16.3	9.3	32.7	26.5	18.2
65+	3.0	1.2	3.9	11.4	4.6
Total males	44.1	31.7	48.1	44.8	43.3
Number)	(578)	(51)	(25)	(176)	(830)
(Percent of 830)	(69.7)	(6.1)	(3.0)	(21.2)	(100.0)
Females, Ages:					
15–24	6.1	9.9	3.9	1.0	5.3
25–44	24.8	32.9	13.4	7.6	21.7
45–64	21.4	23.6	32.7	29.0	23.4
65+	3.6	1.9	1.9	17.6	6.3
Total females	55.9	68.3	51.9	55.2	56.7
(Number)	(732)	(110)	(27)	(217)	(1,086)
(Percent of 1,086)	(67.4)	(10.1)	(2.5)	(20.0)	(100.0)
Total	100.0	100.0	100.0	100.0	100.0
(Number)	(1,310)	(161)	(52)	(393)	(1,916)
(Percent of 1,916)	(68.4)	(8.4)	(2.7)	(20.5)	(100.0)

A group of 1,916 adult examinees who had not seen a physician within one year and who asked for a multiphasic checkup were classified as shown in Table 17-3. Those classified as well comprised 68.4 percent, as worried-well 2.7 percent, as asymptomatic-sick 8.4 percent, and as sick 20.5 percent. In this group, "health" care was indicated for 71 percent (well and worried-well) and "sick" care for only 29 percent (sick and asymptomatic-sick). This shows how an MHTS can be used to evaluate health status and to separate out those who need health care from those who need medical or sick care. Each patient can then be referred for followup care in accordance with his individual needs.

2.   Yield Rates of MHTS

a.   MHTS phases.   The yield rate of positive findings from a given test depends upon the prevalence of the abnormality in the population being tested and upon the sensitivity and specificity of the test.[30,31] Yield sometimes is applied to previously undetected abnormalities, but herein it refers to all positive cases. The yield rate for a test is defined as the number of positives, as a percentage of the total number of patients tested. Table 17-4 shows how the yield rate of electrocardiogram abnormalities is greatly influenced by the age of the examinees and slightly affected by sex. The definition of "abnormal" is also critical. In this table

Table 17-4. Percentage of Electrocardiograms Reported With Some Abnormality

Age Group	Female	Male
20–29	9.3	9.6
30–39	11.7	12.4
40–49	15.6	17.6
50–59	20.7	24.9
60–69	29.7	35.1
70+	41.2	52.2
All ages	17.8	20.8

17 percent of all examinees were reported to have clinically important abnormalities (atrial flutter or fibrillation; first-, second-, or third-degree A-V block; ST-T variations; left or right intraventricular conduction delay; left or right ventricular hypertrophy; atrial abnormality; short P-R interval; Wolff-Parkinson-White syndrome; probable recent or old myocardial infarct; or prolonged QT or QTA). This group also includes an additional 2 percent with reports of borderline or nonspecific changes, sinus tachycardia or bradycardia, and supraventricular premature beats.

The yield rates for some commonly included MHTS tests are shown in Table 17-5 (shown as percent positive for each age group specified). The yield rate, or percent positive, essentially determines the referral rate of patients to physicians for followup care.

One can predict the yield by knowing the prevalence of the conditions that produce a positive test, and the sensitivity and the specificity of the test. The yield will be the sum of the true positives and the false positives. For a sample of N persons, one can predict the yield (y) of positive cases from MHTS. If the population being tested has a disease with a prevalence (p) and the test has a sensitivity (a) and a specificity of (b), then

$$y = Np(a) + N(1 - p)(1 - b).$$

For example (as modified from Flagle[34]), the predicted yield for hypertension from examining a group of 1,000 elderly adults in which the prevalence is 10 percent, for which the testing by sphygmomanometry detects 95 percent of true hypertensives and 98 percent of nonhypertensives, would then be

$$y = (1,000 \times 0.10 \times 0.95) + (1,000 \times 0.90 \times 0.02) = 113 \text{ ``positives.''}$$

This yield would result in a referral to the hypertension clinic of 95 true hypertensives and 18 whom the physicians would not confirm to be hypertensive (false positives).

If a population group of young adults were selected wherein the prevalence of this disease was only 1 percent, then

$$y = (1,000 \times 0.01 \times 0.95) + (1,000 \times 0.99 \times 0.02) = 30 \text{ ``positives,''}$$

or 10 true positives and 20 false positives would be referred. This clearly demonstrates the relatively high costs of testing for low-prevalence diseases, owing to the large proportion of the case yield who are false positives.

As the criteria change for a specific diagnosis, owing to new scientific data, then

Table 17-5. Cost Per Positive Test, According to Test and Age Group*

		All Ages		20–39 Yr		40–59 Yr		60–79 Yr	
Test	Unit Cost ($)	Percent Positive	Cost/ Positive Case ($)	Percent Positive	Cost/ Positive Case ($)	Percent Positive	Cost/ Positive Case ($)	Percent Positive	Cost/ Positive Case ($)
Mammography	5.00	1.2†	417	—	—	1.1‡	455	1.4	357
Chest x-ray	1.45	7.4	20	2.1	69	7.4	20	19.2	8
Electrocardiography	0.90	17.3	5	10.2	9	17.7	5	31.5	3
Blood pressure	0.35	4.1	9	0.4	88	4.3	8	11.5	3
Respirometry	0.65	2.2	30	2.0	32	2.3	28	2.7	24
Visual acuity	0.55	15.8	3	10.6	5	16.1	3	26.3	2
Tonometry	0.75	0.3	250	0.2	375	0.4	187	0.5	150
Audiometry	0.60	16.2	4	5.2	11	17.6	3	36.4	2
Hemoglobin (men)	0.55	3.1	18	1.9	29	3.1	18	5.6	10
Hemoglobin (women)	0.55	10.3	5	12.6	4	10.1	5	5.5	10
White cell count	0.55	2.2	25	2.6	21	2.2	25	1.7	32
Serum glucose (1 hr)	1.00	5.7	18	4.6	22	5.6	18	8.3	12
Serum cholesterol	0.40	2.4	17	1.7	24	2.7	15	3.0	13
Serum uric acid	0.40	4.5	9	3.4	12	4.8	8	6.0	7
Serum calcium	0.40	1.3	31	1.4	29	1.3	31	1.5	27
Serum creatinine	0.40	1.4	29	0.8	50	1.4	29	2.7	15
Serum transaminase	0.40	4.2	10	3.6	11	4.6	9	4.5	9
VDRL	0.30	1.5	20	0.8	37	1.9	16	2.3	13
Urine glucose	0.20	8.2	2	7.6	3	8.9	2	7.3	3
Urine protein	0.20	6.4	3	7.2	3	5.6	4	7.0	3
Urine culture (men)	0.30	0.4	75	0.1	300	0.3	100	1.0	30
Urine culture (women)	0.30	3.3	9	3.3	9	3.2	9	4.0	8

*Modified from Collen, et al.[28]
†Women 50 years of age and older.
‡Women 50 to 59 years of age only.

the sensitivity and specificity of the test will change. For example, if the screening limits remain the same but the criterion for the diagnosis of hypertension changes from a diastolic blood pressure of 90 mm (mercury) to 88 mm or to 85 mm, then the yield increases, and the numbers of false positives decrease and false negatives increase.

b.   Diagnoses reported following MHTS.   The final diagnoses reported by the physicians following the MHTS and physical examination comprise the conventional measure for evaluating the effectiveness of MHTS in health surveillance, disease detection, and disease monitoring of a population group, since these diagnoses are an indication of (a) whether the physicians decided that the positive test was a true or false one, and (b) whether they thought the positive test was clinically important (i.e., warranted therapy). In one group of 2,000 new examinees (see Table 17-3) only one-fourth had clinically important abnormalities (asymptomatic-sick or sick). Table 17-6 shows that for another group of more than 30,000 examinations (for which the criteria were not identical and some persons had more than one examination) some clinically important abnormality was reported in almost two-thirds of examinations. The most common diagnosis was obesity and the second most common was hypertension.

Table 17-5 shows that 1.2 percent of all women over age 50 had a positive mammogram reported as "suspicious of cancer." However, only one in five of these women proved by followup surgical biopsy to have cancer of the breast. Accordingly, the yield rate of true positives (i.e., validated by final diagnosis) for breast cancer detection for women over age 50 was 0.24 percent.

Similarly, the yield rate for abnormal serum glucose tests taken one or two hours following a 75 gm glucose challenge dose was 5.7 percent. However, only about one-half of these (3.3 percent) were ultimately confirmed to have diabetes mellitus (see Table 17-6).

3.   Effects of false positives and false negatives.   MHTS tests are selected with a sufficient sensitivity to detect an acceptable proportion of patients who have the disease (true positives), but if the test is too sensitive it will produce some test results that may identify a person as having the disease (or abnormality) when in fact he does not (false positives). Similarly, the test selected will have sufficient specificity to identify an acceptable proportion of patients who do not have the disease, but if it is too specific it will miss too many who do (false negatives). A frequent criticism of MHTS has been that it produces an excessive number of false positive test results, thereby increasing costs by generating secondary screening tests, using more doctors' and patients' time and increasing patient anxiety. Accordingly, it is important to consider in detail the effects of false positive (and false negative) tests when evaluating a MHTS. (See also F of this chapter, where it is shown that the issue of increased costs of MHTS from false positive and false negative tests is not a significant one.)

a.   Source and prevalence of false positives and negatives.   The validity of a screening test is the measure of the frequency with which its result is confirmed by an acceptable diagnostic procedure—i.e., the ability of the test to separate out accurately those who have the condition sought from those who do not. Applying a screening test to a population will produce four categories of results, provided

Table 17-6. Thirty Most Frequent Diagnoses Found in 30,000 Consecutive MHTS Examinations*

		Percent		
Rank	Diagnosis	New	Old	Total
1	No significant abnormality	—	—	35.0
2	Obesity	4.3	13.0	17.3
3	Hypertension, primary	2.1	5.5	7.6
4	Anxiety state	2.2	5.1	7.3
5	Osteoarthritis	0.8	3.0	3.8
6	Diabetes mellitus	0.9	2.4	3.3
7	Fibrocystic disease, breast (females only)	1.0	2.3	3.3
8	Varicose veins	0.8	2.3	3.1
9	Psychophysiological reaction, gastrointestinal	0.9	2.1	3.0
10	Benign prostatic hypertrophy (males only)	1.1	1.9	3.0
11	Deafness	0.7	2.0	2.7
12	Menopausal syndrome (females only)	0.7	1.2	1.9
13	Chronic dermatitis†	0.6	1.0	1.6
14	Hay fever	0.4	1.1	1.5
15	Depression	0.5	1.0	1.5
16	Ischemic heart disease	0.2	1.2	1.4
17	Duodenal ulcer	0.1	1.3	1.4
18	Low back pain	0.5	0.9	1.4
19	Migraine	0.2	1.1	1.3
20	Rhinitis or sinusitis	0.4	0.9	1.3
21	Testes absent or atrophic (males only)	0.3	1.0	1.3
22	Hypochromic microcytic anemia	0.5	0.7	1.2
23	Emphysema	0.3	0.8	1.1
24	Renal glycosuria	0.6	0.5	1.1
25	Hypothyroidism	0.3	0.8	1.1
26	Kyphosis or scoliosis	0.2	0.8	1.0
27	Bronchial, asthma	0.2	0.8	1.0
28	Irritable bowel syndrome	0.3	0.7	1.0
29	Hiatus hernia	0.2	0.7	1.0
30	Bronchitis, chronic	0.2	0.7	0.9

*Modified from R. Feldman, "Multiphasic Screening in Medical Group Practice," in *Early Disease Detection* (Miami: Halos & Assoc., 1970).
† Condition not otherwise specified.

that the whole population is also examined definitively to establish the actual prevalence of the disease. These four categories, shown in Table 17-7, have been discussed in detail by Sproul,[30] Grant,[31] Thorner,[32] Flagle,[34] Blumberg,[35] and others.

An ideal test would, of course, detect only those persons in a population suffering from the condition looked for (as defined by standard diagnostic criteria) and would not fail to detect any of them. However, no test will perform with 100 percent accuracy.

Table 17-7.   Categories of Screening Test Results*

Screening Test Results	Patient's Health Status		Total Test Results
	Sick	Well	
Positive (+)	True +'s to test	False +'s to test	Total + tests
Negative (−)	False −'s to test	True −'s to test	Total − tests
Total category	Total sick	Total well	Total patients tested

$$\text{Sensitivity } (\%) = \frac{\text{True +'s}}{\text{Total sick}} \times 100$$

$$\text{Specificity } (\%) = \frac{\text{True −'s}}{\text{Total well}} \times 100$$

*Modified from Thorner and Remein.[32]

The accuracy with which a screening test can detect positives and negatives can be expressed in terms of the test's sensitivity and specificity. The sensitivity is the probability of correctly identifying a positive case; it measures the ability to correctly screen as positive the truly diseased cases, and corresponds to the percentage of true positives detected. The error with which the test fails to detect as positive the truly diseased patients—that is, the false negatives—is ordinarily the kind of error more important to avoid, since this represents an "under-referral" of sick patients, and for potentially disabling or life-threatening conditions may cost the patient his health or even his life.

Specificity is the probability of the test's correctly identifying a negative case; it measures the ability to screen out as negative the well (nondiseased persons). The error with which the test fails to identify as negative the well person—that is, the false positives—is usually the less important error to avoid, but it represents an "over-referral" of patients to the physicians, will cost the patient time, dollars, and anxiety, and is disturbing to the physicians and patients.

For quantitative and semiquantitative tests it is possible to vary the sensitivity and specificity by changing the screening level at which the test is considered to be positive. However, changing the screening level to increase the sensitivity will decrease the specificity, and a change to increase specificity will correspondingly decrease sensitivity.

For each disease, clinicians establish test limits outside of which they will consider the patient to be sick and will prescribe treatment. Such limits are not standardized nor agreed upon by all physicians. In Table 17-6, not a single condition listed has specific diagnostic criteria agreed upon by 100 percent of physicians. For example, there is no universal definition of obesity. Some physicians treat primary hypertension patients at diastolic blood pressure exceeding 90 mm mercury, and others begin treatment at 95 mm. The diagnosis of diabetes mellitus has many criteria advocated by several different schools. Accordingly, what is a true positive test for diabetes for one physician may be a false positive for another.

Furthermore, for each specific disease being tested, the physician tends to establish in his mind some general percentage error to limit the frequency of false negatives that he will accept. For some tests, such as the chest x-ray to screen for pulmonary tuberculosis, he will not wish to miss any cases, owing to the high costs of tuberculosis to the individual and to the community, so he will want to limit false negatives to less than 0.1 percent. In others, such as fasting blood sugar for diabetes mellitus, he might tolerate as high as 5 percent false negatives. Accordingly, the percent of true positives detected, or the desired sensitivity of the screening test for pulmonary tuberculosis, would be 99.9 percent, and for diabetes mellitus would be 95 percent.

It is obvious that a decrease in the percentage of false negatives is paid for by an increase in the percentage of false positives. Although false positives usually are a less serious kind of error than false negatives, the relative importance of these two kinds of errors for each disease must obviously be balanced.

False positive and false negative tests may be due to instrumental errors that produce an inaccurate measurement, or they may result from an accurate measurement that for the particular patient is a borderline value between a statistically derived norm and an agreed-upon clinical abnormality. Such borderline values— as, for example, slightly elevated blood glucose—may be viewed as hyperglycemia or prediabetes by physicians interested in preventive medicine, and they may alert the patient to future possible medical problems; but the internist who may be primarily interested in clinically overt diabetes mellitus may consider this as a "false" positive test if the standard glucose tolerance test does not fulfill his clinical criteria for a diagnosis of diabetes.

The difficult problems of establishing "normal" screening levels is also considered in Chapter Nineteen.

b. Costs of false positives.   Attempts to evaluate and quantify the costs of false positives[37] involve comparisons of the expected value of treatment with the expected value of nontreatment in a group of patients with known disease prevalence, the value (costs) of treating the sick, the value (costs) of reassuring the nonsick, the costs of working up the nonsick, and the costs of not treating the sick who, if not tested, would have gone undetected. These types of cost benefit studies are extremely difficult to carry out. (See F.2.a.)

The costs of false positives must be shared by those who benefit by having the disease detected early and by those who are reassured by the fact that they do not have the disease. The value of detecting the disease early is, of course, influenced by the ability of the treatment to alter the natural history of the disease and prevent or postpone overt disability.

For example, there is now convincing evidence that the higher the blood pressure, the shorter the life. In order to treat hypertension earlier and decrease the subsequent incidence of stroke, there is increasing support for early detection of asymptomatic hypertension—especially since hypertension is a relatively high-prevalence disease (it exceeds 7 percent of the adult population; see Table 17-6).

Although for lower-prevalence diseases the problem of false positives is relatively more costly, again, the potential disabling capabilities of the disease are a basic consideration. For example, the prevalence of breast cancer or cervical cancer is low, but the case for mammography for women over age 50 or for

Papanicolaou smears seems to be established.[38] The rate of detection of cervical cancers on initial or first examinations of asymptomatic women is about two per 1,000; the rate for recheck examinations, however, is only about two per 10,000. It is generally recommended, however, that every woman should have at least one or two Pap smears in her lifetime.

The pursuance of automatic secondary testing and online computerized advice rules will tend to decrease the referral rate to physicians for false positives. Examples of automatic secondary testing are routinely performing quantitative serological tests for all with positive VDRL tests, or routinely doing urine cultures with bacterial species identification for positive bacteriuria screening tests in women. An advice rule that arranges a standard morning glucose tolerance test for all patients with an elevated serum glucose on the primary screening test will identify those with diabetes mellitus and eliminate most false positives from the clinicians' considerations.

MHTS have been criticized for raising anxiety with false positive findings. It has been suggested that the tenet of "innocent until proven guilty" should apply not only to law but also to medical screening.[39] No physician should alarm the patient or begin treatment of an asymptomatic person on the basis of one abnormal test result: the physician should repeat the test and require additional corroborative evidence of disease before initiating treatment.

c. Costs of false negatives. A false negative is a more serious error if the condition missed is potentially a disabling one. For example, failing to detect early pulmonary tuberculosis by the screening chest x-ray has always been a great concern to the radiologist, whether the screening program was only for a single disease, tuberculosis, or whether in a multiphasic program it was for several conditions including tuberculosis.

Failing to detect by mammography an early nonpalpable cancer of the breast may cost the patient a possible cure if she does not come in until she palpates a lump in the breast or axilla.

Since it is unlikely that any program has sufficient resources to achieve 100 percent sensitivity and specificity, the actual expenditures will be limited by the program's goals and the community's rate of malpractice suits. The increasing impact of medical liability (malpractice) settlements upon the practice of medicine has generated the concept of "defensive medicine."[40] This results in a physician's ordering additional tests, procedures, and consultations that he deems necessary to support or defend, if challenged, the diagnosis and treatment he has provided his patient. Defensive medicine requires the physician to more completely document his management of the patient. The increasing accountability of a physician for false negative diagnoses that he may generate in his practice significantly influences the average physician's mode of practice. For each patient he must judge the potential cost and damage from a false negative that the patient will accept before he brings suit, and this will greatly affect the utilization and cost of medical services. If we assume that the current standard of practice will accept a physician's missing a certain life-threatening diagnosis in 2 percent (false negatives) of examinees, the costs of reasonable diagnostic services can be estimated. If, however, a patient wishes to decrease this error rate to 1 percent, he will require the physician to order more test procedures and consultations, which may perhaps double the cost of the original workup. If the patient is not willing to accept even a 1 percent error rate and wishes to cut this in half, he may again double the utilization of services and the cost of care, and so forth. Since it is not possible to achieve a 100 percent accuracy in diagnosis, or a zero percent error rate, the cost of defensive medicine will essentially be that which will be acceptable to the community that financially supports its physician.

A cost comparison of MHTS evaluation of patients as compared to the traditional physician's health examination is given in F.4, and Table 17-13 clearly shows the significantly lower costs for the MHTS group for the initial workup and 12 months followup care. These data do not indicate any increased costs due to excess false positives in the MHTS group, and they even suggest that the higher costs in the traditional workup may be due to excess false negatives.

d.   Value of finding a positive test for non-life-threatening conditions.   Many of the problems for which patients request a health checkup or come to see the primary care physician have little or no direct demonstrable disability or mortality associated with them—such as hearing and visual impairments, dental problems, arthralgias and backache, psychosocial problems-in-living, etc., and it is difficult to apply strict cost benefit criteria to them, since the value of identifying a positive test and correcting these conditions is basically in improving the quality of life. For example, how can one express the benefits to an elderly retired person with impaired vision and hearing who with corrective glasses and a hearing aid can now read the newspaper and listen to the radio?

e.   Value of finding a negative test.   It is difficult to objectively evaluate the worth of finding a negative test. We know how to express the value to the patient and to the physician of telling one in 12 to 14 adults that he has hypertension, in terms of decreased likelihood of future disability and mortality; and one in 500 women over age 50 that she has a breast cancer, in similar terms. On the other hand, how do we express the value of a negative test, that of telling 92 to 93 percent of adults that they do *not* have hypertension or 499 women that they do not have breast cancer? Surely the reassurance and avoidance of the costs associated with a positive test to the patient, to the family, to the community, and to the health care system has some value, perhaps even more value than the finding of a positive test, and perhaps eventually expressible by some measures of the quality of life, if such are ever developed.

Garfield has stated[41] that the accentuation of the negative by evaluation of multiphasic health testing on its yield of sickness rather than its yield of health is a product of preoccupation with sickness that has historically prevailed throughout medicine. He asserts that this misplaced emphasis produces reports that read, "It costs $2,000 to detect by mammography one true positive cancer of the breast in 500 women," rather than the alternative, "It costs $5 each to assure 499 women there is no evidence of breast cancer by mammography and $5 to detect one cancer that through early surgery may have a better prognosis." It should be recognized that there is a positive value in detecting health. The patient gains security and can plan his life accordingly.

f.   Importance to patient of all findings, negative and positive.   There is even a value (benefit) to the patient, his family, and his community in earlier detection of already irreversible conditions (cancer, nephritis, etc.) in that it not only provides palliation to the patient but permits him to plan for his limited future by giving him a longer lead time for terminal arrangements. For a man with several dependents, the earlier he learns of impending catastrophe, the more time he has to arrange his estate and take care of his children. For an executive in an organization, it permits earlier replacement planning. It is, of course, impossible to quantify such costs and benefits to the family or to society.

In view of the recognized inadequacies in all types of health examinations, it is well to advise patients of the limitations of the ability of health checkups (including MHTS) to detect all early asymptomatic disease—no examination test is 100 percent perfect—and they should be cautioned to seek assistance promptly for any new symptoms that may develop between scheduled periodic examinations.

Much of the controversy on false positives and negatives is a result of the confusion of the real role of MHTS in health care, simply as an alternative process designed to decrease costs and save doctors' time in periodic health examinations. False positives and false negatives can occur with any type of health checkup.

The physician interested in preventive health maintenance must not become discouraged by the inability of the present data to satisfy the strict requirements to beneficially alter the natural course of disease or to be cost-effective. In 1960 these requirements could not be satisfied by the existing data concerning the routine taking of blood pressure; in 1975, only 15 years later, this screening test was universally recommended. Similarly, it is predictably just a matter of time when better data and more effective treatment will justify many of the other tests routinely done in the usual MHTS.

Horvath[42] has emphasized that health care means *caring* for the patient, in addition to altering the natural course of his problem; and if the problem is a psychosocial problem with somatic symptoms, then reassuring and counseling the patient is *good care* even though the basic course of the patient's psychosocial problem has not been altered. Such "caring" processes and outcomes are impossible to quantify except as they affect patient satisfaction, which to the patient is a real outcome. A health-care-oriented MHTS must concern itself with education and prevention, even though currently the cost effectiveness of every procedure is not yet demonstrable. Very few problems in the real world have simple, quantifiable, and provable cost-effective solutions. MHTS for *health* care is a psychosocial-medical program, affecting not only every medical and psychological outcome of the individual but also the social outcome in the family and in the community, thus MHTS is not a simple solution to a simple problem. On the other hand, very few problems in our society have effective solutions, much less simple solutions. So we must evaluate MHTS in the context of medical, health, psychological, and social outcomes; and good methods for evaluating cost effectiveness of health, psychological, and social measures are not as yet available.

E. EFFICIENCY OF MHTS

1. Introduction

In evaluating a physical system, the engineer defines efficiency as the ratio of output to input. In health care systems, the evaluation of program efficiency was similarly defined by Deniston et al.[43] as the ratio between an output (net attainment of program objectives) and an input (program resources expended, usually expressed as average dollar costs). Often this ratio has been inverted and expressed, for example, as dollar cost per positive case for multiphasic screening.[44]

2. Cost Per Positive Test

In evaluating the efficiency of an MHTS to achieve its objective of providing a disease detection and monitoring program, it is necessary to measure costs to identify clinically important conditions for the various MHTS phases. In such a study, it is essential to establish accurate cost centers to provide reliable unit costs, and to define precisely what clinically important test results or findings are considered to be positive. (See D, above.) Such a study provides useful information as to which tests will be most efficient in planning the examinations for a specified population. (See Chapter Three, E.)

Using the cost analysis for 1973 reported in D, the MHTS costs for reception, supervision, data processing, and overhead (subtotal $6.41) were included in the unit costs for the individual tests considered below by proportionately distributing these common costs back into each test phase. Table 17-5 shows the cost per positive test for young, middle-aged, and older persons, and for the group as a whole. (See page 500.)

a. Mammography. Cephalocaudal and lateral x-ray views of each breast were provided to women age 48 years and older, and interpreted by a radiologist, at a cost per examinee in 1973 of $5.00. In 1.2 percent of all women age 50 and older a positive mammogram was reported as "suspicious for cancer." The cost per positive case was then $5.00/.012 or $417. Mammography in women age 60 years or older yielded 1.4 percent positives, resulting in a somewhat decreased unit cost of $357 per positive mammogram. This is often the most expensive test in an MHTS.

b. Chest x-ray. In 7.4 percent of all examinees, clinically important abnormalities were reported, including suspicious density or lung lesion, lung fibrosis, hyperlucent lung, mediastinal abnormality, hilar enlargement, hiatus hernia, dilated thoracic aorta, prominent left cardiac contour, cardiac enlargement, other cardiovascular abnormality, or bone lesion. Not included were the following conditions (reported in 15.9 percent of examinees): lung calcifications, fibronodular or fibro-calcific lesion, pleural thickening or adhesions, blunted costrophrenic angle, rib anomaly, scoliosis, previous chest surgery, mastectomy, calcific or tortuous aorta.

Table 17-5 shows for chest x-rays the tenfold increase in frequency of clinically important abnormalities reported in adults over age 60 as compared to those under age 40. The unit cost per positive chest x-ray for a clinically important abnormality in the 60-years-or-older group was $8. Because of the low prevalence and high unit cost per positive test for chest x-rays for young adults, many MHTS are eliminating chest x-rays for this group.

c. Electrocardiography. The unit cost per six-lead electrocardiogram, including interpretation by a cardiologist, was $0.90. In 17 percent of all examinees, clinically important abnormalities were reported (see D on yield rates), so the cost per positive ECG test was only $5. Owing to the greatly increased prevalence of abnormal ECGs in older patients, the cost per positive test of $3 for people age 60 to 79 years is very low. However, even in young adults (20 to 39 years) 10 percent had a clinically important abnormality reported at a cost per positive case of $9.

d.   Blood pressure.   Sphygmomanometry was performed by automated instruments read by technicians, at a cost of $0.35 per examinee. In 4.1 percent of all examinees the systolic blood pressure was 160 mm Hg or more *and* the diastolic was 90 or more. This definition resulted in a cost of $9 per positive case. Only 0.4 percent of persons under the age of 40 years had an elevated systolic and diastolic pressure, which produced a unit cost of $88. This prevalence increased tenfold to 4.3 percent for ages 40 to 59, markedly decreasing the unit cost to $8 per positive. Furthermore, in those 60 years of age and over, 11.5 percent were positive, at the low unit cost of $3.

If *either* an elevated systolic *or* diastolic blood pressure were accepted as abnormal, then 15.8 percent of all adult examinees would be reported as positive, at a unit cost of $2.

e.   Respirometry.   The one-second and total forced expiratory vital capacity were measured by an automated spirometer, at a cost of $0.65 per test. Both of these measurements were found to be abnormal in 2.2 percent of all examinees, which gives a cost of $30 per positive case. Table 17-5 shows an increase in positive cases with age.

f.   Visual acuity.   In 15.8 percent of all examinees a visual acuity of 20/40 or less in one or both eyes was reported, at a unit cost of $3 per positive. Table 17-5 shows that 10.6 percent of young adults and 26.3 percent of the oldest group had impairment of visual acuity, again demonstrating the marked increase in frequency with age.

g.   Tonometry.   Ocular tension was measured by a registered nurse using a Schiotz tonometer with a 7.5 gm weight. For all age groups, 0.3 percent had an elevated ocular pressure of 5 units or less (equivalent to 25 mm Hg or more) at a unit cost of $250 per positive case. In persons under 40 years of age the frequency of positive cases was lowest (0.2 percent), resulting in a cost per positive case of $375; accordingly, ocular tension is often not included in MHTS for people less than 40 years of age. The prevalence of elevated ocular tension increases with age, so that for individuals age 60 or more, a frequency of 0.5 percent positive was found, at a unit cost of $150 per positive.

h.   Audiometry.   A clinically important hearing loss was defined as one in which there was a deficit totaling 60 decibels or more at the frequencies of 1,000 and/or 2,000 and/or 3,000 cycles per second. Such a hearing loss was reported for 16.2 percent of all examinees, at a cost per positive case of $4. Important loss of hearing acuity was reported for 5.2 percent of young adults, increasing markedly with age to 36.4 percent of examinees age 60 or more.

i.   Hemoglobin and white cell count.   These two blood tests were measured by an automated hemocytometer at a cost of $0.55 per test. Table 17.5 shows that 3.1 percent of all men (at $18 per positive case) had a hemoglobin less than 13 grams percent; and 10.3 percent of all women ($5 per positive case) had less than 12 grams. Only 1.9 percent of young men had a low hemoglobin, in contrast to 12.6

percent of young women. Over the age of 60 both men and women have a similar prevalence (5.5 to 5.6 percent) of low hemoglobins (at a cost of $10 per positive case).

In 2.2 percent of all examinees a white cell count less than 4,000 *or* greater than 12,000 cells per cubic millimeter was found, at a cost per positive case of $25. Table 17-5 shows that the frequency of abnormal white counts decreased slightly with increasing age.

j. Serum Chemistries.   Eight serum chemistries were determined by automated (AutoAnalyzer) methods:

Serum glucose was tested one hour after ingesting 75 gm glucose solution. The upper normal limit for men and women was similar, but directly related to patient age. In addition, a correction was made whenever a patient had eaten a meal within three hours before ingesting the challenge dose of glucose as follows:

Age Group	Three hours or less since last food
Under 30	210
30–39	220
40–49	235
50 and older	240

For four or more hours since last food, the upper limit was $230 + 0.66 \times$ age.

The one-hour value was above normal limits in 5.7 percent of all examinees, at a cost per positive case of $18. In such positive cases a two-hour serum glucose was also routinely performed with the two-hour test upper normal limit of 150 mg percent. The proportion of examinees with positive one- *and* two-hour tests was 3.5 percent.

Serum cholesterol also had age-related normal limits:

Men: Age	Upper Limit
Under 30	265
30–39	295
40 and older	300

For women the upper limit was $242 + 1.4 \times$ age.

An abnormally high value occurred in 2.4 percent of all examinees, at a unit cost per positive test of $17. The frequency of positive tests increased with age.

Serum uric acid had age-related upper normal limits for women as follows: $(3.5 + 0.02 \times$ age$) + 2.0$. For men, any value greater than 8.1 mg percent was considered to be a positive test. An elevated uric acid was reported in 4.5 percent of all examinees at a unit cost of $9 per positive test. The frequency of positive tests also increased with age.

Serum calcium was considered to be elevated when greater than 10.5 mg percent in women and $11.0 - 0.01 \times$ age for men. In 1.3 percent of adults these values were exceeded; cost per positive test was $31.

Serum creatinine was elevated (i.e., more than 1.3 mg percent in women and more than 1.6 mg percent in men) in 1.4 percent of all persons, at a cost of $29 per positive test. The prevalence of positive tests was only 0.8 percent in young adults; it increased with age to 2.7 percent in the oldest age group, who had a cost per positive case of $15.

Serum glutamic oxaloacetic transaminase (SGOT) was found to be elevated (i.e., more than 41 units) in 4.2 percent of persons, at a cost of $10 per positive case.

k. VDRL Test for Syphilis. The Venereal Disease Research Laboratory (VDRL) test for syphilis was performed at a unit cost of $0.30. A positive test was reported in 1.5 percent of all examinees, at a cost per positive of $20.

l. Urinary Sugar and Protein. Urinalysis for sugar (one hour after a glucose load) and protein was performed by using enzyme "dipstick" paper strips, at a cost of $0.20 each test. Any one-plus reading was considered a positive test. Positive tests for urine sugar were reported in 8.2 percent (at a unit cost of $2 per positive) and urine protein in 6.4 percent of adults including menstruating females (at a unit cost of $3 per positive).

m. Urine Culture for Bacilluria. Midstream "clean catch" urine specimens were collected and incubated at 37°C for six hours with triphenyltetrazolium chloride (TTC) at a cost of $0.30 per test. The development of a pink color in six hours was a positive test, corresponding to a 100,000 or more bacilli per cubic millimeter by colony count. A positive test (for both TTC and colony count of 100,000 or more) was reported in 3.3 percent of women (at a cost of $9 per positive case).

In men the prevalence of bacilluria was very much less, and only in men over age 60 did the frequency of positive tests reach 1 percent.

n. Summary. It must be emphasized that the unit costs herein reported were critically related to an MHTS patient load of about 2,000 per month. If only 1,000 persons were examined monthly, the cost per patient would probably double. If 3,000 persons could be tested per month, the unit cost would probably decrease by about one-third. (See Figure 17-1.)

These data clearly demonstrate how the prevalence of an abnormal test depends upon the specific population examined, especially as related to its age-sex composition.

To illustrate, if one examines only young adults (age less than 40 years) in this population, 0.4 percent of men and 3.3 percent of women will have a positive urine culture. The cost to identify this abnormality in young men would be $300 per positive case, as compared to only $9 per positive in young women. On the other hand, if the group examined were limited to those age 60 years or more, the cost to identify a positive male patient with bacilluria would be $30 and for a positive female patient only $8. This clearly demonstrates how the cost per positive case is directly related to the age and sex of the target population. Thus one could decide for this population that urine cultures as a screening test would be justified for all women, and for only those men age 60 or more.

Finally, it is important to emphasize that in order to evaluate the true efficiency of this method of case detection, this study must be extended to determine the cost per proven "true" positive case, which requires expensive followup confirmatory and validating procedures to determine both the sensitivity and specificity of each test. For example, although the cost per positive mammogram was $417, since only about one in every five of these women with positive mammograms were subsequently confirmed by surgical biopsy to have cancer of the breast, the cost per "true" positive case was approximately $2,000.

One can say that in this program, since it costs about $25 to test an adult, and since about two-thirds of them are well (see Table 17-3), for about $75 one can reassure two persons that they are indeed well and identify one person who has a clinically significant abnormality.

Thus the efficiency of the MHTS process for disease detection depends upon the unit cost to do the tests and the prevalence of the abnormalities in the target population. The generation of data on the cost per positive test is one of the most useful analyses of a MHTS program.

3.   Optimal Content of MHTS Examinations

The criteria for optimal test selection for MHTS depend upon the sensitivity and specificity of the test, cost per test, prevalence in the group being examined, and utility of the test to the physicians in their management of patients. (See Chapter Three.) If costs can be reduced by varying the content of the examination for each examinee (i.e., selective screening), it seems likely that MHTS programs will evolve in the direction of providing just the tests needed for each person, given his age, sex, occupation, habits, present symptoms, past medical history, and previous test findings. (See Chapters Two and Three.) The small amount of research done on the effects of altering MHTS test content has made one principle evident: the more tests that are done, the more abnormalities will be reported—leading to more followup tests and referrals, more diagnoses, and more therapy.[45]

Some do not consider this a benefit. They justify a negative attitude to a comprehensive battery of tests on the basis that if one provides 15 to 20 tests, then purely on a statistical basis half of all randomly selected adults will have at least one abnormal test. Rather than being concerned about this finding, we may find reassuring that "normal" limits provide such a good sensitivity. Since most adults have some chronic impairment (even though slight and asymptomatic), and as no one is physically perfect, a good diagnostician who does enough tests can find some "abnormality" in everyone. Not only is finding an abnormal test by MHTS in one-half of a group of randomly selected adult examinations reasonable, but Table 17-6 shows that significant abnormalities are predictable in two-thirds of MHTS examinations.

F.   COST EFFECTIVENESS OF MHTS

1.   Introduction

A very useful method of evaluating an MHTS system is by comparing its costs to some alternative process for achieving the same specified objectives. This method of comparing inter-program (or even no-program) costs to achieve the same objectives does not require putting dollar values on the changes in health status or other patient outcomes that may be affected.

2. Cost Effectiveness of MHTS Test Phases

An important evaluation for an MHTS is to evaluate each testing phase as to its costs and its effectiveness in detecting the target condition, as compared to (1) no testing at all (that is, the traditional custom of waiting for patients to come in with a complaint), or (2) some alternative testing method. Since this is a very time-consuming and expensive process, it is usually not done for every phase.

a. Mammography.   As an example of this evaluation process, the cost effectiveness of our mammography experience for the detection of breast cancer will be discussed (modified from Kodlin[46]). Assume 20,000 women age 50 or more, (a) one-half receive mammography and (b) the other half seek conventional care with breast palpation only. Assume 20 early breast cancers per 10,000, 16 (80 percent) detectable by mammography, 12 (60 percent) detectable by palpation, and 8 (40 percent) both palpable and detectable by mammography. Also assume a mammography test costs $5 (see Table 17-5), physical examination by physician costs $50, and a breast biopsy costs $150. Then diagnostic costs for the two groups are:

(a)   Total diagnostic tests for the 10,000 women (age 50 and over) receiving mammography:

10,000 mammographies $\times$ \$5	= \$50,000
16 (true positive) $\times$ (50 + 150)	= 3,200
104 (false positive) $\times$ 50 + (3* $\times$ 150)	= 5,650
(*assumes 3 had biopsy)	
4 (false negative) $\times$ 50 + (4** $\times$ 150)	= 800
(**assumes delayed biopsy)	

Total diagnostic costs   = \$59,650

(b)   Total diagnostic tests for 10,000 women (age 50 and over) assuming 1,000 (10 percent) sought conventional care for a breast complaint and 48 had biopsies:

1,000 examinations $\times$ 50	= \$50,000
12 (true positive) $\times$ 150	= 1,800
36 (false positive) $\times$ 150	= 5,400
8 (false negative) $\times$ (50* + 150)	= 1,600
(*assumes delayed biopsy)	

Total diagnostic costs   = \$58,000

Thus, the total diagnostic costs could be almost the same for the two groups, depending upon the frequency with which women over age 50 seek conventional examinations of the breast, and upon the comparative costs of mammography and physical examination. However, to completely evaluate the cost effectiveness of breast cancer detection requires determination of its impact on the referral services in the health care delivery system (even if patient outcomes are not considered). Accordingly, assume treatment cost for a simple mastectomy and hospitalization for an early breast cancer without axillary node involvement is $750, and a radical mastectomy, hospitalization, and radiation therapy for an advanced breast cancer is $1,700. Then immediate treatment costs for the two groups are:

```
(a)  16 (true +):  12 early ×   750    =  $ 9,000
                    4 late   × 1,700    =    6,800
      4 (false −):  4 late   × 1,700    =    6,800
                                            ───────
                    Total costs         =  $22,600

(b)  12 (true +):   6 early ×   750     =  $ 4,500
                    6 late   × 1,700    =   10,200
      8 (false −):  8 late   × 1,700    =   13,600
                                            ───────
                    Total costs         =  $28,300
```

Furthermore, assume 80 percent of late-treated cases will require subsequent extensive hospitalization and treatment for metastases and terminal care at an average cost of $5,000 each. Then late-treatment costs are:

```
(a)   6 × 5,000     =  $30,000
(b)  11 × 5,000     =  $55,000
```

Then total diagnostic and treatment costs for the two groups are:

	(a) Mammography group	(b) Conventional group
Diagnostic costs	$ 59,650	$ 58,800
Immediate treatment	22,600	28,300
Late treatment	30,000	55,000
Total costs	$112,250	$142,100

These data indicate that routine mammography testing of women age 50 or over, in our experience, is more cost-effective than the conventional complaint-response mode. However, as Kodlin[46] emphasized, such cost effectiveness studies are fraught with considerable uncertainties, and all data must be carefully derived from the actual population being tested, since costs and rates vary widely from study to study. To add on the estimated costs and benefits from the viewpoint of the patients complicates even further the evaluation process.

   b. Evaluation of computer-generated advice rules. Another example of evaluating the cost effectiveness of a single-phase function is the following study on advice rules. Since 1964, the Oakland Kaiser-Permanente MHTS has provided "automated" screening by the use of advice (decision) rules programmed into the computer. At the last multiphasic station, while the patient was waiting (i.e., online), his machine-readable test cards were read into the computer. The computer processor had been programmed with various test limits, decision rules and algorithms, based upon the age and sex of the individual patient. From these limits and decision rules the computer provided a preliminary report containing advice as to any additional procedures the physicians wished to have completed before the patient's followup visit for physical examination and diagnosis. For example, if the urine analysis showed proteiniuria, the computer printed out instructions to the receptionist to ask the patient to return to the laboratory with a first morning specimen for retest.

A one-year study[47] was conducted to evaluate the extent to which these online computer-generated advice rules achieved their desired objectives, arranging as many indicated secondary and supplemental tests as were reasonable before the patient saw the physician, so as to (1) conserve physician time on the first routine followup examination visit, (2) decrease the number of second followup contacts with the physician by phone calls or office visits, and (3) decrease the number of followup diagnostic or evaluative laboratory tests provided by the outpatient clinical laboratory.

Accordingly, in the Oakland multiphasic program the followup care patterns of two groups of tested individuals with abnormal laboratory findings were reviewed from their medical records,* namely:

Group 1—"With Advice": those eligible for an online computer-generated advice rule who received it.

Group 2—"Without Advice": those eligible for an online advice rule who did not receive it because of equipment failure or who failed to wait for it.

Table 17-8 shows that the rate of routine first followup visits (for physical examination and diagnosis by a physician) was significantly greater (i.e., better followup compliance) for the group receiving advice rules (96 percent) than for the group not receiving them (88 percent).

The number of additional physician followup office visits required to evaluate the multiphasic test abnormality that generated the online advice rule is also shown in Table 17-8. The efficiency of the automated MHTS process with advice rules in conserving physician time was demonstrated by the fact that 90 percent of all patients had their health examinations completed with only the first routine physician office visit. The online advice rule resulted in a significant decrease in the number of additional physician office visits. For patients without computer advice rules, approximately twice as many additional office visits occurred (19.5 percent vs. 9.6 percent). It is also evident from Table 17-8 that a significantly greater number of telephone calls were required when an online advice rule was not available (14.1 percent vs. 4.4 percent).

Only 11.8 percent of examinees with multiphasic test positives who received an online advice rule required one or more physician-ordered laboratory tests (that is, in addition or supplemental to the computer-ordered laboratory test), compared to 37.3 percent of individuals processed without online advice rules. Almost one-third (32 percent) of those not receiving an advice rule had the test identical to that of the advice rule ordered by the physician, as compared to only 9.8 percent identical retesting for those receiving the rule.

In summary, the addition of computer online advice rules permitted 10 percent more patients to complete their health examination in one physician office visit, decreased the number of additional physician office visits required to evaluate MHTS-detected abnormalities, and significantly decreased the number of

---

*Data collected and analyzed by M. Goldberg, M.D.

Table 17-8. Effect of MHTS Computer-Generated Advice Rules on Frequency of Followup Procedures

Advice Rules	Number of Patients	Percent With Routine Followup	Percent With 1 or More Added MD Visits	Percent With Followup Phone Advice	Percent With Added Lab. Tests	
					Relevant to MHTS Abnormal	Identical to Approp. Rule
With	495	96.0	9.6	4.4	11.8	9.8
Without	441	88.0	19.5	14.1	37.3	32.0

*Modified from Collen.[47]

physician-patient telephone calls and physician-ordered laboratory tests related to the multiphasic test abnormalities. These measures of decreased utilization of resources can readily be converted to equivalent costs.

3.   Cost Effectiveness of Providing Health Examinations

In addition to evaluating each phase, it is important to determine the cost effectiveness of the MHTS program as a whole. The evaluation of the cost effectiveness of providing single or periodic health examinations as compared to not providing such examinations is a measure of the extent to which one achieves the objective of sufficiently decreasing disability and mortality so that the increased earnings of nondisabled survivors more than compensate for the costs of the examinations. Such a study has been carried out,[48] and the results in a group of 45- to 54-year-old men will be summarized herein.

A study group of approximately 1,229 men who were Kaiser Health Plan members, initially ages 45 to 54, were urged to undertake annual MHTS examinations. A control group of similar composition and size were not so urged but were followed up in a similar fashion for each subject's health experience. Since all benefits to patients were not measurable, this is not a cost benefit study. This Multiphasic Checkup Evaluation Study has been under way since late 1964, and a detailed description appears in the next chapter. The group described herein constitutes the one age-sex subgroup in whom a favorable effect on disability was found.

Expenses associated with health-related events were compiled for the study and control groups. It was assumed for these calculations that the event rates for approximately one-fifth of the subjects in both groups lost to followup by the end of 1971 were the same as those for men who remained under observation.

Medical care utilization was measured in the study and control group subjects in the health plan. Disability rates were measured in subjects who remained in the Kaiser plan and responded to mailed questionnaires. For purposes of determining expenses, however, these event rates were adjusted so as to relate to the initial population as of January 1, 1965. In this way the various expenses could be expressed as costs per man entering the program.

Table 17-9 depicts the earnings in the study and control groups. Row A contains the proportions of survivors with no disability and partial disability, adjusted to relate to the initial population, so as to take into account the effect of mortality. "No disability" was defined in the survey questionnaire as a present state of health enabling one to do one's usual work with no limitation. "Partial disability" was defined as a present state of health that caused one to limit or cut down on the amount or kind or work one was doing.

It was learned from a telephone survey that partial disability was associated, on the average, with a 25 percent reduction in earning capacity—that is, a 25 percent earnings loss either to the disabled individual or to the institution providing his compensation. Thus for purposes of computing earnings the partial disability figures were weighted by a factor of 0.75 (row B). It was assumed that the disability prevalence rates remained essentially unchanged throughout each year. Average annual individual earnings estimates (row C) were obtained from results of a survey of health plan members performed in 1971, with figures for the preceding

Table 17-9. Cost Effectiveness of Periodic MHTS Examinations in Men (Ages 45–54 At Entry)*

		1965	1966	1967	1968	1969	1970	1971	1965–1971 Total
A.	Percent of initial group with								
	1. No disability — Control‡	86.8	83.9	81.0	78.6	76.2	73.1	70.1	
	Study†	87.5	85.5	83.2	82.2	81.2	77.8	74.2	
	2. Partial disability — Control	10.4	11.4	12.5	13.2	14.0	15.2	16.4	
	Study	10.3	11.1	11.9	11.2	10.6	11.3	12.1	
B.	Economic equivalent percent of initial groups with no or partial disability (A1 + 0.75A2) — Control	94.6	92.5	90.4	88.5	86.7	84.5	82.4	
	Study	95.2	93.8	92.1	90.6	89.2	86.3	83.3	
C.	Estimated average annual earnings/man — Control and Study	$7,440	$7,710	$8,130	$8,870	$9,540	$10,270	$11,250	
D.	Average annual earnings/man in initial groups (B × C) — Control	$7,038	$7,132	$7,350	$7,850	$8,271	$8,678	$9,270	
	Study	$7,083	$7,234	$7,488	$8,036	$8,510	$8,863	$9,371	
E.	Average earnings difference/man — Study minus Control	$45	$102	$138	$186	$239	$185	$101	$996
F.	Average annual MHTS expense/man — Control	$9	$9	$9	$9	$8	$8	$10	
	Study	$18	$28	$34	$38	$34	$35	$36	
G.	Average difference/man in MHTS expense — Control minus Study	−$9	−$19	−$25	−$29	−$26	−$27	−$26	−$161
H.	Net difference in economic impact of the health-related events/man (in the initial groups) — Study minus Control	$41	$78	$113	$157	$210	$155	$68	$822

*Modified from Collen, et al.[48]
†Study group of 1,229 men (in 1965) urged to have an MHTS examination every year.
‡Control group of 1,364 men (in 1965) not so urged, but voluntarily could obtain such MHTS examinations.

years derived by extrapolation, using percentage of annual income changes for industrial workers published by the United States Department of Labor, Bureau of Labor Statistics.

The combined proportions of living men with no disability and partial disability (row B) were multiplied by the annual income estimates (row C) to give the average annual earnings per man in the initial populations (row D). The study-control group differences, shown in row E, represent the differences in average annual earnings per man in the initial populations due to differences in disability prevalence and mortality. For every year the earnings were higher in the study group.

The result of the urging procedure undertaken by the Multiphasic Evaluation Study was that MHTS utilization rates were substantially higher in the study group. After adjustment to relate the figures to the initial populations, the utilization rates were multiplied by the MHTS costs. There were two components to the MHTS cost: the first was the multiphasic fee charged to health plan nonmembers, which was $30; the second was the earnings loss incurred by one-half day's work absence while undergoing the multiphasic health checkup (1/470 of the estimated annual individual earnings). The product, the average annual MHTS expense per man, appears in row F. To the MHTS costs in the study group were added an additional $4, representing the estimated annual cost per man of contacting the study group subjects and urging them to come in for the checkup. When the total MHTS costs in the study and control groups were compared, there was, as expected, an excess expenditure for the study group every year (row G).

In Table 17-9 the study-control group differences in earnings, the outpatient clinic expenses, which do not form a part of the MHTS itself, and MHTS expenses are combined in row H. Hospital usage costs were slightly higher in the control group, but not significantly, and would not have materially affected these results. It can be seen that the total economic impact favored the study group every year. The total difference for the seven-year period is over $800 per man. It can therefore be concluded that urging 45- to 54-year-old men to have an MHTS examination every year is cost-effective. It should also be pointed out that the savings associated with greater MHTS exposure apply to men in the middle income range, who formed the majority of the subjects in this study. For men with higher incomes the difference would be greater; for men with lower incomes, it would be less. We have not been able to demonstrate, however, that multiphasic health checkups are cost-effective for other groups, such as 35- to 44-year-old males or 35- to 54-year-old females.

4. Cost Effectiveness of Alternative Health Examination Modes

If it is necessary to respond to the public's demand for periodic health examinations, or if an organizational decision is made to provide health examinations to a group of people, the question then arises as to which is the most cost-effective examination method. The following study compared, for "new" patients, the costs of health examinations provided by MHTS (with and without nurse practitioner physical examinations) to the traditional health examinations provided by physicians.[28,49] (See Figure 2-4.)

The Kaiser-Permanente Oakland Medical Center's MHTS, described in prior chapters, provides a systemized battery of tests and a self-administered history. The MHTS group of patients received an MHTS examination followed up by a 15-minute scheduled visit for a physical examination by a physician in the medical department.

Patients who completed the MHTS could also receive an immediate physical examination by trained nurse practitioners, supervised by a physician (the MHTS-RN group). These nurse practitioners provided the physical examinations (including pelvic examinations in women, with cervical smears for cancer detection) in a specially designed health evaluation section located adjacent to the multiphasic testing laboratory. Supervising physicians validated nurses' findings, were available to the nurses for consultation, and participated in final decisions as to the referral followup to other specialty departments.[49] (See Chapter Ten.)

Also available was a "traditional" medical checkup (the TMC group) provided by the same medical department physicians, who, during a 30-minute scheduled visit, took a history and did a physical examination. The physicians who provided care in the traditional medical department were the same internists who did followup MHTS physician physical examinations and who supervised the nurse practitioners.

After the physician saw the patient in any of the above modes, he or the nurse practitioner, or both, would refer the patient to appropriate specialty clinics for "examination followup" clinical laboratory tests, x-rays, EKGs, and other special diagnostic procedures as necessary to arrive at a final diagnosis.

This study was conducted in 1972–74, comparing 6,285 similarly selected patients receiving (1) traditional medical checkups (TMC), (2) multiphasic health checkups (MHTS) with physician physical examinations, or (3) multiphasic checkups with nurse practitioner physical examinations (MHTS-RN). Their health status was determined by chart review and they were classified as well, asymptomatic-sick, worried-well, or sick. (See Chapter Two.) All data were then adjusted so that both groups were comparable by age, sex, and health status. Since the same physicians provided the examinations and arranged followup care for all three groups, the quality of care was assumed to be similar.

Table 17-10 shows the use and cost of services for the initial examination visit by the three modes. The costs shown are costs to the health plan for the services provided to its members; they do not represent fees or charges that would have been paid by nonmember patients (e.g., MHTS cost to the health plan for a member was $17.46, as shown in Table 17-10, but the charge to a nonmember patient would have been $30 to $40). The multiphasic panel of tests replaced the individually selected tests, which were ordered by the physicians in the traditional mode. The great decrease in physician time for the initial physical examination was obviously the main saving in both MHTS and MHTS-RN.

Table 17-11 shows the followup visits and tests ordered by the physicians to complete the health examination. Many patients did not have their health examination fully completed at the initial visit, since the detection of possible variations from normal required further diagnostic tests (clinical laboratory, radiology, ECG, etc.) or physician specialist consultation visits (internal medicine, opthalmology, gynecology, dermatology, etc.) to confirm the validity of the finding or for further diagnostic evaluation. The final report of the health examination was provided to the patient as a followup return visit; or if the entire examination was

Table 17-10. Comparative Use and Cost of Services for Initial Health Examinations Per Patient (Adjusted for Age, Sex, and Health Status)*

	TMC		MHTS		MHTS-RN	
	(N = 2,040)		(N = 1,916)		(N = 2,329)	
	No.	$	No.	$	No.	$
Physician (min)	30.0	28.52	15.0	14.75	3	2.95
Nurse practitioner (min)	0	0	0	0	30	8.22
MHTS	0	0	1	17.46	1	17.46
Clinical laboratory (tests)	6.45	10.71	0	0	0	0
X-ray (films)	0.87	3.60	0	0	0	0
ECG, etc.	0.13	0.71	0	0	0	0
Total		$43.54		$32.21		$28.63

* Modified from Collen, et al.[49]

essentially negative, i.e., there were no clinically significant abnormalities to report to a well patient, this might be handled by a telephone call or a letter. (The costs of phone calls and letters were not included in this study, since they are not significant.)

MHTS and MHTS-RN patients used less medical department M.D. followup time than did patients who took the traditional examination. All patients, on the average, used similar amounts of referral specialist services in other departments (ophthalmology, gynecology, orthopedics, surgery, dermatology, etc.). The costs for ancillary services (clinical laboratory, radiology, ECG, and other diagnostic procedures) used for the followup evaluation workups also are shown in Table 17-11. The impact of the more comprehensive initial testing of MHTS is shown here by comparing the sum of clinical laboratory plus radiology plus special diagnostic procedures for followup evaluations ($7.06 for TMC, $5.14 for MHTS,

Table 17-11. Comparative Use and Cost of Services for Examination Followup Per Patient (Adjusted for Age, Sex, and Health Status)*

	TMC		MHTS		MHTS-RN	
	No.	$	No.	$	No.	$
Medical department MD (min.)	12.2	9.39	8.7	5.61	9.3	6.64
Other departments MD (min.)	1.4	1.43	1.8	1.84	1.5	1.54
Paramedical (min.)	0	0	0	0	1.8	1.25
Clinical laboratory (tests)	3.14	5.21 ⎤	1.48	2.45 ⎤	1.78	2.96 ⎤
X-ray (films)	0.31	1.27 ⎥ 7.06	0.38	1.57 ⎥ 5.14	0.32	1.30 ⎥ 5.04
ECG, etc.	0.10	0.58 ⎦	0.20	1.12 ⎦	0.14	0.78 ⎦
Total		$17.88		$12.59		$14.47

*Modified from Collen, et al.[49]

and $5.04 for MHTS-RN). Do false positive tests generated from the initial MHTS examination produce excessive followup tests and increasing total costs of care? These data show that the issue is not a significant one. (See page 504.)

The total physician time (initial and followup), represented by scheduled minutes, used for each of the three health examination modes was very different. The traditional (TMC) examination method, based upon the required use of physicians for both the initial examination and the followup visits, used a total of 43.6 minutes of physician time, on the average. The MHTS mode reduced the physician time used in the initial examination by one-half, and decreased somewhat the physician time used for followup evaluation, so that the MHTS health examination used on the average a total of only 25.5 minutes, or 42 percent less physician time than the traditional health examination. The MHTS-RN approach further decreased the use of the *initial* physician time to only that for supervising the nurse practitioners who performed the routine physical examinations. As a result, the total physician time used for the MHTS-RN mode of health examination was only 13.8 minutes, or 68 percent less than TMC and 46 percent less than MHTS.

Table 17-12 compares the total costs for providing health examinations by the three methods tested. The total cost for a health examination is the sum of the resources used on the initial examination visit and on the evaluation followup visits. The average total cost for a health examination by the traditional (TMC) physician mode was $61.42. As an alternative, by first providing a multiphasic health testing battery of tests, followed by either a physician (MHTS) or nurse practitioner (MHTS-RN) physical examination, the total costs for a health examination were decreased to $44.80 and $43.10, respectively, for an average savings of $16.62 and $18.32 per examination (or a decrease in total costs of 27 percent and 30 percent, respectively). Since the total costs for testing (MHTS, clinical laboratory, x-ray, and ECG) were similar for all three modes (about $22), the cost differences are due entirely to saving of physician time.

Of additional importance was the finding that the initial increased comprehensiveness of the MHTS examination, when serving as the entry mode to a health care system, had a significant economic impact on the subsequent followup care for at least one year. Table 17-13 compares the total resource costs utilized per 1,000 patients for 12 months beginning with the health evaluations. These costs include all physicians plus all supporting personnel, overhead and facilities costs,

Table 17-12. Summary of Total Costs, Per Patient, for a Health Examination (Initial and Followup) (Adjusted for Age, Sex, and Health Status)*

	TMC		MHTS		MHTS-RN	
MD visits	$39.34		$22.20		$11.13	
Paramedical visits	0		0		9.27	
MHTS	0		17.46		17.46	
Clinical laboratory	15.92	22.08	2.45	22.60	2.96	22.50
X-rays	4.87		1.57		1,30	
ECG, etc.	1.29		1.12		0.78	
Total	$61.42		$44.80		$43.10	

*Modified from Collen, et al.[49]

Table 17-13. Comparison of Impact on 12-Month Total Service Costs $/Yr/1,000 Examinees, Adjusted for Age, Sex, and Health Status*

	TMC	MHTS	MHTS·RN
MD costs	$ 93,673	$ 68,714	$54,683
(percent of TMC)		(73.4)	(58.4)
Total costs	$131,179	$105,966	$98,629
(percent of TMC)		(80.8)	(75.2)

*Modified from Garfield, et al.[28]

etc. Patients who received the more comprehensive multiphasic health checkup (MHTS group) saved $25,213 per 1,000 patients per year as compared to those who received initially a traditional medical checkup (TMC). Contrary to statements that multiphasic testing increases cost of care, total cost of care for the MHTS group over 12 months was only 80.8 percent of traditional care, and with the additional nurse practitioner examinations (MHTS-RN) was only 75.2 percent of traditional care. This decrease of 19 percent in total care costs per year was due primarily to saving in physicians' time, and this savings generally applied to all health status categories of patients.

Lyle[51] reported that for a fee-for-service group practice of seven internists, the implementation of an MHTS improved physician productivity so that the number of new patient examinations seen by the same physicians increased 32.9 percent.

Oszustowicz[52] reported that the adoption of MHTS within a general hospital resulted in a savings in the salaries of interns who prepared admission patient histories, a decrease in bed occupancy, a savings in medical record room labor, and improved medical records. He also found a savings in physician and nursing work after admission, because availability of more detailed quantitative patient data permitted the physician and nursing staff to concentrate more on treatment than on data gathering. The detection of unexpected medical problems at admission sometimes warranted postponement of surgery. Okelberry[33] also reported that preadmission testing shortened length of hospital stay.

5. Optimal Interval Between Health Checkups

Much research is still needed to determine the optimal interval between health checkups. If an asymptomatic patient were examined every day, this would clearly permit detection of new disease at the earliest possible time and daily reassurance of good health; but costs and inconvenience obviously make such an approach ridiculous. At the other extreme, examining patients once every 30 years would be very inexpensive but might result in long and harmful delays in the detection of disease. These extreme examples are given to show that the question of the optimal interval between checkups is a relative matter, which eventually comes down to weighing costs vs. benefits (however defined). To determine the optimal interval between tests, more information is needed for each test concerning the rate over time at which a normal or acceptable value moves into an abnormal range that requires action.

That periodic health checkups should be given to all persons annually has been generally assumed by most persons and medical care providers in the United

States. Yet, given the limitations of medical care resources in this country, serious questions can be raised about providing annual checkups to all persons, and Kaiser-Permanente has never made such a recommendation. For young adults between the ages of 20 and 35, it seems in our experience excessively costly to provide annual checkups to such healthy asymptomatic individuals. We feel that every five to ten years may well be a reasonable interval for general health examination for such young adults, since the incident rate of disease is very low. After age 35, however, the studies referred to in the next chapter show a significant decrease in mortality due to potentially postponable conditions; accordingly, it would appear to be advisable to recommend health evaluations for the 36- to 45-year-olds every two to three years. After age 45, however, the combined effects of aging and chronic impairments warrant MHTS every year or two. The study reported in F.3 supports the significant cost benefits to middle-aged men from multiphasic health checkups every year or two. Perhaps after age 65,.owing to the increasing incident rate of abnormalities, health examinations should be provided oftener than once a year. (See also Chapter Three, E.)

G. PHYSICIAN ACCEPTANCE OF MHTS

The acceptability of an MHTS and its support by physicians has many facets, including the increased physician time and costs incurred by false positives and negatives (see F) and the ethical and legal aspects of acquiring unsolicited data on patients. (See Chapter Two, F.)

Questions have been raised concerning the time physicians spend performing followup evaluations for false positive tests. Our experience suggests that (1) physicians are quite accustomed to the need for "ruling out" preliminary and presumptive diagnoses, (2) much of this work can now be taken over by paramedical personnel, and (3) programmed secondary testing can decrease the proportion of false positives referred to the physician. In fact, as shown in the prior section, the amount of physician time spent in examination followup is less for MHTS patients than for patients who receive traditional health examinations. (See Table 17-11.)

Generally speaking, periodic health checkups are considered to be routine work by the primary care physician. As already stated, MHTS is merely one alternative to providing periodic health checkups by conserving physician time. Since there is an increasing public demand for checkups, it is most efficient for those responsible for providing care to large numbers of people to utilize the multiphasic health testing mode to provide checkups of good quality at low cost.[53] When the physician is satisfied that MHTS can provide a good-quality checkup to his patient at a lower cost, the physician will accept and support the MHTS.[36]

Mechanic[54] points out that medical decisions are influenced by the physician's willingness to assume risks involved in the decision-making process. Physicians usually adopt a conservative decision rule, which makes it a more serious error to dismiss a sick patient than to retain a well person; accordingly, a large part of the differential diagnostic process is involved in ruling out possible diseases that also might account for the patient's symptoms. However, since it is the basic concept of MHTS to comprehensively screen for important symptoms and physical examination signs, and to take a large number of laboratory tests, physicians tend to be overwhelmed by the relatively large numbers of "abnormalities" for which they must rule out diseases. They are uncomfortable with the possible positive or negative effects of the alternatives of ordering or not ordering secondary testing and of treating or not treating borderline abnormalities or asymptomatic diseases. Accordingly, there is a great variability of medical practices, differing greatly in utilization of medical resources and prescriptive management of patients.

Bates[55] surveyed 417 physicians to ascertain their acceptance and followup of multiphasic screening tests; he confirmed the lack of responsiveness of practitioners in confirming an abnormal test or initiating management of detected abnormalities. Bates suggested that (1) MHTS was of value to the physician in providing new diagnoses, providing data for the physician that, even for normal tests, may make other tests unnecessary and furnish baseline information against which to compare future test results; and (2) since physician behavior constitutes the "major block" in patient followup, three choices appear open: (a) improve followup through physician education, (b) make alternate arrangements for followup, or (c) delete the test from MHTS because followup is not carried out.

Williamson,[56] in an ingenious study of physician responses to screening test results, found that only 35 percent of physicians showed any response to unexpected abnormalities on hospital admission screening tests, as determined by a retrospective chart review. A subsequent staff educational program increased this response rate to 45 percent. A strip of fluorescent tape was then used to cover the laboratory test results, and it was found that 78 percent of charts contained some physician responses to unexpected abnormalities; six months after discontinuing the fluorescent tape, responses were evident in only 60 percent of charts reviewed. Williamson suggested that the failure of physicians to respond to screening tests may be a widespread problem, and he offered three reasons:

(1) Physicians may not be consciously aware of the large number of unexpected abnormal screening test results reported. Possibly their attention is focused on symptomatic disease, or laboratory slips may not reach the chart before the patient is discharged.

(2) Physicians who are aware of these reports may believe that only striking abnormalities are significantly correlated with pathology; thus they ignore the majority that are minimally to moderately abnormal.

(3) Physicians, whether or not they are aware of these reports, may believe that if abnormalities are found, potential benefit to the patient may not be worth the effort involved in diagnosis and treatment.

Since educational effects are often short-lived, a continuing cyclic effort seems essential if desired levels of performance are to be achieved and maintained.

The acceptance by physicians of MHTS is clearly influenced by ethical and medico-legal considerations. McKeown[57] emphasized the unconventional impact of screening on the physician's usual practice when the screened patient appears before the physician following MHTS examination. In those instances where a public health authority or an organization has initiated the screening procedures and not the patient, McKeown raises ethical questions as to what is the physician's responsibility. The American Medical Association in its guidelines[58] has attempted to formulate ethical principles for MHTS. (See Chapter Two, F.)

Medico-legal aspects of MHTS primarily result from false negative test results, as in failing to detect pulmonary tuberculosis on chest x-rays and breast cancer on mammography. (See D.3.) Any claims from false positives arise from the anxiety generated by the report. Letters to screenees must be worded with great care and should stress the positive aspects of MHTS; primarily they should notify those people who should see a physician for a particular finding and advise the rest to seek general health counseling.

Personal economics undoubtedly has some role in the acceptability of MHTS by physicians. Medical checkups are often an important source of income for internists, general practitioners, and other primary care physicians. Such physicians, in losing a part of the work they do or control to an MHTS program, are concerned that they may undergo financial loss. Experience has shown that the referral of patients from MHTS often increases physician income.

On the other hand, many physicians find that giving checkups or routine physical examinations is rather uninteresting. They are glad to turn over health assessment activities to MHTS and nurse practitioners or other paraprofessionals so that they can devote most of their time to the care of the sick.

H. SUMMARY OF MHTS SYSTEMS EVALUATION

Since MHTS is still an evolving component of health care delivery, its objectives are still developing and its applications are becoming more diversified. Accordingly, its evaluation must be a continuing and iterative process. However, as of 1977, the extent to which MHTS has achieved its objectives within a health care system can be summarized as follows:

From the viewpoint of the patient, MHTS:

(1) Decreases waiting time for appointments for health checkups and/or for entry to a health care system (especially if the physical examination is provided by nurse practitioners) by eliminating the constraint of the traditional physician first visit.

(2) Greatly decreases the length of time necessary to complete a health checkup.

(3) Is significantly less costly.

(4) Is very acceptable, achieving a high level of satisfaction with services. (See the next chapter.)

(5) Effectively detects disease before symptoms appear, evaluates the patient's health status, and appropriately refers him for followup care for any abnormalities found.

(6) Improves long-term outcome by decreasing mortality of potentially postponable conditions (see the next chapter), and for middle-aged men decreases days lost due to disability, thereby increasing net earnings.

From the viewpoint of the physician, MHTS:

(1) Serves as a referral center for his patients for good-quality health status evaluation at a low cost; provides admission workups for his ambulatory hospital patients.

(2) Effectively detects previously unknown disease and monitors status of known disease, thereby identifying those who need further diagnostic study.

(3) Improves quality and personalization of health checkup by providing (a) normal values individualized for each patient by age, sex, etc., (b) comparisons with prior test results for trend comparisons, and (c) greater accuracy by use of automated equipment and better quality control.

(4) Saves physician time by transferring many routine repetitive tasks to allied health personnel and automated instruments.

(5) Can improve the data base available to physicians, thereby decreasing the amount of time spent in routine data gathering for diagnosis and allowing more time with the patient for therapy.

(6) Provides a comprehensive health profile of patients in a uniformly formatted record.

(7) Stores data in computerized files for subsequent clinical, epidemiological, and health services research.

From the viewpoint of the medical facility administrator, MHTS:

(1) Provides a "health center" component to a medical facility for health care and personal preventive health maintenance services by efficiently determining health status of examinees, detecting early disease, and monitoring the status of known disease.

(2) Can be customized with test phases for the medical needs of the population that uses his facility, including its outpatient clinics, hospital, and surrounding community physicians.

(3) Provides a good-quality, effective health examination process at the lowest cost per examination for ambulatory outpatients or hospital admissions.

(4) When used for hospital admissions, reduces the length of hospital stay by processing admission workups more rapidly and efficiently.

From the viewpoint of the health care systems planner, MHTS:

(1) Is effective and efficient for early disease detection (case finding), health surveillance, and disease monitoring. Based upon our experience with a representative middle- and working-class population, it can be expected that in two-thirds of all adult examinations some clinically important abnormality will be reported by their physicians (see Table 17-6). In 17 percent a significant abnormality will be reported on the electrocardiogram, and in 7 percent on chest x-ray (see Table 17-5). Seven percent of all adults will have hypertension. Five percent of women will have anemia. Three percent of all adults will have diabetes mellitus; two percent will have deafness; and one percent glaucoma. One in every 500 women over age 50 will have breast cancer, and one in every 5,000 adults will have a parathyroid tumor.

(2) Provides the most efficient method of furnishing health examinations to a large population, if health maintenance is one of the health care systems objectives.

(3) Can effectively provide periodic health examinations and, for middle-aged males, can demonstrate cost benefits from promoting annual health examinations.

(4) Increases accessibility to and decreases costs of primary care services by

replacing entry visit to physician, especially if physical examinations, determinations of patient health status, and triage to needed services are performed by nurse practitioners.

(5) Improves quality and individualization of testing data.

(6) Can provide health education and counseling so as to increase patient compliance with referrals to health and preventive maintenance.

In summary, although it is not yet possible to quantify all the benefits of multiphasic health examinations to patients, evidence is now accumulating of improved outcome to some middle-aged groups; effective reassurance to the well and worried-well, who constitute the majority who seek health checkups; effective early disease detection and disease monitoring; improved quality of testing; and overall improved cost effectiveness of health care delivery for all health status groups when multiphasic health checkups serve to provide the entry mode to primary care. Systemized multiphasic type health examinations can be used to provide effective, economical, and acceptable health examinations of the entire population.

REFERENCES

1. Zemach, R. "Program Evaluation and System Control." *Am. J. Pub. Health* 63(1933):607–609.

2. Collen, M. F., et al. *Provisional Guidelines for Automated Multiphasic Health Testing Services,* Vol. 1, 1970. N.T.I.S. Report No. PB 195654; and Zucker, L. W., et al. "Cost and Cost Analysis Guidelines," Part IV, *Provisional Guidelines for Automated Multiphasic Health Testing Services,* Vol. 3, DHEW Publ. No. (HSM) 72-3011, 1970, U.S. Govt. Print. Off., Washington, D. C.

3. Cochrane, A. L. *Effectiveness and Efficiency: Random Reflections on Health Services.* Nuffield Provincial Hospital Trust, 1972.

4. Grimaldi, J. V. "The Worth of Occupational Health Programs. A New Evaluation of Periodic Physical Examinations." *J. Occup. Med.* 7(1965):365–373.

5. Emlet, H. E. "A Preliminary Exploration of Cost Benefits of Multiphasic Health Screening." Presented at Engineering Foundation Research Conference on Engineering in Medicine, Andover, N. H., August 6, 1968.

6. Klarman, H. E. "Application of Cost-Benefit Analysis to Health Systems Technology." Presented at Conference on Technology and Health Care Systems in the 1980s, San Francisco, Calif., January 19-20, 1972, pp. 225–250, also in *J. Occup. Med.* 16(1974):172–185.

7. Lave, J. R., et al. "Economic Impact of Preventive Medicine." Report of Task Force 7, National Conference on Preventive Medicine, pp. 675–714 in *Preventive Medicine USA.* New York: PRODIST, 1976.

8. Thorner, R. M. "Health Program Evaluation in Relation to Health Programming." *HSMHA Tech. Health Rep.* 86(1971):525–532.

9. Bay, K. S., Flathorn, D., and Westman, L. "The Worth of a Screening Program: An Application of a Statistical Decision Model for the Benefit Evaluation of Screening Projects." *Am. J. Pub. Health* 66(1976):145–150.

10. Emlet, H. E. "Progress in Analysis of the Costs and Benefits of Multiphasic Health Screening." Proceedings of the Engineering Foundation Research Conference in Engineering in Medicine. *Multiphasic Screening III.* Deerfield, Mass., 1969.

11. Phillips, R. M., and Hughes, J. P., "Cost Benefit Analysis of the Occupational Health Program: A Generic Model." *J. Occup. Med.* 16(1974):158–161.

12. Kuh, C. "Periodic Health Examination Versus Early Sickness Consultation." *Permanente Foundation Med. Bull.* 3(1945):12–21.

13. Siegel, G. S. "An American Dilemma: The Periodic Health Examination." *Arch. Environ. Health* 13(1966):291–294.

14. Roberts, N. J. "The Values and Limitations of Periodic Health Examinations." *J. Chron. Dis.* 9(1959):95–116.

15. Burr, H. B. "Westinghouse Management Health Examinations and Their Investment Value." *J. Occup. Med.* 2(1960):80–91.

16. Clark, T. W., Schor, S. S., Elsom, K. D., Hubbard, J. P., and Elsom, K. A. "The Periodic Health Examination in Evaluation of Routine Tests and Procedures." *Ann. Int. Med.* 54(1961):1209–1222.

17. Schenthal, J. E. "Multiphasic Screening of the Well Patient." *J.A.M.A.* 172(1960):51–54.

18. Schor, S. S., Clark, T. W., Parkhurst, L. W., Baker, J. P., and Elsom, K. A. "An Evaluation of the Periodic Health Examination." *Ann. Int. Med.* 61(1964):999–1005.

19. Wade, L., Thorpe, J., Elias, T., and Bock, G.: "Are Periodic Health Examinations Worthwhile?" *Ann. Int. Med.* 56(1962):81–93.

20. David, W. D. "The Usefulness of Periodic Health Examinations." *Arch. Environ. Health* 2(1961):339–342.

21. Spitzer, W. D., and Brown, B. P. "Unanswered Questions about the Periodic Health Examination." *Ann. Int. Med.* 83(1975):257–263.

22. Forst, B. E. "An Economic Investigation of Periodic Health Examination Programs." *Inst. Naval Studies Res. Contrib.* 203, November 1971, National Technical Information Service.

23. Smillie, J. "An Important Message Regarding Health Examinations." Kaiser Foundation Hospitals. *Planning for Health Bulletin* 1(1971):2.

24. Collen, M. F., Kidd, P. H., Feldman, R. F., and Cutler, J. L. "Cost Analysis of a Multiphasic Screening Program." *New Eng. J. Med.* 280(1969):1043–1045.

25. Deniston, O. L., Rosenstock, I. M., and Getting, V. A. "Evaluation of Program Effectiveness." *Pub. Health Rep.* 83(1968):323–335.

26. Berg, R. L., ed. *Health Status Indexes.* Chicago: Hospital Research and Educational Trust, 1973.

27. McKeown, T. "Validation of Screening." Chapters 1 and 13 in *Screening in Medical Care.* Nuffield Provincial Hospital Trust. New York: Oxford Univ. Press, 1968.

28. Garfield, S. R., Collen, M. F., Richart, R. H., Feldman, R., Soghikian, K., and Duncan, J. H. "Evaluation of a New Ambulatory Medical Care Delivery System." *New Eng. J. Med.* 294(1976):426–431.

29. Richart, R. H., Duncan, J. H., Garfield, S. R., and Collen, M. F. "An Evaluation Model for Health Care System Changes." J. Med. Systems 1:1977.

30. Sproul, A. "Influence of Conditional Probability on the Effectiveness of Mass Screening Programs." *J.A.M.A.* 196(1966):103–106.

31. Grant, J. A. "Quantitative Evaluation of a Screening Program." *Am. J. Pub. Health* 64(1974):66–70.

32. Thorner, R. M., and Remein, Q. M. "Principles and Procedures in the Evaluation of Screening for Disease." *Pub. Health Monograph* 67. Pub. Health Serv. Pub. No. 846, U. S. Govt. Print. Off., 1961.

33. Okelberry, C. R. "Preadmission Testing Shortens Preoperative Length of Stay." *Ambulatory Care* 49(1975):71–74.

34. Flagle, C. D. "A Decision Theoretical Comparison of Three Procedures of Screening for a Single Disease." In LeCam, L., and Neyman, J., *Fifth Berkeley Symposium on Mathematical Statistics and Probability,* pp. 887–901. Berkeley: University of California Press, 1967.

35. Blumberg, M. J. "Evaluating Health Screening Procedures." *Operations Res.* 5(1957):351–360.

36. Bennett, A. E., and Fraser, I. G. P. "Impact of Screening Programme in General Practice. A Randomized Controlled Trial." *Uses of Epidemiology in Planning Health Services.* Proc. Sixth International Meeting I. E. A., Primosten, Yugoslavia, 1971.

37. Scheff, T. F. "Preferred Errors in Diagnosis." *Med. Care* 2(1964):166–172.

38. Breslow, L. "Early Case Finding Treatment and Mortality from Cervix and Breast Cancer." *Prev. Med.* 1(1972):141–152.

39. Haga, E., ed. *Computer Techniques in Biomedicine and Medicine,* pp. 231–233. Philadelphia: Auerbach Pub. Inc., 1973.

40. Bergen, R. P. "Defensive Medicine Is Good Medicine." A.M.A. Office of the General Counsel. *J.A.M.A.* 228(1974):1188–1189.

41. Garfield, S. R. "Multiphasic Health Testing and Medical Care as a Right." *New Eng. J. Med.* 283(1970):1087–1089.

42. Horvath, W. J. "Obstacles to the Applications of Operations Research Techniques in the Health Field." Chapter 5 in Shuman, L. J., Spears, R. D., and Young, J. P., eds. *Operations Research in Health Care.* Baltimore: The Johns Hopkins Univ. Press, 1975.

43. Deniston, O. L., Rosenstock, I. M., Welch, W., and Getting, V. A. "Evaluation of Program Efficiency." *Pub. Health Rep.* 83(1968):603–610.

44. Collen, M. F., Feldman, R., Siegelaub, A. B., Crawford, D. "Dollar Cost Per Positive Test for Automated Multiphasic Screening." *New Eng. J. Med.* 283(1970):459–463.

45. Friedman, G., Goldberg, M., Ahuja, J., Siegelaub, A., Bassis, M., and Collen, M. "Biochemical Screening Tests: Effect of Panel Size on Medical Care." *Arch. Intern. Med.* 129(1972):91–97.

46. Kodlin, D. "A Note on Cost-Benefit Problem in Screening for Breast Cancer." *Meth. Inform. Med.* 4(1972):242-247.

47. Collen, M. F. "Computer Algorithms for Clinical Data Collection." In Kallstrom, M., and Yarnell, S., eds., *Design and Use of Protocols,* pp. 91–98. Seattle: Medical Computer Services Assoc., 1975.

48. Collen, M. F., Dales, L. G., Friedman, G. D., Flagle, C. D., Feldman, R., and Siegelaub, A. B. "Multiphasic Checkup Evaluation Study. 4. Preliminary Cost Benefit Analysis for Middle-Aged Men." *Prev. Med.* 2(1973):236–246; and Dales, L. G., Friedman, G. D., and Collen, M. F. "Evaluation of a Periodic Multiphasic Health Checkup." *Meth. Inform. Med.* 13(1974):140–146.

49. Collen, M. F., Garfield, S. R., Richart, R. H., Duncan, J. H., and Feldman, R. "Cost Analyses of Alternative Health Examination Modes." *Arch. Int. Med.* 137(1977)73–79, and Collen, M. F., Garfield, S. R. "New Medical Care Delivery System, Final Report, January 1975." National Technical Information Service (NTIS) P.B. 246–630.

50. Taller, S. L., Feldman, R. "The Training and Utilization of Nurse Practitioners in Adult Health Appraisal." *Med. Care* 12(1974):40–48.

51. Lyle, C. B., Citron, D. S., Sugg, W. C., and Williams, O. D. "Automated Multiphasic Health Testing as an Adjunct to Internal Medicine." Chapter 19 in Abernathy, Sheldon, and Prahalad, *The Management of Health Care.* Cambridge, Mass.: Bullough Pub. Co., 1974.

52. Oszustowicz, R. J. "An Economic and Operational Analysis of Automated Health Testing and Screening in a Community Hospital." *Proceedings of the Symposium of the International Health Evaluation Association,* 1971.

53. Collen, M. F. "Multiphasic Testing as a Triage to Medical Care." In Ingelfinger, F. J., et al., *Controversy in Internal Medicine II,* pp. 85-91. Philadelphia: W. B. Saunders Co., 1974.

54. Mechanic, D. "Factors Affecting the Acceptance of AMHTS Among Consumers and Providers." In *Provisional Guidelines for AMHT,* Vol. 3, pp. 235–253. DHEW Pub. No. (HSM) 72-3011, 1970; and Mechanic, D., and Newton, M. "Social Considerations in Medical Education." Chapter 3 in Millon, T., *Medical Behavioral Science.* Philadelphia: W. B. Saunders, 1975.

55. Bates, B., and Yellin, J. A. "The Yield of Multiphasic Screening." *J.A.M.A.* 222(1972):74–78.

56. Williamson, J. W., Alexander, M., and Miller, G. E. "Continuing Education and Patient Care Research—Physicians' Response to Screening Test Results." *J.A.M.A.* 201(1967):118–122.

57. McKeown, T. "Unvalidated Procedures Have No Place in Screening Programs." Chapter 3 in Ingelfinger, F. J., et al., *Controversy in Internal Medicine II,* pp. 92–98. Philadelphia: W. B. Saunders Co., 1974.

58. *Statement on Multiphasic Testing.* Chicago: American Medical Association, 1972.

CHAPTER EIGHTEEN

Effects of MHTS on Patients

Gary D. Friedman

A. INTRODUCTION

As indicated in the previous chapter, MHTS can be evaluated from many points of view. Those of the physician, the health care administrator, the public health official, and the patient all are important. Each concerned individual and group has particular aims and goals to be achieved by MHTS. Evaluation usually seeks to determine how well these goals are being met, at what cost, and with what additional consequences. While there may be disagreement on areas of emphasis, responsible spokesmen for each point of view agree that MHTS should promote the health and satisfaction of the patient. Effects of MHTS on patients will be the focus of this chapter.

In judging the merits of MHTS programs, it is well to keep in mind the uses to which they are being put. (See also Chapters Two and Three.) Among their suggested and actual uses are:

(1) Screening for disease in a population not previously tested.

(2) Testing for disease as an outside adjunct to regular care by a private physician.

(3) Testing for disease within an established medical care program or health maintenance organization.

(4) Collection of baseline data on patients entering a medical care program.

(5) Assessing health status of persons being followed for known chronic disease.

(6) Screening for potentially complicating problems in patients to be admitted to hospitals for elective surgery.

(7) As a health testing and triage mechanism to aid in efficient care delivery to members of an established medical care program or health maintenance organization.

Without consideration of the specific use or uses to which MHTS is to be put, blanket praise or blanket condemnation is inappropriate. MHTS may be very desirable for a particular purpose and undesirable for another. Furthermore, even for a specific purpose, MHTS may work out well in one setting and not in another. For example, the yield of previously unrecognized disease may be much higher if MHTS is applied to an indigent population getting substandard medical care than if it is used in a population already getting frequent care of high quality.

A medical program can be initiated and carried on because health care professionals believe that it benefits patients, or because patients come to believe in the program's efficacy and value and continue to request it. Accepted treatments and programs, having been established without thorough and objective evaluation, may later be shown to be of no value or even harmful. History is replete with preventive or therapeutic approaches that were thoroughly subscribed to by physicians and heatedly demanded by patients, only to be rejected later.

In the case of MHTS, which can be put to many uses, some of these uses have become accepted by physicians and demanded by patients with little objective evidence that they are of value or worth the costs they entail. Thus, a concern with the welfare of patients dictates that evaluation of MHTS go beyond cost-effectiveness comparisons of alternative approaches. The underlying health care activity that MHTS is designed to implement must be questioned and evaluated.

B. EVALUATION METHODS

We live in a time of questioning and skepticism. No longer does the belief of a program director or other key individuals in the desirability of a program convince others as to its merits. Hard data must be collected and analyzed in an objective manner. Furthermore, it is not adequate merely to describe the experience and outcomes in those who undergo MHTS or any other health program. There must be a control group or other basis for comparison.

The evaluation design considered ideal in many situations is the randomized controlled trial. The first step is to define the eligibility criteria for the program and identify all individuals who qualify and are willing to participate. Then, by random selection or an equivalent process, these persons are allocated to one subgroup to whom the program is applied and one or more subgroups who serve as controls, either receiving no program or an alternative one. Sometimes a randomized design cannot be carried out. It may be that the program is to be made available to a whole community with no possibility for excluding any residents who want to participate. Then, another similar community may have to be used as a comparison group.

Sometimes all that can be done is a before-and-after comparison. This approach is better than no control at all, but it does have important susceptibilities to misleading results. An apparent improvement or worsening of the situation following the institution of the program may be due to outside factors that happen to be operating at the same time, such as a change in the pattern of medical care delivery, improvements in medical technology, a new disease epidemic in the community, or the aging of the study group. Wherever possible, therefore, comparative before-after studies should also be made of similar groups not affected by the program being evaluated. Readers interested in pursuing further the principles of program evaluation are referred to the articles by Hutchison, Donabedian, and Deniston et al.[1-4]

An important source of bias deserves special emphasis in stressing the need for controlled evaluation studies: this is self-selection. Persons who seek out, or agree to participate in, health-promoting programs such as MHTS are not a representative sample of the general population. Kuller and Tonascia, for example, found that persons participating in a community screening program showed an overrepresentation of persons of high socioeconomic status.[5] Similarly, investigators in our department (Dankward Kodlin and Marshall Goldberg, unpublished data) compared 404 persons who had been urged to come in for annual multiphasic checkups three times in the three-year period, 1964–1967, and had come in only once—the "reluctants"—with 267 persons who had been urged only once but had come in three times, twice on their own volition—the "regulars." All subjects were born in the two decades spanning 1910–1929. Table 18-1 shows some selected findings in the two groups. Despite a similar sex distribution and a tendency for the regulars to be older, the reluctants showed more evidence of certain chronic diseases and more frequently reported serious cardiorespiratory symptoms. Note also that the reluctants showed higher proportions of heavy alcohol drinkers and heavy cigarette smokers and a lower proportion with three or more years of college education.

Apparently, participants and cooperators are, on the average, healthier, more

Table 18-1. Comparison of Selected Characteristics of "Regular" and "Reluctant" Participants in a Program of Annual Multiphasic Checkups

	Percent with Characteristic in Each Group	
Characteristics	"Regular" ($N = 267$)	"Reluctant" ($N = 404$)
Male	42%	42%
Older (born in earlier decade)	59	51
Diagnoses:		
No significant abnormality	51	37
Primary hypertension	7	13
Diabetes mellitus	2	7
Electrocardiogram abnormal	3	9
Symptoms:		
Shortness of breath with usual work or activity	3	8
Repeated chest pain	9	13
Cough almost every day	3	9
Habits and Education:		
Smoked two or more packs of cigarettes per day for over 20 years	3	9
Drink six or more alcoholic drinks per day	3	11
College education, three or more years	19	8

educated, and less apt to have damaging habits such as heavy drinking and smoking. Thus, an evaluation that is based on comparing participants with non-participants is almost guaranteed to show apparent success for the participants even if the program offers no benefits at all.

C. CRITERIA FOR THE VALUE OF DETECTING EARLY DISEASE

In many settings MHTS is used to detect early or asymptomatic disease. This is also the purpose, of course, of screening programs for single diseases such as cancer of the cervix, phenylketonuria, or hypertension. Questions as to the value of such efforts have led several authorities to set forth criteria that should be met before screening is undertaken.[6-10] (See also Chapters Two and Three). Those given by the World Health Organization[8] are among the most stringent and are listed below.

(1) Screening must lead to an improvement in end-results (defined in terms of mortality; physical, social, and emotional function; pain; and satisfaction) among those in whom early diagnosis is achieved or in the other members of the community.

(a) The therapy for the condition must favorably alter its natural history, not simply by advancing the point in time at which diagnosis occurs, but by improving survival, function, or both. The modification of "risk factors" is not sufficient evidence of effectiveness, nor is the fact that the proposed therapy is "commonly accepted." Claims for therapeutic effectiveness must withstand rigorous methodologic scrutiny; and experimental evidence, such as controlled clinical trials, is a prerequisite. The measurement of survival and other end-results must withstand epidemiologic and biostatistical scrutiny.

(b) Available health services must be sufficient both to ensure diagnostic confirmation among those whose screening is positive and to provide long-term care.

(c) Compliance among asymptomatic patients in whom an early diagnosis has been achieved must be at a level to be effective in altering the natural history of the disease in question.

(d) The long-term beneficial effects, in terms of end-results, must outweigh the long-term detrimental effects of the therapeutic regimen utilized and the "labeling" of an individual as "diseased" or "at high risk."

(2) The effectiveness of potential components of multiphasic screening should be demonstrated individually prior to their combination.

(3) If the benefits of screening accrue to the community at large rather than, or in addition to, the individual identified (e.g., disease carriers, specific occupations), the community benefit claimed must withstand scientific scrutiny.

(a) The appropriateness of the mix of screening tests to the target population must be considered, acknowledging that differences in the distributions of two diseases may render the combination of their respective screening tests inappropriate.

(4) The cost-benefit and cost-effectiveness characteristics of mass screening and long-term therapy must be known. This knowledge is considered essential in developing an appropriate mix of manpower and financial resources. Therefore, a mechanism for the formal periodic weighing of costs against benefits or effectiveness should constitute a basic component of the initial screening activities.

(5) The burden of disability for the condition in question (in terms of disease frequency, distribution, severity, and alternative approaches to its detection and control) must warrant action.

(6) The cost, sensitivity, specificity, and acceptability of the screening test must be known, and it should lend itself to the utilization patterns of the target population.

(7) Ideally, an estimate of the social benefit of preventing, arresting, or curing the condition in question should be known.

Item (2), requiring a demonstration of effectiveness of each component before inclusion in a multiphasic screening program, provides a good example of the differing requirements of different points of view. From the point of view of a public health worker wishing to detect and bring under treatment early disease in his community, with limited funds at his disposal, this need to justify the collection of each item of information seems perfectly reasonable in order to reduce unnecessary effort and expenditure. On the other hand, consider the point of view of a physician working in a medical care system. If a patient is brought back acutely ill, perhaps in a coma, the presence in the patient's medical record of an abundance of information may be of great value in determining the probable cause of his difficulty. From the physician's viewpoint the collection of questionnaire data on family history of disease costs nothing but a little extra time of the patient. Similarly, the addition of a few serum chemistry tests to a panel performed by a multichannel analyzer costs little, but can sometimes provide valuable information in an emergency. It may be almost impossible to demonstrate to a public health worker the value of each of these items in a community screening program; but to the physician faced with a difficult clinical problem, a large battery of information generated by a multiphasic examination may be of great help.

The patient also has an interest in the extensiveness of an examination. If a health care program provides a thorough checkup containing an abundance of tests and procedures, the patient finds reassurance in that he has passed many health tests and that the program is doing something substantial for him. Whittling away at a comprehensive checkup by removing tests that are difficult to justify individually may leave a "bare-bones" examination that will not satisfy today's patients, despite reasoned arguments and citations of statistical evidence.

D. STUDIES OF MAJOR AND LONG-TERM HEALTH EFFECTS

In the United States there has been a consistent demand for and belief in regular or even annual checkups for healthy adults. One of the main purposes for MHTS has been to satisfy, in an efficient manner, the demand for checkups. This use of MHTS has, itself, come under careful scrutiny. Despite the widespread belief in the importance of regular checkups, there is a paucity of supporting scientific evidence. (See also Chapters One and Seventeen.)

Periodic health checkups have been claimed to prolong life in studies going back five decades. In 1921 the Metropolitan Life Insurance Company published followup data on almost 6,000 policyholders who had been given physical examinations at company expense at the Life Extension Institute in 1914 and 1915.[11] After an average of 5½ years of observation, 217 deaths were observed, as compared to 303 expected for "persons of this class." This 28 percent reduction in mortality was interpreted as being due to the physical examinations and had a monetary value of $126,000 (presumably in reduced life insurance claims). The examinations cost the company $40,000. It was concluded that all of the company's principal was returned and that there was a profit of about 200 percent. However, later experience indicated that the costs of the examinations to the company were too high in relation to savings in mortality payments to justify their continuation. Indeed, the policyholders who availed themselves of periodic examinations did not experience mortality rates significantly lower than insured individuals who were comparable with regard to type of policy and other pertinent characteristics.[12]

The Heart Disease Epidemiology Study in Framingham, Mass., has been concerned with the identification of factors predisposing to the development of coronary heart disease and other cardiovascular conditions. To attain these objectives, a random sample of two-thirds of the town's inhabitants, age 30 to 59 in 1950, were invited to have a medical examination every two years. The findings were reported to the subjects' physicians, and patients were advised to contact their physicians if serious abnormalities were noted. Of this sample, about two-thirds participated. Of the one-third not invited, 18 percent participated as volunteers in the biennial examination program. To see whether checkups were actually lengthening life, Jungblut et al.[13] compared the mortality over a ten-year period in the two-thirds invited sample with that in the one-third uninvited group, recognizing the existence of some "crossovers" as described above. The average annual death rate was 7.6 per 1,000 in the invited sample and 7.8 per 1,000 in the uninvited group. The difference was not statistically significant. It was concluded that no effect of periodic examinations on mortality could be demonstrated.

Thorner and Crumpacker[14] reported the mortality rates for executives who had received periodic health checkups at the Greenbrier Clinic. Of 451 men followed for an average of 4½ years, 11 deaths were observed as compared to 25 expected, based on white male U.S. life table mortality. An additional 11 executives died at intervals ranging from 17 to 90 months after their last examination at the clinic, but even if these were added to the initial 11, the mortality was still only 88 percent of that expected. Although the main purpose of the paper was to show the favorable mortality experience of executives, it was also stated that "one would like to think that the periodic health examinations received by the group made a positive contribution to their longevity."

Roberts et al.[15] reported on 20,648 men, mostly upper-socioeconomic-level whites working in managerial positions, who participated in periodic health examination programs at eight cooperating clinics. Over an average of almost seven years of followup, mortality rates were observed and compared with those for (1) all U.S. white males in 1960, (2) U.S. white males in comparable professional, technical, and managerial positions, (3) insured male lives, and (4) preferred-risk insured male lives. Mortality was always lower in the examined group, with observed/expected mortality rates ranging from 0.6 to 0.997. Persons examined two or more times had even lower mortality ratios. The authors noted that the data were compatible with a beneficial effect of periodic health examinations and suggested that well-controlled prospective studies should be carried out.

Braren and Elinson[16] reported a nine-year mortality followup of persons receiving a single clinical evaluation in a study of chronic illness in Hunterdon County, N.J. Persons who were ill comprised a much higher proportion of the examined sample than they did of the county population. The average annual mortality rate was lower in the examined group than in those who refused examination, but the difference was not statistically significant. A statistical test comparing the entire group offered the examination with the comparable control group not offered it was not presented.

Another study of the effects of a single health survey examination took place in Värmland County in Sweden. This was a very large-scale program in which 90,000 or 76 percent of all persons age 25 and over were screened.[17] Of the subjects, 8.6 percent were referred for physician followup examination. A total of 6,804 diagnoses were recorded in 5,539 persons, of which 75 percent were suggested by the screening. Fifty-nine percent of the diagnoses suggested by the screening were previously unrecognized. Anemia, hypertension, diabetes, and hypercholesterolemia were the most frequent conditions of importance. No impact of the examination on mortality in the county during and shortly after the survey was detected.

Another Swedish study provided a followup of about 1,000 persons aged 45, 50, 55, 60, and 65 years who participated in a single multiphasic health screening carried out in 1964 in Eskilstuna.[18] Some 83.5 percent of the screened group plus an unscreened control group were examined five years later. It was concluded that about one-third of the screened group had benefited from the screening with regard to conditions newly detected or preexisting conditions where treatment was resumed or changed. However, no statistically significant difference in health status could be demonstrated between the screened and control groups at the followup examination.

Kuller and Tonascia described the 12-year mortality experience of 984 persons who had undergone multiphasic screening as part of a study of chronic illness in Baltimore.[5] The screenees were compared with persons who were also offered the screening but did not participate. The screened group had a lower death rate, especially women and subjects age 40 to 49. Compared to the general population, screenees had a slightly lower death rate, whereas those who refused had a slightly higher death rate. As mentioned before, it was noted that a higher proportion of screenees were from the upper socioeconomic level.

Such differences between screened and unscreened persons underscore the problem of self-selection bias in evaluating the results of checkups. Fortunately, at least three controlled trials are under way to assess the effects of periodic multiphasic screening. Trevelyan[19] reported one such study to determine the effects of multiphasic screening within a general practice in Britain. Middle-aged individuals registered with two London group practices were randomly divided into two groups of approximately 3,400. Biennial multiphasic screening was offered to one of the groups. The study, not yet complete, will look into the effects of screening on physical state, anxiety about health, disability, demand for health services, and yield of previously unknown disease.

Another controlled followup study is in progress in Titograd, Yugoslavia.[20] Over 13,000 persons aged 30 to 49 in the entire city were randomly divided into an unscreened group and a group that would receive biennial checkups. Outcomes to be measured during a six-year followup include mortality, morbidity, absence from work, and utilization of inpatient and outpatient services. Still another controlled trial of periodic multiphasic checkups is described below.

E.   LONG-TERM MULTIPHASIC CHECKUP EVALUATION STUDY[21-25]

MHTS has been used as part of a regular checkup in the Kaiser-Permanente San Francisco and Oakland outpatient clinics since 1964. The effects of such regular checkups have been evaluated by a controlled trial sponsored by research grants from the U.S. Department of Health, Education and Welfare. This investigation was initiated by M. F. Collen. Other senior investigators have been John L. Cutler, Savitri Ramcharan, Loring G. Dales, and the writer. An Advisory Committee who supervised the planning and study design included Lester Breslow, John Clausen, George Dantzig, Hardin Jones, Benno K. Milmore, Lincoln Moses, Jerzy Neyman, Elizabeth Scott, Reuel Stallones, Arthur Weissman, and Jacob Yerushalmy.

When the study began in 1964 a group of about 46,000 health plan members were identified as satisfying the eligibility criteria for the study. The age range chosen was 35 to 54, with the expectation that in ten or so years of followup, chronic diseases would develop or progress in a substantial proportion of persons in this age group, who might therefore be benefited by periodic multiphasic health checkups (MHCs). Eligible persons also had to be in the health plan for at least two years. It was known that such persons tended to stay with the plan, dropping out at a rate of only 3 to 4 percent per year, whereas a greater fraction of shorter-term members would leave and, for a longitudinal study, be lost to close followup. Residence near the Oakland or San Francisco facilities was also required.

The MHC has consisted of a visit to the MHTS laboratory followed by an appointment with an internist for a physical examination and report of MHTS test results. (Very recently, some of the physical examinations have been performed by a nurse practitioner under physician supervision.) A gynecological examination and Pap smear are also recommended for women, and a sigmoidoscopy is recommended for all persons age 40 and over.

Using certain digits in the medical record number (equivalent to random selection), 5,156 persons were drawn from the eligible subjects and assigned to the "study group," who were to be urged to have annual MHCs. Another 5,557 were assigned to the "control group," who were to be left alone. Members of the research staff have phoned each study group subject every year and attempted to schedule an appointment for an MHC.

Like most studies of human subjects in a free society, this could not be an ideal experiment, where all members of the study group received MHCs every year and all members of the control group received none. On the average about 60 to 65 percent of study-group subjects actually arrived at the MHTS laboratories each year. Then, too, control group subjects could not be denied MHCs, since these were part of their rightful benefits as subscribers to the Kaiser Foundation Health Plan. On the average about 20 percent of control-group subjects received checkups each year.

Nevertheless, the urging program did effect a substantial difference in dosage of MHCs between the two groups. By mid-1973, for example, the average number of MHCs per study-group member was 4.5; for the control group it was 1.7. Looked at in another way, by that time 44 percent of the control group had never received a checkup, compared to only 17 percent of the study group.

As expected, the additional checkups in the study group led to additional labeling of its members with diagnoses. As shown in Figure 18-1, review of a sample of medical charts revealed almost identical numbers of newly recorded diagnoses in the two groups during the baseline years 1962–1964. In 1965 and beyond, study-group subjects received, on the average, substantially more new diagnoses. Computerized prescription-dispensing data for samples of subjects revealed slightly more frequent receipt of prescriptions by the study group.

Although the above differences are interesting, the main purpose of the study was to assess long-term effects of regular checkups on health. One measure we have had of health status was self-reported disability obtained through biennial mailed questionnaire surveys. Each study subject still in the health plan has been asked whether "your health is such that you can *not* do your usual work (job or housework) at all," which we have considered to represent complete disability, whether "you can work, but have to limit or cut down on the amount or kind of work, or other physical exercise," representing partial disability, or whether "you are not limited in any of these ways," representing no disability. Through

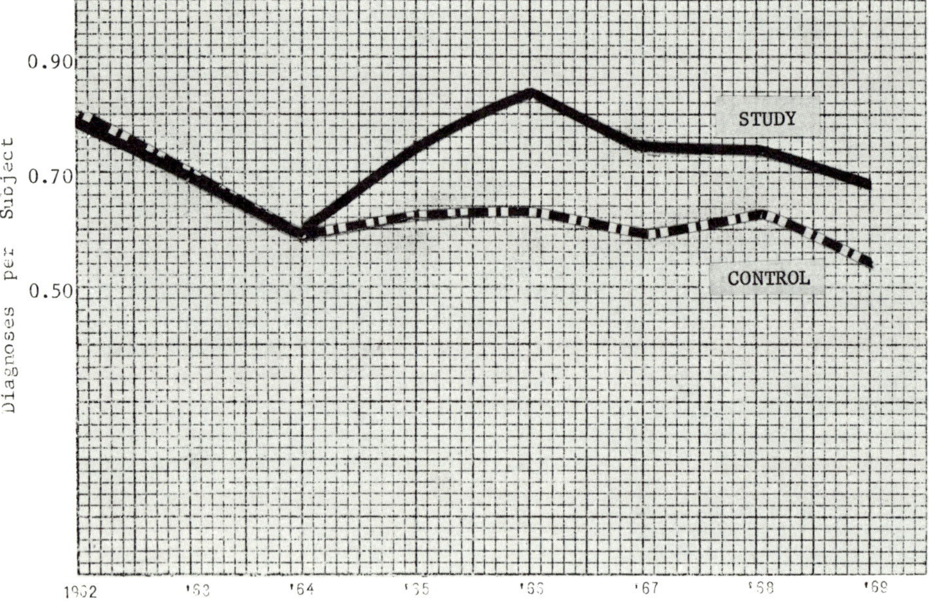

Figure 18-1. Mean annual numbers of newly recorded diagnoses per subject for the years 1962–1969.

the years, as expected, the percentage of completely and partially disabled subjects in the study and control group has been increasing as the subjects age.

The total study and control groups have shown about equal proportions with disability (see Figure 18-2). We also looked at four age-sex subgroups, men and women age 35 to 44 and 45 to 54 when the study began. Among both younger groups disability prevalence has been quite similar. Among the older men, substantially less disability has been present in the study group since 1969, and the differences were significant in 1969 and 1973 using conventional statistical tests. Among the older women the trend since 1969 has been in the opposite direction, with less disability in the control group, but none of the differences has reached statistical significance.

Because it is in a subgroup, the difference in the older men (and the statistical significance test results) is not as persuasive as would be a lower rate of disability in the entire study group. Therefore, we have been following the groups closely both for further evidence of disability differences and for other evidence tending to confirm or deny the apparent benefits of the additional checkups received by the study group. For example, reduction of disability by checkups in the older men would be strongly confirmed if similar study-control group differences were to be observed in the younger men when they got to be ten years older.

Hospitalizations are important as health-related events, because they generally result from serious illness and are the most costly form of medical care. Although checkups might generate extra hospitalizations over the short term by detecting conditions that need hospital-based diagnostic testing or therapy, checkups could perform a very useful service if, over the long run, they diminished a person's need for hospital care. Thus, the study has paid close attention to hospitalizations in the two groups under surveillance (see Figure 18-3). Considerable year-to-year

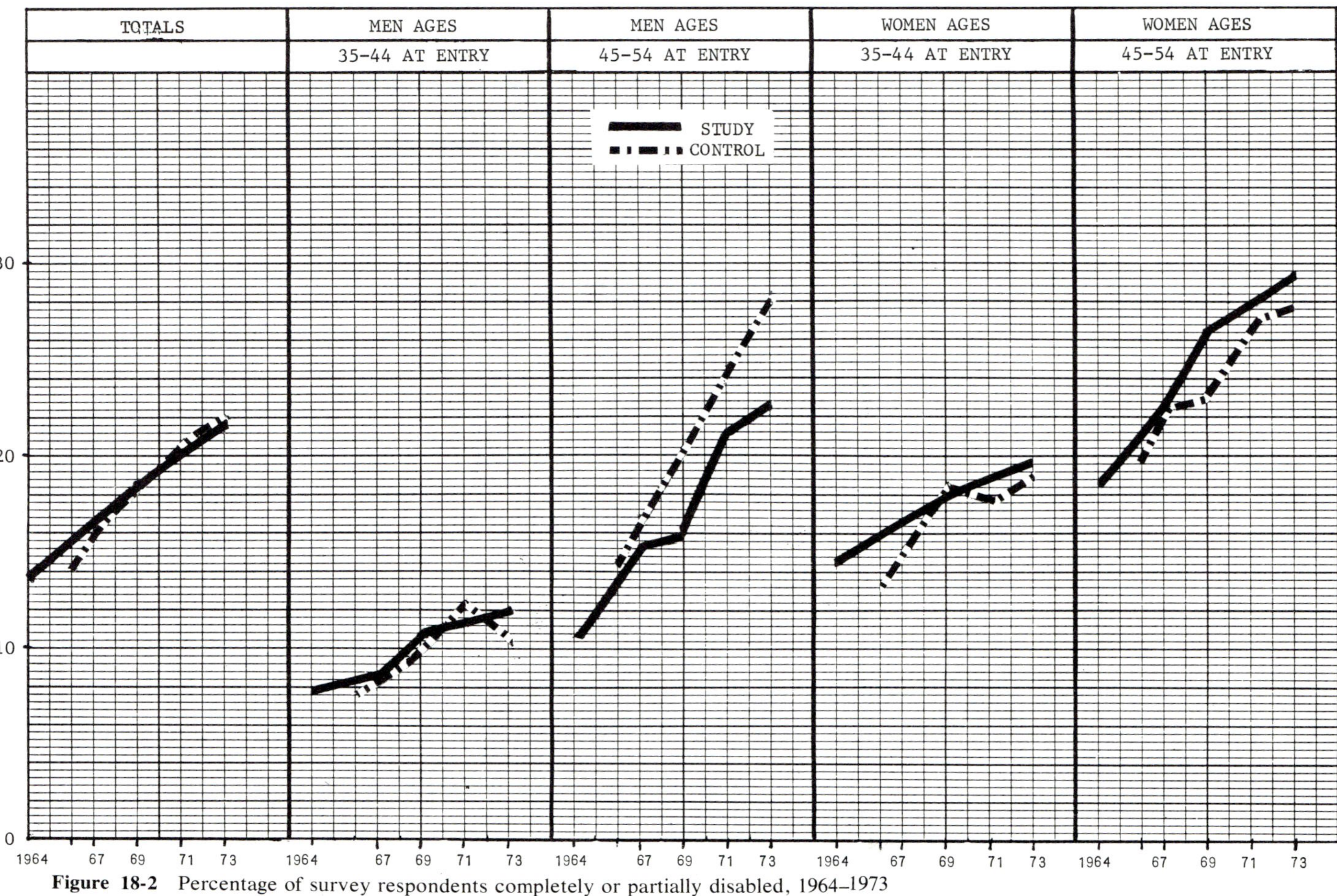

Figure 18-2 Percentage of survey respondents completely or partially disabled, 1964–1973

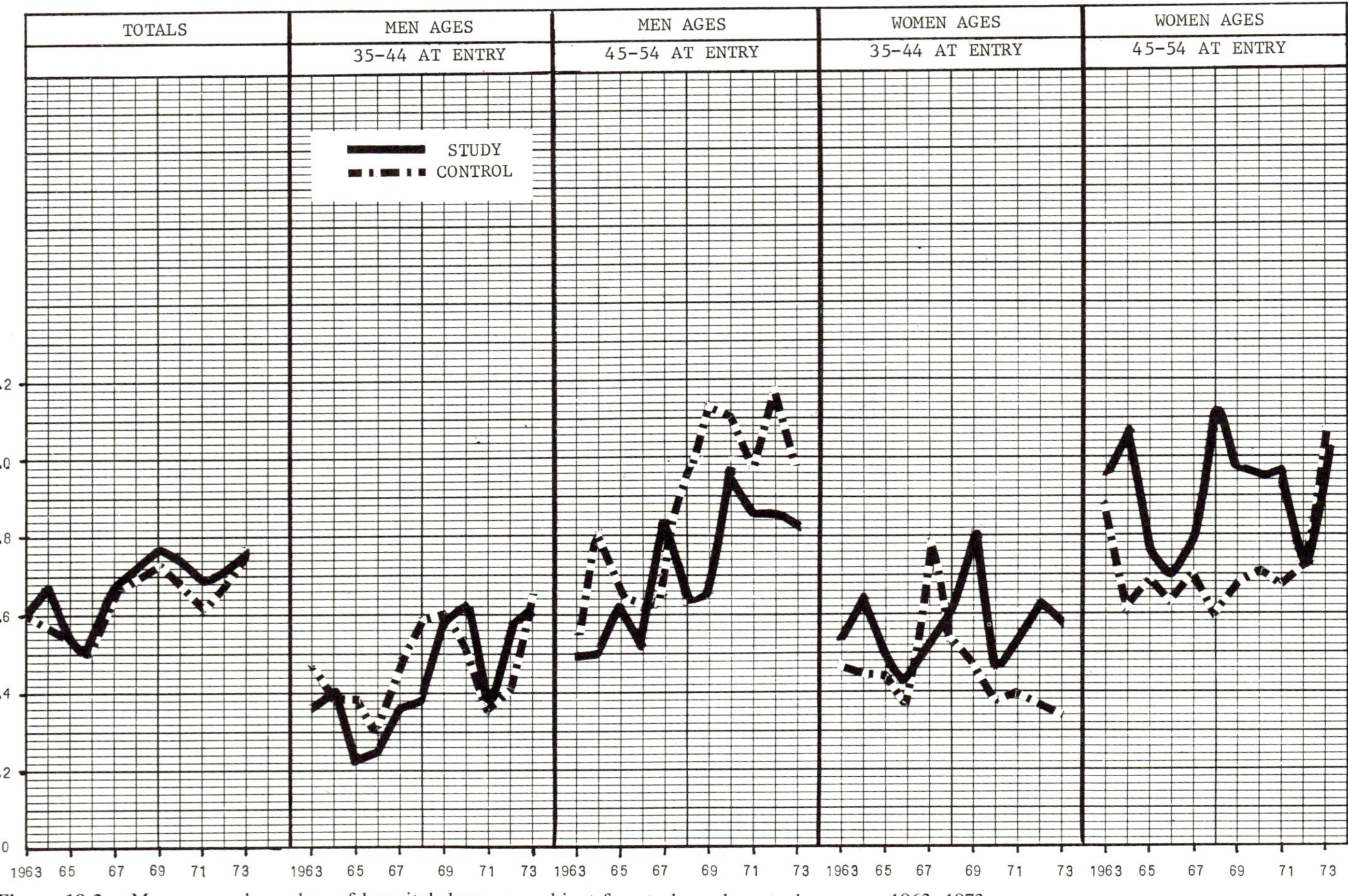

Figure 18-3. Mean annual number of hospital days per subject for study and control groups, 1963–1973.

fluctuation in hospital usage is apparent. Nevertheless, in the older men there appears to be a trend toward higher utilization by the control group starting in 1968. In women of both age decades the opposite trend appears to hold—that is, greater use by the study group. It is not surprising, therefore, to find the year-to-year hospital usage to be similar in the total groups. Outpatient care, both office visits and laboratory tests, has been of similar quantity in the two groups, if the visits for MHCs are not counted.

Mortality followup has been an essential part of the study. Through 1973 both groups had similar death rates, although mortality was slightly lower in the study group than in the control group (53.7 vs. 55.1 per thousand in nine years). Of interest, however, is that before the data were analyzed, three physicians selected a group of "potentially postponable" conditions in which there was the greatest likelihood of preventing or postponing death by periodic MHCs and the care that would result. These consisted of hypertension and closely related conditions, and of frequently lethal cancers that could readily be detected during checkups. This group of conditions, although accounting for only a small fraction of deaths, did show a lower mortality rate in the study group (see Table 18-2). Both older men and older women accounted largely for the excess deaths in the control group.

Among the many conditions looked at, there were significantly ($p < .05$) higher death rates in the study group for suicide and for neoplasms of the lympho-hematopoietic system. To help determine whether these were chance findings to be expected when so many conditions were studied, or represented possible fatal "adverse reactions" to checkups, we reviewed the medical charts of the people dying from these conditions. In only one case could a reasonable link be made between multiphasic checkup and the death. This was a 56-year old study group man who had an MHC in August 1967. High blood pressure was found and he was placed on reserpine therapy. In his checkup questionnaire he indicated no worries, depression, or insomnia. In February 1968 he began complaining of stomach pain, nervousness, and weight loss, and apparently was still taking reserpine. A medical workup was started, but he committed suicide early in March 1968, to the surprise of his physician, who commented that there had been no undue depression or anxiety evident. Since reserpine is known to produce emotional depression in some patients, it is possible that the suicide was related to reserpine therapy, started because of findings at an MHC.

As of this writing (January 1976) the study is still in progress. Study-group subjects are still being invited to have annual MHCs. Both the study and control groups are being followed up in identical fashion for health outcome. Emphasis is currently being placed on elucidating the process or mechanism by which MHCs might have reduced disability in older men and the death rate from potentially postponable conditions. Extensive reviews of the subjects' medical charts are being made for this purpose and to assure that random selection resulted in no important differences between the two groups in baseline status. We are also attempting to translate the findings of this study into economic terms to whatever extent possible, and to compare the overall costs of the MHCs with any economic benefits that are found. An example of a preliminary economic evaluation for older men can be found in the previous chapter.

Table 18-2. Deaths and Death Rates in Study and Control Group Subjects, 1965–1973*

	Number of Deaths		Death Rate (per 1,000 for the 9-year period)		Chi-Square Value
	Study	Control	Study	Control	
Potentially postponable causes	35	59	6.8	10.7	4.51†
Cancer of colon and rectum	3	14	0.6	2.5	6.34†
Cancer of breast (women only)	12	11	4.3	3.8	0.10
Cancer of cervix and uterus (women only)	0	2	0.0	0.7	0.46
Cancer of prostate (men only)	0	1	0.0	0.4	0.00
Cancer of kidney	1	0	0.2	0.0	0.00
Hypertension, hypertensive cardiovascular disease, and hemorrhagic cerebrovascular disease with hypertension	10	22	2.0	4.0	3.65
Hemorrhagic cerebrovascular disease without hypertension	9	9	1.8	1.6	0.00
Other Causes					
Infectious and parasitic disease	5	1	1.0	0.2	2.98
Cancer of buccal cavity and pharynx	0	1	0.0	0.2	0.00
Cancer of esophagus	5	2	1.0	0.4	1.52
Cancer of stomach	3	4	0.6	0.7	0.07
Cancer of pancreas	4	8	0.8	1.5	1.05
Cancer of bronchus and lung	16	17	3.1	3.1	0.00
Cancer of ovary and tube (women only)	4	4	1.4	1.4	0.09
Cancer of brain	2	1	0.4	0.2	0.41
Metastatic cancer, primary site unknown	3	6	0.6	1.1	0.79
Lympho-hematopoietic cancer	13	3	2.5	0.5	7.03‡
Other cancer	7	3	1.4	0.5	1.92

Endocrine, nutritional, and metabolic disease	4	3	0.8	0.5	0.22
Blood and blood-forming organ disease other than cancer	0	0	0.0	0.0	0.0
Mental, nervous system, and sense organ disease	2	4	0.4	0.7	0.36
Ischemic heart disease unassociated with hypertensive cardiovascular disease	74	76	14.4	13.7	0.08
Nonhemorrhagic cerebrovascular disease	6	3	1.2	0.5	1.31
Other circulatory system disease	12	13	2.3	2.4	0.00
Respiratory system disease	10	14	2.0	2.5	0.40
Cirrhosis of the liver	19	29	3.7	5.2	1.41
Other gastrointestinal disease	4	8	0.8	1.5	1.07
Genitourinary system disease	5	7	1.0	1.3	0.20
Skin and subcutaneous tissue disease	0	1	0.0	0.2	0.00
Musculoskeletal system disease	3	3	0.6	0.5	0.00
Suicide	14	5	2.7	0.9	4.97†
Other injuries and poisoning	26	30	5.1	5.4	0.06
All Causes	276	305	53.7	55.1	0.09

* Populations alive as of January 1, 1965; Study, 5,138; Control, 5,536.

† $p < .05.$ ‡ $p < .01.$

F. ACCEPTABILITY OF MHTS TO PATIENTS

The experience at Northern California Kaiser-Permanente facilities strongly supports the view that MHTS is acceptable to patients. Over the years we have found that the majority of patients who request MHCs indicate that they do so of their own accord out of a desire for a regular checkup. Furthermore, most patients who have had one checkup come back again. Of 35,488 persons who had an MHC during the first year MHTS was in operation, 76 percent came back at least once during the next eight years. Many of these patients return quite frequently. It is not surprising, then, to find that at some facilities the demand for MHCs outstrips the capacity of the system and a considerable waiting period for appointments can develop.

K. Soghikian and F. B. Collen[26] surveyed 1,754 patients taking MHCs at the Oakland facility during February 1969 to measure their attitudes toward the MHTS tests and personnel. Ninety-five percent of the patients regarded the staff as helpful and courteous. Survey subjects were requested to indicate whether they found each screening test "very upsetting," "slightly upsetting," or "not upsetting." Table 18-3 shows the percentages of those reporting taking each test who found the test at least slightly upsetting (recomputed from the original data). Complaints centered chiefly around the glucose ingestion, which can produce nausea or vomiting, tonometry, which can be uncomfortable, and the blood tests, which involve a single venipuncture. The complaints about questionnaire items

Table 18-3. Percentages of MHTS Patients Who Found Test Phases Slightly or Very Upsetting. $n =$ Number Who Reported Taking Each Test Out of 1,743 Total Subjects.*

Test	Percent	Test	Percent
Tonometry (n = 1,396)	25.8	Interval history question box (n = 1,622)	5.1
Glucose ingestion (n = 1,575)	23.7	Electrocardiogram (n = 1,663)	4.4
Blood tests (n = 1,623)	18.9	Urine tests (n = 1,629)	3.5
Neuromental question box (n = 1,260)	10.6	Blood pressure (n = 1,630)	2.6
Audiometry (n = 1,619)	8.8	Visual acuity (n = 1,541)	2.6
Spirometry (n = 1,229)	8.0	Anthropometry (n = 1,407)	1.9
Mammography (n = 414)	6.0	Chest x-ray (n = 1,485)	1.8

*Modified from Soghikian and Collen.[26]

centered chiefly about having to answer them again after having done so on previous MHCs.

The patients were also asked to check any of a series of descriptive comments that they thought applied to MHTS. As shown in Table 18-4, most of the patients checked the favorable comments. Often, when critical comments were checked, favorable comments were also checked by the same individual. Combinations such as "impersonal" and "worth the time" or "assembly line" and "pleasant" were not infrequent.

Table 18-4. Percentage of 1,743 MHTS Patients Who Checked the Following Comments*

Comment	Percent	Comment	Percent
Worth the time	82	Not enough tests	6
Thorough	76	Too time-consuming	6
Efficient	73	Dehumanized	4
Pleasant	46	Too many tests	2
Assembly-line	27	Rushed	2
Personalized	22	Confusing	2
Impersonal	17	Worrisome	1
Unpleasant	8	Inefficient	1
Limited	6	Disturbing	1
Too tiring	6		

*Modified from Soghikian and Collen.[26]

It would seem that patients' main objections to the procedure are the "assembly-line" and "impersonal" aspects. One wonders, however, if many are not at least equally impressed with the automatic machines and technology that are evident in this assembly-line process. Certainly, courteous concern for the individual by the testing personnel and the examining physician or nurse practitioner can do much to soften the impression of the assembly-line characteristics of MHTS that are so necessary to hold down costs. (See also discussion of patient acceptability of multiphasic adjunctive services in Chapters Eleven, Twelve, and Fifteen.)

In assessing patient attitudes toward checkups, attention must also be paid to the characteristics of the patients themselves. Mechanic[27] has discussed the various population attributes that play a role in the acceptability of MHTS, as found in several relevant studies. Socioeconomic status is an important variable. Persons at higher levels are, on the average, more interested in preventive medical care and more receptive to "scientific" as opposed to "folk" medicine than persons at lower levels. Nevertheless, careful attention to particular reasons for unfavorable attitudes of various population subgroups can do much to increase their participation in preventive care. (Factors affecting patient compliance are also discussed in Chapters Two and Eleven.)

One of the very positive gratifications that most patients appear to get from thorough checkups comes from learning that there is nothing seriously wrong with them. Many feel that a multiphasic checkup provides extensive testing of their health. If this results in a good report, considerable reassurance and relief of anxiety may be obtained. In measuring the economic costs and values of MHTS, it would appear, therefore, that too much emphasis has been placed on positive findings. Dividing the costs of all tests among only those with a positive result implies that only a positive finding is worthwhile. Sidney Garfield, founder of the Kaiser-Permanente Medical Care Program, has frequently stressed that the benefits of testing accrue to those with both positive and negative results.[28] Perhaps if we had more faith in our bodies and our environment, we would not need this reassurance. But in today's climate of anxiety the value to patients of negative results cannot be denied.

REFERENCES

1. Hutchison, G. B. "Evaluation of Preventive Measures." In *Preventive Medicine*, D. W. Clark and B. MacMahon, eds., pp. 39–54. Boston: Little, Brown, 1967.

2. Donabedian, A. "Evaluating the Quality of Medical Care." *Milbank Mem. Fund Quart.* 44(1966):166–206.

3. Deniston, O. L., Rosenstock, I. M., and Getting, V. A. "Evaluation of Program Effectiveness." *Public Health Rep.* 83(1968):323–335.

4. Deniston, O. L., Rosenstock, I. M., Welch, W., and Getting, V. A. "Evaluation of Program Efficiency." *Public Health Rep.* 83(1968):603–610.

5. Kuller, L., and Tonascia, S. "Commission on Chronic Illness Follow-up Study: Comparison of Screened and Nonscreened Individuals." *Arch. Environ. Health* 21(1970):656–665.

6. Wilson, J. M. G., and Jungner, G. "Principles and Practice of Screening for Disease." *Public Health Papers*, No. 34, pp. 26–27. Geneva: WHO, 1968.

7. McKeown, T. "Validation of Screening Procedures." In Nuffield Provincial Hospital Trust, *Screening in Medical Care*, pp. 1–13. London: Oxford University Press, 1968.

8. "Mass Health Examination as a Public Health Tool." Technical Report No. A24, pp. 50–51. Geneva: WHO, 1971.

9. Cochrane, A. L., and Holland, W. W. "Validation of Screening Procedures." *Brit. Med. Bull.* 25(1971):3–8.

10. Whitby, L. G. "Screening for Disease: Definitions and Criteria." *The Lancet* 2(1974):819–821.

11. "The Value of Periodic Medical Examinations." *Metropolitan Life Ins. Co. Stat. Bull.* 2, 11(1921):1–2.

12. Seltzer, F. (Assistant Actuary, Metropolitan Life Insurance Company). Personal communication, May 11, 1976.

13. Jungblut, E. J., Enterline, P. E., and Dawber, T. R. "Study of the Effect of Periodic Physical Examinations on Mortality Rates." Paper presented at the annual meeting of the American Public Health Association, November 1, 1960.

14. Thorner, R. M., and Crumpacker, E. L. "Mortality and Periodic Examination of Executives." *Arch. Environ. Health* 3(1961):523–525.

15. Roberts, N. J., Ipsen, J., Elsom, K. O., Clark, T. W., and Yanagawa, H. "Mortality Among Males in Periodic-Health-Examination Programs." *N. Eng. J. Med.* 28(1969):20–24.

16. Braren, M., and Elinson, J. "Relationship of a Clinical Examination to Mortality Rates." *Am. J. Pub. Health* 62(1972):1501–1505.

17. *The Värmland Survey.* Socialstyrelsen Redovisar 23. Stockholm, 1971.

18. Sjukvardens Och Socialvardens Planeringes-Och Rationaliseringsintitut (SPRI). *Follow-up Study of Health Screening in Eskilstuna.* Rapp. 9/72. Stockholm, 1972.

19. Trevelyan, H. "Study to Evaluate the Effects of Multiphasic Screening Within a General Practice in Britain: Design and Method." *Prev. Med.* 2(1973):278–294.

20. Thorner, R. M., Djordjevic, D., Vuckmanovic, C., Pesic, B., Culafic, B., and Mark, F. "A Study to Evaluate the Effectiveness of Multiphasic Screening in Yugoslavia." *Prev. Med.* 2(1973):295–301.

21. Cutler, J. L., Ramcharan, S., Feldman, R., Siegelaub, A., Campbell, B., Friedman, G. D., Dales, L. G., and Collen, M. F. "Multiphasic Checkup Evaluation Study: 1. Methods and Population." *Prev. Med.* 2(1973):197–206.

22. Ramcharan, S., Cutler, J. L., Feldman, R., Siegelaub, A. B., Campbell, B., Friedman, G. D., Dales, L. G., and Collen, M. F. "Multiphasic Checkup Evaluation Study. 2. Disability and Chronic Disease After Seven Years of Multiphasic Health Checkups." *Prev. Med.* 2(1973):207–220.

23. Dales, L. G., Friedman, G. D., Ramcharan, S., Siegelaub, A. B., Campbell, B. A., Feldman, R., and Collen, M. F. "Multiphasic Checkup Evaluation Study. 3. Outpatient Clinic Utilization, Hospitalization, and Mortality Experience After Seven Years." *Prev. Med.* 2(1973):221–235.

24. Collen, M. F., Dales, L. G., Friedman, G. D., Flagle, C. D., Feldman, R., and Siegelaub, A. B. "Multiphasic Checkup Evaluation Study. 4. Preliminary Cost Benefit Analysis for Middle-Aged Men." *Prev. Med.* 2(1973):236–246.

25. Dales, L. G., Friedman, G. D., and Collen, M. F. "Evaluation of a Periodic Multiphasic Health Checkup." *Methods Inform. Med.* 13(1974):140–146.

26. Soghikian, K., and Collen, F. B. "Acceptance of Multiphasic Screening Examinations by Patients." *Bull. N.Y. Acad. Med.* 45(1969):1366–1375.

27. Mechanic, D. "Factors Affecting the Acceptance of Automated Multiphasic Health Testing and Services Among Consumers and Providers." *Provisional Guidelines for Automated Health Testing and Services,* Vol. 3, *Proceedings of the Invitational Conference on AMHTS,* January 21–23, 1970. U.S. Department of Health, Education and Welfare, DHEW Publication No. (HSM) 72-3011, 1972, pp. 235–253.

28. Garfield, S. R. "Multiphasic Health Testing and Medical Care as a Right." *N. Eng. J. Med.* 283(1970):1087–1089.

CHAPTER NINETEEN

Research Applications of MHTS

Abraham B. Siegelaub, Gary D. Friedman, Morris F. Collen,
& Dankward Kodlin

A. Reference Data from an MHTS Data Base (A. B. Siegelaub)
B. Derivation of Normal Values (G. D. Friedman & M. F. Collen)
C. Health-Hazard Appraisal and Counseling (D. Kodlin)
D. Identifying High-Risk Groups and Optimal Screening Intervals (D. Kodlin)
E. Computer-Aided Diagnosis (D. Kodlin)
F. Epidemiological Research (G. D. Friedman)

A. REFERENCE DATA FROM AN MHTS DATA BASE

1. Frequency of Multiphasic Examinations

As described in Chapter One, the Kaiser-Permanente Multiphasic Health Testing Services (MHTS) was begun in July 1964, providing multiphasic health checkups (MHC) to members of the Kaiser Foundation Plan in the Oakland and San Francisco areas. The Kaiser-Permanente Health Care Program serves an average of 18 percent of the entire population in these areas. Although, in this general population, women tend to be older than men by three to five years, among Kaiser-Permanente members and MHTS users men and women differ in age by less than one year. On the average, MHTS users are older by as much as nine years than either the general population or Kaiser-Permanente members age 15 and over. Utilization of the Oakland and San Francisco MHTS is shown for a "typical" year (Tables 19-1, 19-3, and 19-4), for each of the nine years (Tables 19-5 and 19-6), and for the entire nine years since its inception (Table 19-2). During this "typical" year (July 1970 to June 1971) exactly 50,000 individuals had an MHC. For the entire nine years from July 1964 to June 1973, 204,537 persons had at least one MHC.

Table 19-4 shows that, for that typical year, an average of 37 percent had their first examination, 18 percent had their second examination, and 45 percent had a third or more multiphasic examinations. However, this varies markedly from age to age. Furthermore, for the 1970–71 year (See Table 19-5), new (first MHC) users had a median age of 33.5 years, while those having a second MHC were almost ten years older (43.1), and those having a third or greater MHC were almost twenty years older (52.4) than new users.

For each of the nine years since its inception, Tables 19-5 and 19-6 show age and frequency of MHCs for users. The date on which an individual became a Kaiser-Permanente Health Plan member was not available; therefore, all persons were not present to take an MHC at the same time and thus were not subject to having the same possible total number of examinations.

Table 19-5 further shows that:

(1) First-time users decreased from 46.1 years of age in the first year to 31.5 years in the ninth year.

(2) Second-time users decreased from 50.7 years of age to 40.2 years.

(3) Third-time or more frequent MHC users remained at approximately 52 years of age through this period.

Table 19-6 shows that:

(1) First-time users decreased from 100 percent in the first year to 36 percent in the sixth year and increased to 42 percent in the ninth year.

(2) Second-time users decreased from 27 percent to 16 percent in this period.

(3) Third-time or more frequent MHC users increased from 14 percent to 42 percent during this same period.

It appears that the proportion of first-, second-, and third-time or more frequent MHC users may tend to become relatively stable after the sixth to seventh years. The tables also show that once a person has taken a first MHC, he or she tends to return at some regular interval. Further, by the ninth year of the MHTS, new (first-time) MHC users with a median age of 31.5 years are much younger (by 8.7

Table 19-1. Number of Persons Receiving a Multiphasic Health Checkup (MHC) in a Typical Year (July 1970–June 1971)

	By Sex and Age in This Year									Median
Age	15–19	20–24	25–34	35–44	45–54	55–64	65–74	≥ 75	Total	Age
Totals	1,474	3,461	10,039	9.361	11,886	9,220	3,824	686	50,000	45.5
Men	663	1,202	4,863	4,754	5,475	4,248	1,624	328	23,172	45.2
Women	811	2,259	5,176	4,607	6,411	4,973	2,200	358	26,821	45.9

Table 19-2. Number of Persons Receiving a Multiphasic Health Checkup (MHC) in Nine Years (July 1964–June 1973)

	By Sex and Age at First MHC									Median
Age	15–19	20–24	25–34	35–44	45–54	55–64	65–74	≥ 75	Total	Age
Totals	10,788	21,007	53,525	43,944	38,891	24,929	9,299	1,437	204,537	38.7
Men	4,650	6,798	25,368	21,495	18,016	11,612	4,477	776	93,530	39.5
Women	6,138	14,209	28,157	22,449	20,873	13,317	4,822	661	110,989	38.0

Table 19-3. Percent of Those Receiving a Multiphasic Health Checkup (MHC) by Sex in a Typical Year (July 1970–June 1971)

Age	By Age in This Year (From Table 19-1)								Total
	15–19	20–24	25–34	35–44	45–54	55–64	65–74	≥ 75	
Totals	100.0	100.0	100.0	100.0	100.0	100.0	100.0	100.0	100.0
Men	45.0	34.7	48.6	50.8	46.1	46.1	42.5	47.8	46.4
Women	55.0	65.3	51.4	49.2	53.9	53.9	57.5	52.2	53.6

Table 19-4. Percent of Persons by Frequency of Multiphasic Health Checkups (MHC) in a Typical Year (July 1970–June 1971)

Age	15–19	20–24	25–34	35–44	45–54	55–64	65–74	≥ 75	Total	Median Age
Number	1,474	3,461	10,039	9,361	11,886	9,220	3,824	686	50,000	45.5
Percent	100.0	100.0	100.0	100.0	100.0	100.0	100.0	100.0	100.0	
1st MHC	88.7	77.7	61.8	35.3	22.7	19.5	13.1	12.2	37.3	33.5
2nd MHC	9.4	15.3	21.0	22.4	17.7	15.0	13.0	12.0	17.9	43.1
3rd–13th	1.9	6.9	17.2	42.3	59.6	65.5	73.9	75.8	44.8	52.4

Table 19-5. Median Age of Persons by Frequency of Multiphasic Health Checkups (MHC) and by Year (July–June) Since Inception of MHTS

Calendar year	64–65	65–66	66–67	67–68	68–69	69–70	70–71	71–72	72–73
Exam year	1	2	3	4	5	6	7	8	9
Median age	46.1	45.7	46.0	45.8	45.5	46.1	45.5	44.1	43.1
1st MHC	46.1	43.5	41.7	38.7	35.5	34.7	33.5	32.7	31.5
2nd MHC	—	50.7	48.4	47.1	45.3	44.2	43.1	41.5	40.2
3rd–13th	—	—	52.6	51.8	50.5	52.3	52.4	53.0	53.2

Table 19-6. Percent of Persons by Frequency of Multiphasic Health Checkup (MHC) by Year (July–June) Since Inception of MHTS

Calendar year	64–65	65–66	66–67	67–68	68–69	69–70	70–71	71–72	72–73
Exam year	1	2	3	4	5	6	7	8	9
Total (100%)	35,488	42,719	43,317	45,471	43,579	42,937	50,000	52,310	54,448
1st MHC	100.0	72.9	52.2	43.1	38.6	35.8	37.3	41.8	42.2
2nd MHC	—	27.1	34.1	27.6	22.3	20.0	17.9	16.2	16.1
3rd or more	—	—	13.7	29.3	39.1	44.2	45.8	42.0	41.7

years) than second-time MHC users, whose median age is 40.2 years, who are in turn younger (13 years) than frequent (third-time or more users, who have a median age of 53.2 years.

For the entire nine years, 204,537 individuals took 414,519 MHCs, or an average of 2.03 per person. This was similar for men and women and varied by age in the following manner:

Age	Mean Number of MHCs Per Person
15–19	1.3
20–24	1.4
25–34	1.6
35–44	2.3
45–54	2.6
55–64	2.5
65–74	2.4
75 or older	1.8

2. Test Results

For all those taking one or more MHCs from mid-1964 to mid-1968, data for selected tests from their first examination are shown in Tables 19-7 to 19-18. Some 110,000 persons were selected in this manner. As part of these analyses, results for all persons by race (skin color), sex, and age are presented. These test values can be used for the derivation of normal values (see B).

a. Serum chemistry. Serum chemistry determinations were performed on samples of venous blood drawn one hour after ingestion of 75 grams of glucose. Subjects were asked to refrain from eating at least four hours prior to examination. The tests were done on an eight-channel AutoAnalyzer. The analytic methods for each of the tests reported here were as follows: serum glucose: potassium ferrocyanide; cholesterol: Lieberman-Burchard reaction; creatinine: alkaline picrate; calcium: cresyl phthalein dye; SGOT: DPN reduction; and uric acid: phosphotungstate and cyanide. Race (skin color)-sex-age specific mean (and standard deviation) levels are presented, together with the number of persons tested in each such group. Numbers vary from table to table because of occasional inoperability of test equipment.

(1) *Serum Glucose* (Table 19-7)

(a) Levels for blacks were much lower at all ages than those for whites and yellow persons.

(b) Yellows were highest, with whites slightly lower, except in the decade 60 to 69.

(c) Levels for women tended to be the same or lower than men's at younger ages, but women were higher at older ages, particularly in the age bracket 60 to 69.

(2) *Serum Cholesterol* (Table 19-8)

(a) Women showed lower levels than men up to age 40 to 49, but these levels became increasingly higher thereafter.

Table 19-7. Serum Glucose (one hour after 75 gm glucose solution), Mean Value and Standard Deviation in Mg/100 Ml, by Skin Color, Age, and Sex

(a) White

| Age | 15–19 | | 20–29 | | 30–39 | | 40–49 | | 50–59 | | 60–69 | | 70–79 | | Total | |
Sex	Men	Women	Men	Women	Men	Women	Men	Women	Men	Women	Men	Women	Men	Women	Men	Women
Number	1,198	1,453	5,622	8,842	8,693	4,004	10,032	11,694	8,166	10,195	4,575	5,887	1,403	1,476	37,689	48,545
Mean	148.2	152.9	161.0	160.5	170.7	173.2	180.0	179.4	186.1	188.6	190.4	196.9	192.8	201.2	177.2	178.7
Std. Dev.	40.7	41.3	43.0	41.4	44.8	44.6	47.0	47.7	49.8	51.2	52.6	54.2	51.6	55.6	48.4	49.4

(b) Black

| Age | 15–19 | | 20–29 | | 30–39 | | 40–49 | | 50–59 | | 60–69 | | 70–79 | | Total | |
Sex	Men	Women	Men	Women	Men	Women	Men	Women	Men	Women	Men	Women	Men	Women	Men	Women
Number	186	318	880	1,691	1,328	1,814	1,669	2,156	946	1,077	278	255	43	17	5,330	7,328
Mean	128.3	132.6	140.7	142.1	154.9	150.0	159.7	157.5	167.9	168.1	167.6	172.7	172.7	168.4	156.2	153.1
Std. Dev.	33.3	37.1	37.3	37.4	44.3	40.9	44.6	43.7	48.5	48.3	46.4	51.6	50.9	60.5	45.1	43.6

(c) Yellow

| Age | 15–19 | | 20–29 | | 30–39 | | 40–49 | | 50–59 | | 60–69 | | 70–79 | | Total | |
Sex	Men	Women	Men	Women	Men	Women	Men	Women	Men	Women	Men	Women	Men	Women	Men	Women
Number	45	55	251	459	646	829	623	660	290	224	134	65	18	7	2,007	2,299
Mean	154.8	160.0	169.0	168.4	176.7	175.3	183.0	178.7	187.5	191.4	190.3	190.1	234.7	145.8	180.2	176.4
Std. Dev.	49.8	41.9	45.9	44.8	48.2	47.6	50.2	49.6	61.1	55.4	64.6	64.2	63.0	44.0	52.6	49.3

Table 19-8. Serum Cholesterol, Mean Value and Standard Deviation in Mg/100 Ml, by Skin Color, Age, and Sex

(a) White

Age Sex	15–19		20–29		30–39		40–49		50–59		60–69		70–79		Total	
	Men	Women	Men	Women	Men	Women	Men	Women	Men	Women	Men	Women	Men	Women	Men	Women
Number	1,130	1,346	5,197	8,174	8,049	8,284	9,344	10,781	7,609	9,327	4,256	5,406	1,319	1,374	36,904	44,692
Mean	178.7	188.4	199.7	200.1	216.5	208.1	227.0	221.4	230.7	242.8	229.9	252.4	228.2	254.1	220.5	223.3
Std. Dev.	32.1	32.8	35.7	35.4	38.5	35.7	39.9	39.0	38.7	42.1	40.0	43.9	42.6	45.5	40.7	43.8

(b) Black

Age Sex	15–19		20–29		30–39		40–49		50–59		60–69		70–79		Total	
	Men	Women	Men	Women	Men	Women	Men	Women	Men	Women	Men	Women	Men	Women	Men	Women
Number	179	272	823	1,581	1,245	1,697	1,564	2,007	886	1,011	263	231	37	17	4,997	6,836
Mean	179.1	185.3	199.9	200.9	215.5	211.1	227.1	227.3	229.1	244.6	228.2	258.7	236.3	261.2	218.5	219.1
Std. Dev.	26.9	31.9	35.6	33.5	38.6	38.2	42.5	41.6	39.5	44.4	39.9	47.5	38.9	43.2	41.3	43.1

(c) Yellow

Age Sex	15–19		20–29		30–39		40–49		50–59		60–69		70–79		Total	
	Men	Women	Men	Women	Men	Women	Men	Women	Men	Women	Men	Women	Men	Women	Men	Women
Number	42	52	229	408	604	750	562	597	257	198	121	56	16	7	1,831	2,068
Mean	185.6	189.5	204.9	198.6	219.2	205.6	231.0	220.5	231.0	243.7	238.6	244.4	249.6	260.4	223.5	213.0
Std. Dev.	27.7	32.4	33.7	33.8	40.5	38.1	42.6	36.8	39.5	41.5	39.6	40.3	39.3	42.7	41.5	39.9

(b) Levels of the three racial (skin-color) groups were similar at all ages.

(c) For men, mean values increased slowly to age 50 to 59, then leveled off and decreased slightly in the 70s. For women the means increased to the 60s, then leveled off in the 70s.

(3) *Serum Calcium* (Table 19-9)

(a) For this test, for all skin colors and sexes, mean levels decreased from age 15 to 19 to age 40 to 49, then increased at older ages.

(b) Men had higher mean values through the 40s and lower thereafter.

(c) Blacks had highest levels, with whites lower, and yellows lowest.

(4) *Serum Creatinine* (Table 19-10)

(a) Mean levels for men were higher than for women at all ages and for all skin colors.

(b) For men and women, mean levels increased with age.

(c) For all ages and both sexes, blacks were highest, with whites intermediate, and yellows lowest.

(5) *Serum Glutamic Oxalic Transaminase* (SGOT) (Table 19-11)

(a) Mean levels for men were much higher than for women.

(b) Yellows and blacks showed similar levels and were higher than whites.

(6) *Serum Uric Acid* (Table 19-12)

(a) Men had higher mean values than women for all ages and skin colors.

(b) Although mean levels increased with age in both men and women, this increase was greater in women than men, particularly after age 40 to 49.

(c) In both men and women, yellow persons were highest; from age 15–19 to age 40–49, whites were higher than blacks; thereafter blacks were higher than whites, but still lower than yellows.

b. Hematology. Hemoglobin concentration was determined by a hemo-photometer, and leukocytes were counted by an automated hemocytometer.

(1) *Hemoglobin* (Table 19-13)

(a) As expected, men had higher mean levels than women.

(b) Whites and yellows had approximately the same mean values, with blacks having much lower means within each sex.

(2) *White Blood Cell Count* (Table 19-14)

(a) Mean values here were higher in women than men through age 40 to 49, and lower thereafter.

(b) Whites showed the highest mean values, with yellows rather lower, and blacks still lower.

(c) For whites, means increased from 15–19 to 20–29 and then decreased with advancing age. Yellows and blacks showed a decreasing trend with age.

c. Blood pressure. Blood pressures were taken manually with a sphyg-momanometer by a trained technician (Tables 19-15 and 19-16). Systolic and diastolic blood pressure means were highest in blacks. Whites were generally

Table 19-9. Serum Calcium, Mean Value and Standard Deviation in Mg/100 Ml, by Skin Color, Age, and Sex

(a) White

| Age | 15–19 | | 20–29 | | 30–39 | | 40–49 | | 50–59 | | 60–69 | | 70–79 | | Total | |
Sex	Men	Women	Men	Women	Men	Women	Men	Women	Men	Women	Men	Women	Men	Women	Men	Women
Number	1,139	1,413	5,313	8,444	8,195	8,508	9.499	11,178	7,762	9.727	4,327	5,588	1,344	1,413	37,577	46,351
Mean	10.05	9.89	9.99	9.78	9.89	9.72	9.81	9.70	9.76	9.81	9.73	9.80	9.69	9.77	9.84	9.76
Std. Dev.	.48	.45	.48	.45	.50	.47	.49	.48	.50	.50	.51	.50	.52	.55	.50	.48

(b) Black

| Age | 15–19 | | 20–29 | | 30–39 | | 40–49 | | 50–59 | | 60–69 | | 70–79 | | Total | |
Sex	Men	Women	Men	Women	Men	Women	Men	Women	Men	Women	Men	Women	Men	Women	Men	Women
Number	182	311	842	1,621	1,264	1,743	1,598	2,083	893	1,043	263	240	38	17	5,080	7,058
Mean	10.10	9.95	10.05	9.80	9.94	9.77	9.92	9.81	9.86	9.91	9.84	9.86	9.86	10.02	9.94	9.82
Std. Dev.	.23	.22	.20	.24	.24	.23	.25	.25	.22	.25	.21	.20	.23	.19	.23	.24

(c) Yellow

| Age | 15–19 | | 20–29 | | 30–39 | | 40–49 | | 50–59 | | 60–69 | | 70–79 | | Total | |
Sex	Men	Women	Men	Women	Men	Women	Men	Women	Men	Women	Men	Women	Men	Women	Men	Women
Number	44	50	233	427	602	775	580	628	274	211	124	60	17	7	1,874	2,158
Mean	10.04	10.01	9.89	9.74	9.79	9.64	9.74	9.63	9.69	9.66	9.74	9.74	9.89	9.91	9.78	9.67
Std. Dev.	.23	.17	.25	.19	.24	.18	.22	.22	.25	.23	.22	.43	.22	.22	.25	.21

Table 19-10.   Serum Creatinine, Mean Value and Standard Deviation in Mg/100 Ml, by Skin Color, Age, and Sex

(a) White

| Age | 15–19 | | 20–29 | | 30–39 | | 40–49 | | 50–59 | | 60–69 | | 70–79 | | Total | |
Sex	Men	Women	Men	Women	Men	Women	Men	Women	Men	Women	Men	Women	Men	Women	Men	Women
Number	1,132	1,390	5,330	8,355	8,275	8,609	9,586	11,185	7,828	9,779	4,414	5,676	1,349	1,428	37,914	46,422
Mean	1.04	.87	1.08	.87	1.09	.88	1.10	.89	1.11	.92	1.12	.95	1.19	.98	1.10	.90
Std. Dev	.36	.16	.20	.26	.27	.28	.26	.23	.30	.28	.29	.31	.42	.30	.28	.27

(b) Black

| Age | 15–19 | | 20–29 | | 30–39 | | 40–49 | | 50–59 | | 60–69 | | 70–79 | | Total | |
Sex	Men	Women	Men	Women	Men	Women	Men	Women	Men	Women	Men	Women	Men	Women	Men	Women
Number	176	304	841	605	1,257	1,731	1,599	2,067	903	1,039	272	250	41	16	5,089	7,012
Mean	1.07	.88	1.14	.89	1.14	.90	1.16	.94	1.19	.96	1.20	1.01	1.26	.99	1.16	.92
Std. Dev.	.06	.03	.04	.05	.04	.12	.09	.14	.07	.05	.07	.25	.11	.07	.06	.10

(c) Yellow

| Age | 15–19 | | 20–29 | | 30–39 | | 40–49 | | 50–59 | | 60–69 | | 70–79 | | Total | |
Sex	Men	Women	Men	Women	Men	Women	Men	Women	Men	Women	Men	Women	Men	Women	Men	Women
Number	44	52	240	427	606	773	593	612	272	205	123	63	16	7	1,894	2,139
Mean	1.02	.81	1.06	.83	1.05	.81	1.06	.83	1.07	.85	1.08	.88	1.21	.92	1.06	.83
Std. Dev.	.05	.02	.03	.13	.03	.06	.04	.03	.04	.04	.04	.03	.04	.04	.04	.06

Table 19–11. Serum Glutamic Oxalic Transaminase (SGOT), Mean Value and Standard Deviation in Units, by Skin Color, Age, and Sex

(a) White

| Age | 15–19 | | 20–29 | | 30–39 | | 40–49 | | 50–59 | | 60–69 | | 70–79 | | Total | |
Sex	Men	Women	Men	Women	Men	Women	Men	Women	Men	Women	Men	Women	Men	Women	Men	Women
Number	1,145	1,387	5,364	8,309	8,314	8,633	9,633	11,258	7,859	9,835	4,412	5,687	1,358	1,426	38,085	46,735
Mean	21.8	17.5	21.4	17.3	22.8	17.6	23.4	18.2	22.5	20.1	22.6	20.4	21.8	20.7	22.6	18.6
Std. Dev.	11.6	9.6	12.3	9.0	14.5	9.5	15.0	10.4	13.7	13.5	14.5	11.4	11.1	11.4	14.0	10.9

(b) Black

| Age | 15–19 | | 20–29 | | 30–39 | | 40–49 | | 50–59 | | 60–69 | | 70–79 | | Total | |
Sex	Men	Women	Men	Women	Men	Women	Men	Women	Men	Women	Men	Women	Men	Women	Men	Women
Number	180	314	853	1,634	1,276	1,749	1,615	2,087	909	1,039	274	245	42	16	5,149	7,084
Mean	21.0	17.7	22.9	17.4	24.1	18.5	24.0	19.2	23.6	20.4	22.1	19.8	19.1	19.5	23.5	18.7
Std. Dev.	8.9	10.9	15.9	9.1	13.6	10.2	16.4	11.4	16.7	13.5	12.9	9.0	5.3	4.6	15.3	10.9

(c) Yellow

| Age | 15–19 | | 20–29 | | 30–39 | | 40–49 | | 50–59 | | 60–69 | | 70–79 | | Total | |
Sex	Men	Women	Men	Women	Men	Women	Men	Women	Men	Women	Men	Women	Men	Women	Men	Women
Number	44	54	239	432	614	789	503	628	272	212	123	62	17	7	1,872	2,184
Mean	19.9	17.8	23.5	17.9	24.1	18.0	24.7	19.6	23.5	21.1	24.8	23.2	18.8	23.1	24.0	18.9
Std. Dev.	6.0	7.5	14.2	8.2	19.4	9.1	14.5	15.0	12.9	9.3	14.1	31.5	8.3	10.6	15.8	12.1

Table 19-12. Serum Uric Acid, Mean Value and Standard Deviation in Units, by Skin Color, Age, and Sex

(a) White

| Age | 15–19 | | 20–29 | | 30–39 | | 40–49 | | 50–59 | | 60–69 | | 70–79 | | Total | |
Sex	Men	Women	Men	Women	Men	Women	Men	Women	Men	Women	Men	Women	Men	Women	Men	Women
Number	1,126	1,377	5,266	8,276	8,156	8,500	9,526	11,134	7,796	9,771	4,366	5,625	1,343	1,412	37,579	46,075
Mean	5.65	4.23	5.74	4.12	5.80	4.18	5.89	4.37	5.91	4.78	5.92	5.01	6.12	5.12	5.86	4.47
Std. Dev.	1.14	1.04	1.21	1.00	1.27	1.02	1.29	1.11	1.34	1.22	1.38	1.27	1.43	1.35	1.30	1.17

(b) Black

| Age | 15–19 | | 20–29 | | 30–39 | | 40–49 | | 50–59 | | 60–69 | | 70–79 | | Total | |
Sex	Men	Women	Men	Women	Men	Women	Men	Women	Men	Women	Men	Women	Men	Women	Men	Women
Number	178	300	842	1,590	1,248	1,723	1,611	2,079	907	1,037	263	245	41	16	5,090	6,990
Mean	5.40	3.78	5.44	3.83	5.61	4.10	5.80	4.41	5.89	4.91	5.98	5.14	6.10	5.18	5.71	4.28
Std. Dev.	1.11	1.01	1.32	.98	1.39	1.14	1.45	1.23	1.51	1.42	1.47	1.46	2.07	1.13	1.43	1.25

(c) Yellow

| Age | 15–19 | | 20–29 | | 30–39 | | 40–49 | | 50–59 | | 60–69 | | 70–79 | | Total | |
Sex	Men	Women	Men	Women	Men	Women	Men	Women	Men	Women	Men	Women	Men	Women	Men	Women
Number	42	51	235	422	599	775	576	619	276	206	119	59	16	6	1,863	2,138
Mean	6.14	4.41	5.84	4.29	5.97	4.31	5.99	4.44	6.12	4.94	6.41	5.47	6.30	6.11	6.02	4.45
Std. Dev.	1.22	.96	1.27	.97	1.35	1.06	1.40	1.07	1.45	1.31	1.49	1.50	1.34	2.13	1.38	1.12

Table 19-13. Blood Hemoglobin, Mean Value and Standard Deviation in Gm/100 Ml, by Skin Color, Age, and Sex

(a) White

| Age | 15–19 | | 20–29 | | 30–39 | | 40–49 | | 50–59 | | 60–69 | | 70–79 | | Total | |
Sex	Men	Women	Men	Women	Men	Women	Men	Women	Men	Women	Men	Women	Men	Women	Men	Women
Number	1,199	1,455	5,622	8,849	8,703	9,019	10,044	11,706	8,180	10,214	4,586	5,891	1,406	1,479	39,740	48,613
Mean	14.75	12.96	14.97	12.98	14.83	12.88	14.66	12.88	14.59	13.20	14.51	13.24	14.33	13.18	14.70	13.02
Std. Dev.	1.14	1.03	1.09	1.08	1.11	1.14	1.15	1.21	1.16	1.12	1.23	1.10	1.31	1.16	1.16	1.14

(b) Black

| Age | 15–19 | | 20–29 | | 30–39 | | 40–49 | | 50–59 | | 60–69 | | 70–79 | | Total | |
Sex	Men	Women	Men	Women	Men	Women	Men	Women	Men	Women	Men	Women	Men	Women	Men	Women
Number	186	318	884	1,694	1,332	1,816	1,672	2,160	944	1,075	278	254	43	17	5,339	7,334
Mean	14.16	12.23	14.50	12.34	14.29	12.25	14.13	12.33	14.01	12.55	13.91	12.51	13.56	12.78	14.20	12.35
Std. Dev.	1.24	1.10	1.20	1.16	1.18	1.21	1.25	1.26	1.27	1.12	1.23	1.14	1.32	1.24	1.24	1.20

(c) Yellow

| Age | 15–19 | | 20–29 | | 30–39 | | 40–49 | | 50–59 | | 60–69 | | 70–79 | | Total | |
Sex	Men	Women	Men	Women	Men	Women	Men	Women	Men	Women	Men	Women	Men	Women	Men	Women
Number	45	55	251	458	648	829	623	662	291	223	135	65	18	7	2,011	2,299
Mean	14.92	13.11	15.01	12.82	14.75	12.67	14.71	12.68	14.70	13.00	14.39	13.20	14.74	13.23	14.74	12.76
Std. Dev.	1.16	1.04	1.18	1.00	1.20	1.19	1.27	1.16	1.22	1.14	1.14	1.12	1.24	.92	1.22	1.14

Table 19-14. White Blood Cell Count, Mean Value and Standard Deviation in Cells Per Cu. Ml, by Skin Color, Age, and Sex

(a) White

| Age | 15–19 | | 20–29 | | 30–39 | | 40–49 | | 50–59 | | 60–69 | | 70–79 | | Total | |
Sex	Men	Women	Men	Women	Men	Women	Men	Women	Men	Women	Men	Women	Men	Women	Men	Women
Number	1,193	1,452	5,592	8,821	8,658	8,983	9,991	11,663	8,121	10,165	4,561	5,866	1,401	1,472	39,517	48,432
Mean	7,803	8,002	7,838	8,324	7,842	8,151	7,832	7,944	7,800	7,540	7,689	7,338	7,469	7,083	7,798	7,869
Std. Dev.	1,673	1,772	1,803	1,936	1,897	1,932	1,939	1,918	1,919	1,892	1,991	1,715	1,883	2,034	1,905	1,928

(b) Black

| Age | 15–19 | | 20–29 | | 30–39 | | 40–49 | | 50–59 | | 60–69 | | 70–79 | | Total | |
Sex	Men	Women	Men	Women	Men	Women	Men	Women	Men	Women	Men	Women	Men	Women	Men	Women
Number	186	318	880	1,690	1,324	1,815	1,665	2,151	937	1,071	277	254	43	17	5,312	7,316
Mean	7,063	7,409	6,971	7,596	6,869	7,311	6,934	7,002	6,643	6,773	6,259	6,709	6,381	6,212	6,838	7,188
Std Dev.	1,754	1,963	1,791	2,093	1,799	1,967	1,854	1,826	1,774	1,788	1,599	1,827	1,874	1,650	1,808	1,949

(c) Yellow

| Age | 15–19 | | 20–29 | | 30–39 | | 40–49 | | 50–59 | | 60–69 | | 70–79 | | Total | |
Sex	Men	Women	Men	Women	Men	Women	Men	Women	Men	Women	Men	Women	Men	Women	Men	Women
Number	45	55	248	453	644	826	619	653	290	222	134	65	18	7	1,998	2,281
Mean	7,669	8,060	7,417	7,708	7,410	7,588	7,385	7,324	7,248	7,060	7,028	7,180	7,456	7,129	7,360	7,483
Std. Dev.	1,650	1,921	1,736	1,818	1,753	1,762	1,703	1,650	1,631	1,685	1,458	1,589	1,756	1,941	1,699	1,746

Table 19-15. Systolic Blood Pressure, Mean Value and Standard Deviation in Mm Hg, by Skin Color, Age, and Sex

(a) White

Age	15–19		20–29		30–39		40–49		50–59		60–69		70–79		Total	
Sex	Men	Women	Men	Women	Men	Women	Men	Women	Men	Women	Men	Women	Men	Women	Men	Women
Number	1,200	1,462	5,626	8,873	8,707	9,039	10,048	11,720	8,179	10,225	4,592	5,896	1,403	1,480	39,755	48,695
Mean	123.3	114.4	126.1	115.9	126.4	117.7	129.4	124.6	137.3	135.9	147.0	148.8	155.2	159.7	132.7	127.8
Std. Dev.	13.5	11.8	13.8	12.3	14.6	13.8	16.6	18.2	20.3	21.5	23.3	23.1	24.4	25.3	19.6	21.9

(b) Black

Age	15–19		20–29		30–39		40–49		50–59		60–69		70–79		Total	
Sex	Men	Women	Men	Women	Men	Women	Men	Women	Men	Women	Men	Women	Men	Women	Men	Women
Number	190	320	885	1,699	1,330	1,824	1,671	2,170	946	1,081	283	256	43	17	5,348	7,367
Mean	122.6	116.0	128.5	120.3	130.5	125.3	137.1	136.4	145.4	149.9	154.5	157.3	162.0	166.5	136.1	131.8
Std. Dev.	13.0	11.9	15.0	14.7	16.1	18.2	20.1	23.4	22.3	26.2	26.0	25.9	22.0	30.3	20.6	23.6

(c) Yellow

Age	15–19		20–29		30–39		40–49		50–59		60–69		70–79		Total	
Sex	Men	Women	Men	Women	Men	Women	Men	Women	Men	Women	Men	Women	Men	Women	Men	Women
Number	46	56	251	461	647	832	623	664	291	224	135	65	18	7	2,011	2,309
Mean	121.2	108.8	123.2	111.1	122.6	114.4	122.6	121.4	135.8	136.9	151.3	148.3	159.3	160.9	128.0	118.9
Std. Dev.	16.0	11.8	14.1	11.8	13.3	14.2	16.8	18.8	20.4	24.3	22.9	25.8	24.0	24.3	18.5	19.1

Table 19-16. Diastolic Blood Pressure, Mean Value and Standard Deviation in Mm Hg, by Skin Color, Age, and Sex

(a) White

Age	15–19		20–29		30–39		40–49		50–59		60–69		70–79		Total	
Sex	Men	Women	Men	Women	Men	Women	Men	Women	Men	Women	Men	Women	Men	Women	Men	Women
Number	1,187	1,456	5,608	8,860	8,699	9,030	10,039	11,711	8,175	10,215	4,587	891	1,402	1,480	39,697	48,643
Mean	66.9	67.7	71.7	69.4	74.4	73.1	79.2	77.8	82.4	82.2	84.5	85.7	85.9	87.0	78.4	77.2
Std. Dev.	13.2	11.4	13.0	11.6	12.6	11.4	12.8	12.3	13.4	12.6	14.0	12.8	13.9	13.8	13.9	13.4

(b) Black

Age	15–19		20–29		30–39		40–49		50–59		60–69		70–79		Total	
Sex	Men	Women	Men	Women	Men	Women	Men	Women	Men	Women	Men	Women	Men	Women	Men	Women
Number	187	320	885	1,698	1,328	1,823	1,670	2,166	945	1,081	282	256	43	17	5,340	7,361
Mean	68.7	69.3	73.8	72.9	78.3	79.4	84.8	85.7	87.7	91.1	89.8	90.7	91.1	97.9	81.6	81.5
Std. Dev.	14.1	12.7	14.3	13,6	14.7	14.2	15.3	14.7	15.6	14.7	16.5	13.8	11.7	23.9	16.1	15.8

(c) Yellow

Age	15–19		20–29		30–39		40–49		50–59		60–69		70–79		Total	
Sex	Men	Women	Men	Women	Men	Women	Men	Women	Men	Women	Men	Women	Men	Women	Men	Women
Number	45	56	250	460	645	832	622	663	291	224	135	65	18	7	2,006	2,307
Mean	69.2	64.6	71.2	68.5	75.5	72.3	79.0	76.7	82.9	82.7	84.0	88.1	86.7	87.4	77.7	74.1
Std. Dev.	13.8	11.2	12.6	10.9	11.5	11.2	12.8	12.9	15.2	14.3	13.9	14.8	15.5	15.1	13.5	13.1

higher than yellows except after age 50 to 59. Again, men were higher than women until age 40 to 49, after which women became higher.

d.   Spirometry.   Respirometry was measured on a Collins spirometer (Tables 19-17 and 19-18). Both forced expiratory volume at one second ($FEV_{1.0}$) and total forced vital capacity (FVC) showed similar trends. Mean values were higher in men than women at all ages and skin colors. Whites were higher than blacks or yellows in both sexes. Blacks and yellows were about the same.

3.   Frequency of Diagnosis

When taking a multiphasic health checkup (MHC), patients also make an appointment to see their physicians at some later time. A summary report of the multiphasic tests is sent to the physician, who after a physical examination completes a diagnosis form. This is a structured marksensed form with 167 diagnoses arranged by organ and system. For one 12-month period (September 1966 to August 1967), Table 19-19 shows those diagnoses which were reported in at least 1 percent of men or women. Also shown are the rates at which these were reported as "old" (known to physician), "new", or new and old (exacerbation of previously known diagnosis). More than one diagnosis may be reported for a particular patient. These diagnoses are ranked separately for men and women by the total rate—that is, without regard to whether they were new or old. (See also Chapter Seventeen, Table 17-6.)

a.   Findings

(1) Approximately one-third of all men and women had no significant (clinical) abnormality (NSA).

(2) Excluding NSA, 20 diagnoses occurred in at least 1 percent of men, and 21 in 1 percent of women.

(a) Obesity was found most frequently both in men and women. The next most frequently found diagnoses were primary hypertension and anxiety state, again in both men and women.

(b) Also in both sexes, the same five diagnoses were reported in the fourth to tenth ranks. In fact, of the 21 most frequently reported diagnoses, 14 were the same in men and women.

(c) Most of these diagnoses were already known to the physician.

(d) Those diagnoses for which the newly found were a majority were, in men and women, renal glycosuria, and in women, migraine, low back pain, urinary infection, and chronic dermatitis.

B.   DERIVATION OF NORMAL VALUES

1.   Concepts and Problems

An MHTS must have a set of "normal" values for each test in order to help separate the sick from the well examinees. At first a set of normal test values needs to be adopted from some reliable source, but eventually each MHTS can derive normal values from its own data base.

Table 19-17. Forced Expiratory Volume, 1 second ($FEV_{1.0}$), Mean Value and Standard Deviation in Liters, by Skin Color, Age, and Sex

(a) White

| Age | 15–19 | | 20–29 | | 30–39 | | 40–49 | | 50–59 | | 60–69 | | 70–79 | | Total | |
Sex	Men	Women	Men	Women	Men	Women	Men	Women	Men	Women	Men	Women	Men	Women	Men	Women
Number	1,160	1,401	5,421	8,503	8,436	8,752	9,774	11,343	7,927	9,835	4,433	5,584	1,345	1,365	38,496	46,783
Mean	3.68	2.61	3.64	2.55	3.40	2.39	3.08	2.16	2.70	1.90	2.29	1.65	2.01	1.45	3.04	2.15
Std. Dev.	.75	.54	.76	.56	.74	.54	.71	.50	.69	.46	.67	.46	.61	.40	.85	.60

(b) Black

| Age | 15–19 | | 20–29 | | 30–39 | | 40–49 | | 50–59 | | 60–69 | | 70–79 | | Total | |
Sex	Men	Women	Men	Women	Men	Women	Men	Women	Men	Women	Men	Women	Men	Women	Men	Women
Number	179	302	849	599	1,278	1,753	1,611	2,079	913	1,014	273	243	41	16	5,144	7,006
Mean	3,05	2.27	3.12	2.22	2.88	2.07	2.59	1.85	2.34	1.65	2.03	1.45	1.89	1.45	2.69	1.96
Std. Dev.	.79	.55	.73	.48	.66	.50	.64	.45	.66	.43	.55	.37	.44	.52	.73	.52

(c) Yellow

| Age | 15–19 | | 20–29 | | 30–39 | | 40–49 | | 50–59 | | 60–69 | | 70–79 | | Total | |
Sex	Men	Women	Men	Women	Men	Women	Men	Women	Men	Women	Men	Women	Men	Women	Men	Women
Number	39	54	245	437	629	800	598	631	276	207	129	57	15	6	1,931	2,192
Mean	3.05	2.24	3.07	2.15	2.90	2.00	2.59	1.86	2.23	1.60	1.90	1.37	1.41	1.33	2.65	1.94
Std. Dev.	.67	.48	.67	.61	.62	.56	.61	.58	.59	.41	.47	.35	.50	.42	.70	.59

Table 19-18. Forced Vital Capacity, Total, Mean Value and Standard Deviation in Liters, by Skin Color, Age, and Sex

(a) White

| Age | 15–19 | | 20–29 | | 30–39 | | 40–49 | | 50–59 | | 60–69 | | 70–79 | | Total | |
Sex	Men	Women	Men	Women	Men	Women	Men	Women	Men	Women	Men	Women	Men	Women	Men	Women
Number	1,158	1,401	5,415	8,504	8,429	8,759	9,770	11,346	7,931	9,845	4,435	5,595	1,348	1,365	38,486	46,815
Mean	4.72	3.26	4.86	3.30	4.62	3.23	4.24	2.95	3.82	2.62	3.35	2.30	3.02	2.03	4.19	2.90
Std. Dev.	.76	.52	.79	.56	.80	.57	.79	.56	.79	.54	.75	.52	.72	.47	.94	.66

(b) Black

| Age | 15–19 | | 20–29 | | 30–39 | | 40–49 | | 50–59 | | 60–69 | | 70–79 | | Total | |
Sex	Men	Women	Men	Women	Men	Women	Men	Women	Men	Women	Men	Women	Men	Women	Men	Women
Number	179	302	849	1,599	1,278	1,754	1,612	2,078	912	1,015	273	243	41	16	5,144	7,007
Mean	3.93	2.80	4.12	2.79	3.88	2.69	3.56	2.45	3.24	2.21	2.95	1.95	2.62	2.04	3.65	2.55
Std. Dev.	.78	.52	.80	.54	.72	.55	.73	.52	.70	.51	.76	.64	.59	.59	.81	.58

(c) Yellow

| Age | 15–19 | | 20–29 | | 30–39 | | 40–49 | | 50–59 | | 60–69 | | 70–79 | | Total | |
Sex	Men	Women	Men	Women	Men	Women	Men	Women	Men	Women	Men	Women	Men	Women	Men	Women
Number	39	54	245	438	630	802	598	630	276	208	129	57	15	6	1,932	2,195
Mean	3.80	2.76	3.98	2.72	3.80	2.65	3.48	2.48	3.06	2.19	2.71	1.84	2.21	1.95	3.53	2.55
Std. Dev.	.72	.49	.69	.45	.67	.48	.65	.55	.65	.47	.60	.46	.67	.69	.76	.53

Table 19-19. Most Frequent Diagnoses for a One-Year Period

| | | Men (13,933) | | | | | | Women (17,910) | | | |
| | | Rate per 100 Men | | | | | | Rate per 100 Women | | | |
Rank	Diagnosis	New	Old	New & Old	Total	Rank	Diagnosis	New	Old	New & Old	Total
	No significant abnormality				35.99		No significant abnormality				34.19
1	Obesity	2.79	10.51	.61	13.91	1	Obesity	4.01	15.00	1.00	20.01
2	Primary hypertension	1.87	5.41	.38	7.66	2	Anxiety state	2.34	6.52	.51	9.37
3	Anxiety state	1.23	3.19	.24	4.66	3	Primary hypertension	1.70	5.51	.34	7.55
4	Diabetes mellitus	.81	3.03	.08	3.92	4	Osteoarthritis	.78	3.82	.16	4.76
5	Deafness	.83	2.53	.09	3.45	5	Varicose veins	.82	2.95	.11	3.88
6	Prostatic benign hypertrophy	1.00	1.88	.09	2.97	6	Psycho-physiol.-reaction gastrointestinal	.73	2.43	.22	3.38
7	Psycho-physiol.-reaction gastrointestinal	.56	1.79	.21	2.56	7	Fibrocystic disease—breast	.92	2.27	.11	3.30
8	Osteoarthritis	.42	2.00	.11	2.53	8	Diabetes mellitus	.86	1.90	.11	2.87
9	Duodenal ulcer	.17	1.96	.09	2.22	9	Depression	.67	1.43	.07	2.17
10	Varicose veins	.51	1.54	.12	2.17	10	Deafness	.49	1.60	.06	2.15
11	Chronic dermatitis	.57	1.32	.10	1.99	11	Hypochromic anemia	.76	1.13	.12	2.01
12	Emphysema	.46	1.41	.08	1.95	12	Menopausal syndrome	.71	1.18	.04	1.93
13	Ischemic heart disease	.20	1.66	.09	1.95	13	Migraine	1.52	.18	.01	1.71
14	Hay fever	.26	1.21	.05	1.52	14	Hypothyroid	.33	1.22	.09	1.64
15	Renal glycosuria	.75	.62	.01	1.38	15	Hay fever	.34	1.08	.11	1.53
16	Rhinitis/sinusitis	.30	.98	.07	1.35	16	Low back pain	.47	.98	.05	1.50
17	Testes, absent/atrophy	.27	1.00	.02	1.29	17	Kyphosis/scoliosis	.25	1.01	.06	1.32
18	Low back pain	.36	.81	.09	1.26	18	Urinary infection	.64	.57	.10	1.31
19	Chronic bronchitis	.28	.89	.07	1.24	19	Chronic dermatitis	.44	.80	.05	1.29
20	Myocardial infarct	.01	1.05	.01	1.07	20	Rhinitis/sinusitis	.38	.79	.11	1.28
21	Bronchial asthma	.17	.75	.06	0.98	21	Irritable bowel	.30	.88	.03	1.21

Unfortunately, much confusion surrounds this area, because the term "normal" has more than one meaning.[1,2] As used above, to separate the well from the sick, it means "good" or "desirable" or "healthy." Another important meaning is "usual" or "frequent." In this sense, it is normal for an older person to have gray hair. This says that the occurrence is common but implies nothing either way about desirability. As if these two definitions did not cause sufficient confusion, there is a third meaning, having to do with the shape of a distribution curve that is often observed in studies of human characteristics. This symmetrical, bell-shaped curve is referred to as the "Gaussian" or "normal" distribution curve.

One method that has been used to define the "normal-healthy" has been to determine the "normal-usual." That is, the particular test is applied to a large population. A cutoff point is applied to one or both ends of the distribution curve so that an arbitrary small percentage, say 5 percent or 1 percent of the population, will be called abnormal. Clearly, by this method, the normal range is merely the usual range; but it is easy to drift into the view that normal-usual means normal-healthy.

This method for determining normal-healthy limits can be improved upon by finding the normal-usual values in a population that is known to be healthy. Unfortunately, the healthy group studied often has been small and select—for example, a group of medical or nursing students. Thus it was hard to be sure whether test values associated with health in these groups would also be associated with health in persons of different ages and circumstances.

Another technique used to find the healthy among the usual has been to identify the part of the distribution that is normal-bell-shaped and assume that this represents the normal-healthy, and that the deformity at one or both ends of the distribution curve is due to the sick persons who have been included in the study population. This method is attractive in its elegant simplicity and it makes sense in that many human measurements not related to illness, such as height, do fit a normal-bell-shaped distribution; and mixtures of well and sick people produce distributions that are mostly normal-bell-shaped, but skewed at one end (such as white cell count or blood sugar). Furthermore, this approach seems to work, since normal-healthy values obtained by this technique in many cases seem to agree well with the clinical standards that have evolved.

Yet, one cannot help but feel uneasy about using normal-bell-shaped curves to determine what is normal-healthy. One of the major contributions of epidemiology in recent years has been to show that people at one end of a normal-bell-shaped distribution are better off than those at the other end of the distribution, and even better off than those in the trusted middle. Serum cholesterol level is probably the best example of this phenomenon. If we consider middle-aged men, there is abundant evidence that three or four times as many persons in the highest quartile of the bell-shaped distribution are going to develop coronary heart disease as in the lowest quartile. Knowing that about one in every five individuals in that highest quartile will develop coronary heart disease in the next ten years, one can hardly call such individuals normal-healthy, especially since there is mounting evidence that medical attention to their diet and living habits may reduce their high risk. There is good reason, then, not to place blind faith in the normal-bell-shaped curve as representing the normal-healthy.

Another problem in attempting to determine the normal-healthy is that there are no compelling reasons for deciding, from observations on healthy persons alone, where to set the upper limit of normal. Clearly, taking two standard deviations from the mean in both directions does not seem appropriate when illness produces changes in only one direction. Even when only one direction is considered, there is no firm basis for deciding to have a cutoff point at two standard deviations from the mean, or at the 95th percentile or the 99th percentile, to pick a few common examples.

Making such a decision would seem to require, in addition, a knowledge of how diseased persons score on the test, keeping in mind that a number of different diseases can cause the same abnormalities. The values for sick persons generally overlap to some degree the values for the healthy. Thus, there will be a gray zone in which a person's value has a reasonable chance of belonging either in the normal-healthy range or in the sick range. Where in this area is the best place to set the upper limit of normal? This question relates to the old problem of determining the sensitivity and specificity of a test. (See Chapters Three and Seventeen.) In the absence of a perfect test, some misclassification will always result, no matter where the decision level is set. If one wishes to make a test more sensitive, so as to detect as many sick individuals as possible, he can move the cutoff point further into the normal range. By doing so he will make the test less specific, so that many who are labeled as sick will be healthy. By shifting the level further into the sick range, he will be making the test more specific but will decrease the sensitivity or ability to detect all of the sick individuals.

Thus, the purpose for performing the test or the situation in which the test is used must enter into a decision to set the upper limit of normal at a given point. Consider uric acid, for example. The Kaiser-Permanente group has selected 8.0 mg percent as a cutoff point for males on the basis of the multiphasic screening experience. This relatively high value has served well as a level for screening. If the level were set much lower, say at 6.5 mg percent, the advantages of detecting a few more potential gout patients would be outweighed by an undesirable result. The Permanente physicians would see many individuals who were labeled as abnormal but for whom there would be little or no particular treatment or advice to offer.

Consider the uric acid level in another setting—this time an arthritis clinic. If a patient appears complaining of acute joint pain and the clinical picture does not permit clear distinction between gout and rheumatoid arthritis, a lower cutoff point may be more appropriate. Knowing that about 7 percent of persons with uric acid between 6.0 and 7.0 mg percent have or will soon develop gout and that far fewer of this group have rheumatoid arthritis, a value of 6.5 might be very suggestive of gout in the clinical circumstances described, whereas it would be much less so in a screening situation. Hence, the importance of considering the test situation is clear.

2. Normal Values from "Healthy" People

The availability of extensive data bases from large MHTS programs provides an opportunity to derive more reliable normal values by age, sex, and race, as is evident from the data presented in Section A.

In addition to analyzing the test results from all examinees who go through MHTS, one can use the test values from those who have been identified as being well and having no clinically significant abnormalities. For example, the physicians who reviewed the test results from the MHTS and provided a physical examination to the patient furnished to the MHTS a final diagnosis. The diagnosis "no significant abnormality" was used as a criterion for identifying well patients.[3]

The following groups of people, then, were analyzed with respect to their laboratory values:

(1) "All MHTS"—All persons examined in the multiphasic laboratory during the period of study, numbering 15,003 males and 18,926 females.

(2) "NSA-once"—Persons who had a doctor's diagnosis of "no significant abnormality": 3,920 males and 4,888 females.

(3) "NSA-twice"—Persons having at least two examinations during the period and who had a doctor's diagnosis of "no significant abnormality" on both examinations: 1,045 males and 1,350 females.

Age- and sex-specific means and standard deviations were computed for each group under study. The means for groups 2 and 3 were each compared to the means for group 1 (All-MHTS) using Student's t statistic to evaluate differences.

Table 19-20 shows the data for uric acid, which represented a good example of values differing significantly between well persons and all examinees. Not only were the mean values generally lower for the well groups, but the variability, as represented by the standard deviations, was also lower in almost all subgroups. Thus, the values derived from persons determined to be well should be more precise in identifying normal healthy people. If serial examinations are used to identify persons who are well over ten years and even longer, the range of normal values will probably be narrower and may serve to identify low-risk persons with high probability for longevity.[4]

C. HEALTH-HAZARD APPRAISAL AND COUNSELING

Health-hazard (risk-factor) appraisal as a motivating and counseling service has been recommended by Sadusk and Robbins,[1] Robbins and Hall,[2] Colburn and Baker,[3] and most recently by LaDou et al.[4]

The principle of such appraisal is simple. Information from various epidemiological studies on risk factors is brought to bear, in an individual counseling session, on a given patient for whom risk factors have just been determined. The 10-year mortality expectation is compared with that of a person without such factors. The display of this contrast, it has been argued, may strongly motivate a person to undertake the required changes of habit. Such attempt at risk-factor control might be more effective than educational approaches directed toward the general public or the traditional counseling of an individual at the time of a medical office visit.

At present, neither the effect on risk-factor control nor that on long-term outcome has been studied, if one disregards the findings of LaDou et al.[4], who failed to include a control group in their analysis. Nevertheless, common sense would suggest that avoidance of apparent hazards should be encouraged, even if the detailed experimental proof of benefits of intervention is still missing.

MHTS programs are ideally suited to health-hazard appraisal (HHA), since most of the required information is likely to be already included in the standard

Table 19-20. Uric Acid for White Persons, by Age, Sex, and Category of Population Studied*

Age	All MHC's			NSA-Once			NSA-Twice		
	No.	Mean	S.D.	No.	Mean	S.D.	No.	Mean	S.D.
				Males					
20–29	1,843	5.49	1.20	586	5.50	1.21	69	5.47	1.15
30–39	2,861	5.58	1.34	943	5.47§	1.23	196	5.49	1.20
40–49	3,958	5.61	1.31	1,152	5.52§	1.19	370	5.48†	1.24
50–59	3,656	5.65	1.36	857	5.52§	1.26	283	5.40§	1.18
60–69	2,039	5.66	1.39	314	5.39§	1.25	109	5.40†	1.25
70–79	676	5.82	1.48	68	5.84	1.47	18	5.71	1.02
Total	15,033	5.61	1.34	3,920	5.50	1.23	1,045	5.46	1.20
				Females					
20–29	3,016	3.93	0.96	1,003	3.87‡	0.93	103	3.68§	0.82
30–39	2,998	3.94	0.98	940	3.82§	0.84	211	3.95	0.82
40–49	4,732	4.09	1.06	1,292	3.96§	0.94	416	3.95§	0.82
50–59	4,638	4.42	1.18	1,063	4.18§	0.96	398	4.16	1.00
60–69	2,763	4.67	1.30	499	4.42§	1.13	189	4.31§	1.00
70–79	779	4.91	1.39	91	4.83	1.20	33	4.79	1.27
Total	18,926	4.24	1.15	4,888	4.02	0.97	1,350	4.06	0.98

*Modified from Cutler, et al.[3]
†$P < .05.$ ‡$P < .01.$ §$P < .001.$

test panels and questionnaire. Thus HHA service may well become a regular part of MHTS in the near future. Since cardiovascular conditions form the leading cause of death from middle age onwards and reliable information on 12-year coronary heart disease incidence is available from the Framingham Study,[5] at Kaiser-Permanente Oakland we have concentrated on the issue of appraising this hazard rapidly, so that the patient can be informed, at the conclusion of the multiphasic examination, and any counseling instituted promptly. Entering, into a small desk calculator programmed for the task, the patient's "relevant variables": sex, age, cholesterol, systolic blood pressure, relative weight, cigarette consumption, and EKG findings (the latter two in the appropriate Framingham code), one may at once obtain the 12-year risk of coronary heart disease for this patient, say *p,* from the "multivariate logistic" formula

$$\log \frac{p}{1 - p} = \alpha + \Sigma \, \beta_i x_i,$$

where α and β_i are the parameters estimated from the Framingham data[5] and x_i are the patient's values. We have performed these calculations on an unselected sample of recent multiphasic records and are impressed with the frequency in which high-risk patients (say, disease probability greater than 25 percent in the next 12 years) appear through this assessment. The patient's current risk, if high, would then be contrasted with a goal value—a risk computed with variables reasonably altered; e.g., "Suppose you would be 20 percent underweight rather than overweight." The difference between current and goal risk would constitute the potential benefit in return for cumbersome changes in life style. These "goal" values (however tentative they must be in view of our uncertainty on the issue of reversibility), would, at the same time, form the basis of a counseling program that would have to be set up for the individual patient. A variety of options exist, exercise and dietary prescriptions, with followup in shorter intervals or referrals to existing health maintenance clinics. To achieve consistency in decision making, these options would have to be formalized in procedural manuals.

The current enthusiasm for HHA is unlikely to sustain itself unless the activity can be shown to have at least a measurable effect on the risk-factor variables. This calls for an evaluation study in the form of a genuine clinical trial, contrasting the subsequent course of risk variables with that in control subjects who do not receive appraisal and counseling. Thus, some time will elapse until a judgment on the merits of HHA can be obtained.

D.   IDENTIFYING HIGH-RISK GROUPS AND OPTIMAL SCREENING INTERVALS

In the preceding section we have briefly outlined the identifying of high-risk groups with respect to coronary heart disease, with a view to screening out subgroups that may benefit from preventive counseling. More generally, one may ask what modifications should be introduced, if any, into the basic uniformity of a screening program. Breast cancer screening, for instance, has always been restricted to older females, other groups with markedly lower incidence giving rather low case finding rates. However, among the older females, epidemiological research has identified a number of factors (race, social class, reproductive history, relative weight, family history, and benign breast pathology) that individually raise the incidence by approximately a factor of two to three and jointly perhaps to much more than that. Should such women be identified and screened more intensively? Should, in general, high-risk groups be screened differently from low-risk ones, a policy that would lead to the principle of selective health testing? The case of breast cancer screening is suitable for quantitative arguments, which, in the absence of empirical information, must be theoretical in nature. To set up a fairly elementary model, we might take the following set of assumptions.

(1) The incidence of "preclinical" cancer identifiable by screening is uniformly distributed, with parameter $1/\beta$, over an interval that is a multiple of the screening interval M, measured in months. The incidence in that interval is thus $M(1/\beta)$.

(2) There is an exponential lag-time distribution, the lag time being the interval between the preclinical and the clinical phase, the latter characterized by symptoms leading to the "traditional" diagnosis of breast cancer. The parameter of the lag-time distribution is given by λ, so that $1/\lambda$ is the mean lag time.

Under these assumptions, y, the yield of cancer in a population screened in intervals of M, is, for this interval,

$$y = (1/\beta)(1/\lambda)(1 - e^{-\lambda M}),$$

giving the probability that a woman will be found (screen-detected) with cancer at the examination before the lag period is over. It should be noted that this lag time is generally longer than the lead time,[1,2] the period between screen discovery and the beginning of the clinical phase. Yield y rises, then, in the form of diminishing return, as M increases. Furthermore, F_M, the fraction of screen-discovered cases among all cases occurring in the interval M, is

$$F_M = \frac{y}{M(1/\beta)} = \frac{1/\lambda}{M}(1 - e^{-\lambda M}).$$

In those terms one may concisely define the purpose of screening as an effort of gaining lead time, with the expectation of effective preclinical intervention. Suppose now that an identifiable high-risk subgroup exists, with proportion f_1, having risk $1/\beta_1$; the remainder, $f_2 = 1 - f_1$, are of low risk with parameter $1/\beta_2$. Under these conditions the yield rate $\bar{y}$ is

$$\bar{y} = f_1 y_1 + f_2 y_2.$$

For instance, with a uniform yearly screening policy of $M_1 = M_2 = 12$ months one would obtain, with $1/\beta_1 = 16.7$ and $1/\beta_2 = 8.35$ per 100,000, corresponding to an annual incidence of $M(1/\beta_1) = 2$ per 1,000 and $M(1/\beta_2) = 1$ per 1,000 and with $1/\lambda = 20$ months, and $f_1 = 0.3$, $f_2 = 0.7$.

$$\bar{y} = (0.3 \times 151 + 0.7 \times 75)10^{-5} = 97.8 \times 10^{-5},$$

corresponding to

$$\bar{F}_M = \frac{\bar{y}}{f_1 M(1/\beta_1) + f_2 M(1/\beta_2)} = \frac{97.8}{130} = 0.75.$$

Thus, three-fourths of all cases with preclinical onset in the interval would be discovered on annual examinations, the remaining one-fourth coming to clinical recognition before the screening date.

Consider now an alternative policy that would screen the high-risk group every six months, while retaining the 12 months policy for the remainder. This would give

$$y = f_1 2 y_{1M_1} + f_2 y_{2M_2}$$

$$= (0.3 \times 2 \times 87 + 0.7 \times 75)10^{-5}$$

$$= 104.7 \times 10^{-5},$$

an increase of 7 percent over the previous value of 97.8. The subscripts M_1 and M_2 are attached to the y's, since the latter cover different periods of M. $\bar{F}_M$ would rise to 0.80.

One recognizes, of course, that this additional achievement of 7 percent is purchased by a considerable increase in cost. Under the uniform policy the average number of annual tests per person is

$$a = f_1 N_1 + f_2 N_2 = 1$$

where N_1 and N_2 are the numbers of examinations per person per year. For the alternative policy, however, we have $N_1 = 2$, $N_2 = 1$, thus $a = 1.3$. There is a cost increase of 30 percent. Of greater interest is the question of what selective screening policies could improve the value of $\bar{y}$ if cost were kept constant—that is to say, if, after we chose M_1 and thus N_1, N_2 were adjusted so that (2) continued to hold. For instance, with $M_1 = 6$, thus $N_1 = 2$, we have from (2)

$$N_2 = \frac{1 - f_1 N_1}{f_2} = 0.57.$$

This would mean that $M_2 = (1/N_2)12 = 21$, the low-risk group being screened only every 21 months. Thus, from (1), $y_2 = 108 \times 10^{-5}$, and since during the same period there would have been 3.5 examinations for the high-risk group,

$$\bar{y} = (0.3 \times 3.5 \times 87 + 0.7 \times 108)10^{-5} \frac{12}{21} = 95.4 \times 10^{-5},$$

the factor $\frac{12}{21}$ being used to make the yield comparable to the previous ones that related to a one-year period. We see that this policy, cost-equivalent with the indiscriminate annual screening policy, is slightly worse in annual yield, the spacing of the low-risk group being excessive. No advantage would be achieved with $M_1 = 8$, giving $N_1 = 1.5$, $N_2 = 0.78$, $M_2 = 15.3$, and $\bar{y} = 98 \times 10^{-5}$, equivalent in yield and cost with the indiscriminate annual screening policy.

The examples may suffice to demonstrate that selective screening policies directed towards high-risk groups, although intuitively appealing, may not necessarily result in spectacular gains.

E.   COMPUTER-AIDED DIAGNOSIS

Like health-hazard appraisal, MHTS appears to be well suited for any of the numerous variants of computer-aided diagnosis, in particular the nonsequential schemes, relying on a predetermined set of variables that have already been measured.[1-6]

In its most elementary form, computer-aided diagnosis may simply consist of comparing a given test value against a mean, or more commonly, against established "normal limits," proving thus a convenient tabulation of abnormalities for a given patient. This feature, commonly found in MHTS reports, is of considerable help in scanning the summary report. On a second level of complexity, so-called advice rules have come into use that single out patients with particular abnormalities or abnormality combinations for specific courses of action. The Kaiser-Permanente program, for instance, has provided critical one-hour serum glucose levels depending on age and hours since last food intake, a computer assuming the tedious task of looking up two-way tables for each patient and screening out "abnormals" for whom medical appointments have to be arranged. Similarly, a more advanced advice rule, selecting patients for immediate attention who are not only 25 percent above the critical level but have also positive urine sugar and acetone findings, replaces the need to visually scan reports for more complex patterns of abnormality.

The third level of workup data, while not yet in practice, has been considered at length. Without attempting differential-diagnostic detail, the procedure should scan a relevant variable set for each of the major categories of the current diagnosis check list and for each patient single out those categories for which the probability of a diagnosis is sufficiently high, say greater than 0.1. Several examples of such a technique have been given.[5-7] Work of this nature requires a fairly large data base unless one wants to take recourse to "subjective" probabilities elicited from experts.

For instance, if one considers, for a given disease such as diabetes, with a prevalence around 3 percent, some 26,000 records derived from one year of MHTS examinations, one obtains about 800 cases for study. It is advisable to split those into a "learning" and a "validation" sample, the latter being retained to demonstrate the performance characteristics (sensitivity and specificity) of any diagnostic decision rules derived from the study of the learning sample. Thus one would be left with some 400 cases from which to derive such rules. If, furthermore, as much as six dichotomized variables (yes-no answers to a questionnaire and positive-negative results from quantitative measurements) were considered, one would have $2^6 = 256$ possible patterns and thus expect to get information also on relatively rare pattern frequencies. It is also, of course, necessary to study nondiseased controls, at least on a sampling basis.

If pattern frequencies for both cases and controls have been established in this way, a probabilistic statement can be made, using Bayes' formula. For instance, if a given examinee has a certain pattern i with respect to variables used for the diagnosis of diabetes, and the frequency of such a pattern among cases is, say, $p_i = 0.6$, while among noncases it is $p_i' = 0.1$, then the probability of that person being a case is equal to

$$\frac{Pp_i}{Pp_i + (1 - P)p_i',}$$

where P is the disease prevalence in the population. With $P = 0.03$, the example would give a disease probability for this patient of 0.16, five times larger than the "unconditional" $P = 0.03$.

In this fashion, then, one could imagine a computerized workup of the patient, briefly listing the probability for each of some 10 to 20 diagnostic classes. Thus, the approach would merely provide an aid to clinicians rather than assuming their function, these probabilities simply stating in quantitative terms what the past "diagnostic behavior" has been with respect to patients with a given complex of findings. Nevertheless, schemes of this nature may also form the basis of vigorously followed decision rules, equivalent to the advice rules mentioned above, directing, for instance, nurse practitioners involved in physical examinations to undertake certain tasks such as retesting or referral, depending on critical values to be set for the Bayes probabilities. In most cases these critical values, now determinants of action concerning patient management, will remain somewhat arbitrary. Formalisms from the area of decision theory[5,8-11] may on occasion be useful in clarifying the value system implicit in alternative courses of action.

F. EPIDEMIOLOGICAL RESEARCH

Data from well-run MHTS programs may prove useful for epidemiologic research, since MHTS can provide extensive health-related data collected in a standardized fashion on large populations. The population to be studied may be one that has been specifically singled out for investigation and brought in for testing because of its unique characteristics. For example, the Kaiser-Permanente multiphasic program has been used to collect standardized data for an epidemiologic study of Japanese-Americans living in the San Francisco Bay Area,[1] and an earlier nonautomated multiphasic checkup was employed for a study of longshoremen.[2] The population studied, on the other hand, may be all of the users of a particular MHTS program.[3] In this case, it is important to determine and describe the population's characteristics and how it happened that the MHTS were provided. If several different reasons for receiving the MHTS were operating (e.g., invited for regular annual checukup vs. came in because of own desire for regular checkup vs. came in because of symptoms or illness), it may be most appropriate to include only one or some of these subgroups in an investigation.

All of the standard epidemiologic study designs—prevalence or cross-sectional, incidence or cohort, and case-control studies—may be used when MHTS data are employed. Each of these approaches will be described and illustrated briefly below.

1. Cross-Sectional Studies

Often one wishes to study the relation between particular attributes. When it seems reasonable that a single measurement of each attribute is adequate, then the findings at a single MHTS examination can be employed. For example, a question arose as to racial differences in serum glucose concentrations. We were able to show in an analysis of over 100,000 examinations that blacks had distinctly lower mean serum glucose levels one hour after a 75-gram oral glucose challenge than did members of the white or yellow races.[4] Similarly, we have related a variety of characteristics measured at these examinations to the patients' smoking habits.[5-8]

2. Cohort Studies

The study of longshoremen previously referred to is an example of a cohort study in which MHTS findings were related to a subsequent outcome in the same group of people. The outcomes usually studied in this manner are the development of one or more diseases, disability, and/or death. Thus, the investigator must have, in addition to the MHTS results, good sources of followup data to determine outcome. Careful surveillance of an identified cohort may require considerable additional data collection efforts.

Where the outcome can be adequately assessed from the MHTS findings, then repeated checkups can be the source of longitudinal followup data. In this way one can supplement findings concerning the cross-sectional relationship of one attribute to another and determine the relationship of *changes* in one attribute to *changes* in the other. Thus, in a primarily cross-sectional study of cigarette smoking and the leukocyte count,[5] we could add longitudinal data on what happens to smokers' leukocyte counts when they quit smoking by observing both smoking status and the count on two successive examinations. It must be remembered that persons with repeated examinations may differ from those with only one, on the basis of self-selection, just as persons with at least one examination may differ from those who have none. (See Chapter Eighteen.)

3. Case-Control Studies

Case-control comparisons can usefully employ MHTS data if a group of cases can be found who have had multiphasic checkups prior to disease development. Controls who have remained free of the disease are then selected from other examinees. The MHTS data must, of course, contain at least some of the variables that one desires to study. MHTS variables can also be used to match controls with the cases if such matching is desired. For example, we were able to conduct a case-control study of myocardial infarction in which members of one of the control groups were matched to the cases for seven different coronary risk factor measurements as well as age, sex, and race. The presence of computer-stored data from about one-quarter million examinations on about 120,000 people made possible the successful matching on this large number of variables.[9]

In choosing between the cohort and case-control methods for studies based on MHTS data, the advantages and disadvantages of each method must be weighed. The cohort approach will permit the direct measurement of risk of disease development in relation to the attributes measured by MHTS and will facilitate the ascertainment of a variety of disease outcomes, including those not originally planned on for study. The case-control approach is simpler and cheaper, since the often laborious and expensive followup efforts for the entire cohort are not required. However, it will yield only measurements of relative, not absolute, risk associated with attributes. The use of standardized MHTS data collected before disease development does overcome a potential bias of case-control studies—that the presence of disease will modify persons' attributes or affect the recollection of past characteristics or events. Being reasonably quick and economical, the case-control method is also well suited for exploratory studies (fishing expeditions) in which a variety of MHTS data are tested for association with a disease in the hope of finding previously unknown predictors or causative factors.[9,10]

4. Problems with MHTS Data

MHTS programs are usually set up with the primary goal of contributing to health care. Therefore neither the scope nor manner of data collection may satisfy the needs of a particular research project for which the MHTS findings are to be used. Here we have a variant of the old problem of trying to use data for a purpose for which they were not originally collected. For example, one may wish to have blood sugar levels determined in the fasting state and find that the MHTS program was set up to collect random sugars. Changes in procedure (e.g., from random to fasting) must also be of concern. Even if it is known that such a change has taken place, it may be difficult to find documentation of the exact date when the instructions to the patients were changed. Questionnaire items may not be stated in just the manner that is desired by the researcher. For example, in our study of myocardial infarction[9] we would have preferred that the duration categories for usual daily physical activity be narrower, since, with the category of 0–1 hour, we could not distinguish between persons getting no regular exercise and those exercising one hour daily. And, of course, particular data essential for an investigation may not have been included at all. Extra efforts may then be required to collect these items if one is to study the MHTS examinees.

5. Health-Care Studies Involving MHTS

Difficult to separate from epidemiologic studies are evaluative studies of health care systems. These may involve health care systems of which MHTS is a part, an MHTS program itself, or portions or modifications of MHTS programs. The principles and methods underlying these studies are discussed in Chapter Eighteen.

REFERENCES (A., B.)

1. Friedman, G. D. *Primer of Epidemiology,* pp. 191–194. New York: McGraw-Hill, 1974.
2. Friedman, G. D. "An Epidemiologist's Assessment of the Reported Laboratory Findings." *Proceedings of Technicon International Congress,* Chicago, June 1969.
3. Cutler, J. L., Collen, M. F., Siegelaub, A. B., and Feldman, R. "Normal Values for Multiphasic Screening Blood Chemistry Tests." *Proceedings of Technicon International Congress,* Chicago, June 1969; and "Determination of Normal Values for Blood Chemistry Tests." *Bull. College of Am. Pathologists,* October 1969, pp. 319–326.
4. Collen, M. F., Siegelaub, A. B., Cutler, J. L., and Goldberg, R. "Aspects of Normal Values in Medicine." *Ann. N.Y. Acad. Sci.* 161(1969):572–580.

REFERENCES (C.)

1. Sadusk, J. F., and Robbins, L. C. "Proposal for Health-Hazard Appraisal in Comprehensive Health Care." *J.A.M.A.* 203(1968):1108–1110.
2. Robbins, L. C., and Hall, J. H. *How to Practice Prospective Medicine.* Methodist Hospital of Indiana, 1970.
3. Colburn, H. N.. and Baker, P. M. "Health Hazard Appraisal in Patient Counseling." *Can. J. Pub. Health* 64(1973):490–492.
4. LaDou, J., Sherwood, J. N., and Hughes, L. "Health Hazard Appraisal in Patient Counseling." *West. J. Med.* 122(1975):177–180.
5. Truett, J., Cornfield, J., and Kannel, W. "A Multivariate Analysis of the Risk of Coronary Heart Disease in Framingham." *J. Chronic Dis.* 20(1967):511–524.

REFERENCES (D.)

1. Hutchison, G. B., and Shapiro, S. "Lead Time Gained by Diagnostic Screening for Breast Cancer." *J. Natl. Cancer Inst.* 41(1968):665–681.
2. Feinleib, M., and Zelen, M. "Some Pitfalls in the Evaluation of Screening Programs." *Arch. Environ. Health* 19(1969):412–415.

REFERENCES (E.)

1. Collen, M. F., Rubin, L., Neyman, J., Dantzig, G. B., Baer, R. M., and Siegelaub, A. B. "Automated Multiphasic Screening and Diagnosis." *Am. J. Pub. Health* 54(1964):741–750.
2. Brodman, K., and van Woerkom, A. J. "Computer-Aided Diagnostic Screening for 100 Common Diseases." *J.A.M.A.* 197(1966):901–905.
3. Van Woerkom, A. J., and Brodman, K. "Statistics for a Diagnostic Model." *Biometrics* 17(1961):299–318.
4. Rubin, L., Collen, M. F., and Goldman, G. E. "Frequency Decision Theoretical Approach to Automated Medical Diagnosis." *Proc. Fifth Berkeley Symp. Math. Stat. Prob.*, Vol. IV, pp. 867–886. Berkeley: Univ. of Calif. Press, 1967.
5. Kodlin, D., and Collen, M. F. "Automated Diagnosis in Multiphasic Screening." In *Proc. Sixth Berkeley Symp. Math. Stat. Prob.*, Vol. IV, pp. 15–23. Berkeley: Univ. of Calif. Press, 1971.
6. Gleser, M. A., and Collen, M. F. "Towards Automated Medical Diagnosis." *Comp. Biomed. Res.* 5(1972):180–189.
7. Kodlin, D. "Two Studies on Automated Diagnosis." In *Automated Multiphasic Health Testing*. New York: Engineering Foundation, 1971.
8. Gory, G. A., and Barnett, G. O. "Experience with a Model of Sequential Diagnosis." *Comp. Biomed. Res.* 1(1968):490–507.
9. Flagle, C. D. "A Decision Theoretical Comparison of Three Procedures of Screening for a Single Disease." In *Proc. Fifth Berkeley Symp. Math. Stat. Prob.*, Vol. IV, pp. 887–901. Berkeley: Univ. of Calif. Press, 1967.
10. Lusted, L. B. "Decision-Making Studies in Patient Management." *N. Eng. J. Med.* 284(1971):416–424.
11. Kodlin, D. "A Note on the Cost-Benefit Problem in Screening for Breast Cancer." *Methods Inform. Med.* 11(1972):242–247.

REFERENCES (F.)

1. Kagan, A., Harris, B., Winkelstein, W., Johnson, K. G., Kato, H., Syme, S. L., Rhoads, G. G., Gay, M. L., Nichaman, M. Z., Hamilton, H. B., and Tillotson, J. "Epidemiologic Studies of Coronary Heart Disease and Stroke in Japanese Men Living in Japan, Hawaii, and California: Demographic, Physical, Dietary and Biochemical Characteristics." *J. Chron. Dis.* 27(1974):345–364.
2. Paffenbarger, R., and Hale, W. E. "Work Activity and Coronary Heart Mortality." *N. Eng. J. Med.* 292(1975):545–550.
3. Friedman, G. D., Seltzer, C. C., Siegelaub, A. B., Feldman, R., and Collen, M. F. "Smoking Among White, Black, and Yellow Men and Women: Kaiser-Permanente Multiphasic Health Examination Data, 1964-1968." *Am. J. Epidemiol.* 96(1972):23–35.
4. Dales, L. G., Siegelaub, A. B., Feldman, R., Friedman, G. D., Seltzer, C. C., and Collen, M. F. "Racial Differences in Serum and Urine Glucose After Glucose Challenge." *Diabetes* 23(1974):327–332.
5. Friedman, G. D., Siegelaub, A. B., Seltzer, C. C., Feldman, R., and Collen, M. F. "Smoking Habits and the Leukocyte Count." *Arch. Environ. Health* 26(1973):137–143.

6. Friedman, G. D., Siegelaub, A. B., and Seltzer, C. C. "Cigarette Smoking and Exposure to Occupational Hazards." *Am. J. Epidemiol.* 98(1973):175–183.

7. Seltzer, C. C., Friedman, G. D., and Siegelaub, A. B. "Smoking and Drug Consumption in White, Black, and Oriental Men and Women." *Am. J. Public Health* 64(1974):466–473.

8. Friedman, G. D., Siegelaub, A. B., and Dales, L. G. "Cigarette Smoking and Chest Pain." *Ann. Intern. Med.* 83(1975):1–7.

9. Friedman, G. D., Klatsky, A. L., Siegelaub, A. B., and McCarthy, N. M. "Kaiser-Permanente Epidemiologic Study of Myocardial Infarction: Study Design and Results for Standard Risk Factors." *Am. J. Epidemiol.* 99(1974):101–116.

10. Friedman, G. D., Klatsky, A. L., Siegelaub, A. B. "Predictors of Sudden Cardiac Death." *Circulation* 51–52, Suppl. III(1975):164–169.

CHAPTER TWENTY

Standard Procedures for MHTS

Michael D. Gahar, Vicki Surdez, & James Duncan

A. Introduction
B. Operations Manual for MHTS Stations

A. INTRODUCTION

It is very important for an operating MHTS to have a standard procedures manual that includes detailed expert instructions as to methods and procedures for personnel for each testing phase (or station). The purpose is to tell all MHTS personnel exactly what is to be done at each station, thus helping to insure a uniform standard of quality of testing and a reproducibility of measurements through time. Those pages of the operations manual that apply to each testing phase should be prominently posted in each station for continual reference by the technicians.

Standardization of procedures does not in itself guarantee uniformity of accomplishment. Standard procedures should be established for man-machine operations once the best methods for accomplishing the objectives of the operations have been determined. An operation that does not involve equipment also requires an operations manual to insure continuity and uniformity of methods.

This chapter contains the Standard Procedures Manual for Kaiser-Permanente Oakland Automated Multiphasic Health Testing (AMHT) as of 1976. (See also Chapter One, F.) The format of the manual, for most of the stations (phases), is as follows:

(1) Brief description of the station's function.
(2) Information process chart for data cards for the station.
(3) Process flow chart for patients, specimens, and data for the station.
(4) The test data cards associated with the station.

Station 14, Health Evaluation Section (HES), does not detail the actual methods used by the medical nurse practitioner (MNP), but rather shows flow charts that depict the flow and interaction of patients in the system.

When new testing equipment has been tested and installed, or when new methods are approved, the standard procedures manual is changed. The method for initiating, approving, and installing new procedures is important. A System Modification Request (SMR), discussed in Chapter Five, illustrates one method for handling such a situation.

The charts shown herein are those posted in each of the AMHT stations. The locations of the fifteen stations are shown in Figure 20-1. The preappointment processing function is identified as Station 0.

B. OPERATIONS MANUAL FOR MHTS STATIONS

Station 0. Preappointment Processing

As shown in Figure 20-2, the computer center prepares preprinted appointment cards for each month by punching and interpreting an appointment date and time on each card. The cards (arranged in time and date order) are sent to Central Appointments. Upon receiving a phone call from a patient requesting a multiphasic, the appointment clerk pulls an appointment card (Figure 20-3) bearing a date and time agreeable to the patient. The clerk completes the appointment card by entering the required information. Completed appointment cards are batched and sent back to the computer center. A header card (Figure 20-4) is punched for each appointment card. When the header cards have been punched, the appointment cards are sent to Central Appointments, which, in turn, mails the appointment card with an instruction sheet to the patient. The header cards are used as the data source in the preparation of labels, pre-lists for the day's appointments, and patient card packs.

Station 1.   Registration for Multiphasic Testing

The registration phase prepares patients to proceed and complete the multiphasic testing. The appropriate forms are prepared and fees collected. The forms and correct patient card pack are placed on a clipboard and given to the patient, who is then directed to the next test phase. Figure 20-5 is a chart diagramming the functions of Station 1, and Figures 20-6a to d are flow charts detailing all procedural steps. (See also Figure 1-15.)

Station 2.   Blood Drawing

The patient arrives at the AMHT laboratory to have blood samples drawn by venipuncture using standard aseptic technique. In accordance with Figures 20-7 and 20-8, after a successful venipuncture the following disposable vacutainer tubes are filled: (1) one lavender top, 3204QS (containing versene anticoagulant for hematology); (2) one large red top, 3218 (for chemistry and VDRL). These tubes are labeled with computer-prepared labels having the following identification data: patient's name, medical record number, code and group, birthdate and sex. The Simplex patient accession number is handwritten on all labels after the blood specimen drawing-processing cycle. After the blood is drawn, a Band-Aid is applied and the patient is instructed to apply pressure to the venipuncture site for five minutes. The AMHT lab cards (Figures 20-9 and 20-10) are assembled with each patient's blood specimens.

Station 3.   Urine Testing

Patients, while in the AMHT laboratory area, are instructed in providing a urine specimen following the blood drawing procedure: the patient's urine is collected and tested for glucose, protein, pH, and hemoglobin using Hema-Combistix reagent strips (Figures 20-11 and 20-12). If glucose is positive with Hema-Combistix, the following are both completed: (1) urine is tested with Clinitest and reported on the test report card (Figure 20-13) as 0, 1+, 2+, 3+, or 4+ by comparing closely to the standard color chart with good lighting; (2) urine is tested for acetone with Keto-stix strips and reported as 0 or +. (See also Figure 1-17.)

Station 4.   Dressing Rooms

Patients prepare themselves for further testing by partially undressing and putting on a disposable gown (Figure 20-14). (Female patients should remove girdles and bras.) (See also Figure 1-18.)

Testing stations that require that patients wear gowns are 5 (electrocardiogram), 6 (height and weight), 7 (chest x-ray), and 8 (mammography).

Male patients and those female patients who are not eligible for mammography

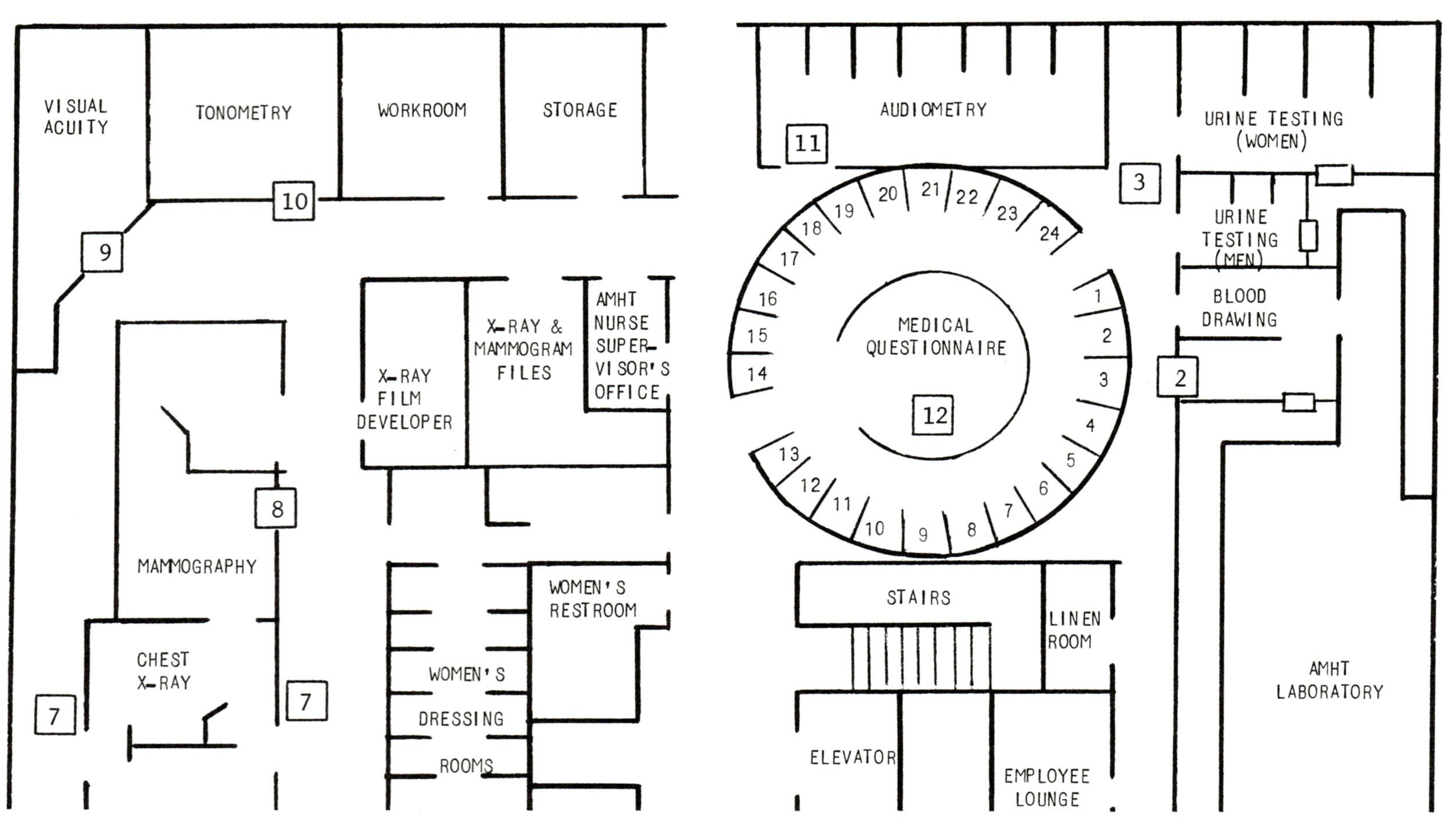

VISUAL ACUITY
TONOMETRY
WORKROOM
STORAGE
AUDIOMETRY
11
URINE TESTING (WOMEN)
3
URINE TESTING (MEN)
BLOOD DRAWING
2
10
9
X-RAY FILM DEVELOPER
X-RAY & MAMMOGRAM FILES
AMHT NURSE SUPER- VISOR'S OFFICE
MEDICAL QUESTIONNAIRE
12
1
2
3
4
5
6
7
8
9
10
11
12
13
14
15
16
17
18
19
20
21
22
23
24
8
MAMMOGRAPHY
WOMEN'S RESTROOM
WOMEN'S DRESSING ROOMS
STAIRS
LINEN ROOM
AMHT LABORATORY
CHEST X-RAY
7
7
ELEVATOR
EMPLOYEE LOUNGE

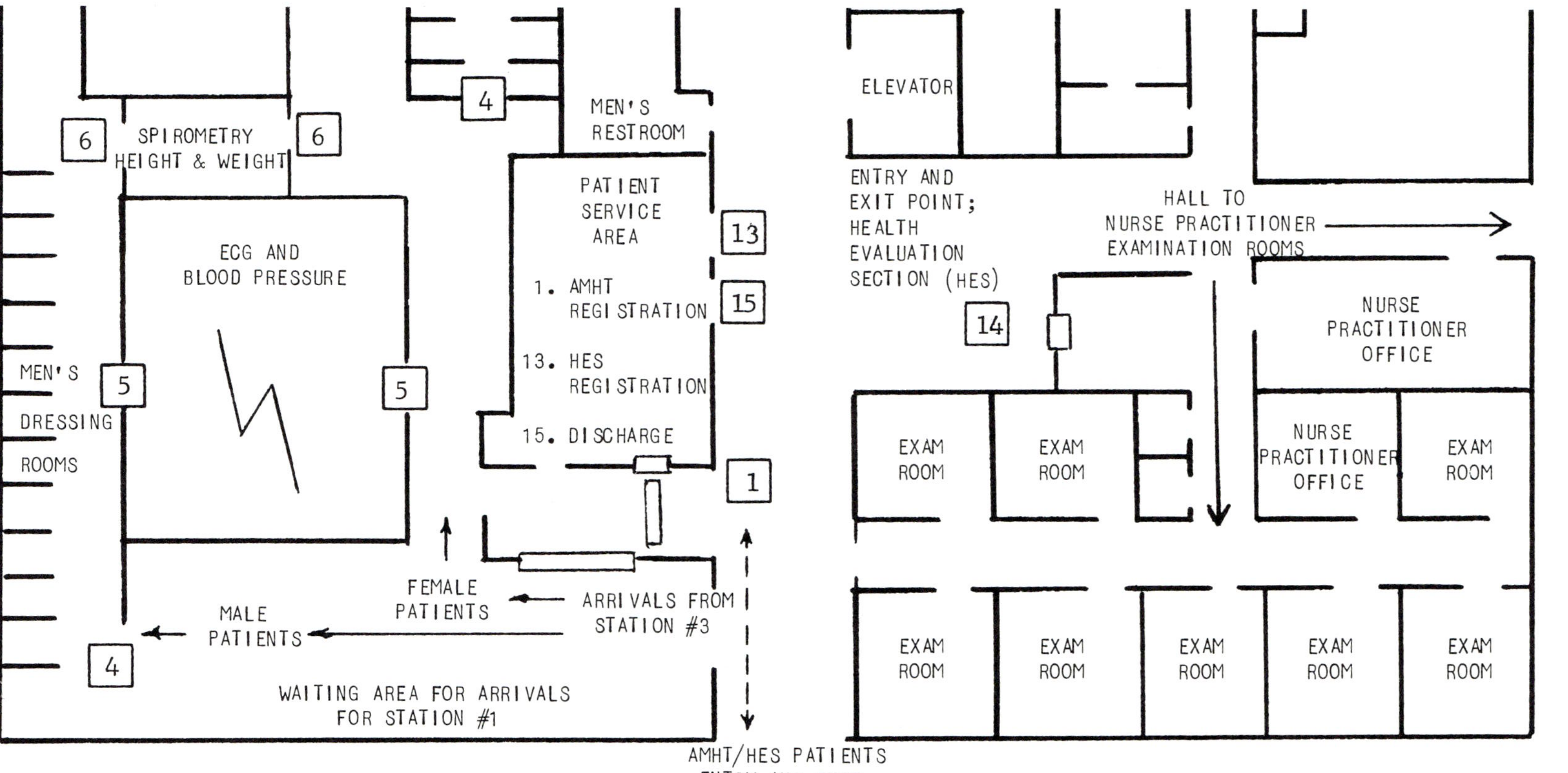

Figure 20-1. Location of Station 1 through 15 in Oakland Automated Multiphasic Health Testing (AMHT) including nurse practitioner Health Evaluation Section (HES).

589

CHART O - 1976

PRE-APPT PROCESSING

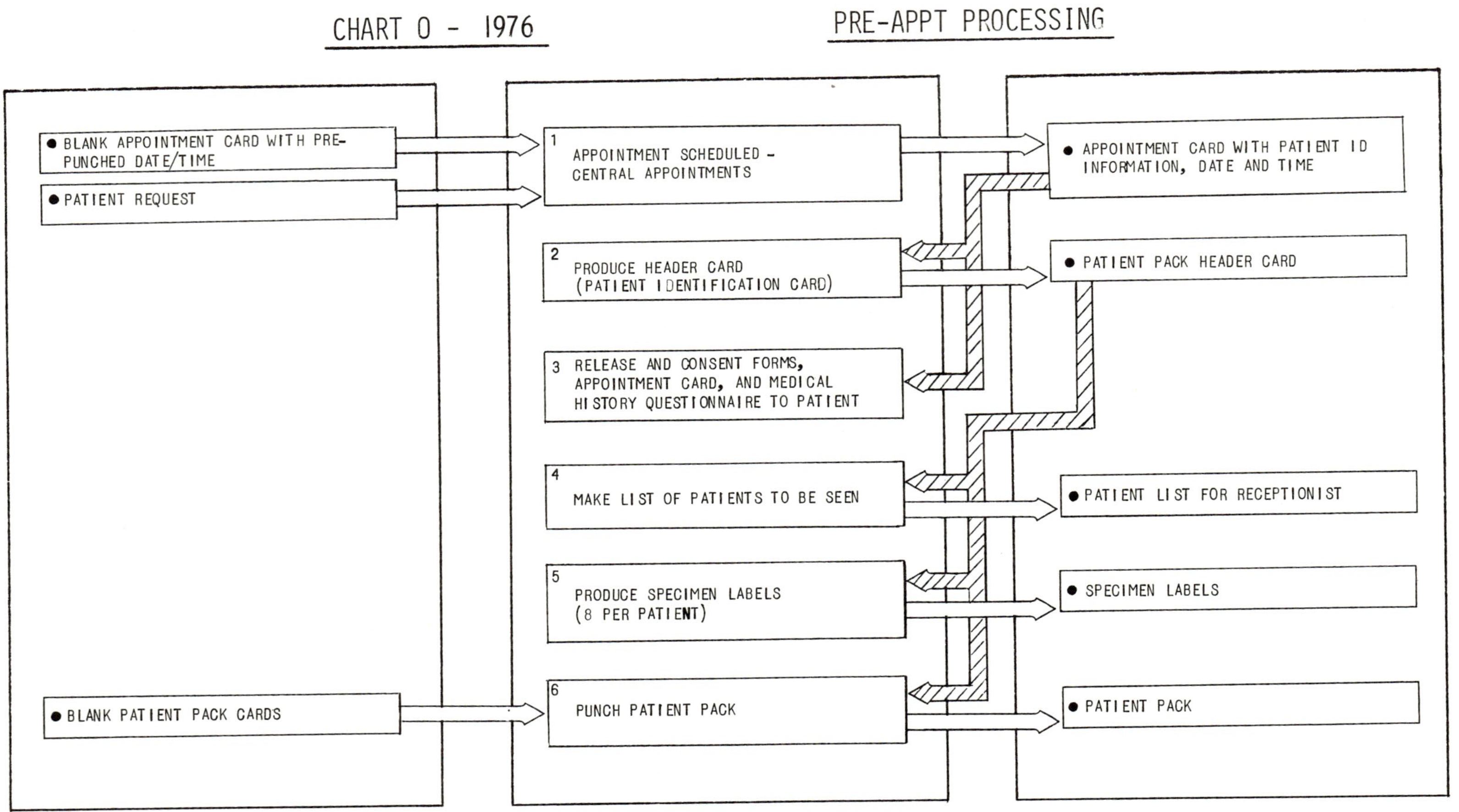

Figure 20-2. Information chart for the preappointment procedures.

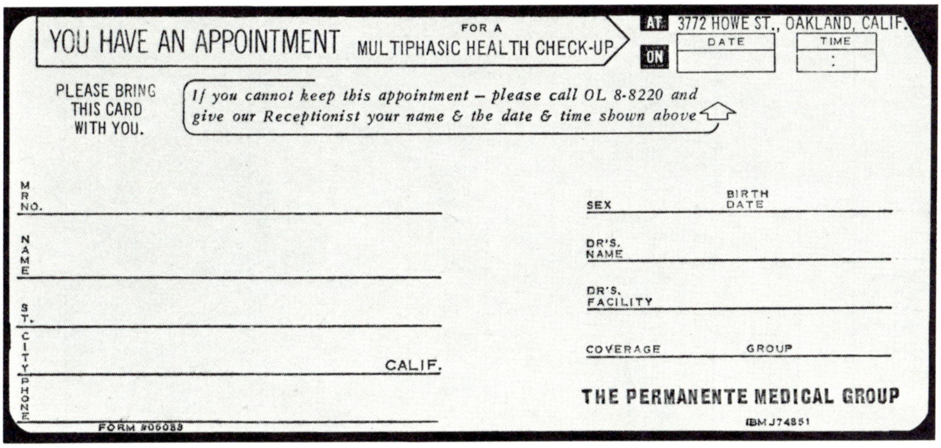
YOU HAVE AN APPOINTMENT
FOR A MULTIPHASIC HEALTH CHECK-UP
AT 3772 HOWE ST., OAKLAND, CALIF.
ON
DATE
TIME
PLEASE BRING THIS CARD WITH YOU.
If you cannot keep this appointment – please call OL 8-8220 and give our Receptionist your name & the date & time shown above
M R NO.
NAME
ST.
CITY
CALIF.
PHONE
SEX
BIRTH DATE
DR'S. NAME
DR'S. FACILITY
COVERAGE
GROUP
THE PERMANENTE MEDICAL GROUP
FORM #06088
IBM J74851

Figure 20-3. Appointment card used for booking of appointments and for generating header card. Five different card colors represent the five days of the week.

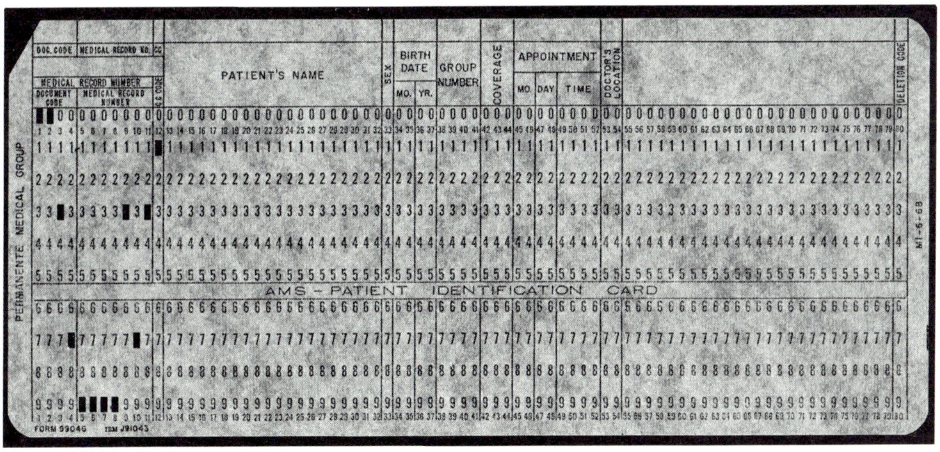
DOC. CODE
MEDICAL RECORD NO.
MEDICAL RECORD NUMBER
PATIENT'S NAME
SEX
BIRTH DATE
MO.
YR.
GROUP NUMBER
COVERAGE
APPOINTMENT
MO.
DAY
TIME
DOCTOR'S LOCATION
DELETION CODE
PERMANENTE MEDICAL GROUP
AMS – PATIENT IDENTIFICATION CARD
FORM 99046

Figure 20-4. Header card containing identifying data used for generating appointment listings.

return to their dressing rooms after completing testing at Stations 5, 6, and 7, re-dress, and are instructed to proceed to Station 9 for visual acuity testing. Female patients requiring mammography return to the dressing rooms after completing testing at Stations 5, 6, 7, and 8 (mammography), re-dress, and are instructed to proceed to Station 9 for visual acuity testing.

Station 5. Electrocardiography and Blood Pressure

Patients arrive wearing paper gowns for electrocardiogram recording. The nine leads (I, II, III, AVR, AVL, AVF, V1, V3, V5) are recorded simultaneously (Figures 20-15 and 20-16). In the event the nine-lead machine is inoperative, a lead I strip is taken with a stand-by machine, and the Electrocardiogram Report card (Figure 20-17) is marked "Lead I only." (See Figure 1-19.)

CHART 1 – 1976

REGISTRATION FOR AMHT

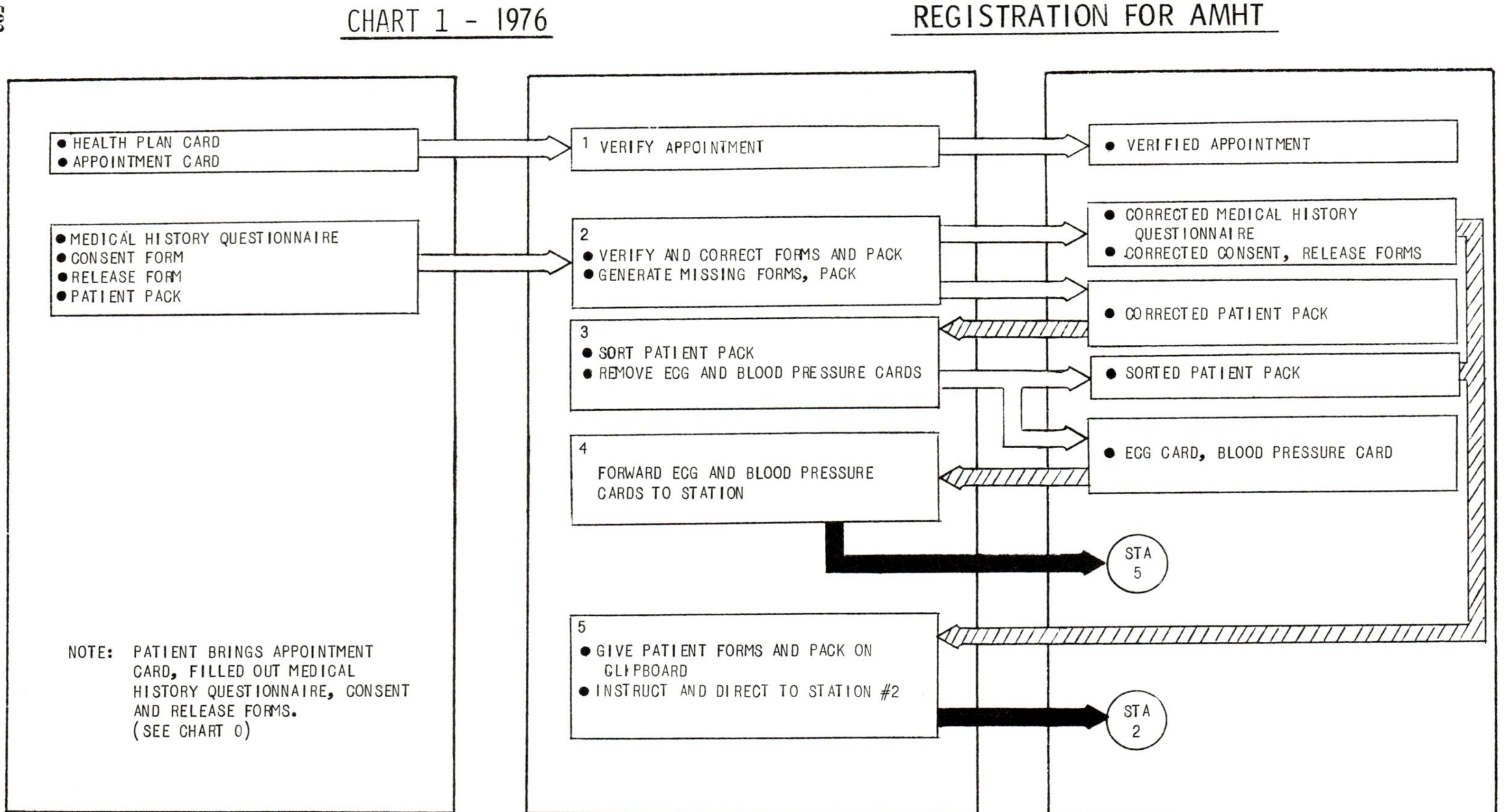

Figure 20-5. Information chart for the registration procedure at Station 1.

STATION 1 - REGISTRATION FOR MULTIPHASIC TESTING

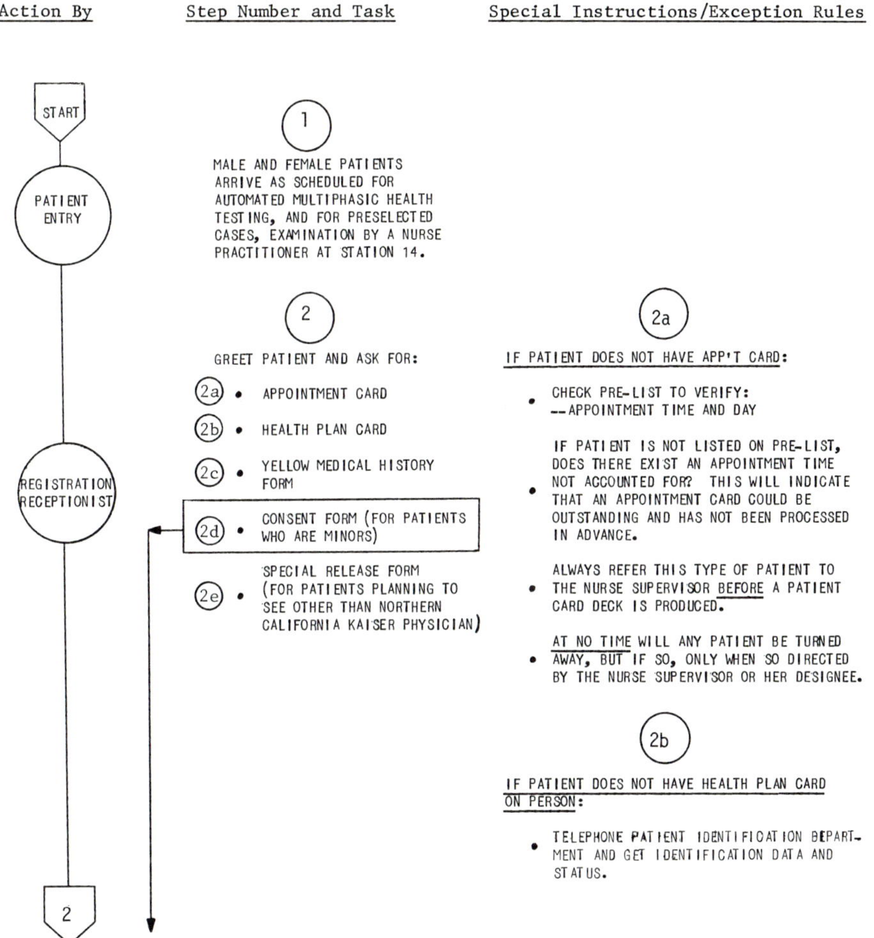

Figure 20-6a. Flow chart for registration for multiphasic testing.

Systolic and diastolic blood pressure readings are obtained and punched automatically into the card (Figure 20-18). (See also Figure 1-20.) Manual measurements are taken in the event of equipment malfunction and punched manually.

Station 6.   Spirometry and Anthropometry

Patients arrive wearing paper gowns to have height, weight, and spirometry measures taken and recorded (Figures 20-19 and 20-20). Height and weight are keypunched into the card (Figure 20-21) by the test operator to the nearest half-pound and tenth of an inch, respectively.

The patient is instructed and encouraged to blow as hard and as fast as possible to yield the spirometry values, which include peak flow, forced expiratory volume for one and two seconds, and vital capacity. The values are punched automatically (Figure 20-21) and a maximum of three test efforts can be recorded. (See also Figure 1-21.)

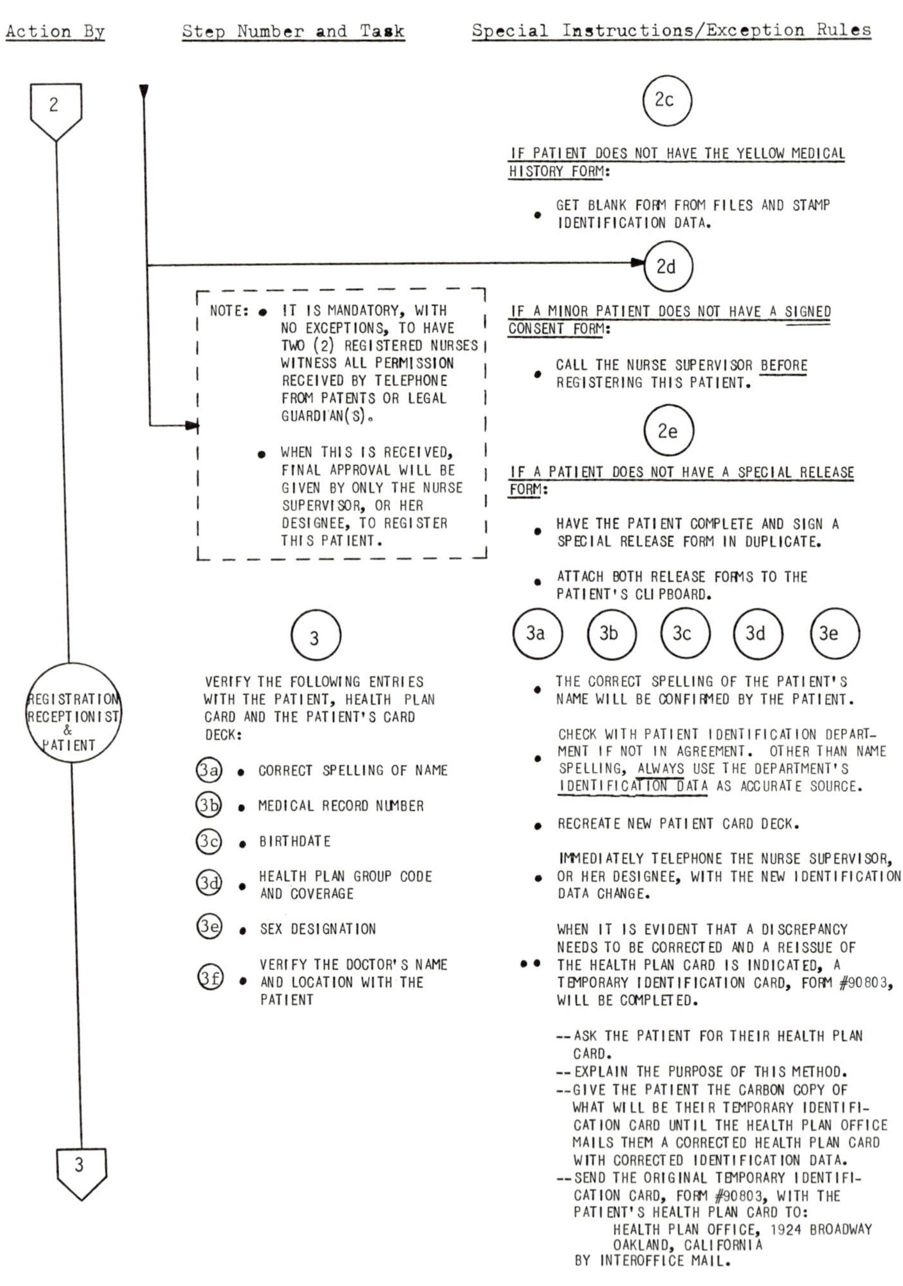
2

2c

IF PATIENT DOES NOT HAVE THE YELLOW MEDICAL HISTORY FORM:

• GET BLANK FORM FROM FILES AND STAMP IDENTIFICATION DATA.

2d

IF A MINOR PATIENT DOES NOT HAVE A SIGNED CONSENT FORM:

• CALL THE NURSE SUPERVISOR BEFORE REGISTERING THIS PATIENT.

2e

IF A PATIENT DOES NOT HAVE A SPECIAL RELEASE FORM:

• HAVE THE PATIENT COMPLETE AND SIGN A SPECIAL RELEASE FORM IN DUPLICATE.

• ATTACH BOTH RELEASE FORMS TO THE PATIENT'S CLIPBOARD.

NOTE: • IT IS MANDATORY, WITH NO EXCEPTIONS, TO HAVE TWO (2) REGISTERED NURSES WITNESS ALL PERMISSION RECEIVED BY TELEPHONE FROM PATENTS OR LEGAL GUARDIAN(S).

• WHEN THIS IS RECEIVED, FINAL APPROVAL WILL BE GIVEN BY ONLY THE NURSE SUPERVISOR, OR HER DESIGNEE, TO REGISTER THIS PATIENT.

3a 3b 3c 3d 3e

• THE CORRECT SPELLING OF THE PATIENT'S NAME WILL BE CONFIRMED BY THE PATIENT.

CHECK WITH PATIENT IDENTIFICATION DEPARTMENT IF NOT IN AGREEMENT. OTHER THAN NAME SPELLING, ALWAYS USE THE DEPARTMENT'S IDENTIFICATION DATA AS ACCURATE SOURCE.

• RECREATE NEW PATIENT CARD DECK.

• IMMEDIATELY TELEPHONE THE NURSE SUPERVISOR, OR HER DESIGNEE, WITH THE NEW IDENTIFICATION DATA CHANGE.

•• WHEN IT IS EVIDENT THAT A DISCREPANCY NEEDS TO BE CORRECTED AND A REISSUE OF THE HEALTH PLAN CARD IS INDICATED, A TEMPORARY IDENTIFICATION CARD, FORM #90803, WILL BE COMPLETED.

--ASK THE PATIENT FOR THEIR HEALTH PLAN CARD.
--EXPLAIN THE PURPOSE OF THIS METHOD.
--GIVE THE PATIENT THE CARBON COPY OF WHAT WILL BE THEIR TEMPORARY IDENTIFI-CATION CARD UNTIL THE HEALTH PLAN OFFICE MAILS THEM A CORRECTED HEALTH PLAN CARD WITH CORRECTED IDENTIFICATION DATA.
--SEND THE ORIGINAL TEMPORARY IDENTIFI-CATION CARD, FORM #90803, WITH THE PATIENT'S HEALTH PLAN CARD TO:
HEALTH PLAN OFFICE, 1924 BROADWAY OAKLAND, CALIFORNIA
BY INTEROFFICE MAIL.

REGISTRATION RECEPTIONIST & PATIENT

3

VERIFY THE FOLLOWING ENTRIES WITH THE PATIENT, HEALTH PLAN CARD AND THE PATIENT'S CARD DECK:

3a • CORRECT SPELLING OF NAME

3b • MEDICAL RECORD NUMBER

3c • BIRTHDATE

3d • HEALTH PLAN GROUP CODE AND COVERAGE

3e • SEX DESIGNATION

3f • VERIFY THE DOCTOR'S NAME AND LOCATION WITH THE PATIENT

3

Figure 20-6b.

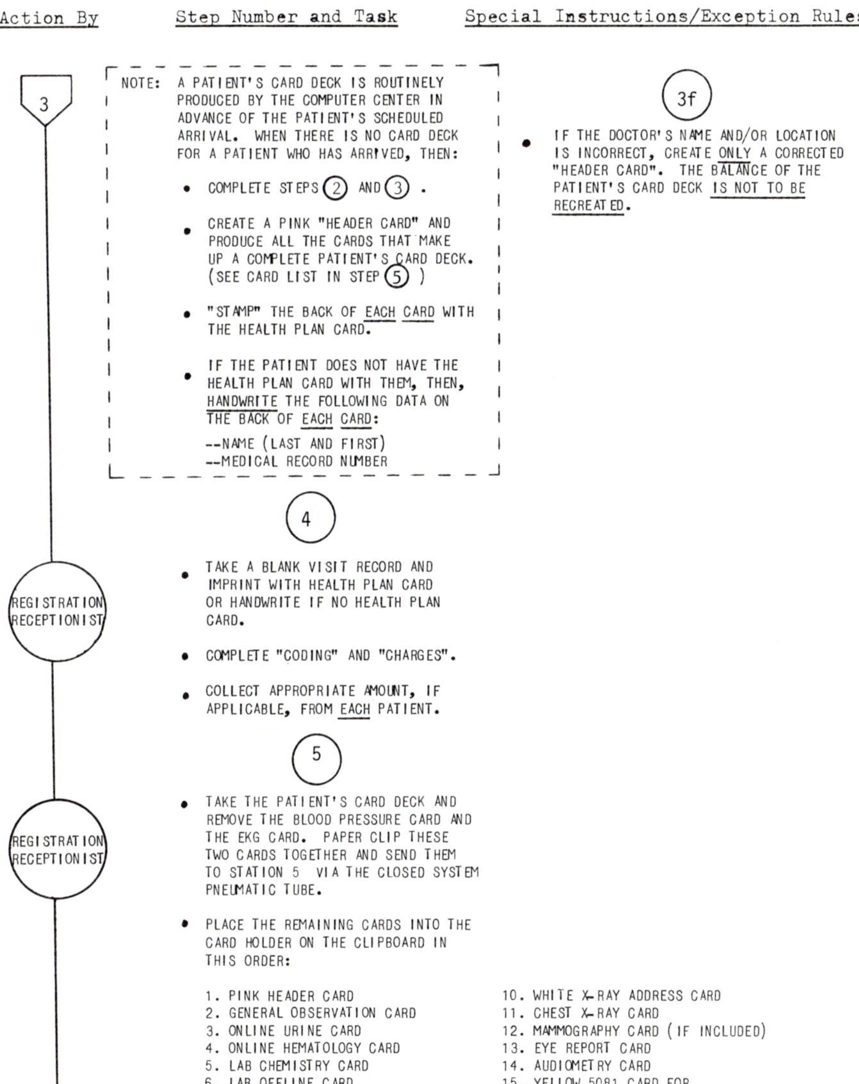

3

NOTE: A PATIENT'S CARD DECK IS ROUTINELY
PRODUCED BY THE COMPUTER CENTER IN
ADVANCE OF THE PATIENT'S SCHEDULED
ARRIVAL. WHEN THERE IS NO CARD DECK
FOR A PATIENT WHO HAS ARRIVED, THEN:

• COMPLETE STEPS 2 AND 3 .

• CREATE A PINK "HEADER CARD" AND
PRODUCE ALL THE CARDS THAT MAKE
UP A COMPLETE PATIENT'S CARD DECK.
(SEE CARD LIST IN STEP 5)

• "STAMP" THE BACK OF EACH CARD WITH
THE HEALTH PLAN CARD.

• IF THE PATIENT DOES NOT HAVE THE
HEALTH PLAN CARD WITH THEM, THEN,
HANDWRITE THE FOLLOWING DATA ON
THE BACK OF EACH CARD:
--NAME (LAST AND FIRST)
--MEDICAL RECORD NUMBER

3f

• IF THE DOCTOR'S NAME AND/OR LOCATION
IS INCORRECT, CREATE ONLY A CORRECTED
"HEADER CARD". THE BALANCE OF THE
PATIENT'S CARD DECK IS NOT TO BE
RECREATED.

4

REGISTRATION
RECEPTIONIST

• TAKE A BLANK VISIT RECORD AND
IMPRINT WITH HEALTH PLAN CARD
OR HANDWRITE IF NO HEALTH PLAN
CARD.

• COMPLETE "CODING" AND "CHARGES".

• COLLECT APPROPRIATE AMOUNT, IF
APPLICABLE, FROM EACH PATIENT.

5

REGISTRATION
RECEPTIONIST

• TAKE THE PATIENT'S CARD DECK AND
REMOVE THE BLOOD PRESSURE CARD AND
THE EKG CARD. PAPER CLIP THESE
TWO CARDS TOGETHER AND SEND THEM
TO STATION 5 VIA THE CLOSED SYSTEM
PNEUMATIC TUBE.

• PLACE THE REMAINING CARDS INTO THE
CARD HOLDER ON THE CLIPBOARD IN
THIS ORDER:

1. PINK HEADER CARD
2. GENERAL OBSERVATION CARD
3. ONLINE URINE CARD
4. ONLINE HEMATOLOGY CARD
5. LAB CHEMISTRY CARD
6. LAB OFFLINE CARD
7. SPIROMETRY/ANTHROPOMETRY CARD
8. ORANGE ADDRESS CARD
9. RECEPTIONIST'S CARD

10. WHITE X-RAY ADDRESS CARD
11. CHEST X-RAY CARD
12. MAMMOGRAPHY CARD (IF INCLUDED)
13. EYE REPORT CARD
14. AUDIOMETRY CARD
15. YELLOW 5081 CARD FOR
MEDICAL QUESTIONNAIRE BOX.

4

Figure 20-6c.

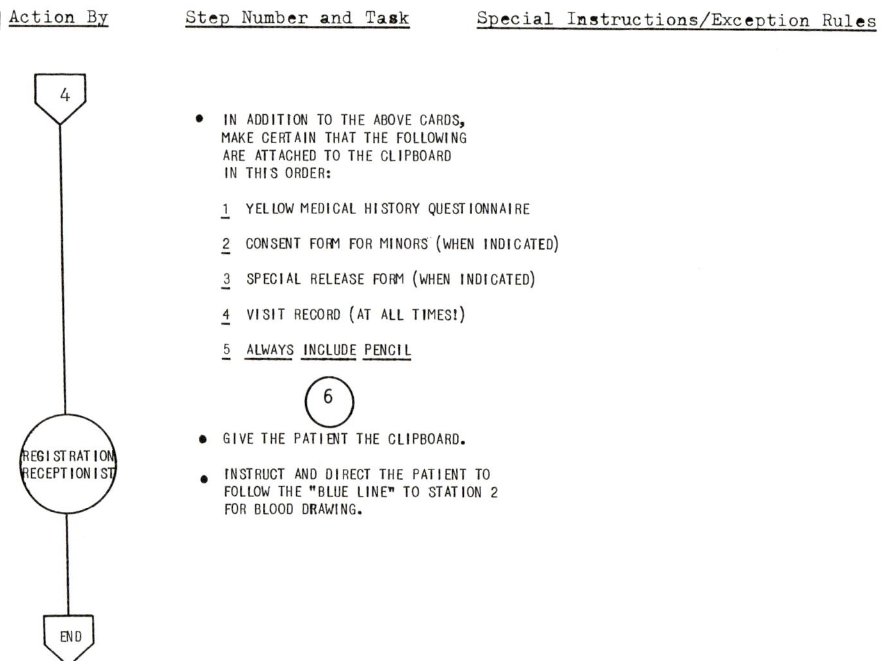

Figure 20-6d.

7. Chest X-Ray Procedure

Patients arrive wearing paper gowns and a 70 mm posterior-anterior chest roentgenogram is obtained (Figures 20-22 and 20-23). Patients who have had a chest x-ray in the past six months and who are pregnant now will not have x-ray taken. Women patients 48 years of age and over and women of any age who have had a mastectomy are screened at this station to determine eligibility for mammography testing at Station 8. If the chest x-ray machine is not working, the chest x-ray card (Figure 20-24) will be marked using an electrographic pencil in the response position, "EXAM NOT DONE." Female patients under age 48, female patients 48 and over and not eligible for mammography, and all male patients are instructed to return to the dressing rooms (Station 4), discard the paper gowns, re-dress, and proceed to Station 9 for vision testing. (See also Figure 1-22.)

8. Mammography

Female patients age 48 years or older and who have not had breast x-rays taken within ten months, and women of any age who have had a mastectomy, will arrive wearing a paper gown to have mammography (Figures 20-25 and 20-26). This consists of cephalocaudal and lateral-tangential views of each breast. If the patient has had a multiphasic breast x-ray before, the mammography card (Figure 20-27) is stamped on the back with prior date given by patient and marked on the patient's preprinted gummed label. (See also Figure 1-23.)

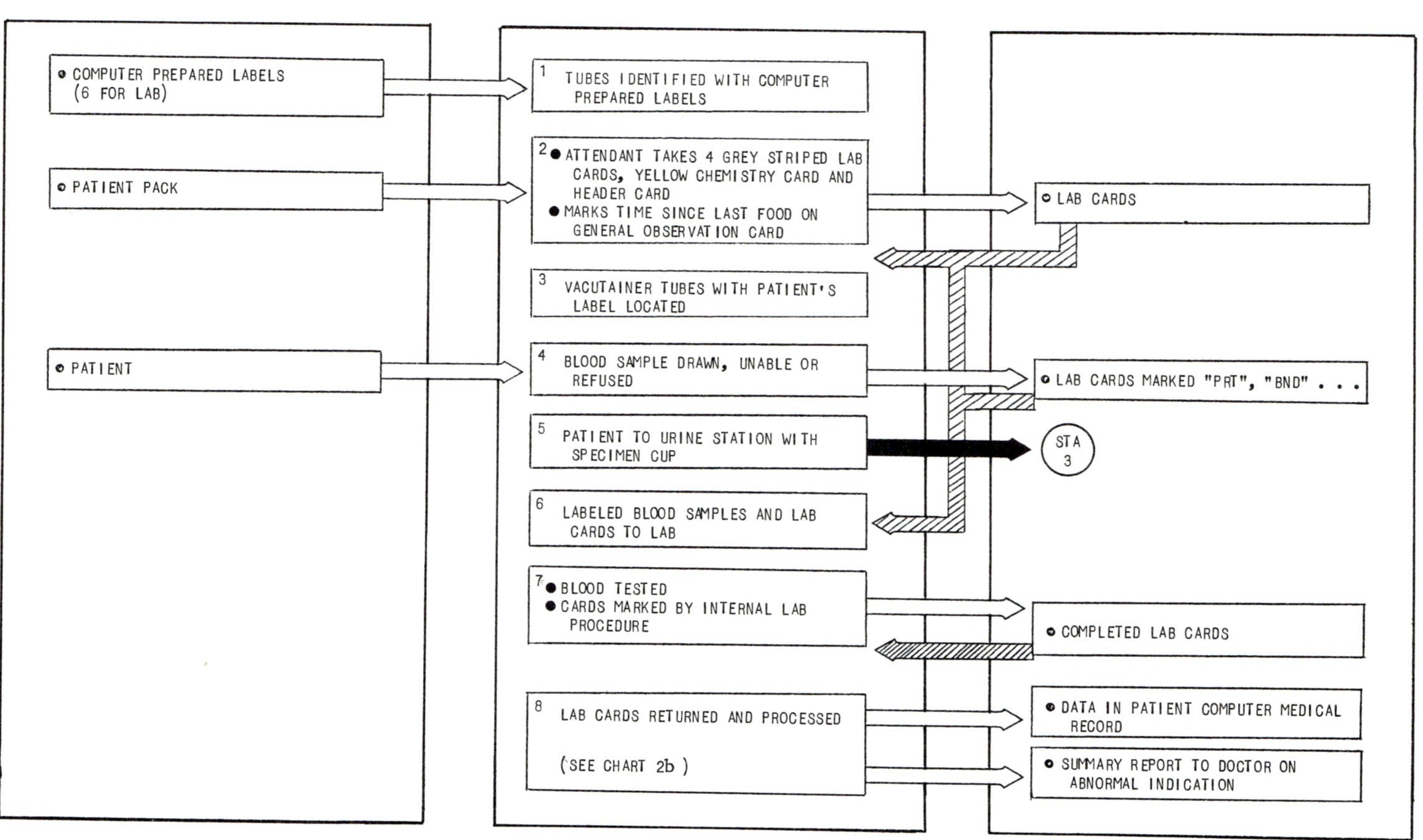

Figure 20-7a. Information chart for blood drawing.

CHART 2b - 1976

BLOOD DRAWING

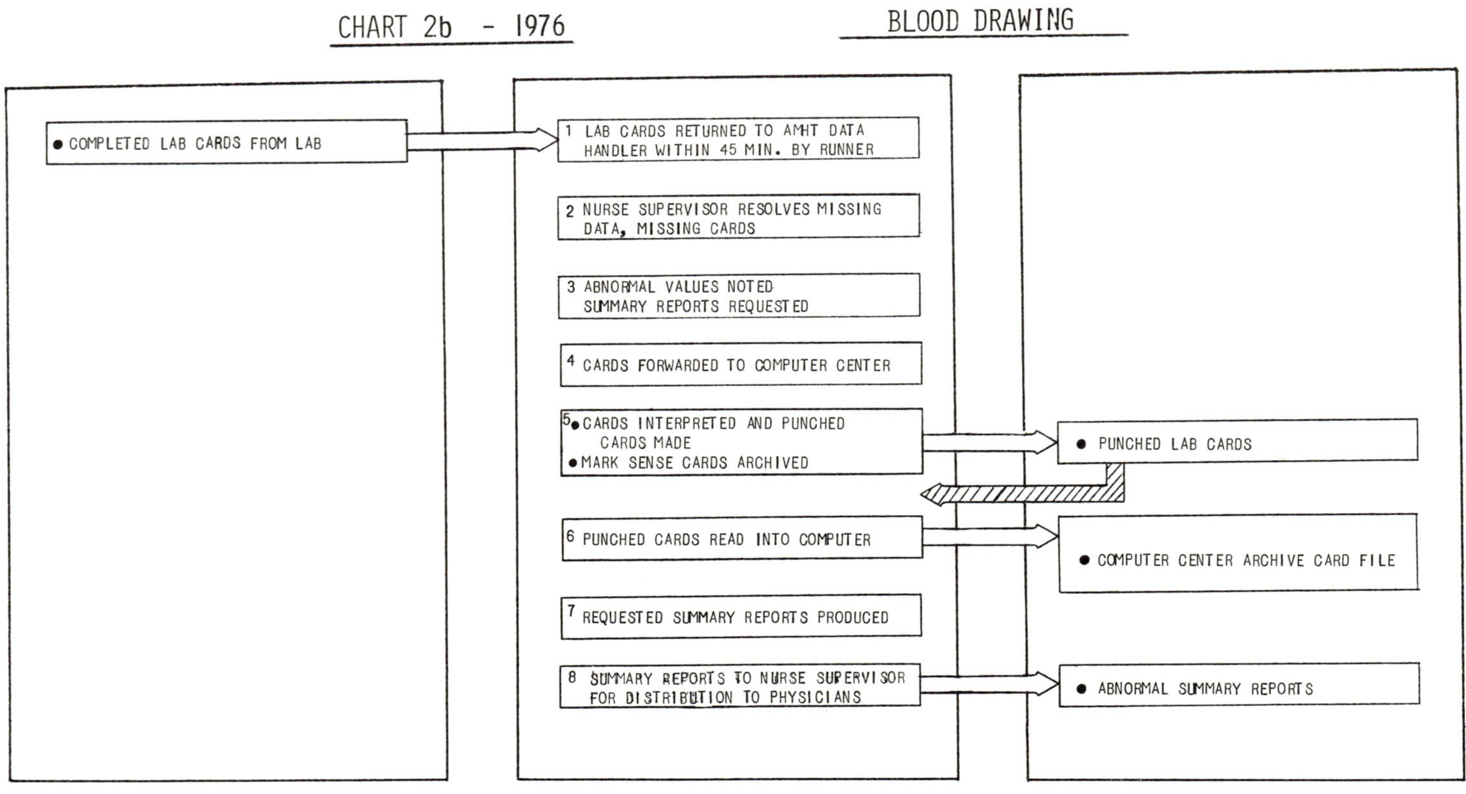

Figure 20-7b.

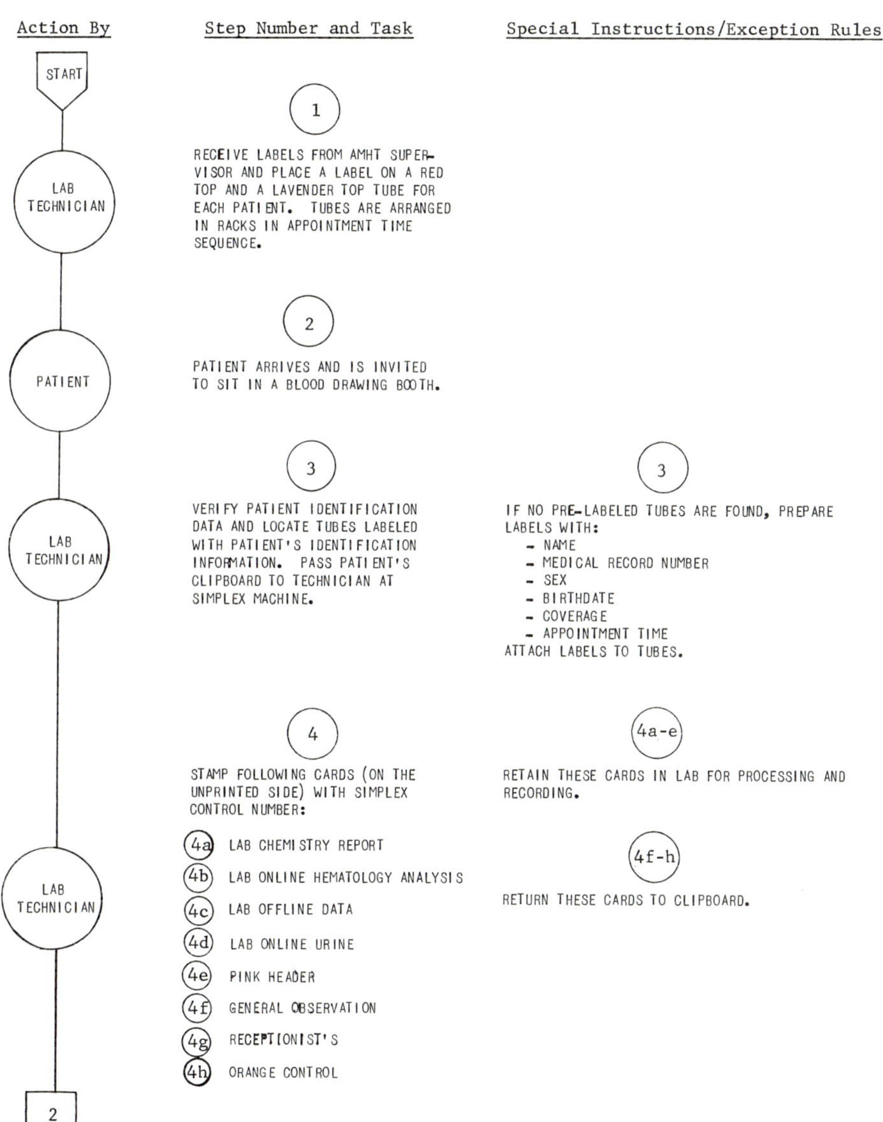

Figure 20-8a.   Flow chart for blood drawing.

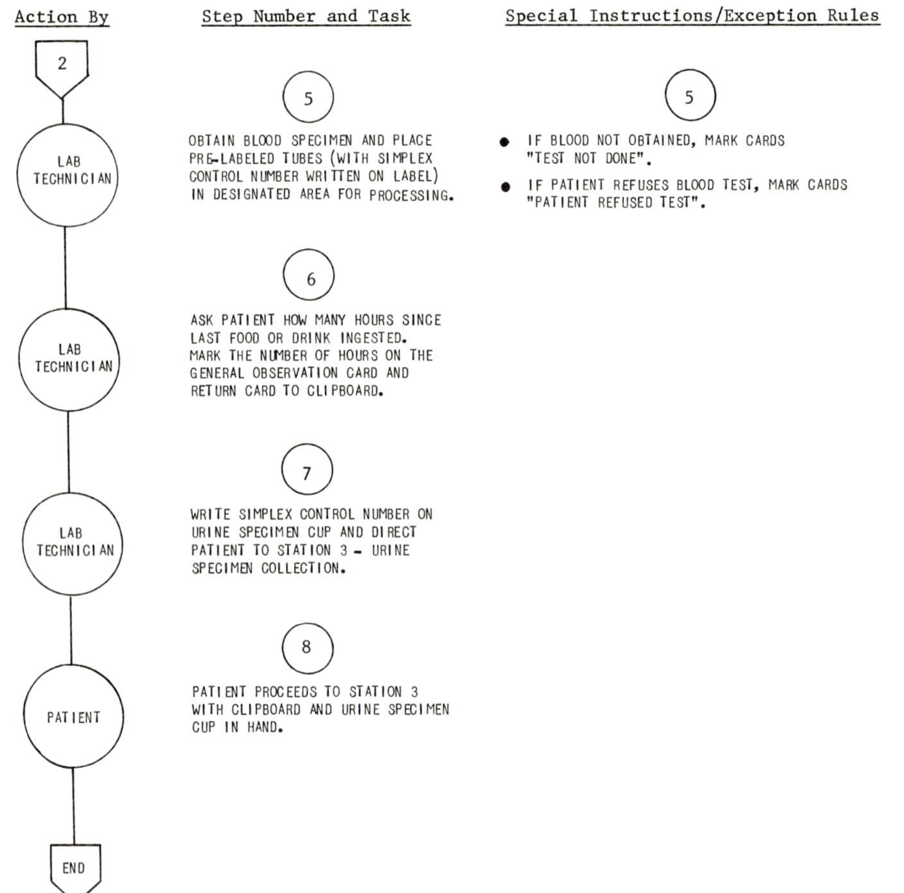

Figure 20-8b.

9. Visual Acuity

Male and female patients arrive from dressing rooms after having re-dressed to have visual acuity checked (Figures 20-28 and 20-29). Identification information is verified and procedure explained to patient. First the right and then the left eye is checked. The number of letters missed with each eye as the patient reads the chart is marksensed on the eye card (Figure 20-30).

10. Tonometry

Patients arrive to be screened for glaucoma. After test eligibility is determined and identification information is verified, a brief explanation of the test procedure is given to the patient (Figures 20-31 and 20-32). The measurement as shown on the digital display on the tonometer is marksensed on the eye card by the test operator (Figure 20-30). (See also Figure 1-24.)

11. Audiometry

The patient arrives to have hearing tested for six frequencies (500, 1,000, 2,000, 3,000, 4,000 and 6,000) in each ear (Figures 20-33 and 20-34). A Rudmose card is

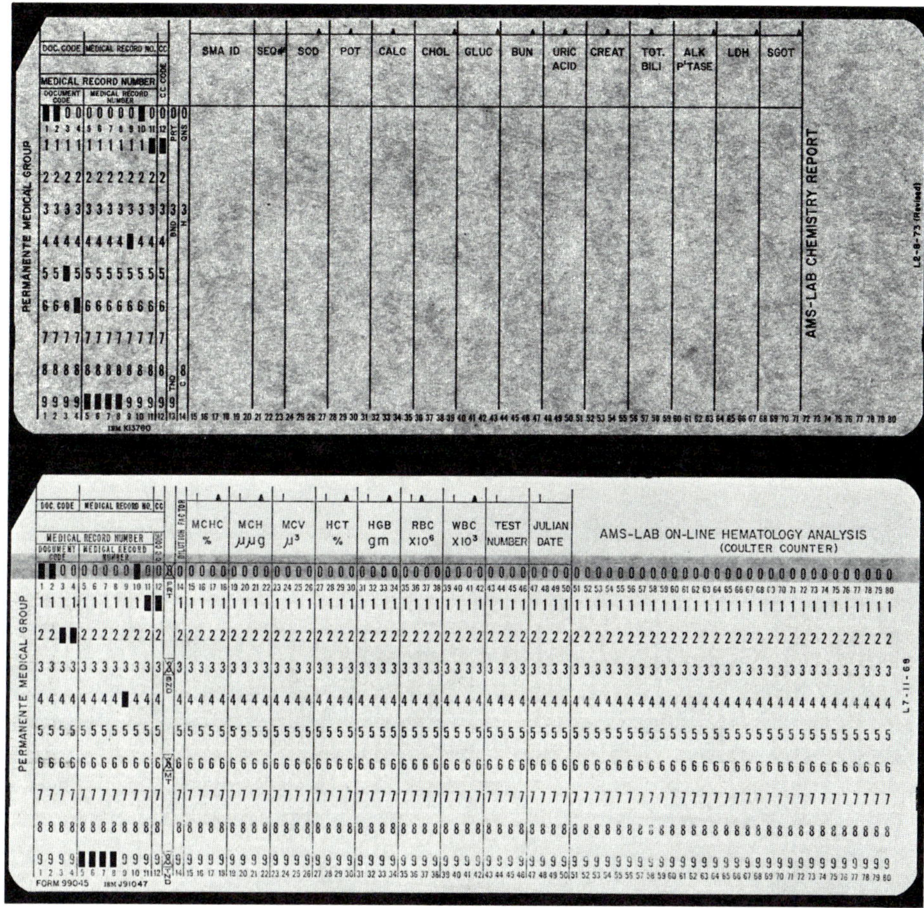

Figure 20-9. AMHT clinical laboratory chemistry and hematology cards.

placed in the audiometer, and the excursions are manually transferred to a marksense readable card (Figure 20-35). The patient is given comprehensive instructions and afforded a test run as a means of understanding his role in relation to the prerequisites for successful testing. Although the patients are tested in groups of six, every attempt is made to personalize the testing by providing individual instructions to minimize any mystique the patient may associate with this testing. (See also Figure 1-25.)

12. Medical History

The patient arrives and identification is verified (Figures 20-36 and 20-37). Medical questions are sorted using a prepunched deck of cards (Figure 20-38) into yes or no responses. Every attempt is made to properly instruct the patient in the effective use of the questionnaire box. The patient's yellow medical questionnaire form is reviewed by the nurse or clinic assistant at the station for completeness and clarity. The patient is afforded the opportunity to clarify vague entries and to review yes or no responses for whatever second thoughts may occur regarding their medical history information. (See also Figure 1-26.)

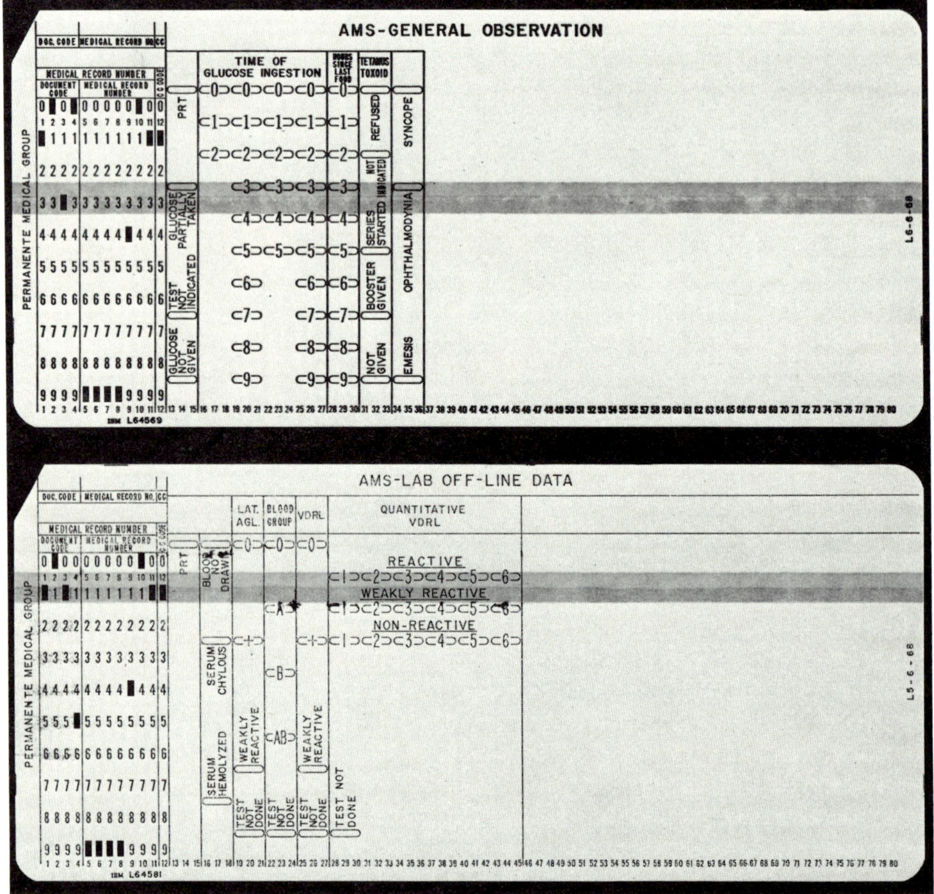

Figure 20-10.   AMHT lab general observation and offline data cards.

13.   HES Registration

Patients to be seen in the Health Evaluation Section (HES) have had their eligibility for nurse practitioner physical examination determined by Central Appointments at the time of multiphasic appointment booking. Therefore, upon completion of the multiphasic testing the patient arrives at the patient service area bearing information indicative of HES eligibility (Figures 20-39 and 20-40). The appropriate forms are prepared, fees collected, and the patient is directed to the appropriate area to await the physical examination by a medical nurse practitioner.

14.   HES Nurse Practitioner Examination

The patient arrives in the HES on a prescheduled appointment basis for a general health evaluation (Figures 20-41 and 20-42). This is performed by a nurse practitioner under the direct supervision of a physician according to physician-developed protocols. The nurse practitioner will be performing the physical examination (and recording data on a physical examination report form), reviewing

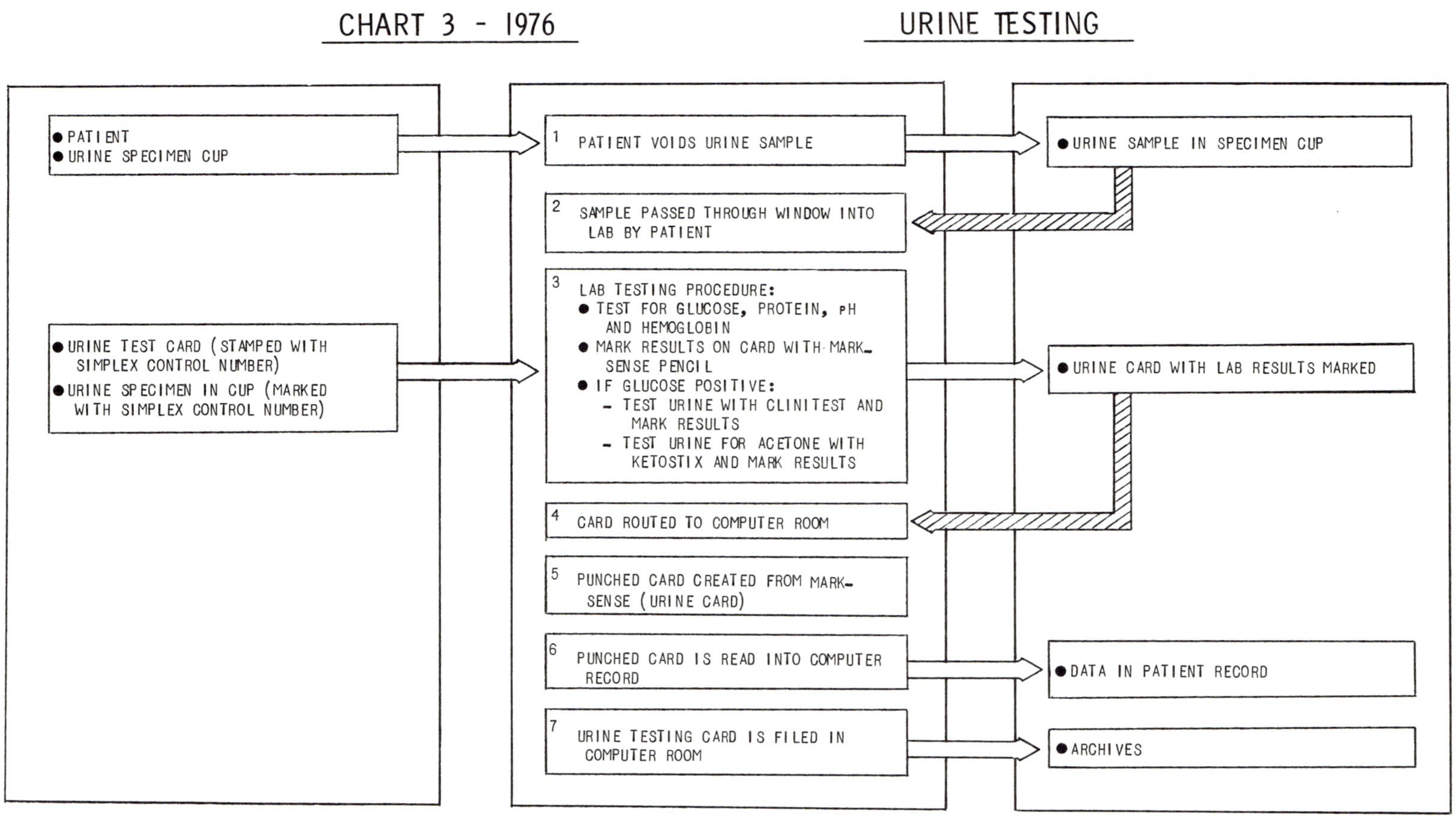

Figure 20-11. Information chart for urine testing.

STATION 3 - URINE TESTING

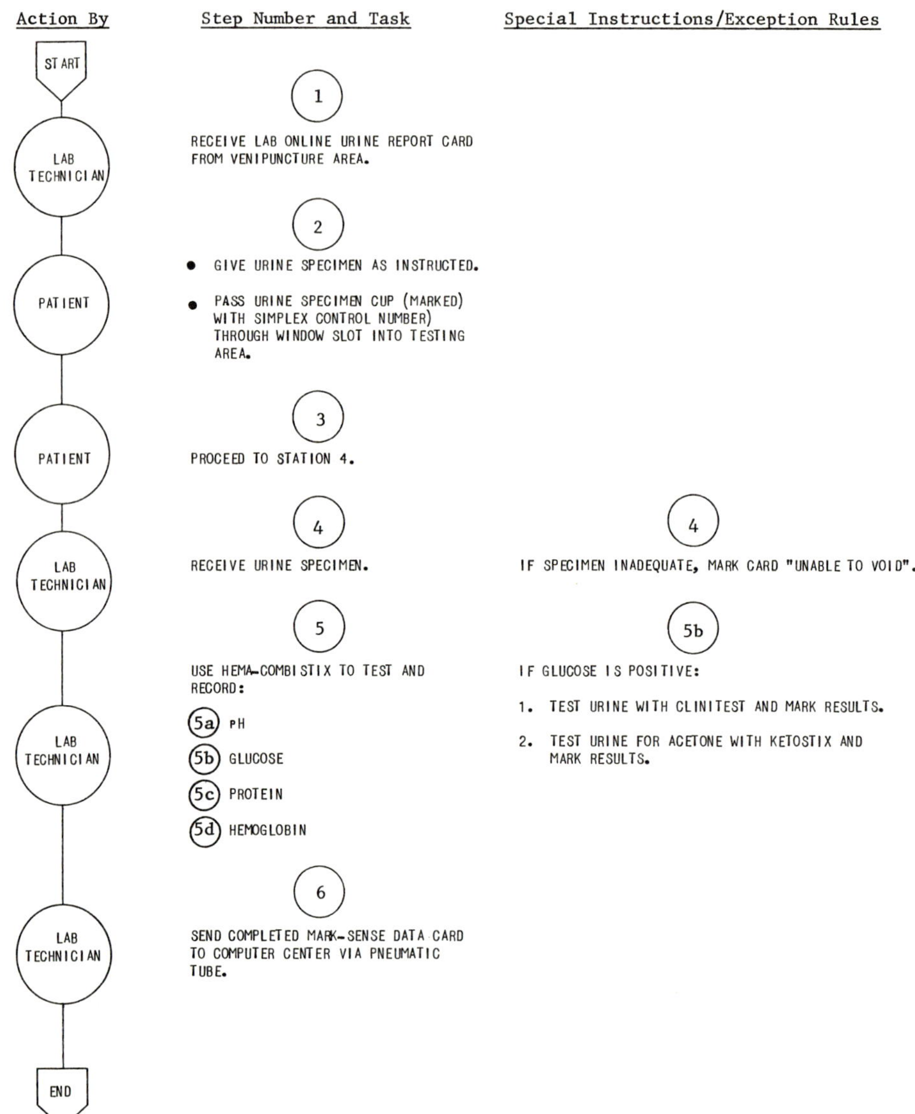

Figure 20-12.   Flow chart for urine testing.

medical history, screening laboratory data, assisting in channeling patients into appropriate divisions of the health care delivery system, and providing appropriate patient counseling in specified health problems. (See also Figure 1-29.)

15.   Discharge and Referral

Patient discharge encompasses review of forms for completeness, collection of any additional charges, and any explanation of final instructions that the patient is to receive (Figures 20-43 and 20-44). Patients arriving to be discharged include

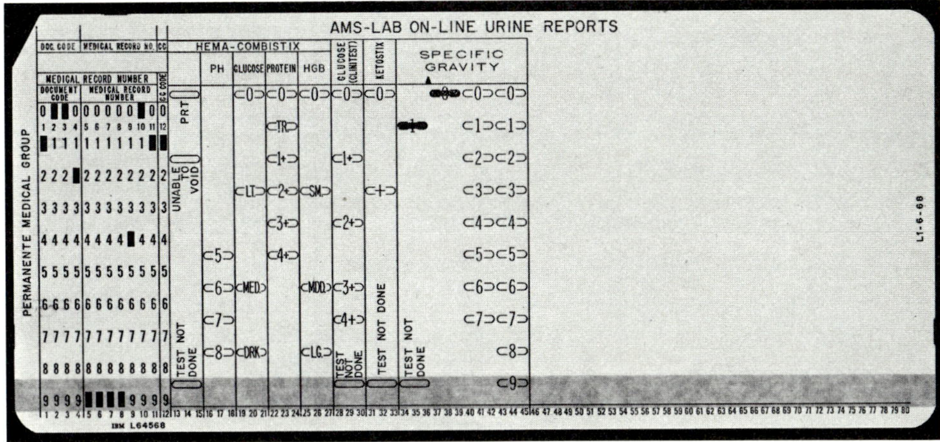

Figure 20-13.   Urinalysis report card.

those who have completed the multiphasic testing and will not be seeing a medical nurse practitioner, as well as those who have already been seen by the nurse practitioner. At this point the patient is relieved of the clipboard, and the materials remaining on it are placed in the designated locations for collection and distribution to the appropriate areas.

Any necessary followup care appointments with physicians are reviewed with the patient. (See also Figure 1-28.)

16.   Post-AMHT Procedures

As needed by the medical nurse practitioners on the day of testing, online summaries are produced from the online data cards received in the computer room (Figure 20-45). These cards are then filed until the offline data card collection is complete (currently an interval of seven days is sufficient). On the seventh day post-AMHT the final summaries are run for the testing day. The entire group of summaries is sent to the chart room, where the carbon copies are sent to the physicians named by the patients and the original copies are filed in the patients' medical charts.

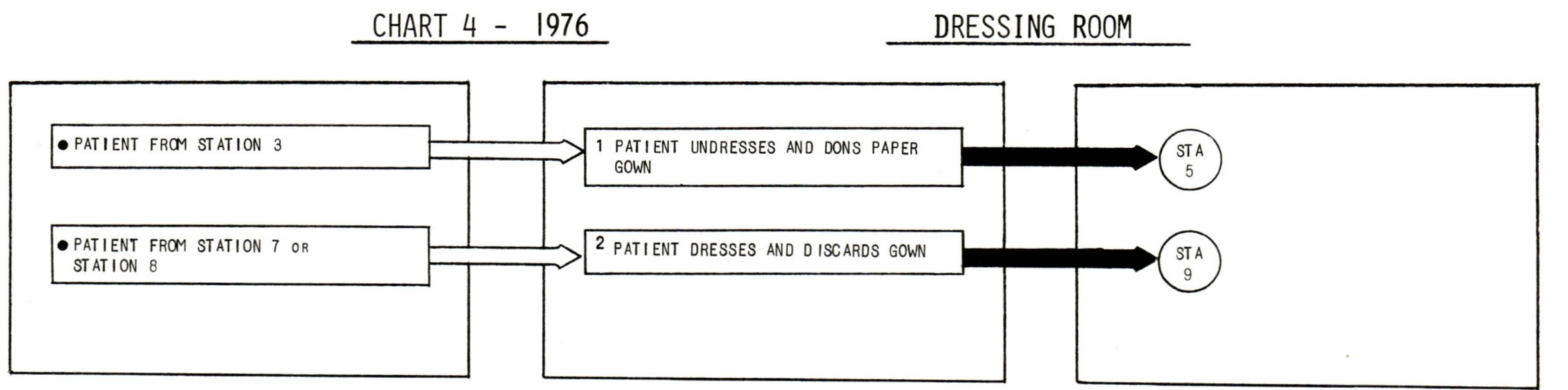

Figure 20-14. Information chart for dressing with disposable gown.

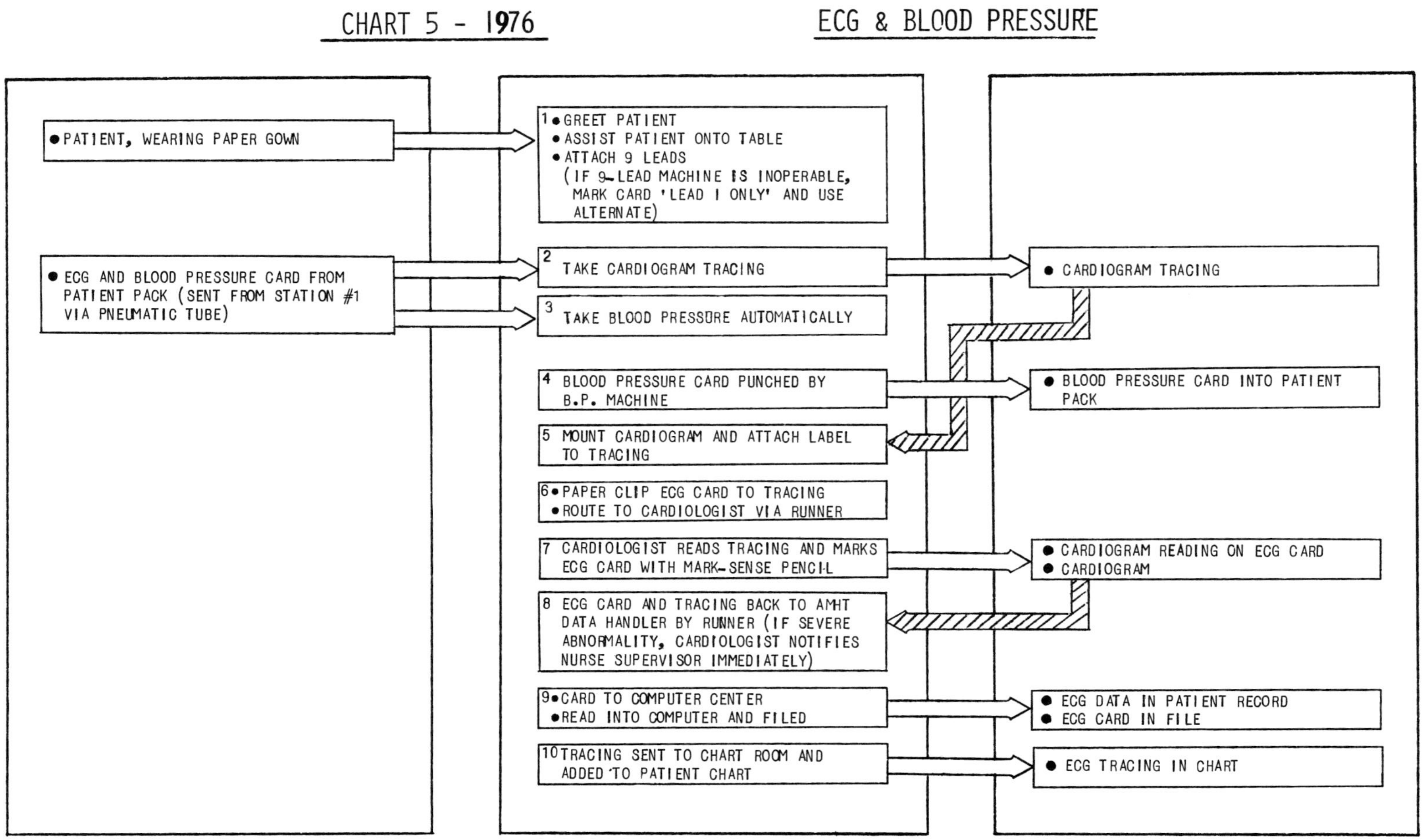

Figure 20-15. Information chart for ECG and blood pressure phases.

STATION 5 - ELECTROCARDIOGRAPHY AND BLOOD PRESSURE

Action By	Step Number and Task	Special Instructions/Exception Rules
START		
RECEPT. & EKG TECH.	1 EKG (DOC. CODE 0045) AND BLOOD PRESSURE (DOC. CODE 0023) CARDS ARRIVE VIA PNEUMATIC TUBE TO EKG AREA. THIS INDICATES PATIENT HAS REGISTERED FOR MHC APPOINTMENT AND WILL BE READY FOR EKG AFTER GOING TO THE LABORATORY AND INTO THE DRESSING ROOM TO PUT ON PAPER GOWN (FOR WOMEN) OR PAPER SHIRT (FOR MEN). CARDS ARE KEPT IN APPOINTMENT TIME ORDER AND PATIENTS CALLED ACCORDINGLY.	1 IF TECHNICIAN IS AWARE THAT PATIENTS ARE READY, BUT CARDS HAVE NOT ARRIVED RECEPTIONIST MUST BE ALERTED TO SEND CARDS. OFTEN A FEW SHARP TAPS ON THE PNEUMATIC TUBE WILL BE SUFFICIENT TO ALERT RECEPTIONIST. IF NOT, GO DIRECTLY TO RECEPTIONIST TO OBTAIN THE CARDS. NOTIFY SUPERVISOR, OR DESIGNEE, IF CARDS CARDS CANNOT BE LOCATED.
EKG TECH.	2 CALL PATIENT INTO ROOM. MALE PATIENTS ARE CALLED FROM DRESSING ROOMS AND FEMALES FROM SEATING AREA OUTSIDE THE TEST STATION.	2 IF PATIENT NOT PRESENT WHEN FIRST CALLED CALL NEXT PATIENT. IF PATIENT NOT THERE AFTER SEVERAL CALLS, CHECK BOTH MALE AND FEMALE DRESSING AREAS AND THEN NOTIFY NURSE SUPERVISOR SO THAT THE PATIENT MAY BE LOCATED (OCCASIONALLY PATIENTS ARE WAITING AT THE WRONG LOCATION TO BE CALLED AND ARE OUT OF HEARING RANGE FROM THE EKG STATION OR A TECHNICAL DIFFICULTY MAY HAVE ARISEN THAT WILL DELAY THE PATIENT'S ARRIVAL TO THE EKG AREA).
EKG TECH.	3 EXPLAIN TO THE PATIENT THAT THE EKG AND BLOOD PRESSURE MEASUREMENT WILL BE PERFORMED. EXPLAIN THE PROCEDURES TO THE PATIENT AND ANSWER ANY QUESTIONS THAT MAY ARISE. FOR MANY PATIENTS THIS MAY BE THE FIRST EKG EXPERIENCE. AS THE ALCOHOL IS READY TO BE APPLIED EXPLAIN THAT IT WILL BE COLD.	
2		

Figure 20-16a. Flow chart for ECG and blood pressure phases.

2

EKG TECH.

EKG TECH.

EKG TECH.

EKG TECH

EKG TECH.

3

4

GATHER INFORMATION:

- ASK IF PATIENT TAKING BLOOD PRESSURE
  OR CARDIAC MEDICATION.

- ASK IF PATIENT HAS HISTORY OF CARDIAC
  OR BLOOD PRESSURE PROBLEMS.

5

POSITION PATIENT ON EKG TABLE AND APPLY CHEST
LEADS.

5

WIPE CALVES AND FOREARMS WITH ALCOHOL AND
POSITION IN LEG AND ARM RESTS WHICH ARE
THE LIMB LEADS.

CHEST LEADS:
    YELLOW – V1
    BLACK – V3
    BLUE   – V5

6

PREPARE BLOOD PRESSURE CUFF AND POSITION
ON PATIENT'S RIGHT ARM.

6

– APPLY SPECIFIED GEL TO SENSOR ON BLOOD
PRESSURE CUFF.
– SENSOR TO BE WIPED WITH ALCOHOL AFTER
EACH USE.
– A WIDE CUFF IS AVAILABLE FOR LARGE ARMS.

7

ACTIVATE BLOOD PRESSURE RECORDER (SEE
OPERATIONS MANUAL FOR DETAILS OF MACHINE
OPERATION).

8

LOCATE PATIENT'S LABELS (2) AND WRITE
IN RED FELT PEN THE FOLLOWING INFORMATION:

8a THE LETTER "P" IN THE MIDDLE OF THE
LABEL IF THE PATIENT IS A PRACTITIONER
PATIENT. THIS IS INDICATED BY THE
LETTERS "HES" ON THE YELLOW QUESTIONNAIRE
AND THE RECEPTION CARD WHICH ARE ON THE
CLIPBOARD.

8b SIMPLEX NUMBER IN LOWER RIGHT CORNER OF
LABEL. SIMPLEX NUMBER STAMPED ON RECEPT-
ION CARD.

8c APPOINTMENT TIME IN UPPER RIGHT CORNER
OF LABEL. APPOINTMENT TIME PRINTED IN
UPPER RIGHT CORNER ON BACK OF EKG AND
BLOOD PRESSURE CARDS.

8

IF NO LABELS ARE FOUND USE BLANKS PRO-
VIDED. WRITE THE FOLLOWING INFORMATION
IN BLACK PEN ON THE LABEL:
  – PATIENT'S NAME
  – MEDICAL RECORD NUMBER
  – SEX
  – BIRTHDATE
  – COVERAGE (PRINTED ON BACK OF EKG AND
    BLOOD PRESSURE CARDS).
  – APPOINTMENT TIME.

Figure 20-16b.

Action By	Step Number and Task	Special Instructions/Exception Rules
3		
EKG TECH.	**(9)** (9a) TURN SWITCH BOX TO CORRECT BED NUMBER AND TAKE EKG. (9b) OBSERVE QUALITY OF EKG GRAPH. WHEN SATISFACTORY GRAPH OBTAINED ATTACH LABEL AT UPPER RIGHT END OF TRACING SO AS NOT TO COVER ANY PART OF THE EKG. (9c) PLACE EKG CARD IN DESIGNATED LOCATION TO KEEP CARDS IN SEQUENCE WITH GRAPHS.	**(9a)** IF MACHINE BECOMES INOPERATIVE: –OBTAIN SINGLE CHANNEL MACHINE (LEAD I) FROM STATION 9 - VISUAL ACUITY. –CONNECT THE MACHINE TO TABLE 2. –RUN LEAD I ONLY. –FILL-IN "LEAD I ONLY" BUBBLE ON EKG CARD. –PROCEED AS USUAL. **(9b)** IF DEXTROCARDIA IS OBSERVED NOTE IT ON THE GRAPH AND ON THE BACK OF THE EKG CARD.
EKG TECH.	**(10)** OBSERVE BLOOD PRESSURE MEASUREMENT.	**(10)** TAKE A SECOND MEASUREMENT IF: –READING IS ELEVATED (SYSTOLIC 160 AND OVER AND/OR DIASTOLIC 90 AND OVER). –MACHINE INDICATES AN INACCURATE READING (SEE OPERATIONS MANUAL FOR DETAILS).
EKG TECH.	**(11)** RECORD BLOOD PRESSURE: (11a) INSERT BLOOD PRESSURE CARD INTO KEY PUNCH WITH PRINTED SIDE UP AND CLIPPED CORNER IN UPPER LEFT DIRECTION. (11b) PRESS "FEED" BUTTON TO MOVE CARD TO THE CORRECT COLUMN. (11c) CHECK THAT AUXILLARY UNIT IS SET FOR THE CORRECT TABLE: TABLE I - CHANNELS 18,19 TABLE 2 - CHANNELS 20,21 (11d) PRESS "ADV" SWITCH TO OBTAIN DESIRED CHANNEL.	**(11c)** IF THE AUXILLARY UNIT IS INOPERATIVE PUNCH BLOOD PRESSURE MANUALLY. -- INSERT B.P. CARD IN KEY PUNCH -- PRESS "FEED" BUTTON (AUTOMATICALLY ADVANCES CARD TO COL. 15) -- TURN THE FLY BACK (TO THE RIGHT) -- BACK SPACE ONE COLUMN TO COLUMN 14 -- HOLD DOWN "NUM" BUTTON, PUNCH THE CORRECT TABLE NUMBER -- TURN FLY BACK (TO LEFT) -- SPACE TO COLUMN 16 -- PUNCH BLOOD PRESSURE -- PRESS "REL" BUTTON TO RELEASE CARD
4		

Figure 20-16c.

Action By	Step Number and Task	Special Instructions/Exception Rules
4		
EKG TECH.	(11e) PRESS THE "TREADLE SWITCH" ONCE TO RECORD SYSTOLIC PRESSURE AND A SECOND TIME TO RECORD THE DIASTOLIC.	(11e) IF MACHINE READING IS: SYSTOLIC OF 160 OR OVER AND/OR DIASTOLIC 90 OR OVER A MANUAL BLOOD PRESSURE MUST BE TAKEN.
	(11f) PRESS THE "REL" BUTTON ON THE KEY PUNCH TO RELEASE THE CARD.	TAKE BLOOD PRESSURE MANUALLY.
	(11g) RETURN THE CARD TO THE PATIENT'S CLIP-BOARD (UNDER THE OTHER DATA CARDS IN THE CARD HOLDER).	RECORD MANUAL READING: -- INSERT B.P. CARD INTO KEY PUNCH -- PRESS "FEED" BUTTON -- PRESS SPACE BAR TO COL. 26 -- PUNCH THE TABLE NUMBER (MACHINE WILL AUTOMATICALLY ADVANCE TO COLUMN 28) -- PUNCH IN THE BLOOD PRESSURE. SYSTOLIC AND DIASTOLIC PRESSURE SHOULD HAVE THREE DIGITS EACH. FOR INSTANCE, IF B.P. IS 90/60 YOU WOULD PUNCH 0,9,0,0,6,0. -- PRESS "REL" BUTTON TO RELEASE CARD. -- IF MANUAL READING IS ELEVATED (160 OR OVER AND/OR 90 OR OVER) MAKE A DUPLICATE USING THE SPECIFIED BLANK CARDS: - INSERT THE CARD TO BE DUPLICATED IN THE KEY PUNCH. - INSERT THE ORIGINAL TO THE LEFT. - PRESS "FEED" BUTTON. - PRESS "DUP" BUTTON. - WHEN COMPLETE PRESS "REL" BUTTON. - COMPARE THE DUPLICATE WITH THE ORIGINAL FOR ACCURACY. - STAMP THE UNPRINTED SIDE OF THE DUPLICATE WITH PATIENT'S HEALTH PLAN CARD AND WRITE THE FOLLOWING INFORMATION IN THE UPPER RIGHT CORNER OF THE PRINTED SIDE: BLOOD PRESSURE MEDICATIONS, IF ANY, PATIENT'S DOCTOR, SIMPLEX CONTROL NUMBER, THE LETTER "P", IF THE PATIENT TO SEE A NURSE PRACTITIONER, APPOINTMENT TIME. -- RETURN THE ORIGINAL BLOOD PRESSURE CARD TO THE PATIENT'S CLIPBOARD (AS IN STEP 11F) -- TAKE DUPLICATE CARD TO DESIGNATED AREA TO ALERT THE MULTIPHASIC SUPER-VISOR.
EKG TECH.	(12) DIRECT PATIENT TO STATION 6, HEIGHT, WEIGHT AND SPIROMETRY.	
END		

Figure 20-16d.

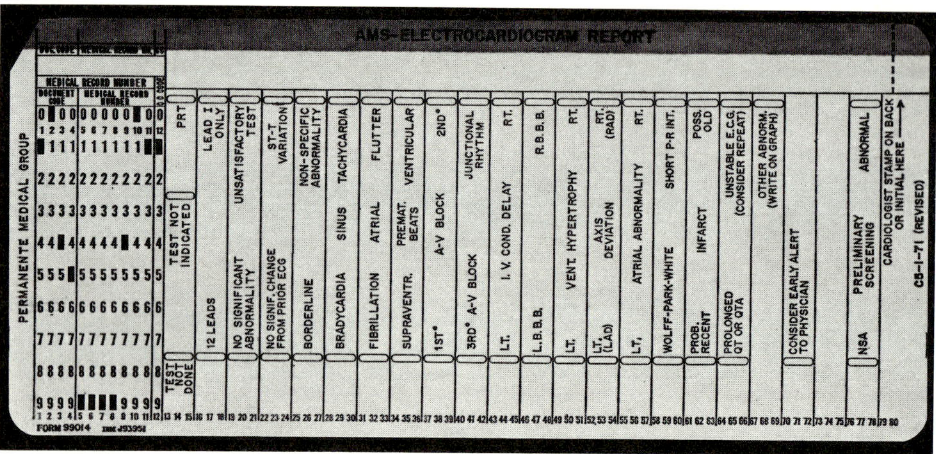

Figure 20-17. Electrocardiogram report card for marksensing cardiologist's interpretations.

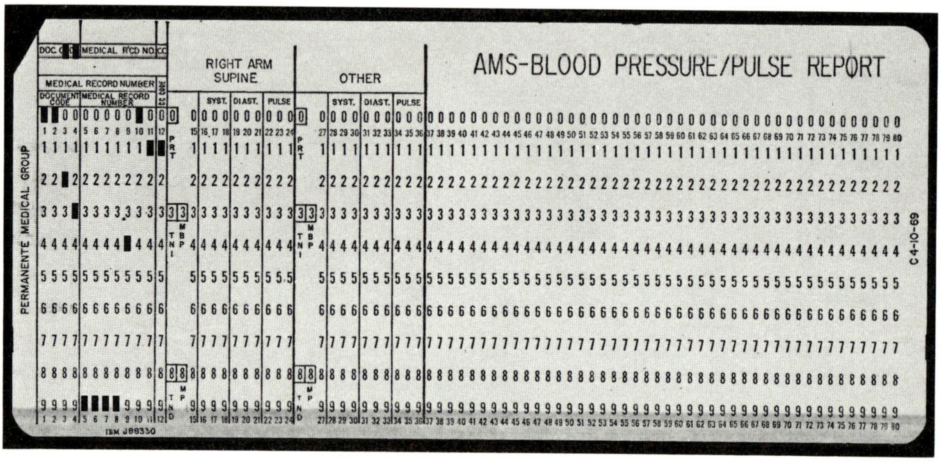

Figure 20-18. Blood pressure card for automated entry of measurements.

SPIROMETRY AND ANTHROPOMETRY

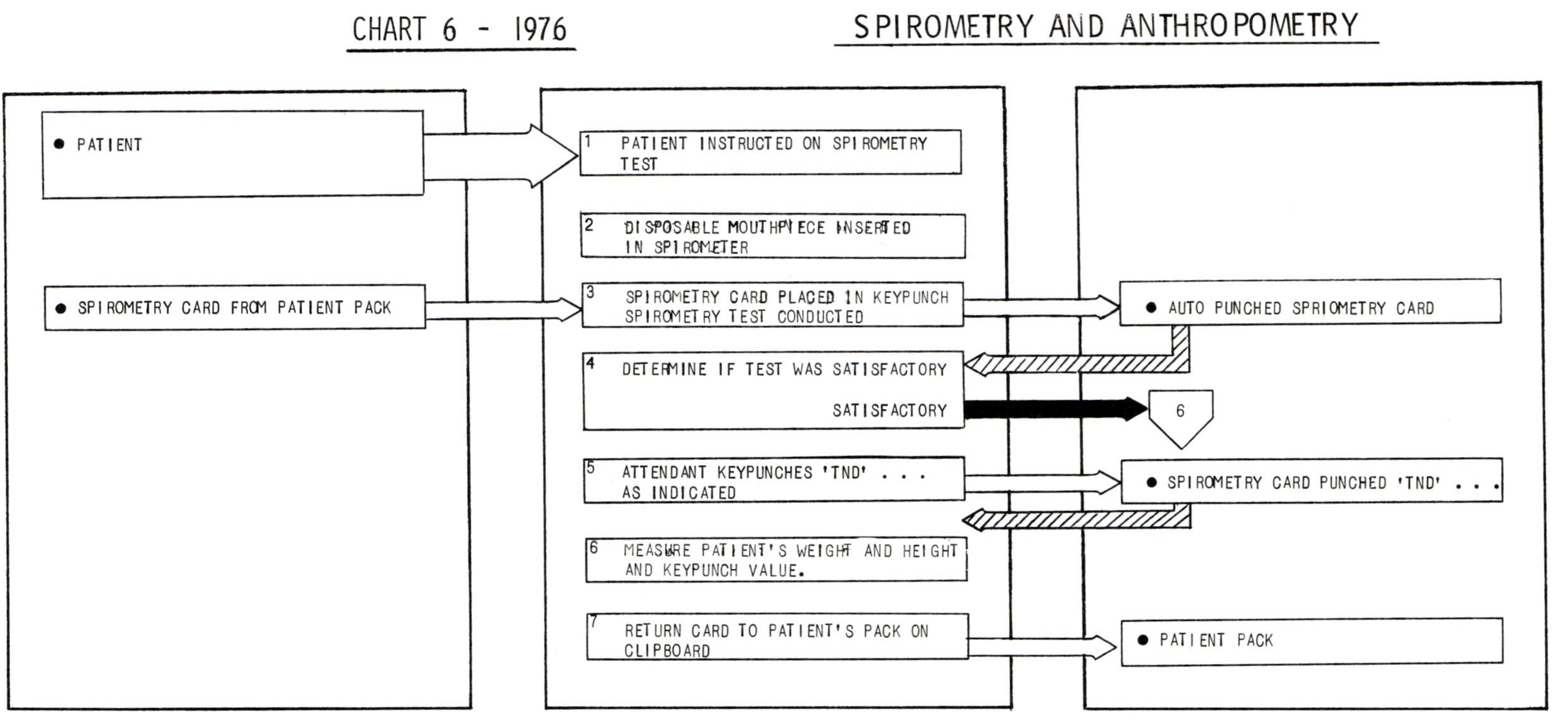

Figure 20-19. Information chart for spirometry and anthropometry.

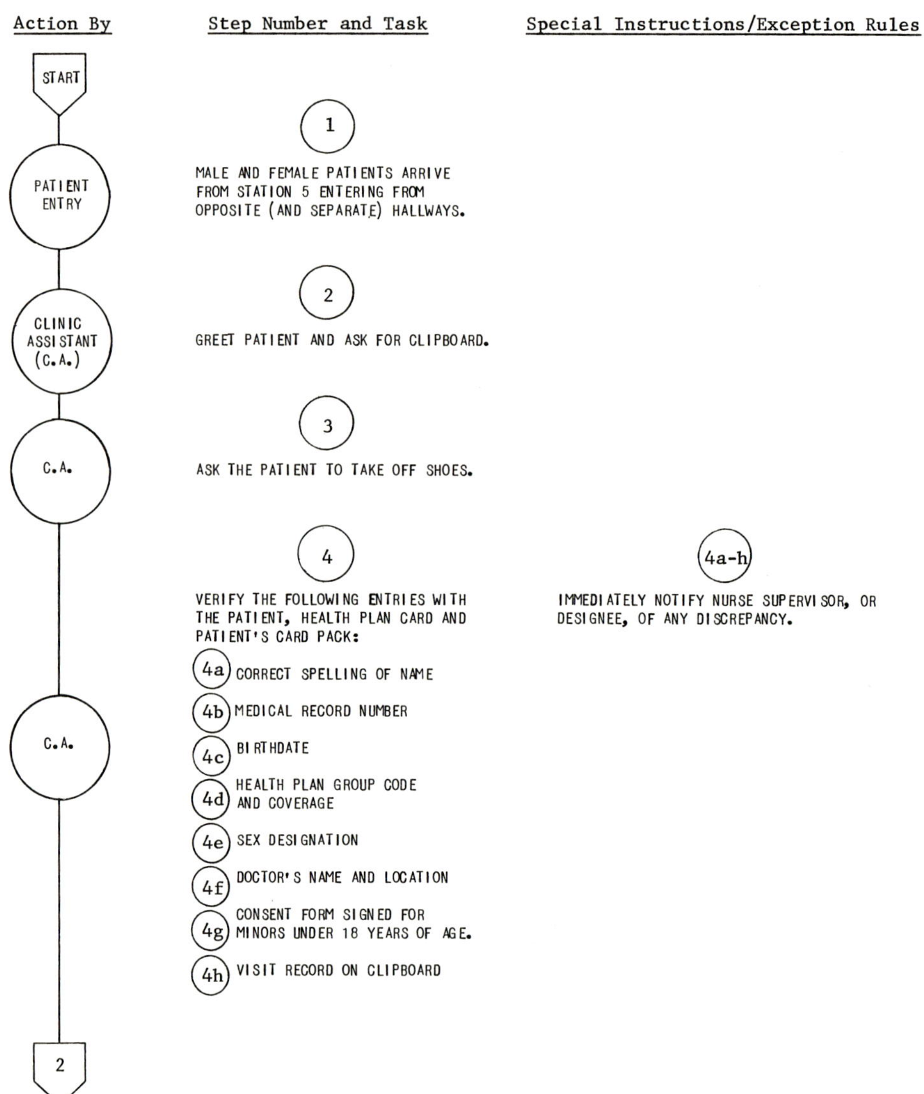

Figure 20-20a.   Flow chart for spirometry and anthropometry.

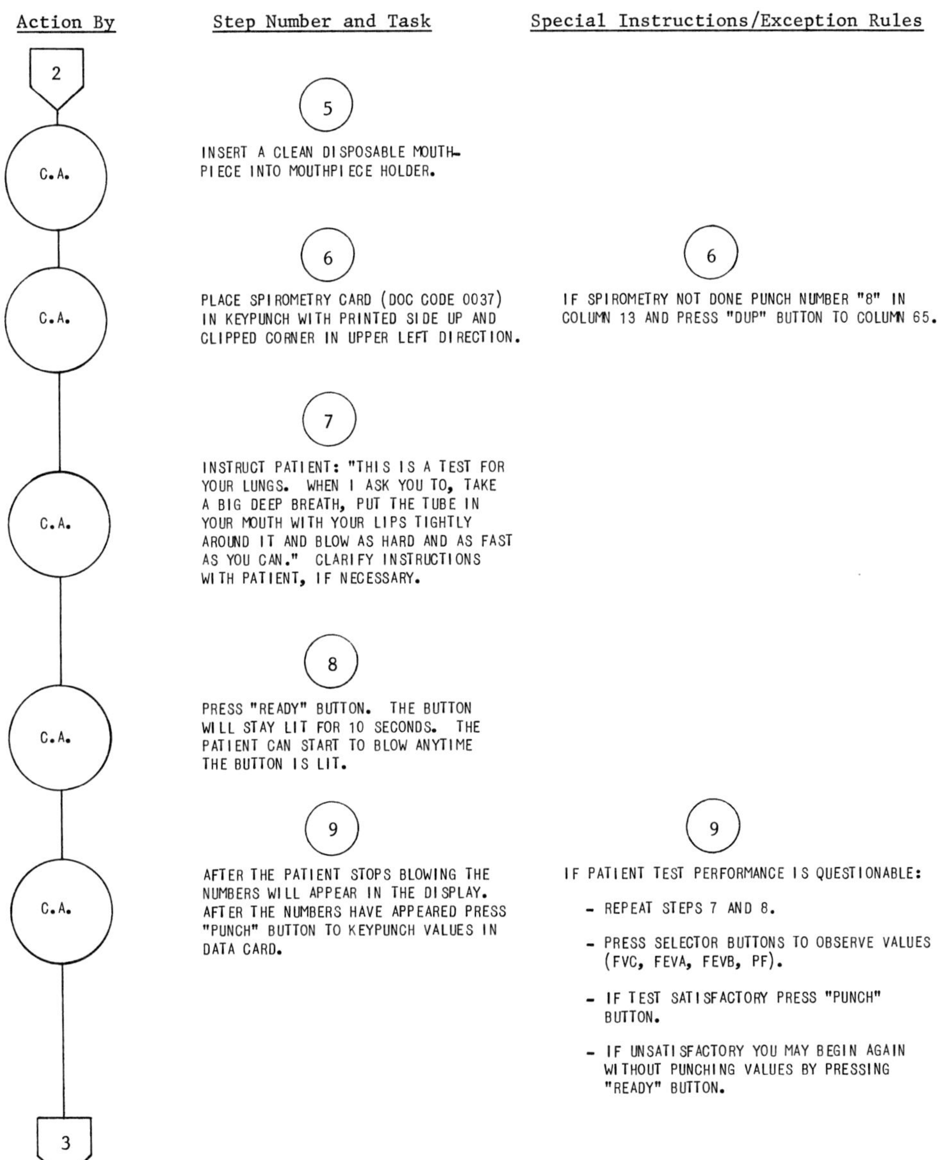

Figure 20-20b.

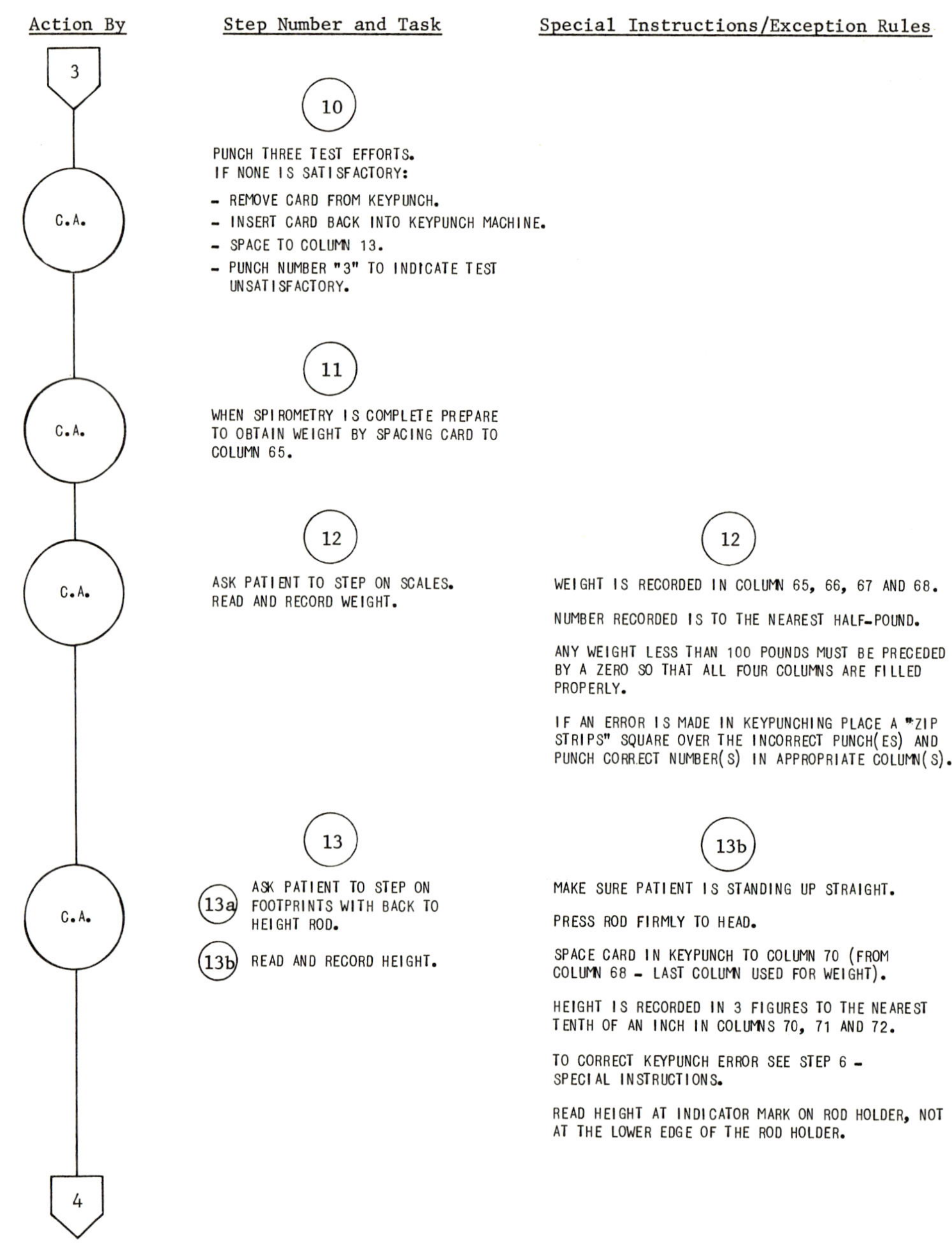

Figure 20-20c.

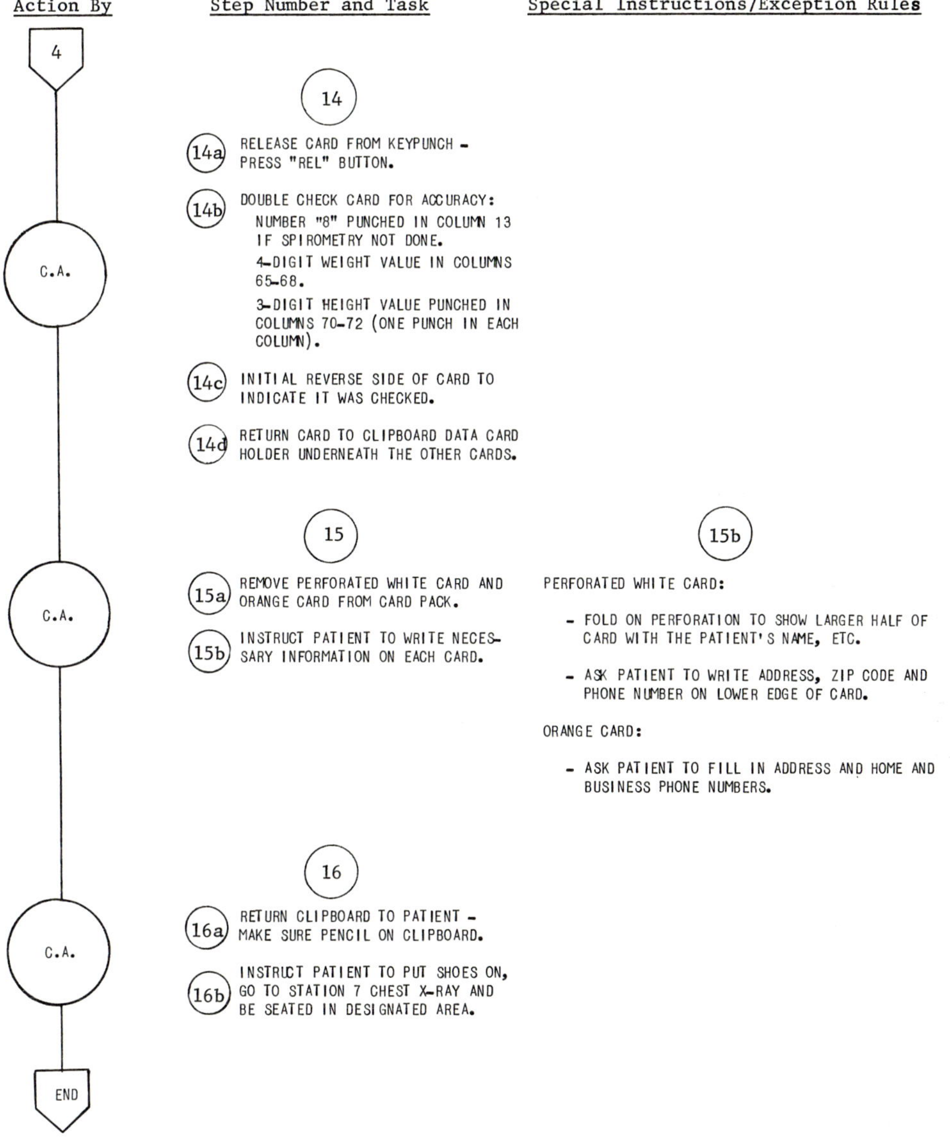

Figure 20-20d.

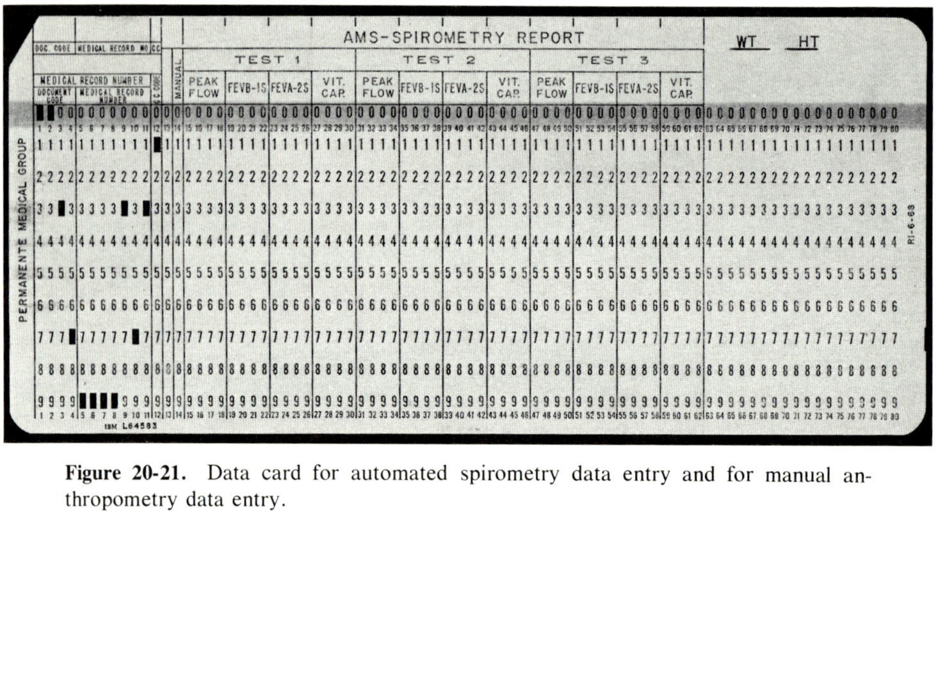

Figure 20-21. Data card for automated spirometry data entry and for manual anthropometry data entry.

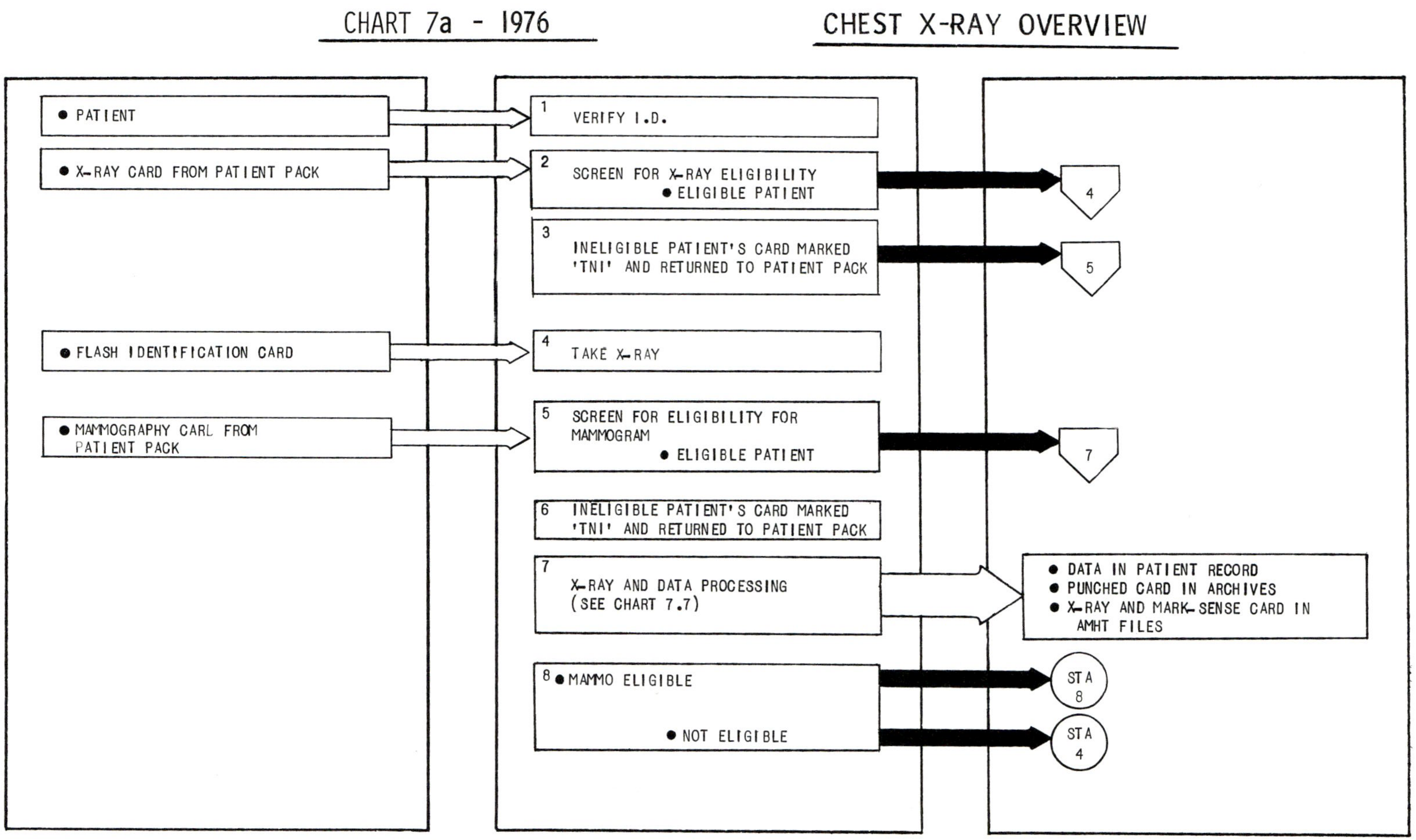

Figure 20-22a. Information chart for chest x-ray station.

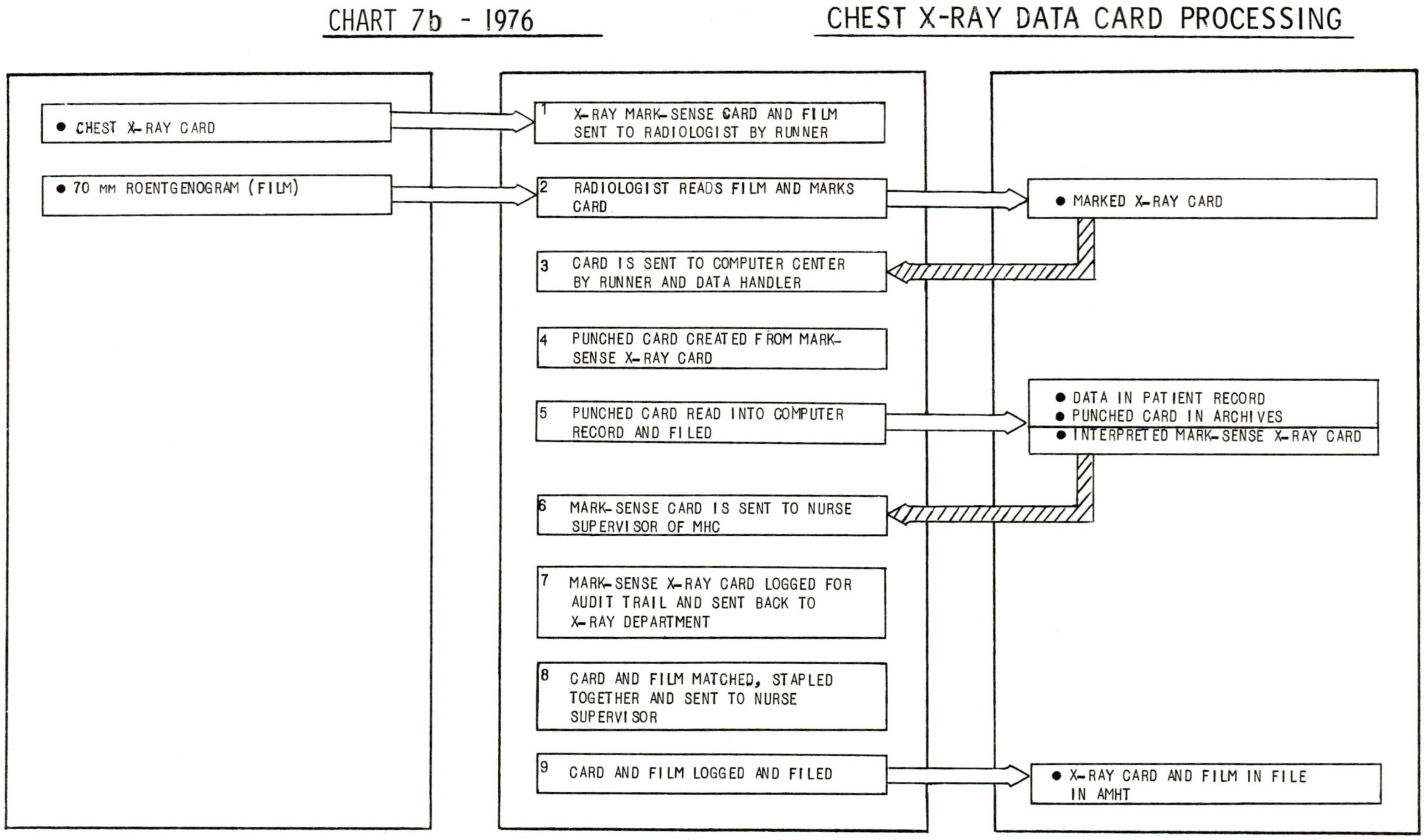

Figure 20-22b.   Information chart for chest x-ray data card processing.

Action By	Step Number and Task	Special Instructions/Exception Rules

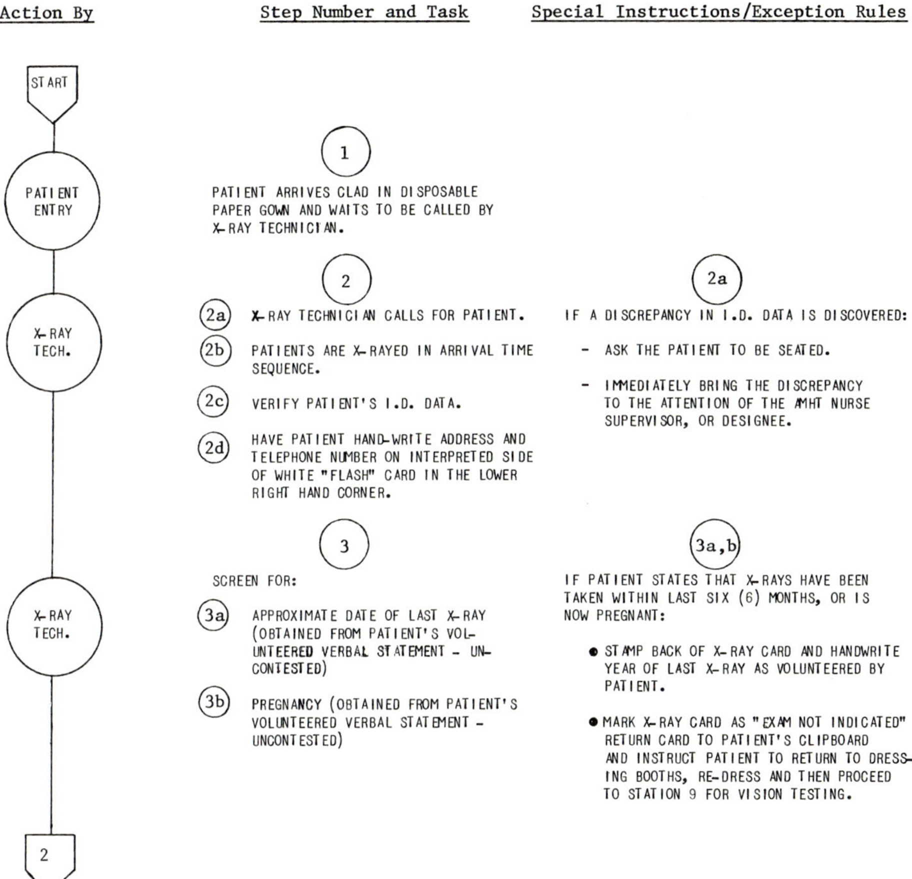

Figure 20-23a. Flow chart for chest x-ray station.

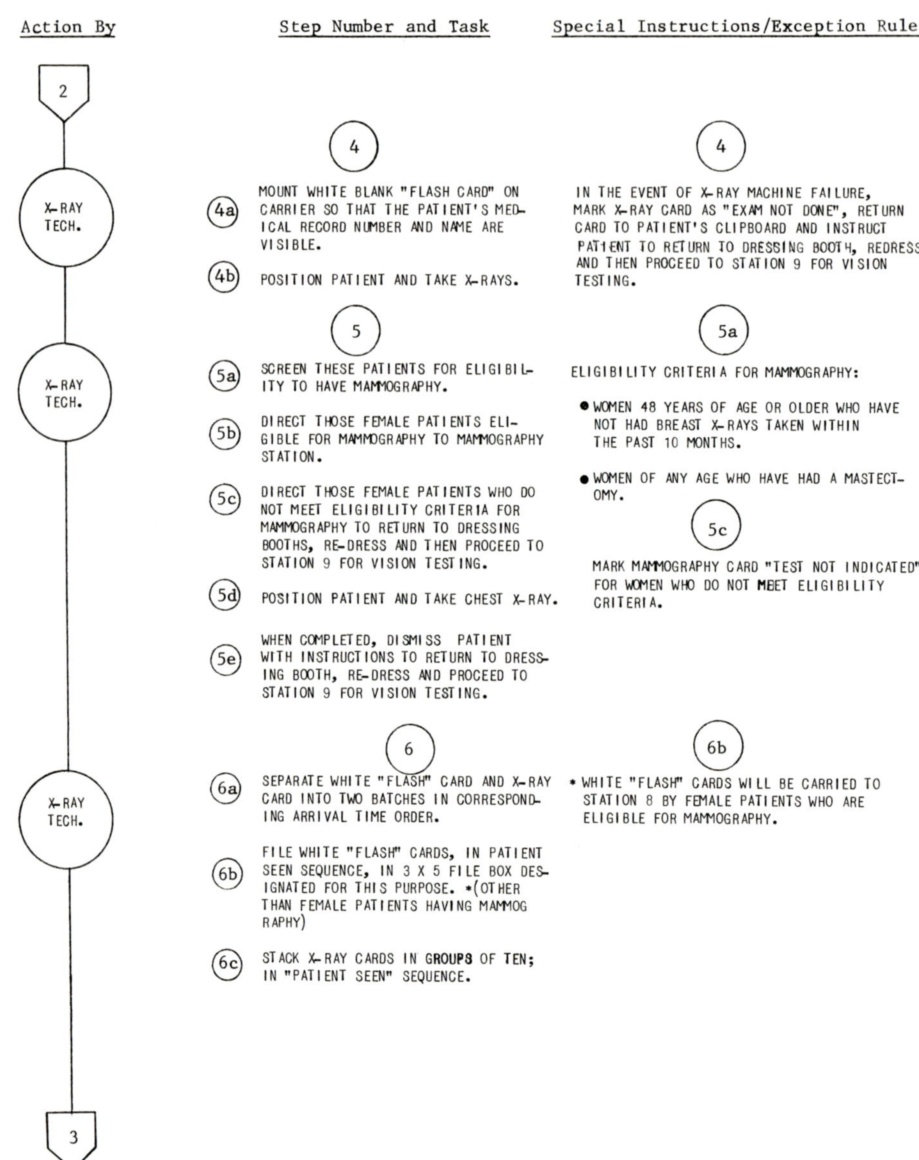

Figure 20-23b.

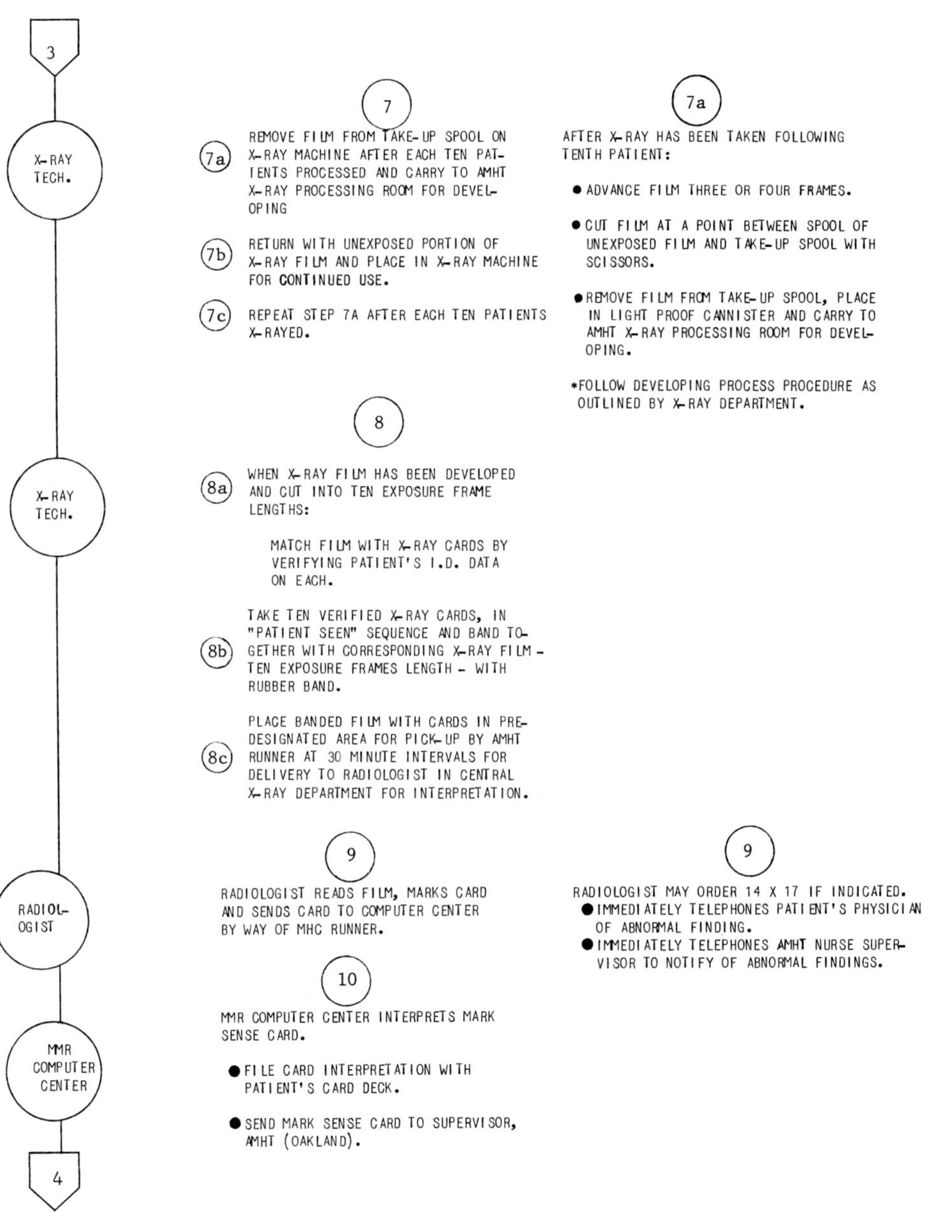

Figure 20-23c.

Action By: AMHT SUPERVISOR

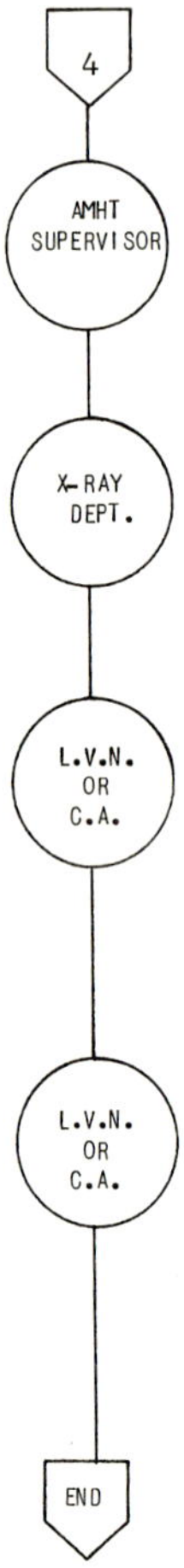

11. SUPERVISOR, AMHT, (OAKLAND) USES LOG-IN PROCEDURE TO CREATE AUDIT TRAIL, SENDS MARK SENSE CARD TO X-RAY DEPARTMENT FOR ATTACHING TO FILM.

Action By: X-RAY DEPT.

12.

12a — X-RAY DEPARTMENT MATCHES MARK SENSE CARD WITH FILM.

12b — FILM WITH MARK SENSE CARD ATTACHED IS RETURNED TO SUPERVISOR, AMHT – OAK.

Action By: L.V.N. OR C.A.

13.

- FILM WITH MARK SENSE CARD ATTACHED IS AUDITED AGAINST LOG TO VERIFY RECEIPT (CHECK AND BALANCE) (SEE STEP 3)

- LOG IS USED TO TRACK FILM NOT RECEIVED FROM X-RAY DEPARTMENT FOR WHICH CARDS HAD BEEN PREVIOUSLY SENT.

Action By: L.V.N. OR C.A.

14.

- FILM WITH MARK SENSE CARD ATTACHED IS FILED BY AMHT IN MEDICAL RECORD NUMBER SEQUENCE BY YEAR.

- RETAINED IN AMHT FILES FOR FOUR YEARS.

- RETIRED TO BERKELEY STORAGE BY X-RAY DEPARTMENT AT END OF FOUR YEARS.

END

Figure 20-23d.

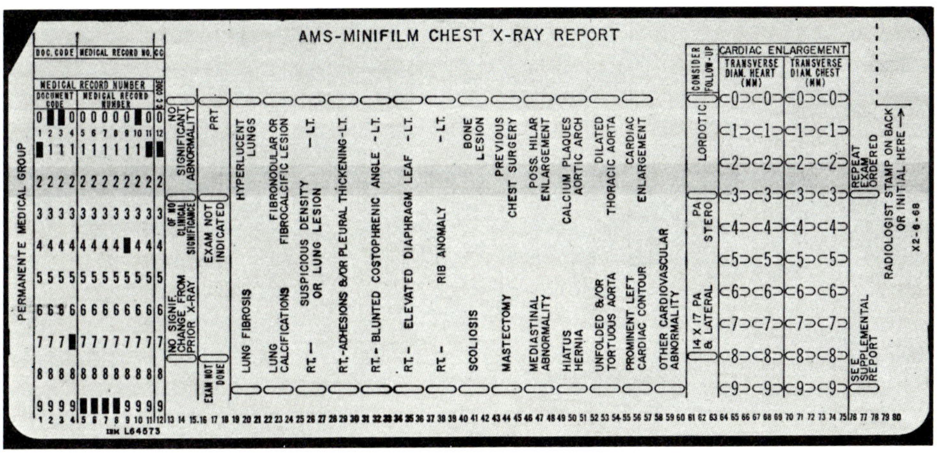

Figure 20-24. Chest x-ray report card for marksensing radiologist's interpretations.

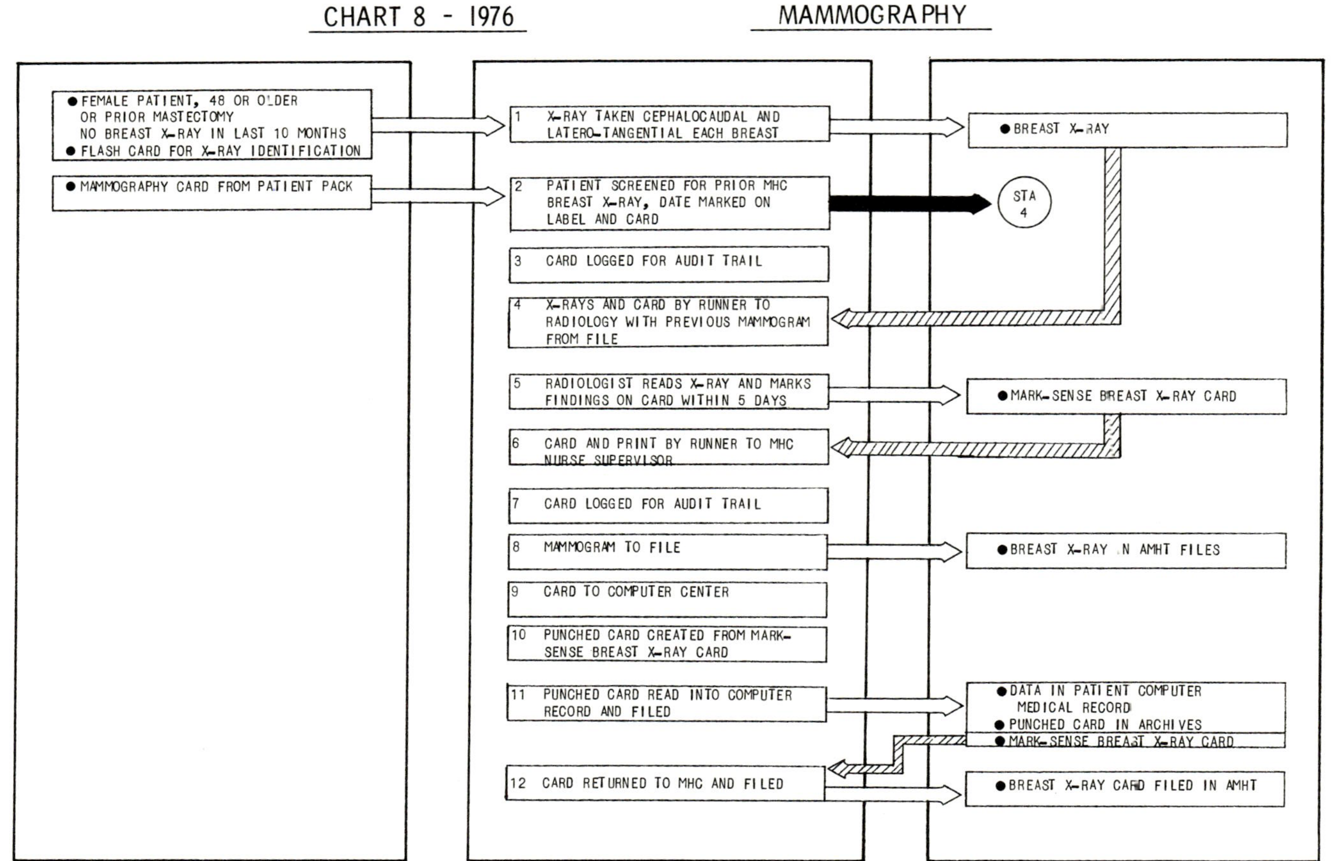

Figure 20-25. Information chart for mammography.

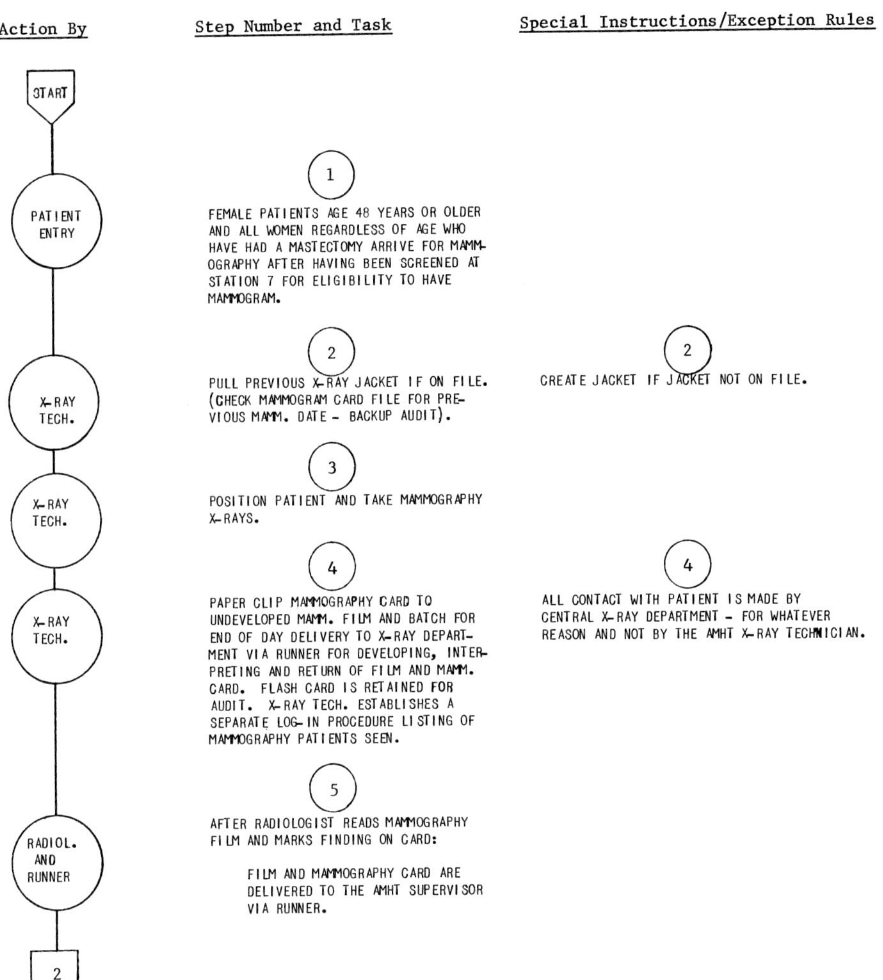

Figure 20-26a. Flow chart for mammography.

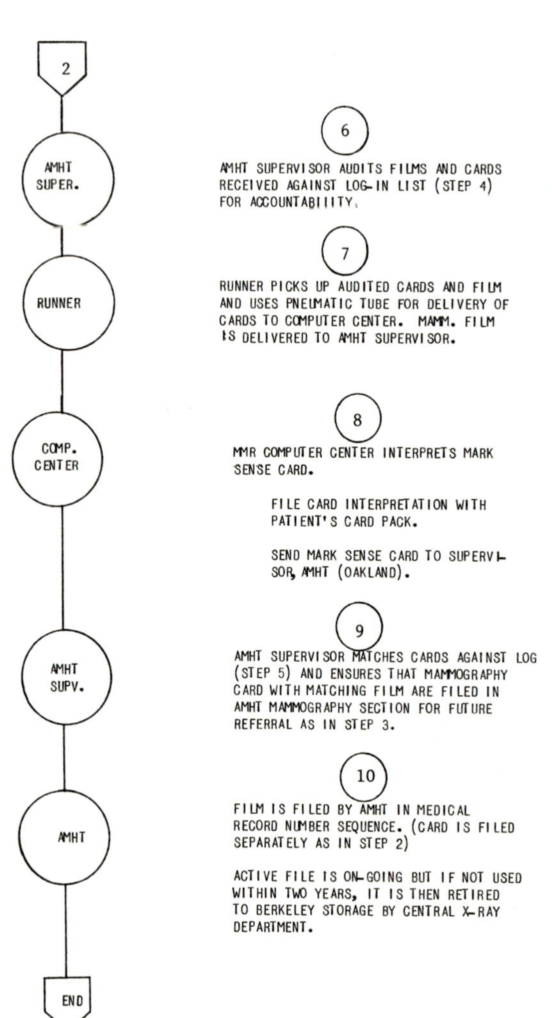

6

AMHT SUPERVISOR AUDITS FILMS AND CARDS RECEIVED AGAINST LOG-IN LIST (STEP 4) FOR ACCOUNTABILITY.

6

IF CARD AND FILM ARE NOT RECEIVED, A TRACER IO INITIATED TO SURFACE THE MISSING CARD AND FILM.

7

RUNNER PICKS UP AUDITED CARDS AND FILM AND USES PNEUMATIC TUBE FOR DELIVERY OF CARDS TO COMPUTER CENTER. MAMM. FILM IS DELIVERED TO AMHT SUPERVISOR.

8

MMR COMPUTER CENTER INTERPRETS MARK SENSE CARD.

FILE CARD INTERPRETATION WITH PATIENT'S CARD PACK.

SEND MARK SENSE CARD TO SUPERVISOR, AMHT (OAKLAND).

8

ALL DISCREPANCIES OF CARD INPUT ARE DIRECTED TO THE AMHT SUPERVISOR.

9

AMHT SUPERVISOR MATCHES CARDS AGAINST LOG (STEP 5) AND ENSURES THAT MAMMOGRAPHY CARD WITH MATCHING FILM ARE FILED IN AMHT MAMMOGRAPHY SECTION FOR FUTURE REFERRAL AS IN STEP 3.

10

FILM IS FILED BY AMHT IN MEDICAL RECORD NUMBER SEQUENCE. (CARD IS FILED SEPARATELY AS IN STEP 2)

ACTIVE FILE IS ON-GOING BUT IF NOT USED WITHIN TWO YEARS, IT IS THEN RETIRED TO BERKELEY STORAGE BY CENTRAL X-RAY DEPARTMENT.

Figure 20-26b.

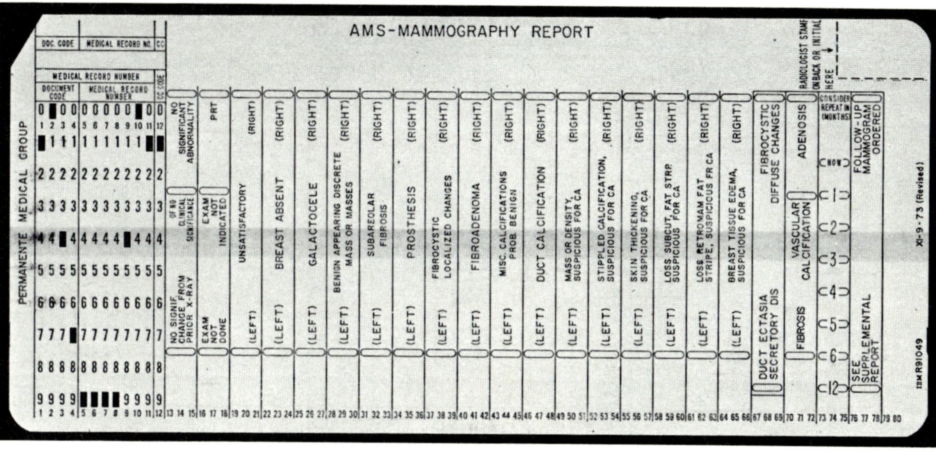

Figure 20-27. Mammography test card for marksensing radiologist's interpretations.

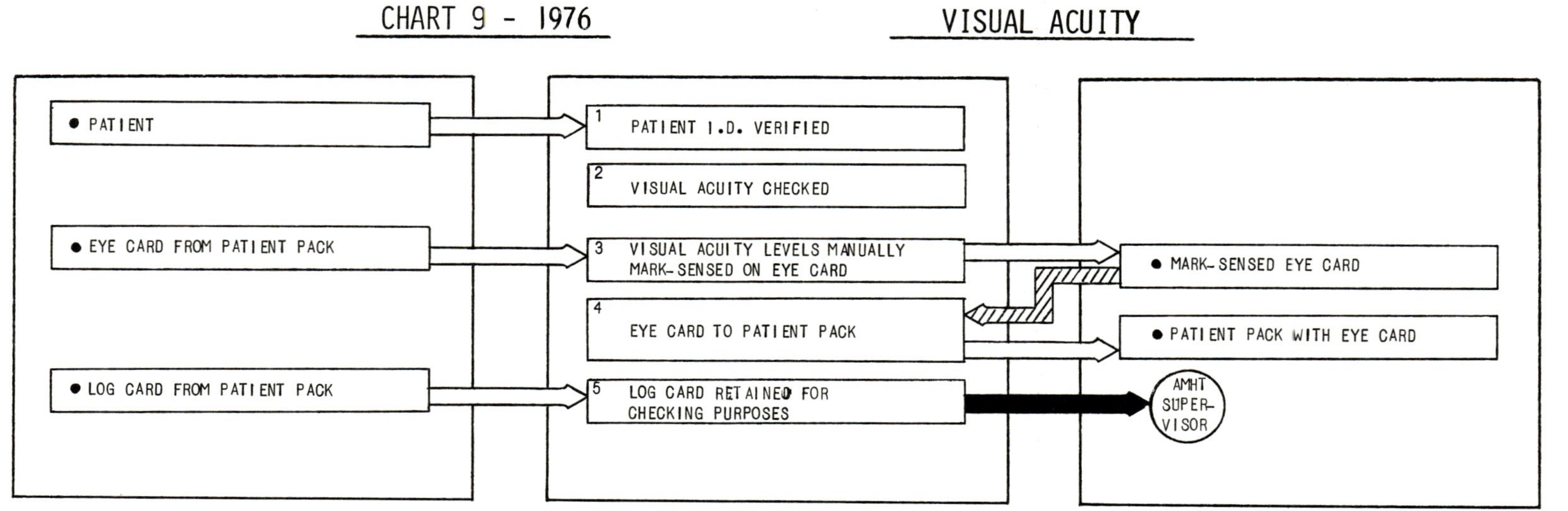

Figure 20-28. Information chart for visual acuity.

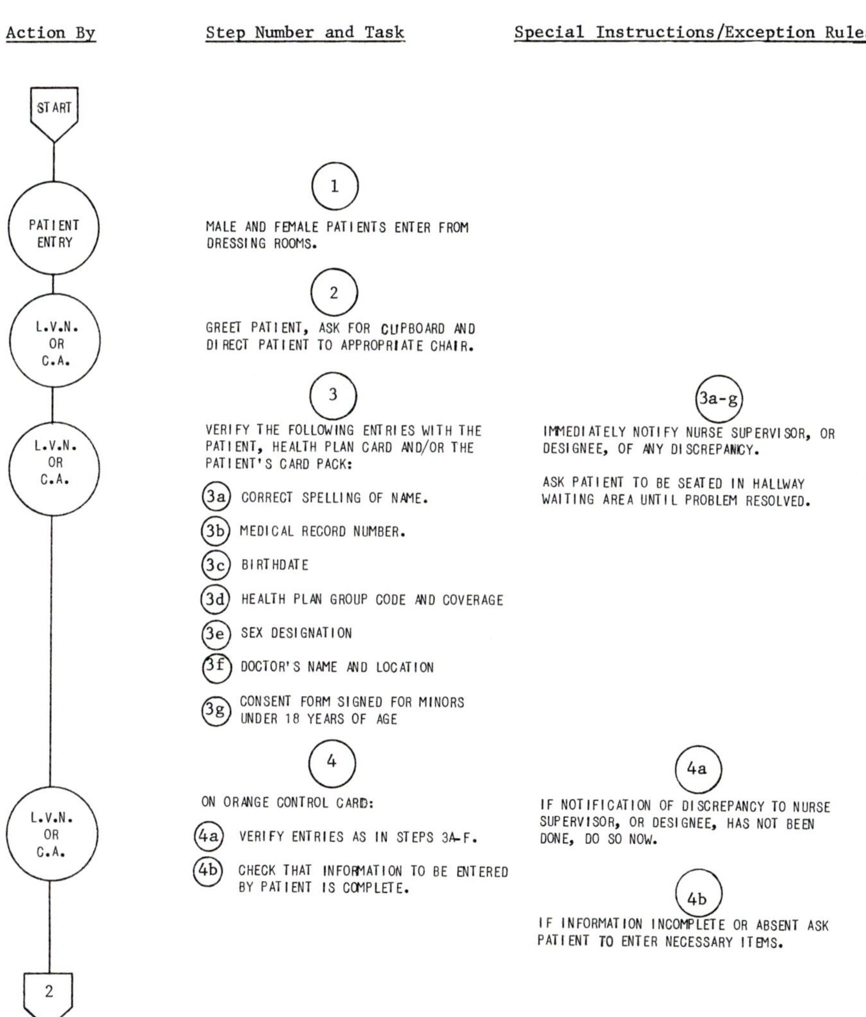

Figure 20-29a.   Flow chart for visual acuity.

<u>Action By</u>   <u>Step Number and Task</u>   <u>Special Instructions/Exception Rules</u>

2

4c IN BLACK PEN OR FELT-TIP PEN WRITE CONTROL NUMBER IN UPPER RIGHT CORNER ON PRINTED SIDE OF CARD.

4d WRITE THE LETTER "P" AFTER THE CONTROL NUMBER IF THE PATIENT MAY SEE A NURSE PRACTITIONER.

4e RETAIN ORANGE CARD. DO NOT PUT IT BACK ON CLIPBOARD.

4c THE CONTROL NUMBER IS A THREE DIGIT NUMBER STAMPED ON THE BLANK SIDE OF THE CARD BY A SIMPLEX MACHINE IN THE LAB.

DOUBLE CHECK THE CONTROL NUMBER ON THE BACK OF THE CARD WITH THE NUMBER ON THE WHITE SLIP OF PAPER. THEY SHOULD AGREE, IF NOT, NOTIFY NURSE SUPERVISOR, OR DESIGNEE.

4d VISIT CODE NUMBERS ARE WRITTEN ON RECEPTION CARD AND YELLOW QUESTIONNAIRE.

PATIENTS WITH CODES 1, 2, 3, 4, 7, 8 MAY SEE THE NURSE PRACTITIONER.

L.V.N. OR C.A.

5 DETERMINE ELIGIBILITY FOR TEST:

5a ASK PATIENT IF HE/SHE HAS SEEN AN EYE DOCTOR (OPHTHAMOLOGIST, NOT OPTOMETRIST) IN THE PAST YEAR.

5b IF YES, ASK WHERE, WHEN AND FOR WHAT.

5c PATIENT FOR SOME REASON REFUSES TEST.

5a IF YES AND IF THE DOCTOR WAS A KAISER DOCTOR FILL IN THE "YES" BUBBLE (IN ELECTROGRAPHIC PENCIL) IN VISUAL ACUITY FIELD OF EYE CARD (DOC. CODE 0010).

IF NO VISIT OR THE DOCTOR WAS NOT A KAISER DOCTOR, FILL IN THE "NO" BUBBLE.

5b ON REVERSE SIDE OF EYE CARD WRITE LOCATION, DATE AND DIAGNOSIS, IF ANY, OF LAST VISIT.

IF A PRIVATE DOCTOR, MAY JUST WRITE "PRIVATE M.D."; IF AN OPTOMETRIST WAS SEEN MAY ABBREVIATE WITH O.D.

5c FILL IN "PRT" BUBBLE.

SEND PATIENT TO NEXT STATION.

6 GATHER INFORMATION FOR THE TEST:

6a DOES PATIENT WEAR CONTACTS?

6a IF CONTACTS ARE WORN FOR THE TEST FILL IN THE "CONTACT LENSES" BUBBLE AND ON BACK OF CARD WRITE "WEARING CONTACTS" TO ALERT TONOMETRY STATION.

IF NOT WEARING CONTACTS FOR TEST, BUT DOES HAVE THEM, WRITE ON BACK OF CARD "WEARS CONTACTS".

L.V.N. OR C.A.

3

Figure 20-29b.

Action By | Step Number and Task | Special Instructions/Exception Rules

3

6b DOES PATIENT WEAR GLASSES FOR DISTANCE (NOT READING)?

6b

ASK PATIENT TO PUT ON DISTANCE GLASSES FOR TEST.

FILL IN "WITH GLASSES" BUBBLE.

IF PATIENT WEARS GLASSES, BUT DID NOT BRING THEM HAVE THE PINHOLE ON HAND. REMIND THE PATIENT TO BRING GLASSES NEXT TIME.

L.V.N. OR C.A.

7

PERFORM VISUAL ACUITY CHECK:

7a ASK PATIENT TO COVER LEFT EYE WITH PAPER (TO CHECK RIGHT EYE).

7b ASK PATIENT TO READ LETTERS IN COLUMN ONE FROM TOP TO BOTTOM.

7c FILL IN BUBBLE FOR NUMBER OF LETTERS MISSED IN COLUMN HEADED "RIGHT" UNDER "NUMBER OF LETTERS MISSED" FIELD OF CARD.

7d REPEAT PROCEDURE TO TEST LEFT EYE. HAVE PATIENT COVER RIGHT EYE, READ COLUMN TWO AND MARK NUMBER MISSED IN COLUMN HEADED "LEFT".

7c,d

PATIENT MISSES MORE THAN 5 LETTERS:

- EXPLAIN TO PATIENT TO LOOK THROUGH THE PINHOLE.
- ASK PATIENT TO READ THE LETTERS IN THE APPROPRIATE COLUMN.
- MARK ON REVERSE SIDE OF CARD "P/H" (TO INDICATE THE PINHOLE WAS USED), WHICH EYE (O.D. FOR RIGHT EYE, O.S. FOR LEFT) AND THE NUMBER OF LETTERS MISSED.
- DO NOT FILL IN THE PINHOLE BUBBLE ON FRONT OF CARD.

L.V.N. OR C.A.

8

FILL IN APPROPRIATE BUBBLES FOR "IRIS COLOR" AND "SKIN COLOR".

L.V.N. OR C.A.

9

DOUBLE CHECK THAT APPROPRIATE BUBBLES ARE FILLED IN AND INTIAL REVERSE SIDE OF CARD IN LOWER RIGHT CORNER.

L.V.N. OR C.A.

10

RETURN CLIPBOARD TO PATIENT AND DIRECT TO NEXT STATION.

END

Figure 20-29c.

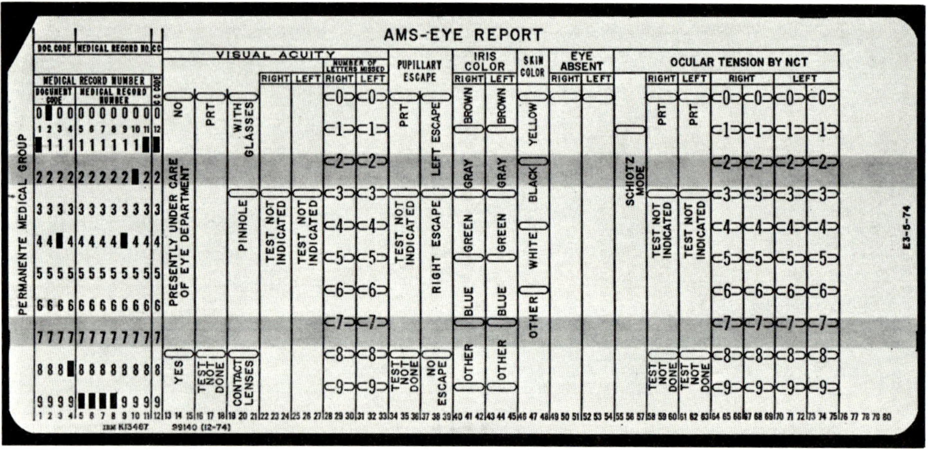

Figure 20-30. Test card for visual acuity.

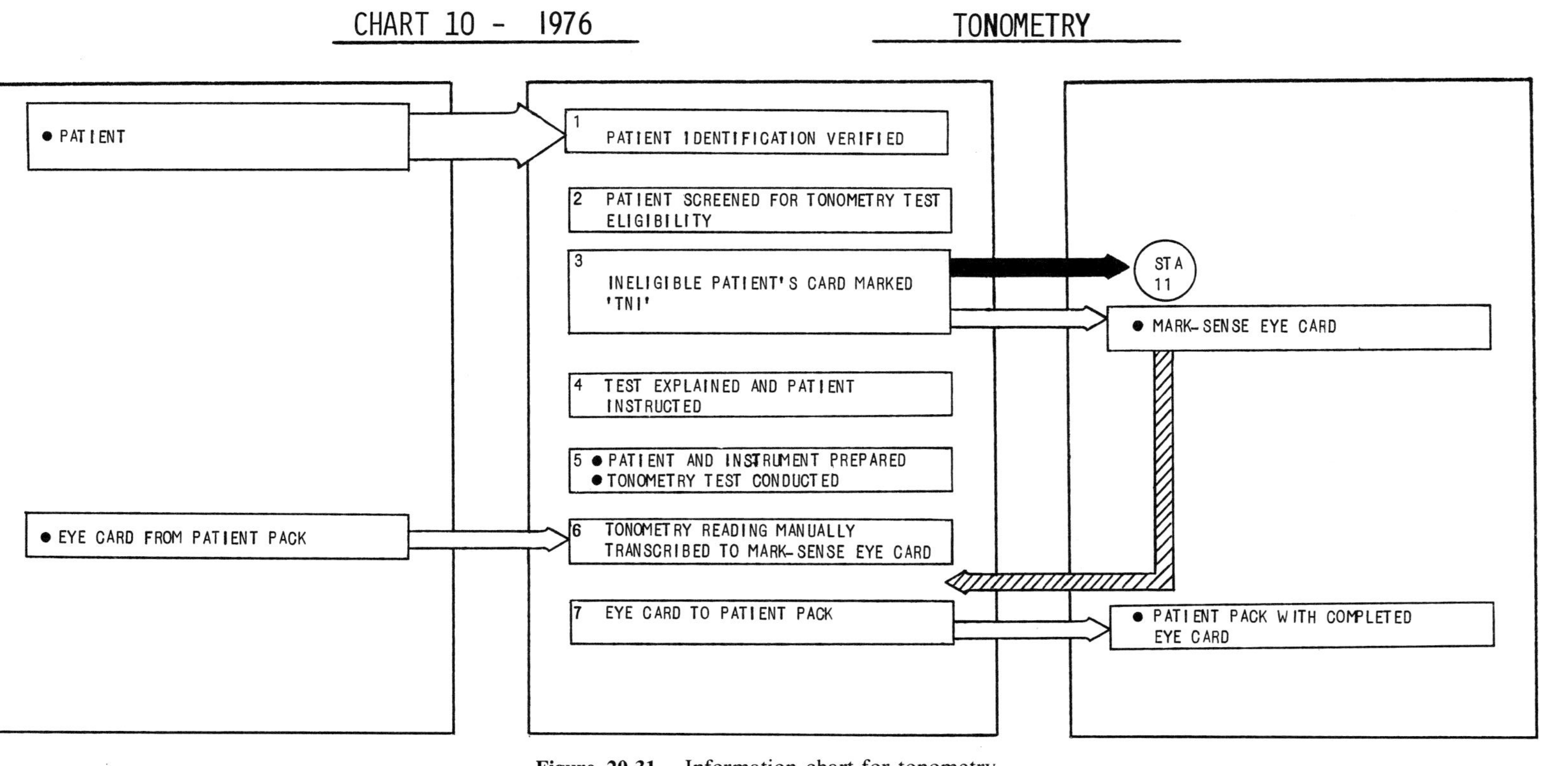

Figure 20-31. Information chart for tonometry.

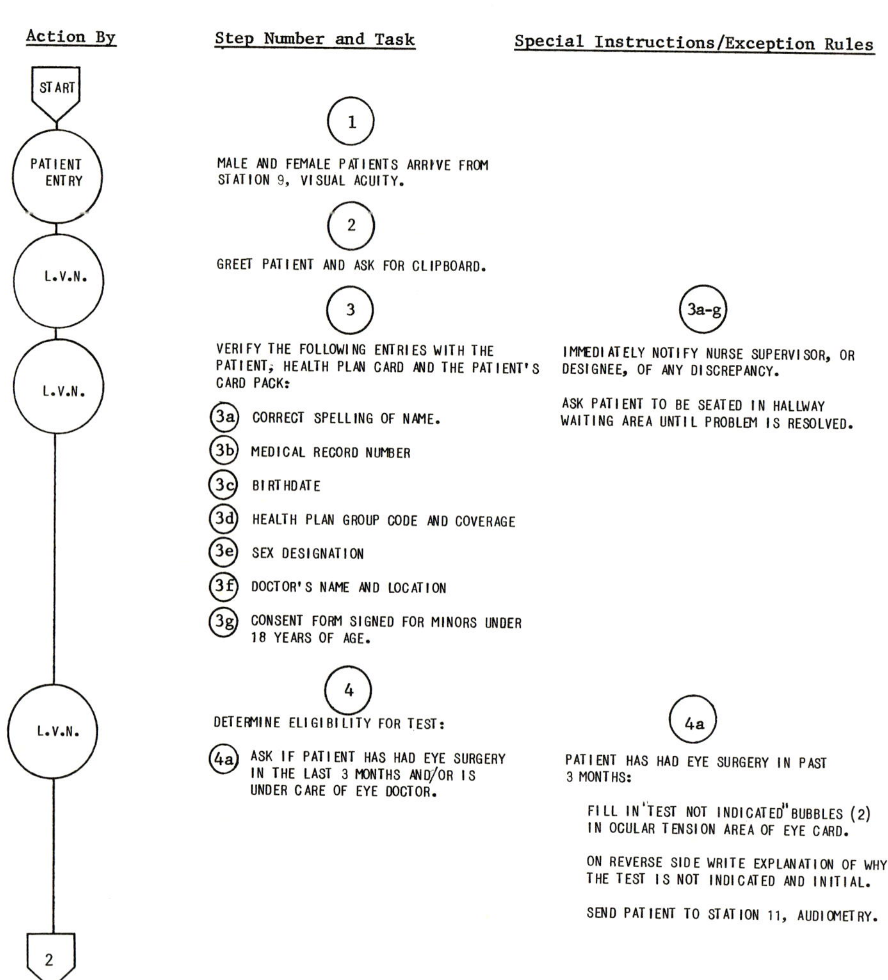

Figure 20-32a.   Flow chart for tonometry.

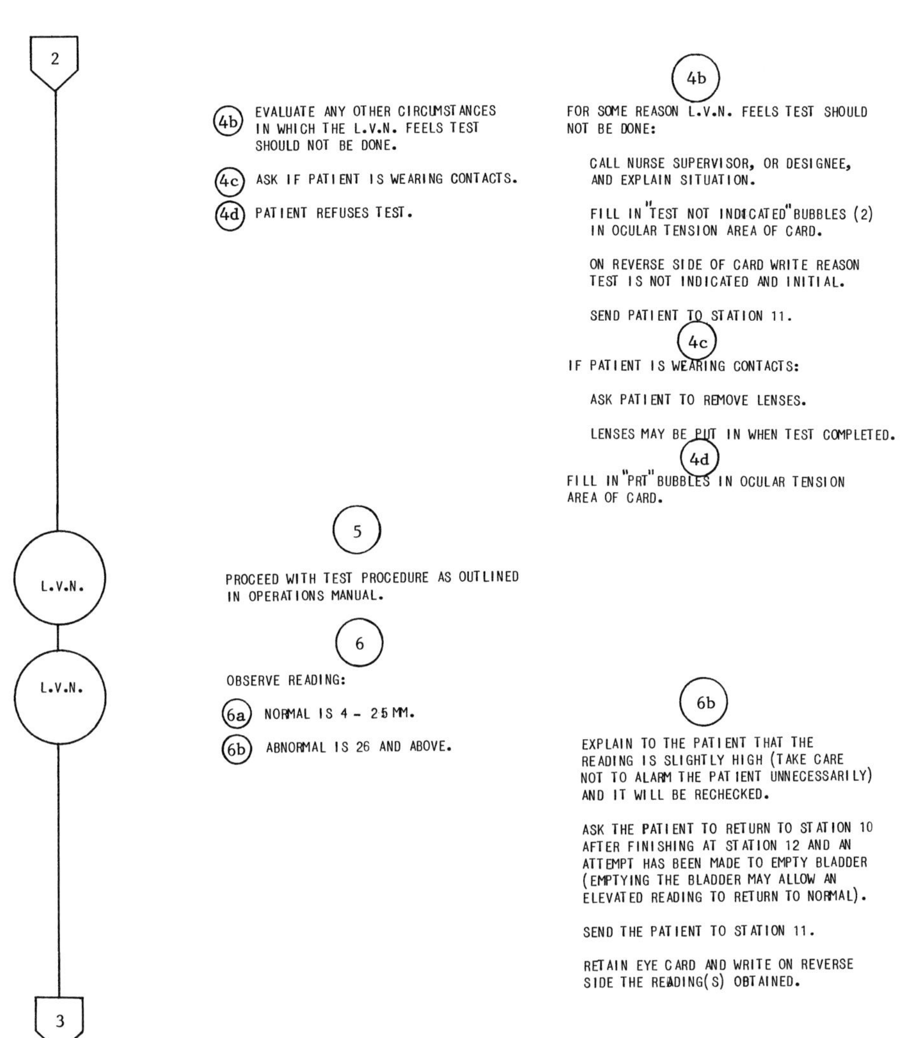

Figure 20-32b.

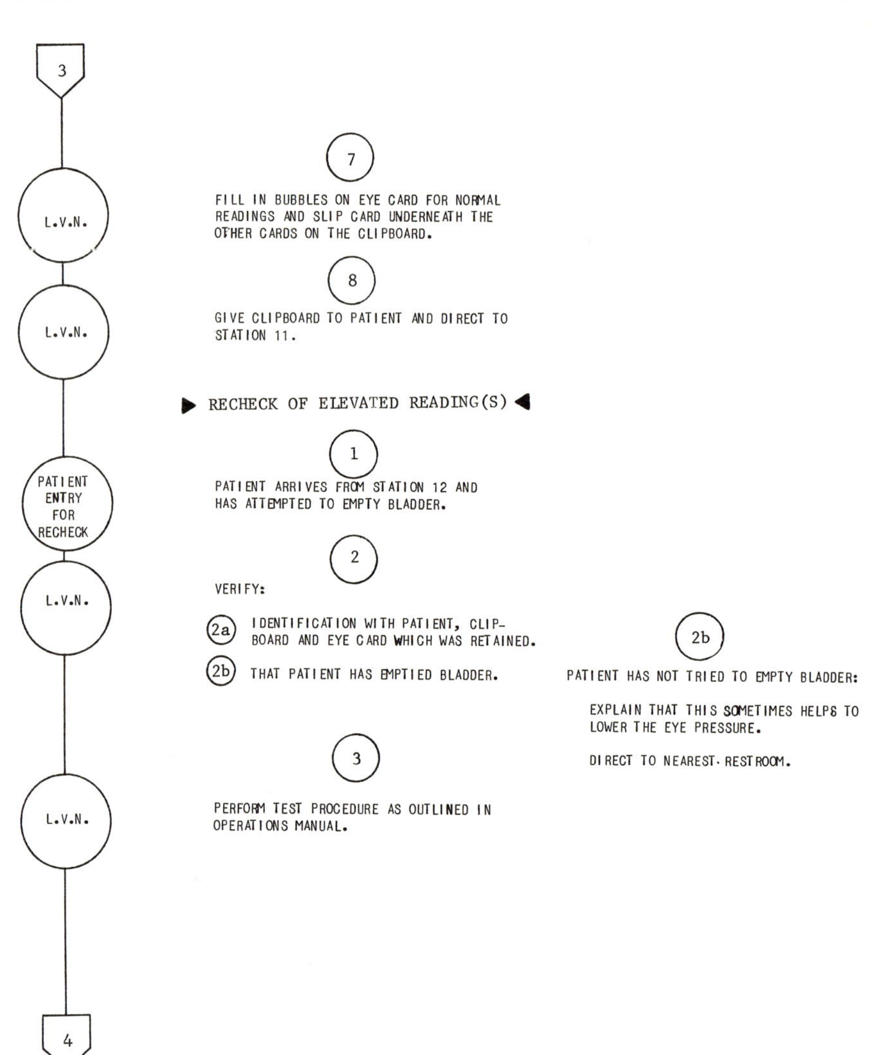

Figure 20-32c.

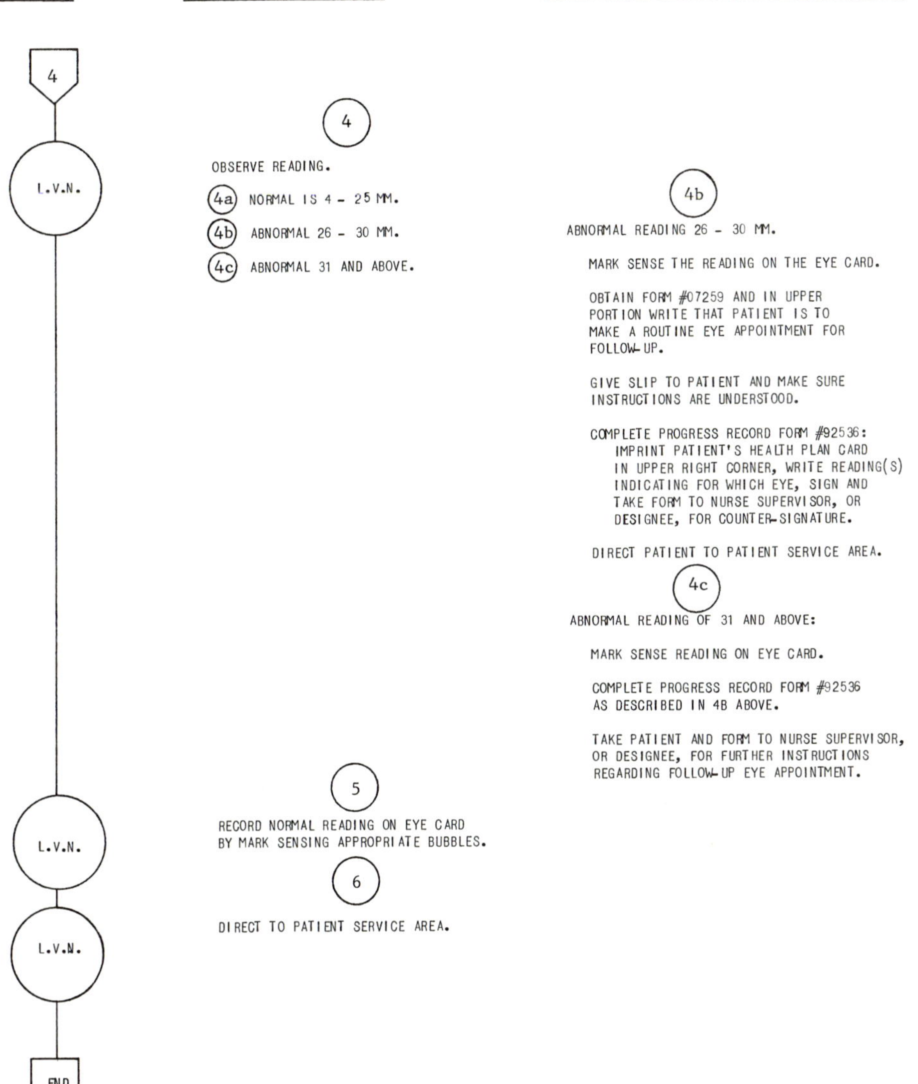

Figure 20-32d.

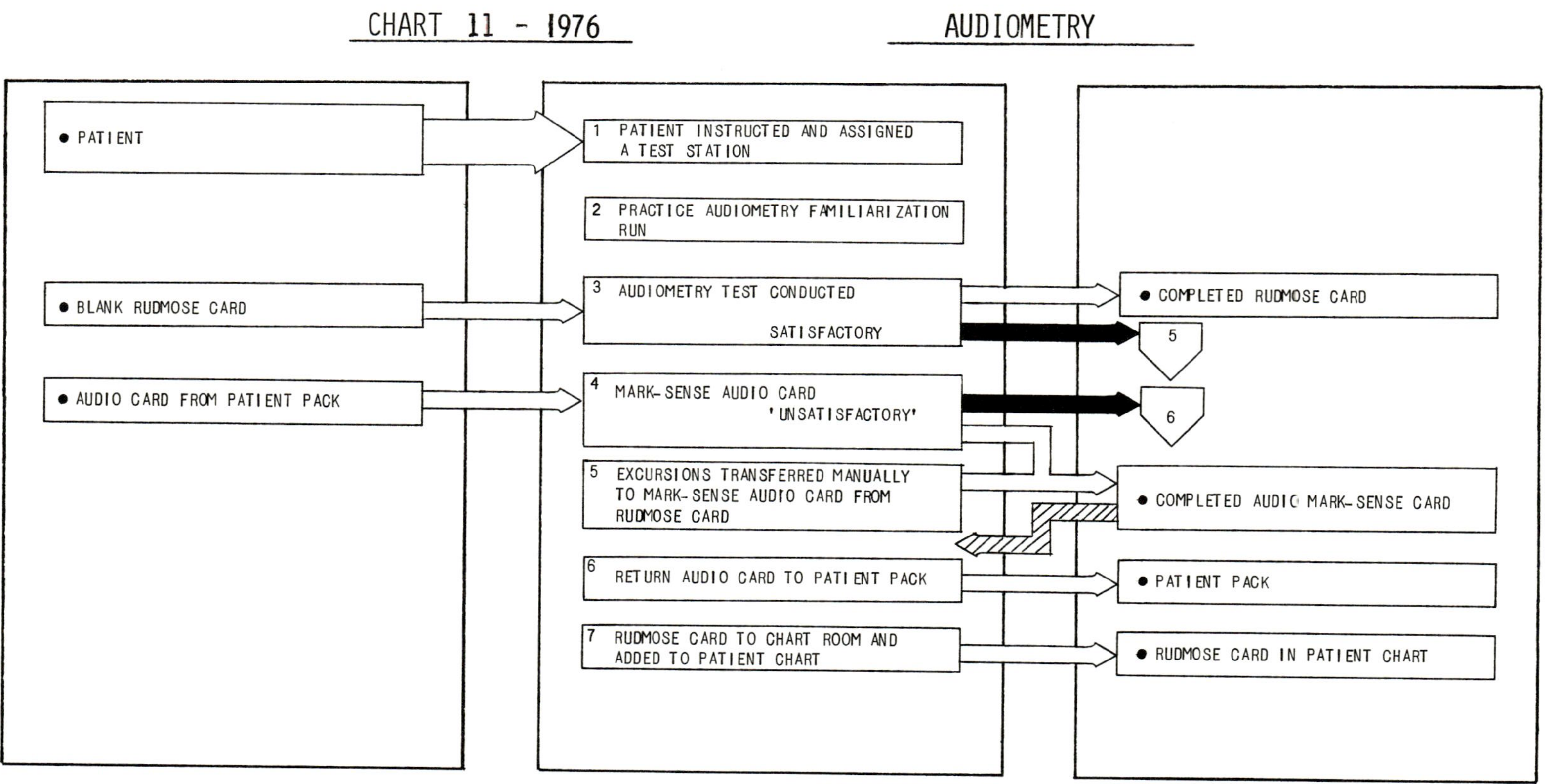

Figure 20-33. Information chart for audiometry.

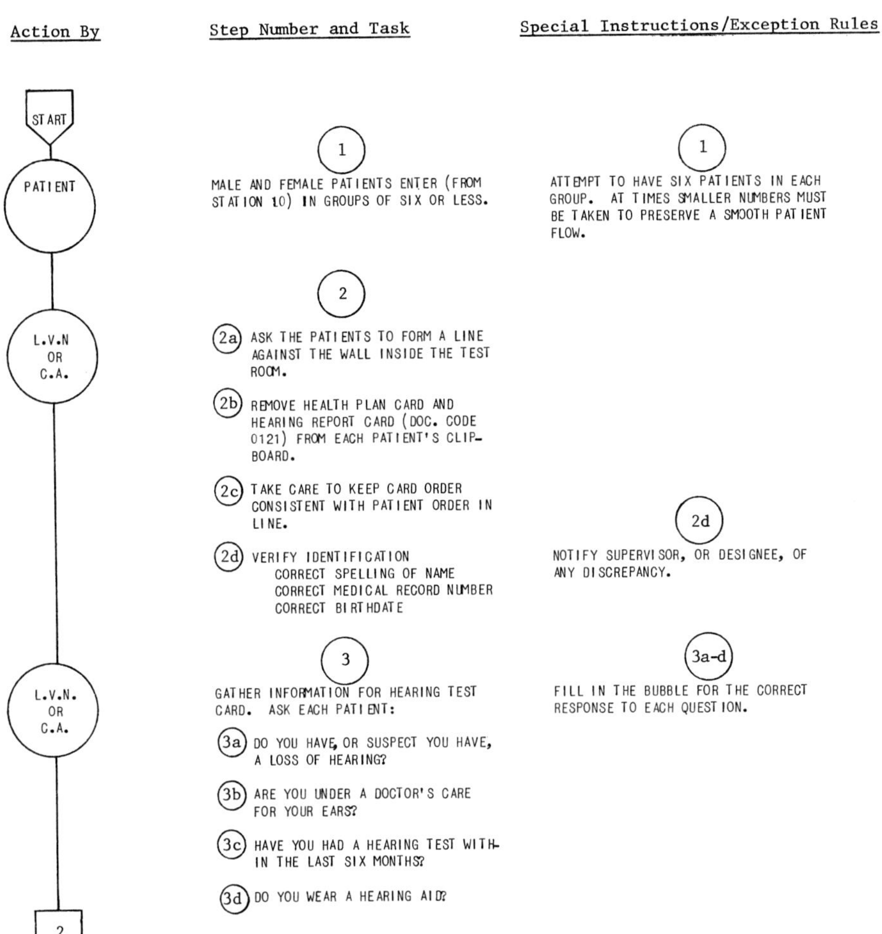

Figure 20-34a. Flow chart for audiometry.

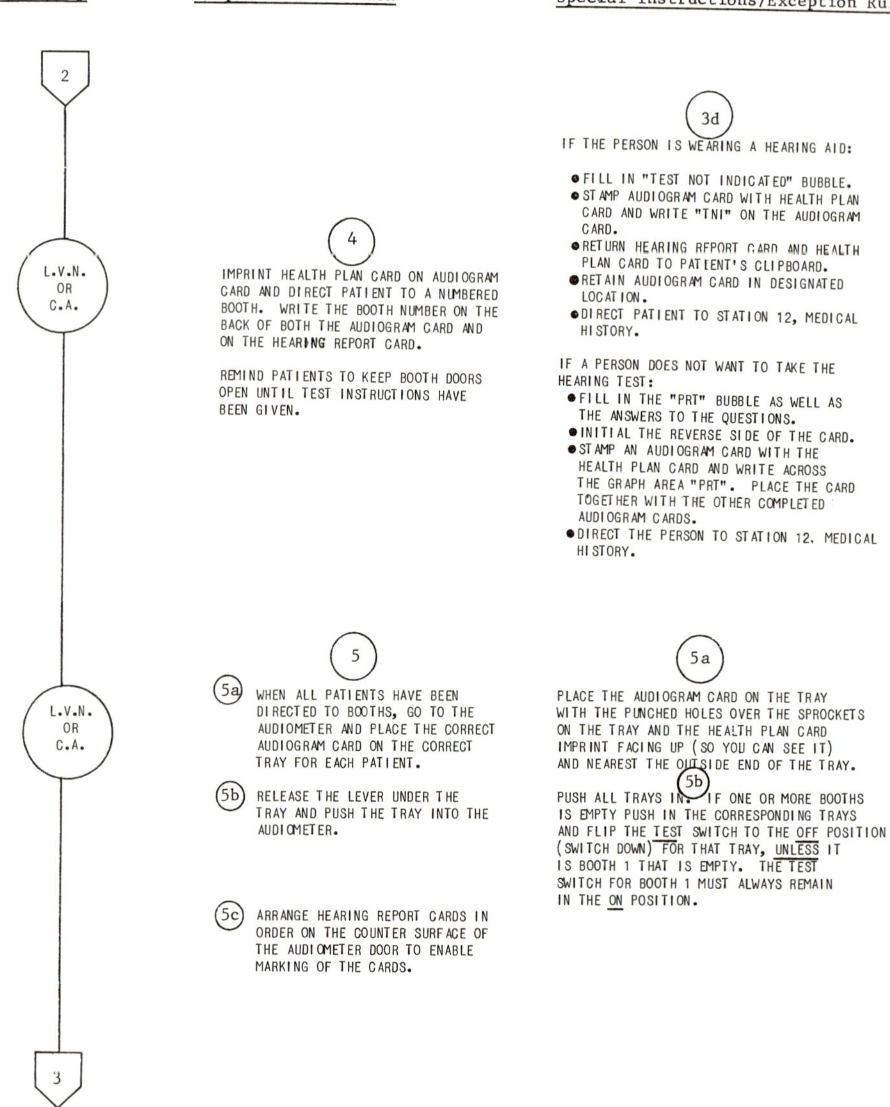

Figure 20-34b.

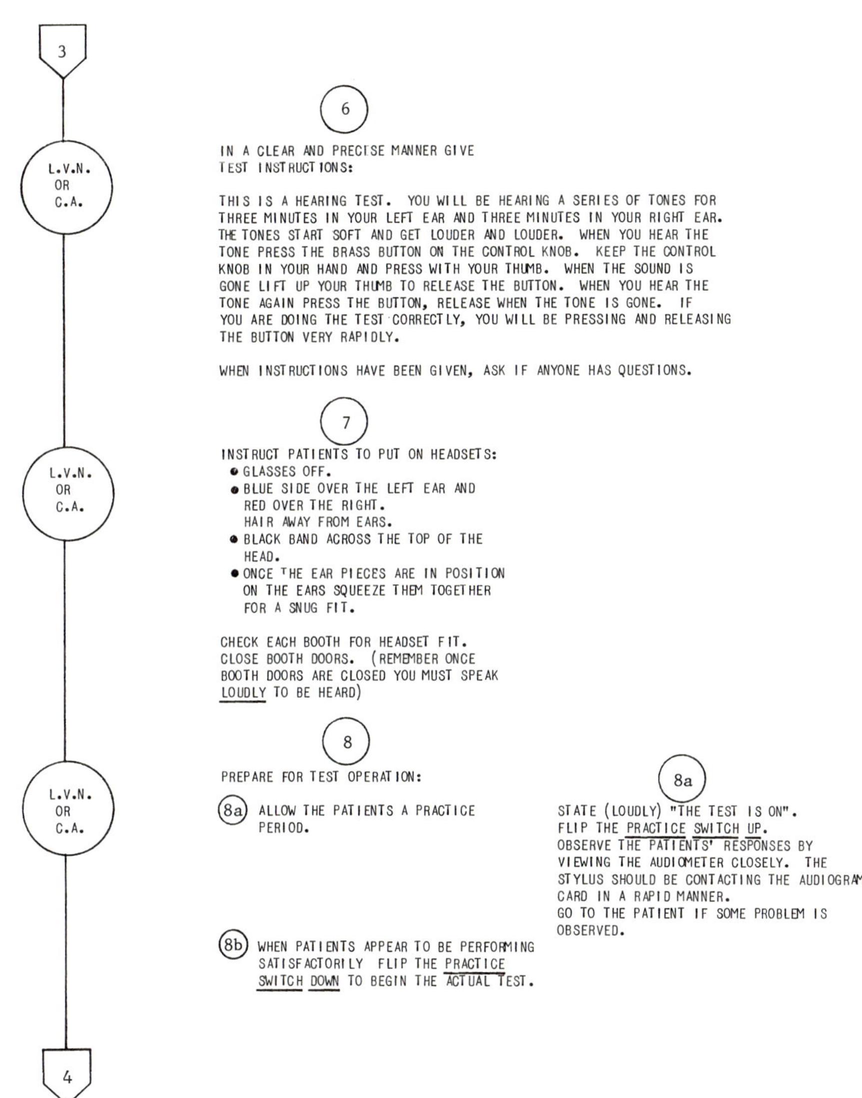

Figure 20-34c.

Action By | **Step Number and Task** | **Special Instructions/Exception Rules**

4
L.V.N.
OR
C.A.
L.V.N.
OR
C.A.
END

9

9a MARK THE HEARING REPORT CARD WITH THE READINGS FROM THE AUDIOGRAM CARD.

9a AS YOU LOOK AT THE AUDIOGRAM CARD AND THE HEARING REPORT CARD THE FREQUENCY COLUMNS EXTEND CROSSWISE AND THE DECIBELS LENGTHWISE.

AS THE AUDIOGRAM CARD MOVES OUT OF THE AUDIOMETER THE <u>LEFT</u> EAR RECORDINGS AT 500, 1000, ETC BECOME VISIBLE. PREPARE TO BEGIN MARKING IN THIS AREA OF THE HEARING REPORT CARD.

OBSERVE THE PINPOINT MARKINGS MADE BY THE STYLUS ON THE AUDIOGRAM CARD. DETERMINE THE NUMBER (0-90) CORRESPONDING TO THE AREA OF HIGHEST CONCENTRATION OF STYLUS MARKINGS AND FILL IN THE APPROPRIATE BUBBLE FOR THAT NUMBER ON THE HEARING REPORT CARD.

9b CONSIDER THE TEST UNSATISFACTORY IF THE STYLUS MARKINGS COVER A RANGE OF 15 DECIBELS OR MORE FOR ONE FREQUENCY (MOST WILL BE WITHIN 10 DECIBELS).

9b WHEN A TEST IS UNSATISFACTORY:

- FILL IN THE TEST UNSATISFACTORY BUBBLE ON THE HEARING REPORT CARD.
- WRITE ON THE REVERSE SIDE OF THE AUDIOGRAM CARD "TEST UNSATISFACTORY".

10

WHEN THE TEST CYCLE IS COMPLETE:

10a TELL THE PATIENTS THE TEST IS OVER AND ASK THEM TO REMOVE THEIR HEADPHONES AND PLACE THEM ON THE HOOKS IN THE BOOTHS.

10b FINISH MARKING THE HEARING REPORT CARDS AND INITIAL THE REVERSE SIDE OF THE CARD.

10c RETURN THE HEARING REPORT CARDS TO THE PATIENTS' CLIPBOARDS. INSERT THE CARD UNDER THE OTHERS IN THE CARD HOLDER.

10d DIRECT PATIENTS TO STATION 12, THE CIRCLE DESK AREA.

10e REMOVE AUDIOGRAM CARDS FROM AUDIOMETER AND PLACE THEM IN DESIGNATED AREA.

Figure 20-34d.

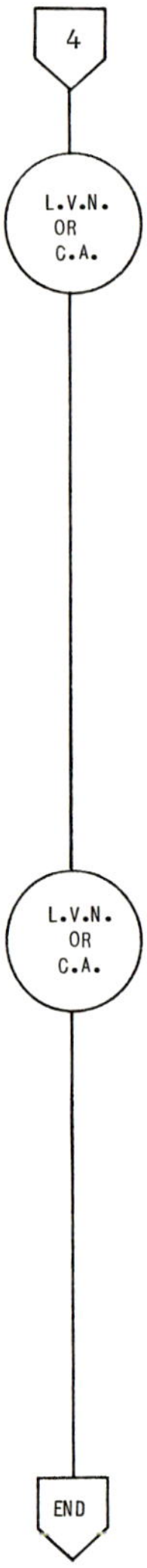

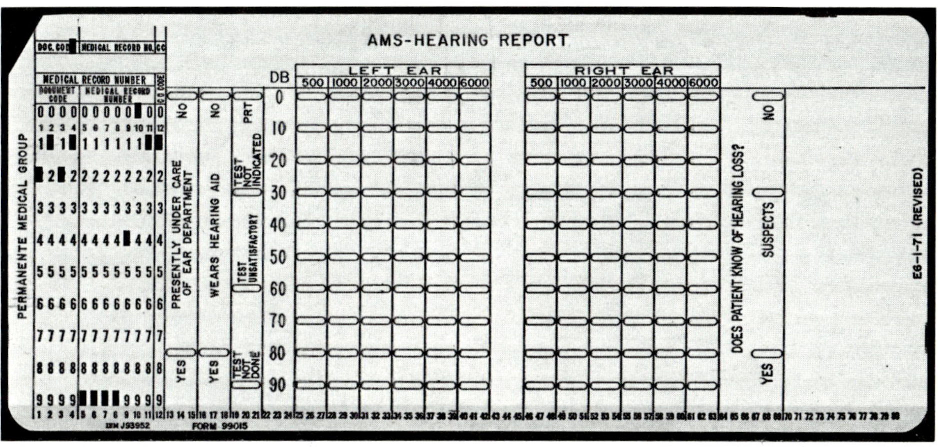

Figure 20-35. Test card for audiometry.

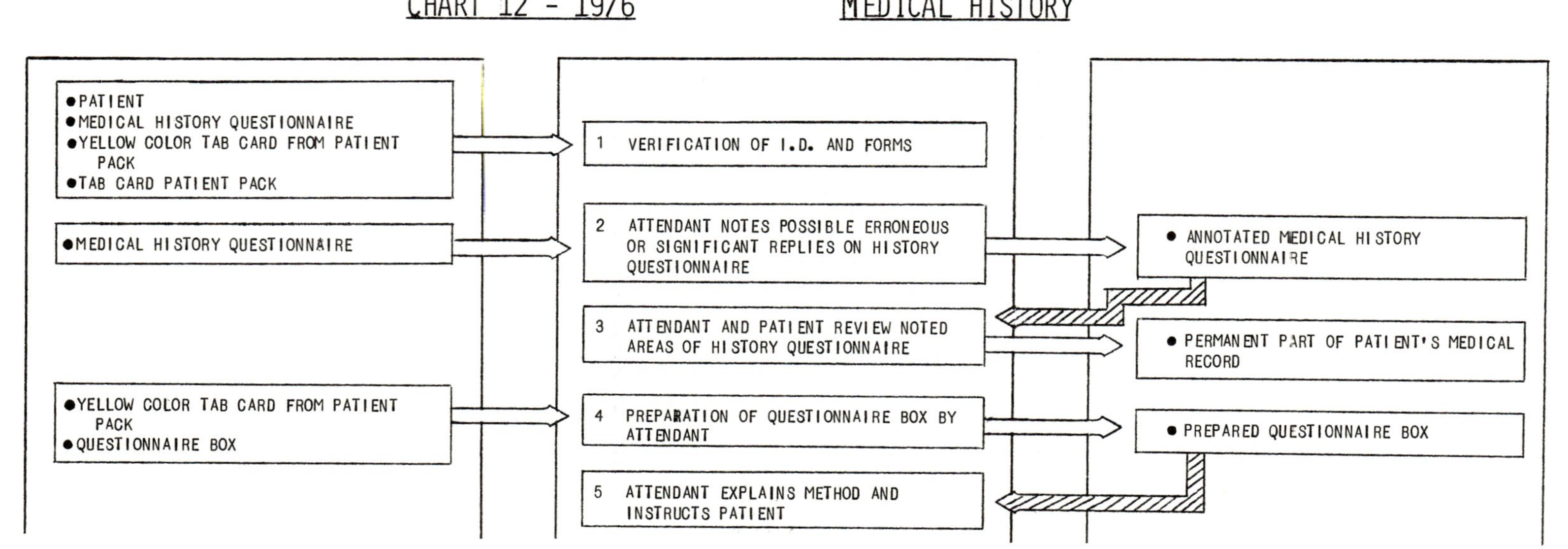
CHART 12 - 1976
MEDICAL HISTORY
PATIENT
MEDICAL HISTORY QUESTIONNAIRE
YELLOW COLOR TAB CARD FROM PATIENT PACK
TAB CARD PATIENT PACK
1 VERIFICATION OF I.D. AND FORMS
MEDICAL HISTORY QUESTIONNAIRE
2 ATTENDANT NOTES POSSIBLE ERRONEOUS OR SIGNIFICANT REPLIES ON HISTORY QUESTIONNAIRE
3 ATTENDANT AND PATIENT REVIEW NOTED AREAS OF HISTORY QUESTIONNAIRE
YELLOW COLOR TAB CARD FROM PATIENT PACK
QUESTIONNAIRE BOX
4 PREPARATION OF QUESTIONNAIRE BOX BY ATTENDANT
5 ATTENDANT EXPLAINS METHOD AND INSTRUCTS PATIENT
ANNOTATED MEDICAL HISTORY QUESTIONNAIRE
PERMANENT PART OF PATIENT'S MEDICAL RECORD
PREPARED QUESTIONNAIRE BOX

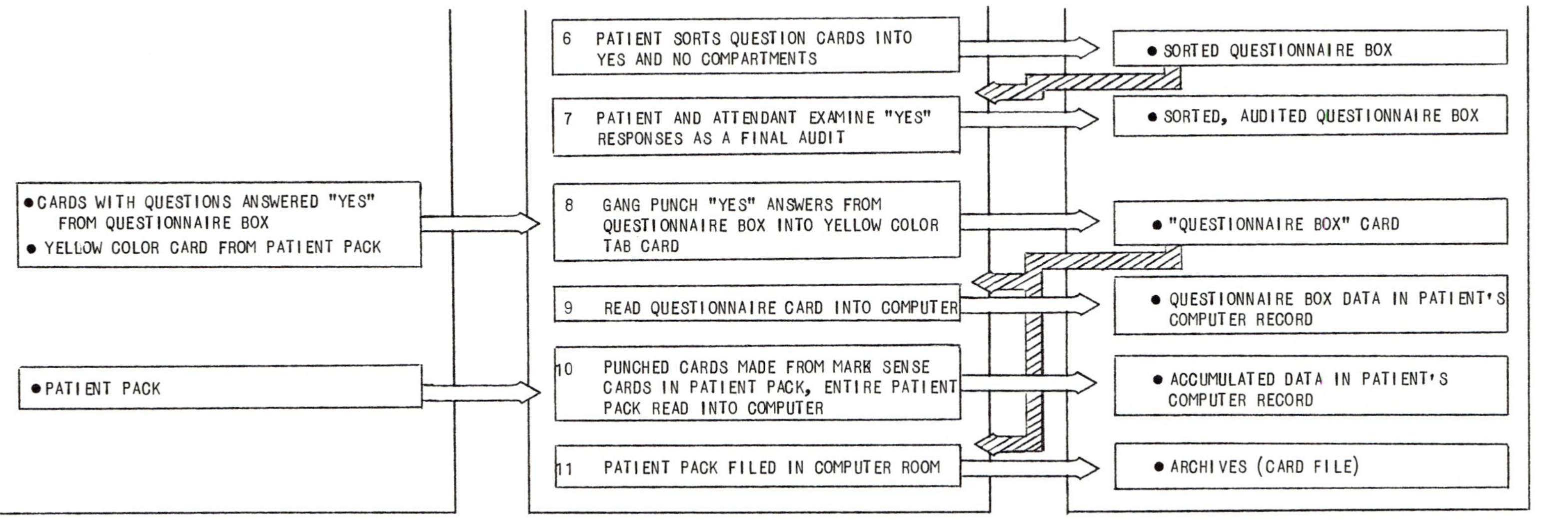

Figure 20-36. Information chart for medical history.

<u>Action By</u>   <u>Step Number and Task</u>   <u>Special Instructions/Exception Rules</u>

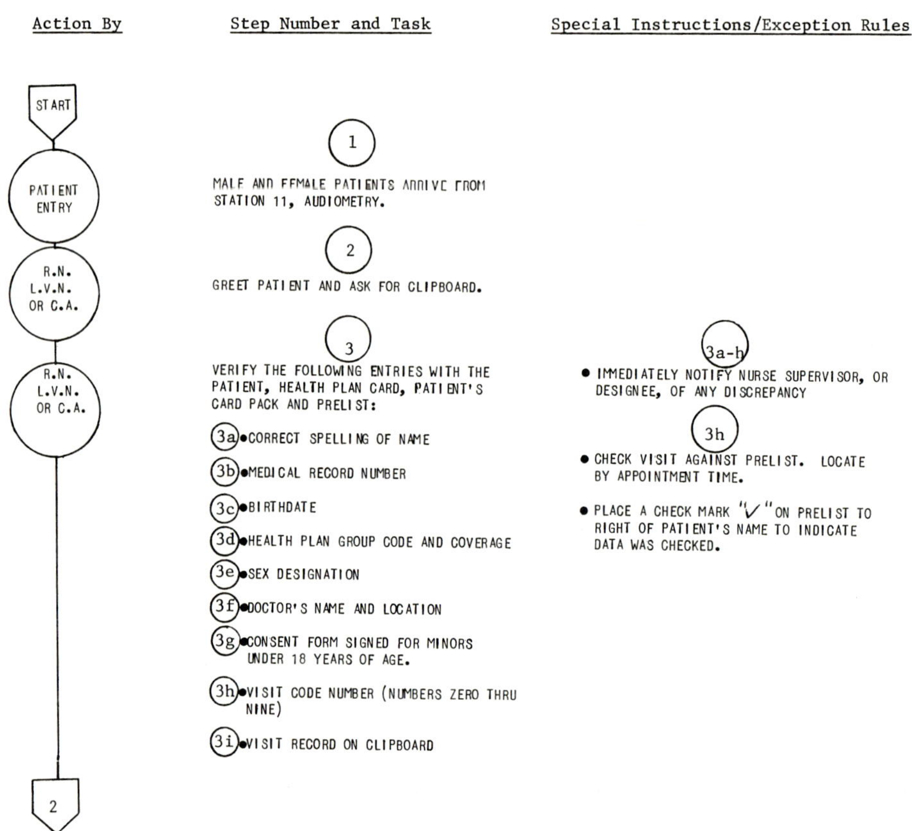

Figure 20-37a. Flow chart for medical history.

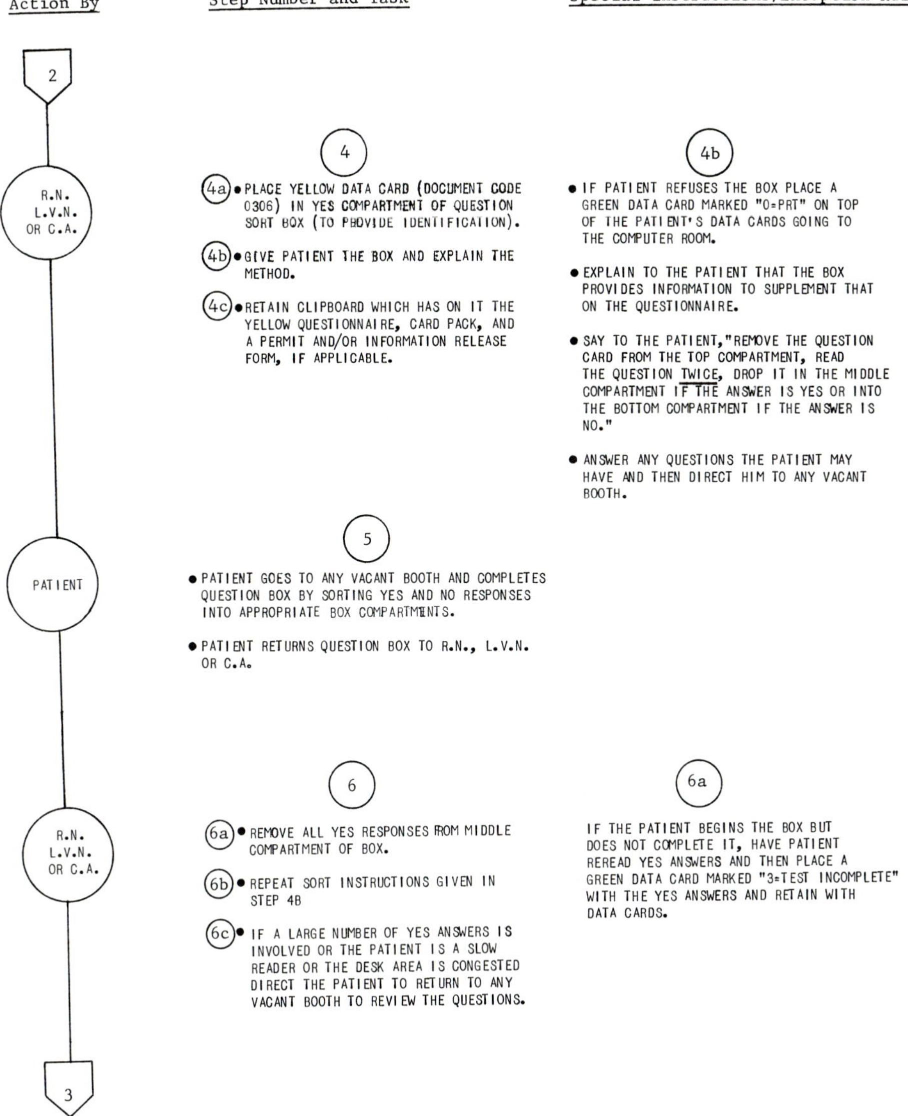

Figure 20-37b.

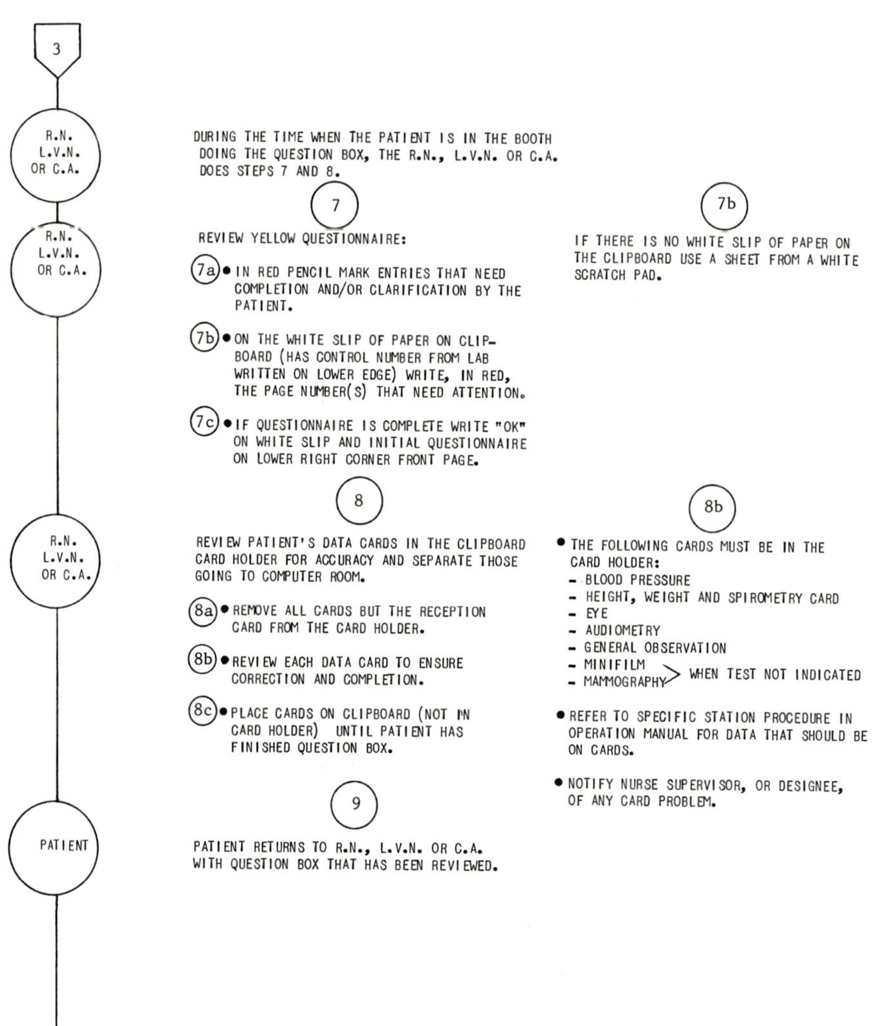

Figure 20-37c.

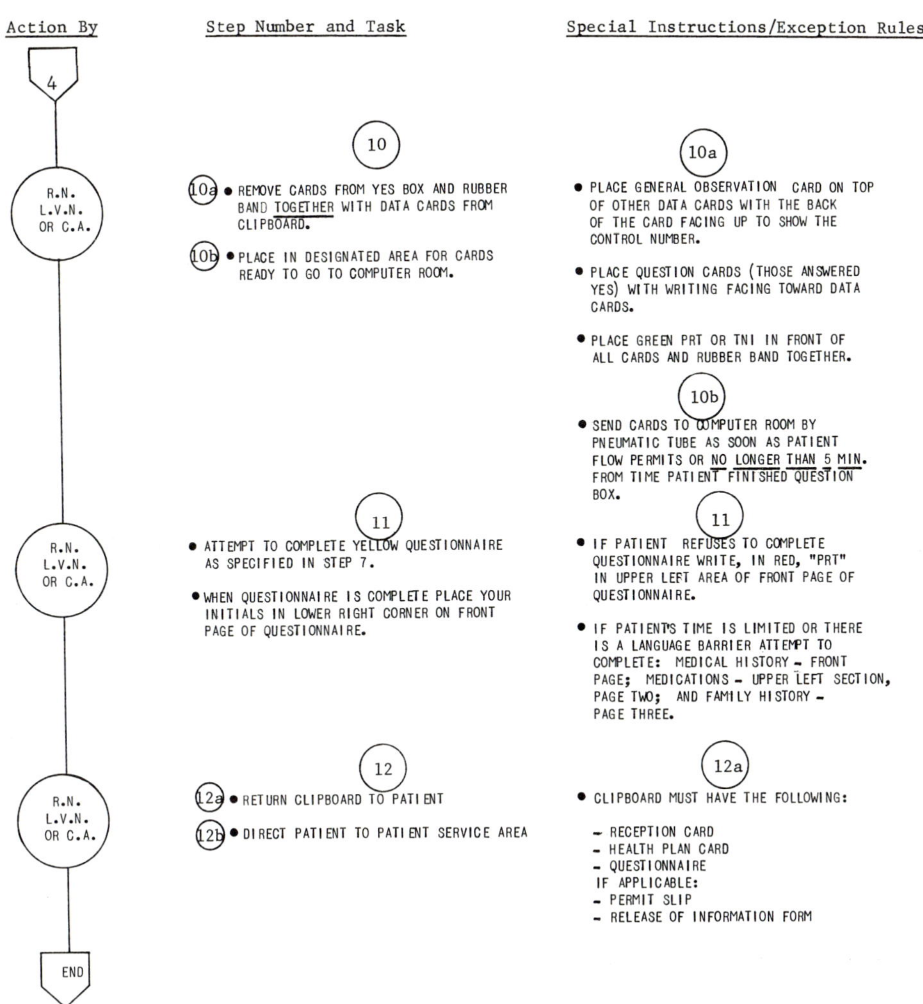

Figure 20-37d.

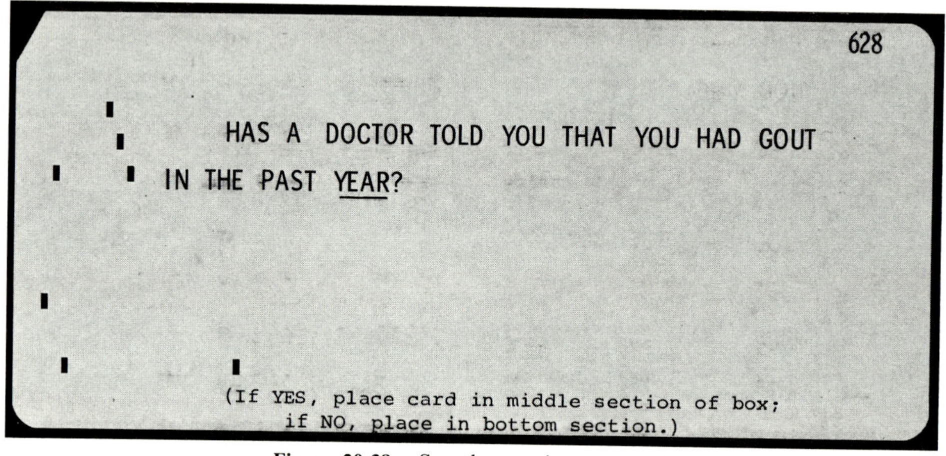

Figure 20-38. Sample question sort card.

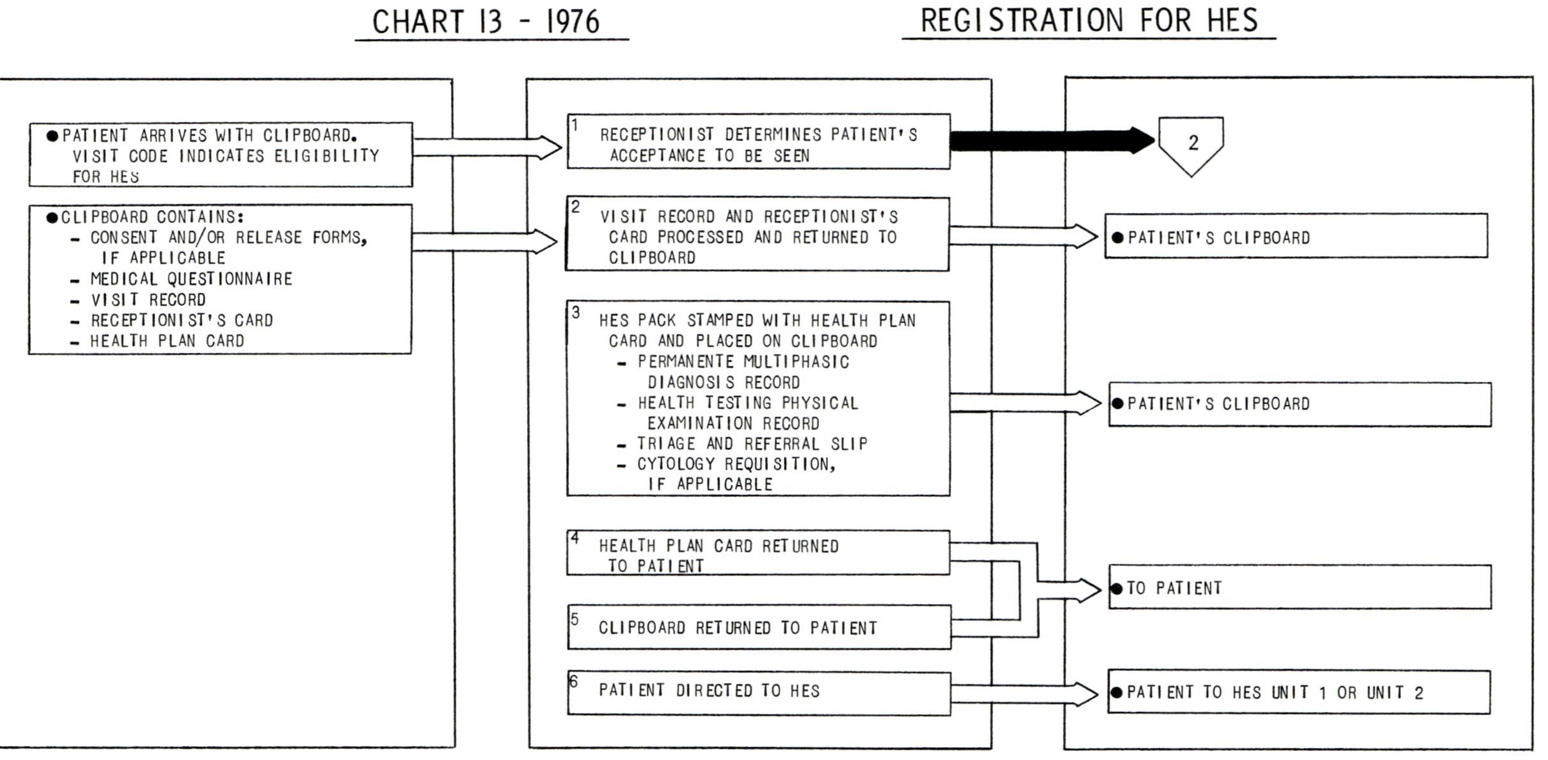

Figure 20-39. Information chart for HES registration.

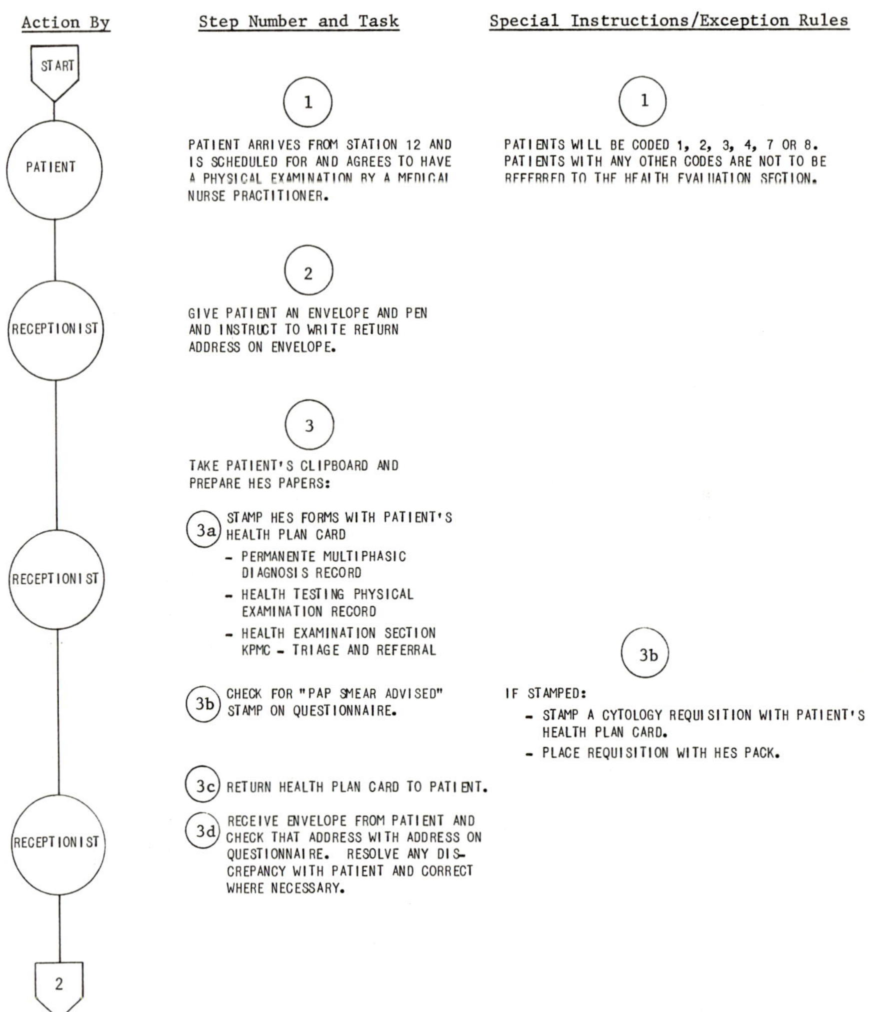

Figure 20-40a.   Flow chart for HES registration.

<u>Action By</u>   <u>Step Number and Task</u>   <u>Special Instructions/Exception Rules</u>

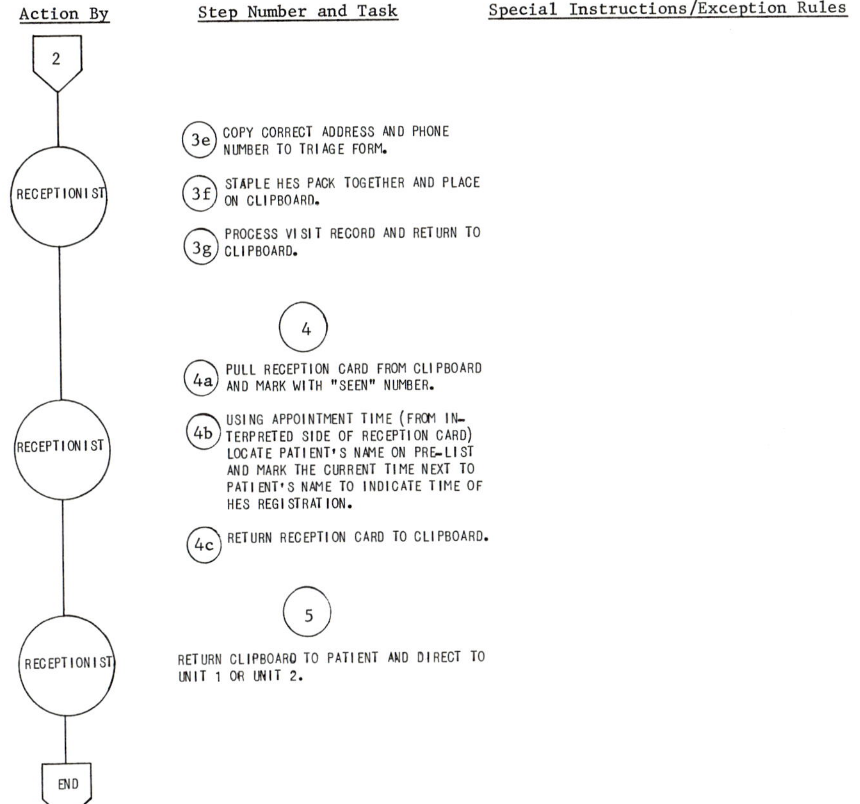

Figure 20-40b.

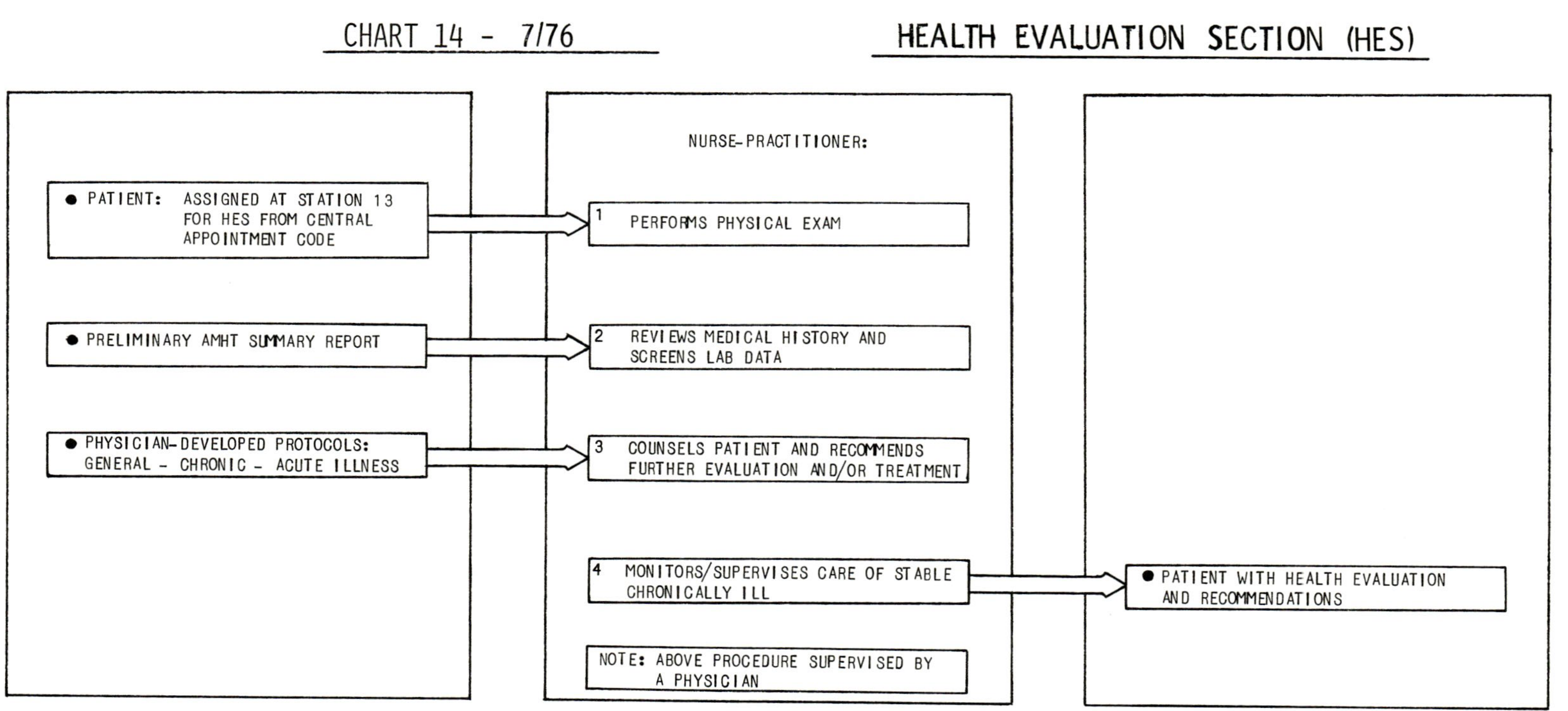

Figure 20-41. Information chart for HES examination.

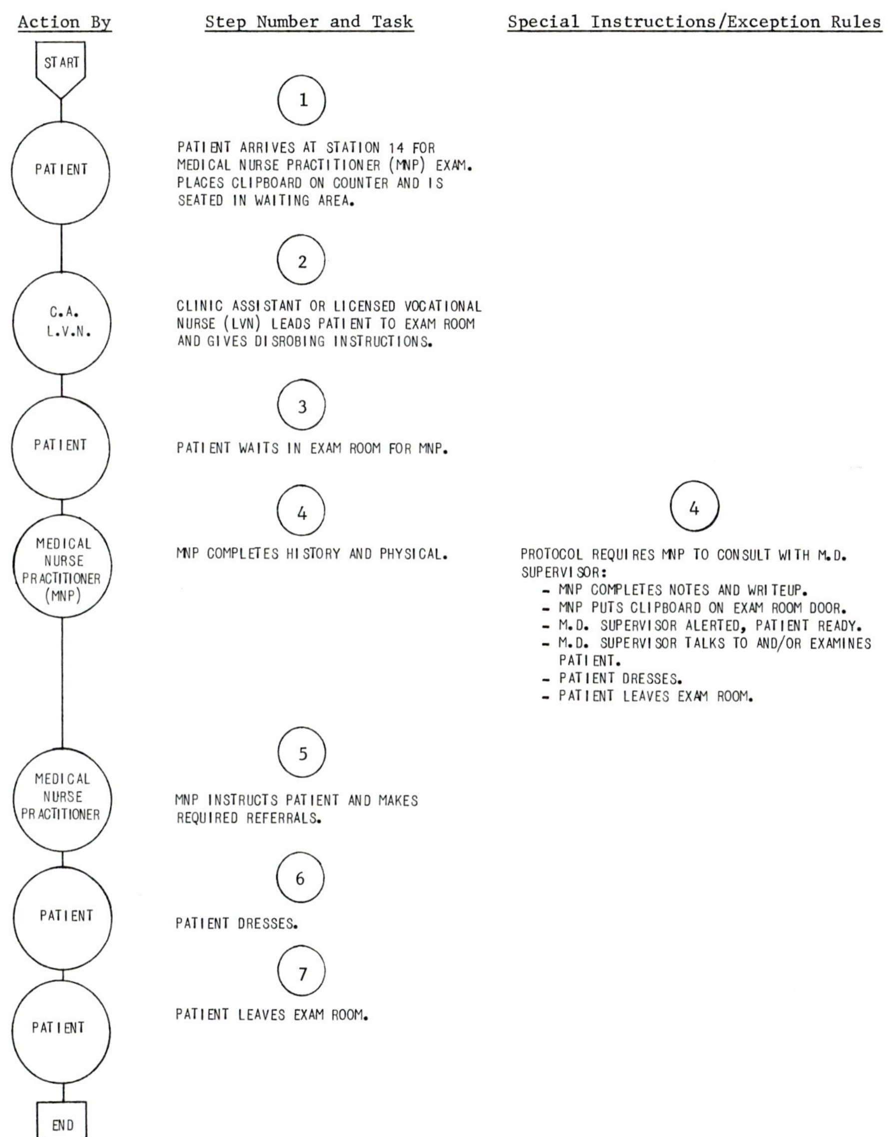

Figure 20-42.   Flow chart for HES examination.

CHART 15 - 1976

PATIENT DISCHARGE & REFERRAL

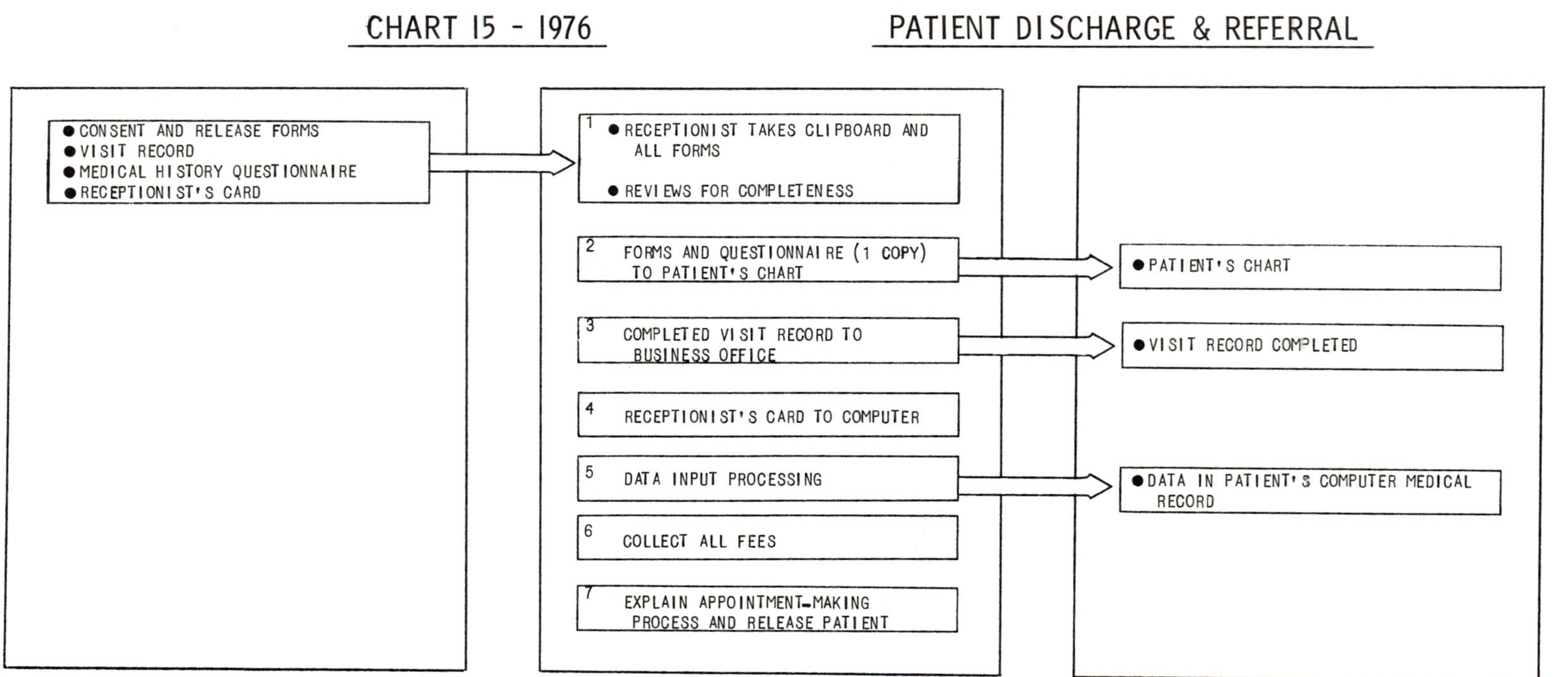

Figure 20-43. Information chart for patient discharge and referral stations.

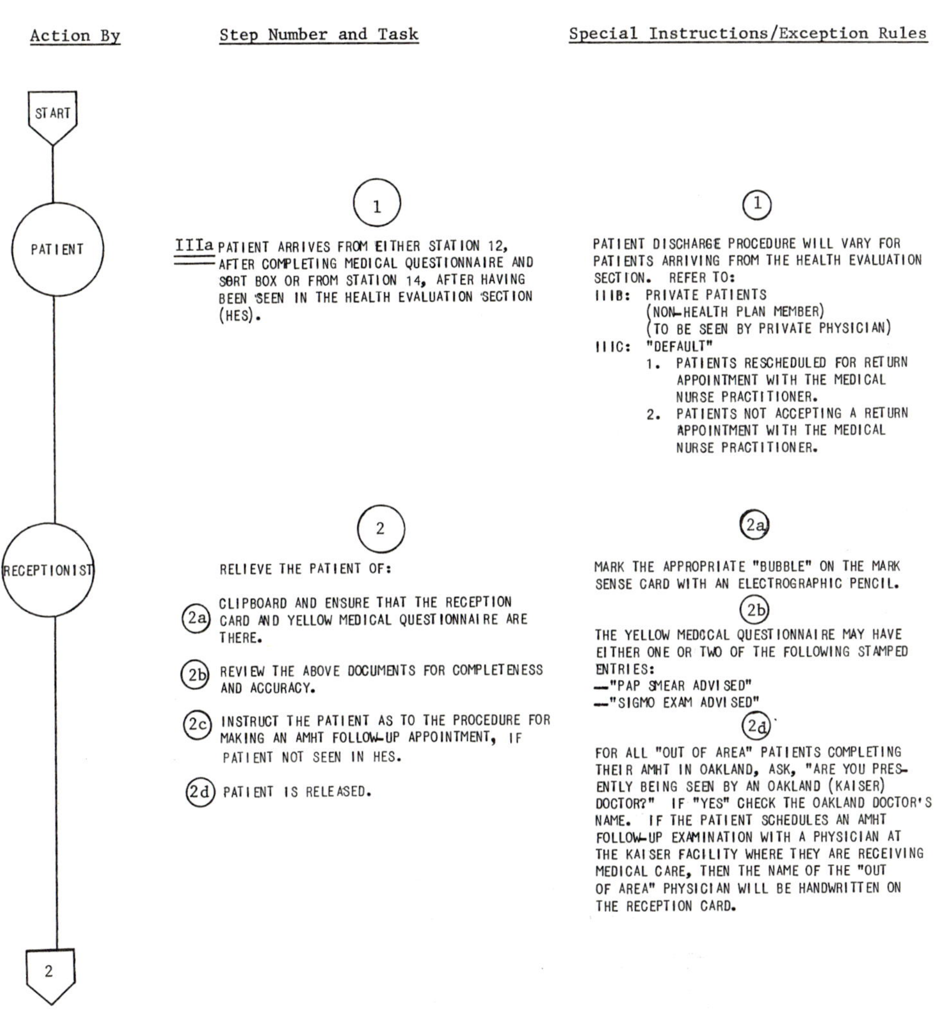

Figure 20-44a. Flow chart for patient discharge and referral.

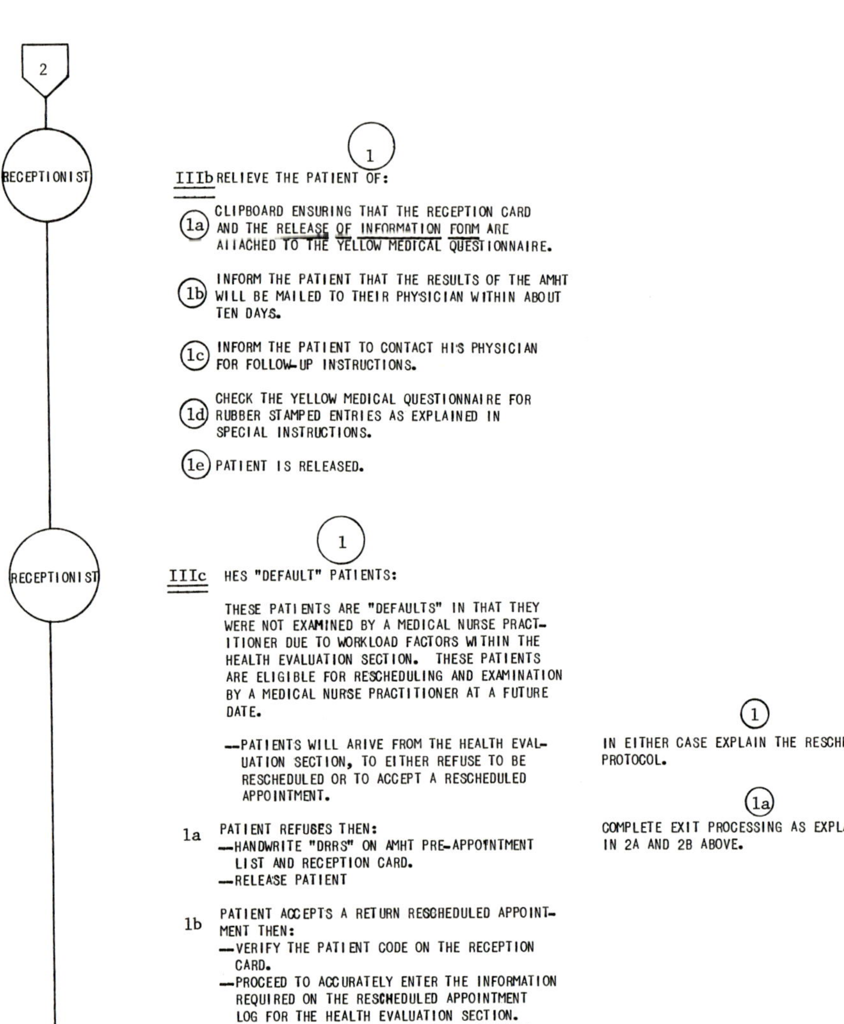

Figure 20-44b.

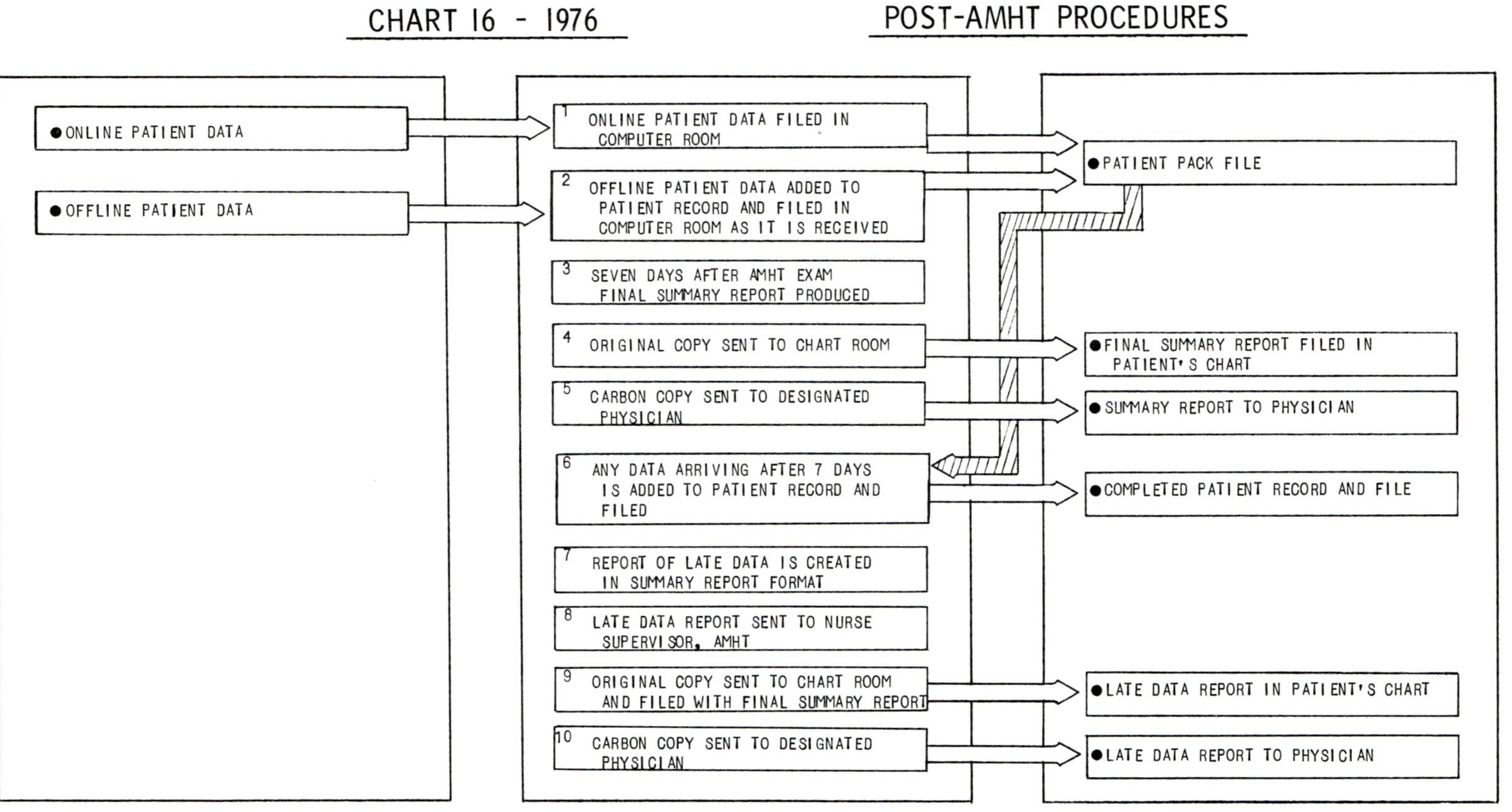

Figure 20-45. Information chart for post-AMHT procedures.

Index